NEW PROSPECTS IN PSYCHIATRY

THE BIO-CLINICAL INTERFACE

Bio-Clinical Psychiatry
Mapping Brain Function

Editors:

J.-P. Macher
M.-A. Crocq
J.-F. Nedelec

British Library Cataloguing in Publication Data
A catalogue record for this book is available from the British Library.

ISBN 2-7420-0110-7

Editions John Libbey Eurotext
127, avenue de la République, 92120 Montrouge, France.
Tél.: (1) 46.73.06.60

John Libbey and Company Ltd
13, Smiths Yard, Summerley Street, London SW18 4HR, England.
Tel.: (01) 947.27.77.

John Libbey CIC
Via L. Spallanzani, 11, 00161 Rome, Italy. Tel.: (06) 862.289.

© John Libbey Eurotext, 1995, Paris

Il est interdit de reproduire intégralement ou partiellement le présent ouvrage — loi du 11 mars 1957 — sans autorisation de l'éditeur ou du Centre français du Copyright, 6 *bis*, rue Gabriel-Laumain, 75010 Paris.

NEW PROSPECTS IN PSYCHIATRY

THE BIO-CLINICAL INTERFACE

Bio-Clinical Psychiatry
Mapping Brain Function

Edited proceedings of the Bio-Clinical Interface conferences, held in Rouffach, France, between 1992 and 1994.

Editors :

J.P. Macher
M.-A. Crocq
J.-F. Nedelec

*Centre Hospitalier
68250 Rouffach, France*

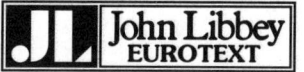

Contents

Addresses of contributors XI

Preface XV

Bio-clinical psychiatry

1. Molecular genetic studies of bipolar illness.
   W.H. Berettini, T.N. Ferraro, H. Choi, L.R. Goldin, S.D. Detera-Wadleigh,
   D. Muniec, W-T. Hsieh, M. Hoehe, J. Guroff, D. Kazuba, J.I. Nurnberger Jr,
   E.S. Gershon 3

2. The question of a «nuclear depressive syndrome».
   O. Doerr-Zegers 19

3. The nuclear depressive syndrome seen from a phenomenology
   of the corporality.
   O. Doerr-Zegers 29

4. A role for CRF in the pathophysiology of affective and anxiety disorders ?
   Laboratory and clinical studies.
   M.J. Owens, C.B. Nemeroff 39

5. Evaluation of anxiety, depression and management of psychotic anxiety in
   schizophrenic patients.
   O. Blin, J.M. Azorin 49

6. Endogenous opioids and their putative role in disturbances of social
   behavior, in particular autism.
   J.K. Buitelaar 57

7. The D_3 dopamine receptor as a target for antipsychotics.
   D. Levesque, P. Sokoloff, J. Diaz, M.-P. Martres, C. Pilon,
   J.-C. Schwartz 69

8. Multihormonal responses to a series of neuroendocrine challenges
   in psychiatry: a multivariate approach.
   F. Duval, M.-C. Mokrani, M.-A. Crocq, M. Jautz, P. Bailey, T. S. Diep,
   E. E. de Andrade, A. de Andrade, J.-P. Macher 77

9. Composite diagnostic evaluation system at the major psychiatric disorders.
   P. Gaszner, T. A. Ban 91

10. **Predictive bio-clinical profiles of antidepressant responses in major depression**
 F. Duval, M.-C. Mokrani, M.-A. Crocq, M. Jautz, P. Bailey, T. S. Diep, E. E. de Andrade, A. de Andrade, J.-P. Macher 99

11. **Late auditory evoked potentials: contribution to diagnosis of schizophrenia and correlations with Andreasen's rating scales (SANS, SPAS).**
 M. Smets, P. Gallois, G.Forzy, P. Hautecœur, C.E. Thomas, J.M. Hennebique 111

12. **First pharmaco-electroencephalographic approach of Euphytose®**
 R. Luthringer, G. Lefrançois, D. Rod, J.-P. Macher 117

13. **Therapeutic sleep deprivation in patients resistant to antidepressants.**
 S. Kasper, S. Ruhrmann, RH. van den Hoofdacker 127

14. **Methodological difficulties in clinical trials in developing countries.**
 D. Moussaoui 139

15. **Value of computerized EEG and evoked potentials in the diagnosis of depressive pseudodementia.**
 P. Morault, E. Palem, M. Bourgeois, J. Paty 145

16. **Phenomenology of aging.**
 O. Doerr-Zegers 157

17. **An ammonia hypothesis of Alzheimer disease.**
 N. Seiler 165

Mapping brain function

18. **Pattern recognition techniques in MRI. Brain diseases diagnosis : a quantified approach.**
 A. Alaux 187

19. **Relevance of psychiatric rating scales : what do they measure ?**
 P.E. Bailey 195

20. **Comparing cerebral blood flow response (FMRI) and neuronal response (MEG) to motor activation.**
 R. Beisteiner, G. Gomiscek, M. Erdler, C. Teichtmeister, E. Moser, L. Deecke 201

21. **Functional MRI studies of spatial working memory and language.**
 A. M. Blamire 207

22. **Parametric imaging : application to Parkinsonism.**
    J.M. Bonny, J.Y. Boire, F. Durif, D. Sinardet, A. Veyre, M. Zanca 213

23. **How to take advantages of gradients ? Fundamentals and some applications.**
    A. Briguet, M. Bourgeois, O. Beuf 223

24. **Neuronal Integrity in the frontal cortex of schizophrenics evaluated by ^{1}H magnetic resonance spectroscopy.**
    G. Calabrese, A. Falini, S. Lipari, D. Origgi, C. Colombo, A. Bonfanti,
    G. Scotti, S. Scarone 229

25. **Evaluation of multiple sclerosis with magnetization transfer.**
    A. Campi 233

26. **Blood oxygenation and NMR signal changes.**
    J. Chambron 243

27. **Visualisation of vein effect in functional imaging using phase gradient methods.**
    G. Cros, F. Hennel, N. Bolo, F. Girard, C. Labadie, J.-F. Nedelec,
    J.-P. Macher, M. Décorps 251

28. **Methodological difficulties in localized spectroscopy.**
    M. Décorps, A. Ziegler, C. Rémy 257

29. **Functional MRI in Parkinson's disease.**
    F. Durif, D. Sinardet, J.M. Bonny, J.Y. Boire, A. Veyre, M. Zanca 263

30. **Functional imaging and functional spectroscopy during motor activation.**
    E. Feifel, N. Bolo, J. Hennig, Th. Ernst, J.F. Nedelec, F. Hennel, G. Deuschl,
    J.-P. Macher... 269

31. **Quantitative assessment of MRI lesion load in multiple sclerosis.**
    M. Filippi 275

32. **2D localised spectroscopy on human brain.**
    B. Gillet, B-T. Doan, D. Wecker, J-F. Nedelec, J-P. Macher, J-C. Belœil 287

33. **^{13}C and ^{1}H NMR studies of glucose transport in the human brain.**
    R. Gruetter 291

34. **Neurofunctional imaging and language.**
    M. Habib, M. Didic, O. Levrier, J.-F. Demonet, P. Sabbah, G. Salamon 299

35. **Proton MR spectroscopy in Parkinsonism.**
    A. Heerschap, J. C.M. Zijlmans, H.O.M. Thijssen, A de Koster,
    M.W.I.M. Horstink 309

36. Functional imaging at 3 Tesla using interleaved EPI.
    F. Hennel, N. Bolo, G. Cros, F. Girard, F. Hodé, J.F. Nedelec, J.P. Macher 317

37. How to improve fast imaging?
    J. Hennig 323

38. Enhanced brain structure delineation in the rodent
    by diffusion weighted imaging.
    P.D. Hockings, D.C. Harrison, D. A. Middleton, D.G. Reid, D.M. Doddrell 329

39. Fluorine MRS in human brain.
    R. A. Komoroski, J. E. Newton, C. Heimberg, C. N. Karson 335

40. Hippocampal metabolite depletion in schizophrenia detected
    by proton magnetic resonance spectroscopy.
    M. Maier, M.A. Ron 343

41. Overcoming field inhomogeneities in MRI.
    D.J.O. McIntyre, R.W. Bowtell, M.-J Commandre, F. Hennel, P. Mansfield,
    P.G. Morris 349

42. *In vivo* metabolic study with NMR spectroscopy in Alzheimer disease.
    G. Mecheri, M. Marie-Cardine 357

43. Effect of spatial resolution on activation ratio in echo-planar functional
    MRI.
    M.-E. Meyer, L. Hertz-Pannier, R.C. Risinger, S. Posse, D. Le Bihan 363

44. Metabolic alterations in Alzheimer's disease using *in vitro* ^{1}H NMR.
    P. Mohanakrishnan, A.H. Fowler, M.M. Husain, J.P. Vonsattel, P.R. Jolles,
    P. Liem, R.A. Komoroski 369

45. Advances in brain MRI and MRS.
    P. Morris, H. Bachelard, K. Bingham, R. Coxon, P. Glover, M. Humberstone,
    J. Hykin, D. McIntyre, G. Sawle, N. Thatcher 377

46. High temporal and spatial resolution in functional MRI.
    E. Moser, R. Beisteiner, E. Müller, C. Teichtmeister, V. Edward 385

47. Methods to improve EEG spatial resolution with implications
    for medical and cognitive science.
    P. L. Nunez 391

48. Localizing sources within the human brain by means of MEG and EEG.
    M. J. Peters, S. P. van den Broek, T. Knösche, F. Zanow 399

49. Automated estimation of metabolite concentrations from
    localized proton MRS.
    S. W. Provencher 405

50. Perils and pitfalls of fMRI: photic stimulation in subjects with schizophrenia.
    P.F. Renshaw, D.A. Yurgelun-Todd, B.M. Cohen 415

51. ^{1}H MR spectroscopy in multiple sclerosis.
    W. Roser, G. Hagberg, I. Mader, E.W. Radü, H. Bruunschweiler,
    L. Kappos, J. Seelig 421

52. Quality control in volume selective spectroscopy.
    K.V. Schenker 429

53. Sensorimotor cortex changes and neurological soft signs in schizophrenia :
    a study with functional magnetic resonance imaging.
    J. Schröder, F. Wenz, R. Niethammer, L.R. Schad, K. Baudendistel, A. Stockert,
    M.V. Knopp, H. Sauer 441

54. Vascular responses in fMRI of motor activity.
    C. Segebarth, C. Delon-Martin, V. Belle, R. Massarelli, J. Decety, J.-F. Lebas,
    M. Décorps 449

55. Combination of MRI and EEG data for realistic source localization.
    L. Soufflet, J-F. Nedelec, N. Bolo, J-P. Macher 455

56. MRS studies on excitotoxic cell damage in brain
    N.M. Thatcher, R.S. Badar-Goffer, P.G. Morris, M.A. McLean, A. Taylor,
    H.S. Bachelard 461

57. Functional MRI of the human cortex : effect of stimulus speed
    and handedness.
    S. van Oostende, P. van Hecke, E. Corthout, A.L. Baert 469

58. Volumetric measurements of the temporal lobes in Alzheimer's disease.
    L.-O. Wahlund, P. Julin 475

59. ^{1}H spectroscopy of the temporal lobes in schizophrenic
    and bipolar patients.
    D.A. Yurgelun-Todd, S.A. Gruber, B.M. Cohen, P.F. Renshaw 481

60. Echo-planar MRI of schizophrenics and normal controls
    during word production.
    D.A. Yurgelun-Todd, P.F. Renshaw, S.A. Gruber, B.M. Cohen 487

Addresses of contributors

ALAUX André, Département de Physique, Institut de Biologie, boulevard Henri-IV, 34060 Montpellier, France.
BAILEY Paul, Secteur 8 du Haut-Rhin, Centre Hospitalier, 27 rue du 4e-R.S.M., 68250 Rouffach, France.
BEISTEINER Roland, Neurological University Clinic, Wahringer Gürtel Strasse 18-20, Vienna, Austria.
BERETTINI Wade, Department of Psychiatry, Thomas Jefferson University, 1025 Walnut Street, 312 College, Philadelphia PA 19107, USA.
BLAMIRE Andrew, MRC Biochemical and Clinical MR Unit, John Radclife Hospital Headington, Oxford OX3 9DU England.
BLIN Olivier, Hôpital de La Timone, Centre de Pharmacologie Clinique et d'Evaluations Thérapeutiques, boulevard Jean-Moulin, 13385 Marseille Cedex 5, France.
BONNY Jean-Marc, Etude Métabolique des Molécules Marquées, INSERM U 71, B.P. n° 184, 63005 Clermont-Ferrand Cedex, France.
BRIGUET André, Laboratoire de Résonance Magnétique Nucléaire, Bâtiment 721, Université Lyon 1, 43, boulevard du 11-Novembre-1918, 69622 Villeurbane Cedex, France.
BUITELAAR Jan, Department of Child Psychiatry, Heidelberglaand 100, NL, 3584 CX Utrecht, The Netherlands.
CALABRESE Giovanna, Dept. of Neuropsychiatry, San Raffaele Hospital, University of Milan, Via Prinetti 29, 20127 Milan, Italia.
CAMPI Adriana, Department Neuroradiology/Neurology, San Raffaele Hospital, Via Olgettina 60, 20132 Milan, Italia.
CHAMBRON Jacques, Institut de Physique Biologique, Faculté de Médecine, 4, rue Kirschleger, 67085 Strasbourg Cedex, France.
CROS Ghislaine, FORENAP, Unité de Résonance Magnétique, Centre Hospitalier, 68250 Rouffach, France.
DÉCORPS Michel, Université Joseph-Fourier, U. 318 INSERM, Pavillon B, Centre Hospitalier Universitaire, B.P. 217 X, 38043 Grenoble, France.
DOERR-ZEGERS Otto, Psiquiatria y Psicoterapia Luis Thayer, OJEDA n° 0115 of 502, CL, Santiago de Chile, Chili.
DURIF Franck, Hôpital Fontmaure, Service de Neurologie, Avenue de Villars, 63407 Chamallières Cedex, France.
DUVAL Fabrice, Secteur 8 du Haut-Rhin, Centre Hospitalier, 27 rue du 4e-R.S.M., 68250 Rouffach France.
FEIFEL Eckert, Klinikum der A.-Ludwig, Universität Radiologische Klinik, Hugstetterstrasse 55, 79106 Freiburg, Germany.
FILIPPI Massimo, St.Raffaele Hospital, Department Neuroradiology/Neurology, Via Olgettina 60, 20132 Milan, Italia.
GASZNER Peter, Orszagos Pszichiatriai és Neurologial Intézet, 116 Hüvösvölgyi, 1021 Budapest, Hungary.

GILLET Brigitte, Institut de Chimie des Substances Naturelles, Laboratoire de RMN Biologique, Avenue de la Terrasse, 91198 Gif-sur-Yvette, France.
GRUETTER Rolf, Abteilung für Magnetresonanz Spectroskopie und METHODIK, MR Center, Inselspital and University, Inselheimmatte, 3010 Berne, Switzerland.
HABIB Michel, Service de Neuroradiologie, Centre Hospitalier Universitaire La Timone, 13013 Marseille Cedex 5, France.
HEERSCHAP Arend, Institute of Neurology and Radiology, University Hospital Nijmegen, 6500 HB Nijmegen, The Netherlands.
HENNEL Franck, Forenap, Unité de Résonance Magnétique, Centre Hospitalier, 68250 Rouffach, France.
HENNIG Jürgen, Klinikum der Albert-Ludwigs-Universität, Radiologische Klinik, Hugstetterstrasse 55, 79106 Freiburg, Deutschland.
HOCKINGS Paul, Biophysical Sciences, SmithKline Beecham Pharmaceuticals, New Frontiers Science Park, 3rd avenue, Harlow, Essex CM19 5AW, UK.
KASPER Siegfried, Universitäts Nervenklinik und Poliklinik Psychiatrie, Sigmund-Freud Strasse 25, 5300 Bonn 1, Deutschland.
KOMOROSKI Richard, University of Arkansas for Medical Sciences, Department of Radiology and Pathology NMR Laboratory, 4301 West Markham Street, Slot 582, Little Rock, 72205-7199 Arkansas, USA.
LEVESQUE Daniel, Unité de Neurobiologie et Pharmacologie, Centre Paul-Broca de l'INSERM, 2 *ter*, rue d'Alésia, 75014 Paris, France.
LUTHRINGER Rémy, Secteur 8 du Haut-Rhin, Centre Hospitalier, 27 rue du 4e-R.S.M., 68250 Rouffach, France.
MAIER Michael, Institute of Neurology, Department of Clinical Neurology, Queen Square, WC1N 3 BG London, England.
McINTYRE Dominick, St Georges Hospital Medical School, Department of Biochemistry, Cranmer Terrace Tooting, SW17 Ore London, England.
MECHERI Gabriel, Centre Hospitalo-Universitaire, Centre Hospitalier Le Vinatier, 69677 Bron Cedex, France.
MEYER Marc-Etienne, Institut de Physique Biologique, 4, rue Kirschleger, 67085 Strasbourg France.
MOHANAKRISHNAN P, University of Arkansas for Medical Sciences, Little Rock, AR 72205, and Brain Tissue Resource Center, McLean Hospital, Belmont, MA, USA.
MORAULT Pierre, Hôpital Pellegrin, Tripode, 33076 Bordeaux Cedex, France.
MORRIS Peter, University of Nottingham Magnetic Resonance Center, Department of Physics, University Park, NG7 2 RD Nottingham, England.
MOSER Ewald, Arbeitsgruppe NMR, Institute of Medical Physics University of Vienna, Währingerstrasse 13, A-1090 Vienna, Austria.
MOUSSAOUI Driss, Centre Psychiatrique Universitaire Ibn Rochd, Rue Tarik Ibn Ziad, Casablanca, Maroc.
NUNEZ Paul L, Department of Biomedical Enginnering, Tulane University, LA 70018 New Orleans, USA.
OWENS Michael J, Emory University School of Medicine, 1639, Pierce Drive, Suite 4000, Atlanta Georgia 30322, USA.

PETERS Maria, Twente University, Faculty of Applied Physic, P.O. Box 217, 7500 AE Enschede, The Netherlands.

PROVENCHER Stephen, Max Planck Institut, Für Biophysikalische Chemie, Amfassberg, Postfach 2841, 37018 Gottingen, Deutschland.

RENSHAW Perry, Imaging Center, McLean Hospital, Admission Building G-79, 115 Mill Street - Belmont MA 02178-9106 Massachusetts, USA.

ROSER Werner, MR-Zentrum der Universität Basel, Klingelbergstrasse 50, 4031 Bašel, Switzerland.

SCHENKER Kurt, Spectrospin AG - Analytik und Medizintechnik, Industriestrasse 26, CH 8117 Faellanden, Switzerland.

SCHRÖDER John, Heidelberg Hospital, Department of Psychiatry, Voss Strasse, 69115 Heidelberg, Deutschland.

SEGEBARTH Christophe, Université Joseph-Fourier, U. 318 INSERM, Pavillon B, Centre Hospitalier Universitaire, B.P. 217 X, 38043 Grenoble, France.

SEILER Nikolaus, Marion Merrell Dow Research Institute, 16, rue d'Ankara, 67009 Strasbourg Cedex, France.

SMETS Marc, Centre Hospitalier Saint-Venant, 62350 Saint-Venant, France.

SOUFFLET Laurent, Secteur 8 du Haut-Rhin, Centre Hospitalier, 27 rue du 4e-R.S.M., 68250 Rouffach, France.

THATCHER Nicola, University of Nottingham Magnetic Resonance Center, Department of Physics, University Park, NG7 2RD Nottingham, England.

Van OOSTENDE Sylvie, University Hospital, Departement Radiology, K.U. Leuven, Belgique.

WAHLUND Lars-Olof, Karolinska Insitute, Department of Clinical Neuroscience and Family Medicine, Division of Geriatric Medicine B56, Stockholm, Sweden.

YURGELUN-TODD Deborah, Brain Imaging Center at McLean Hospital, 115 Mill Street, 02178 Belmont MA, USA.

Preface

This book contains an updated selection of the papers presented at the lastest scientific conferences held in Rouffach, France.

Rouffach, a medieval town located at the crossroads of Europe near Strasbourg in Alsace, is the seat of both our hospital and our research center. The hospital in Rouffach is in charge of the bulk of the psychiatric care in the southern half of the Alsace region. The research center is based in the hospital and includes, among other resources, one of the largest European sleep units, quantitative EEG and high-field 3-Tesla magnetic resonance brain mapping facilities and a modern unit for the study of new drugs in the earliest stages of clinical research.

The yearly conferences, called the « Bio-Clinical Interface », were first started more than a decade ago. The latest conferences were presided by Steven M. Paul (then at the National Institute of Mental Health, Bethesda, USA), Herman M. van Praag (University of Limburg, The Netherlands), and Jorge Alberto Costa e Silva (Director of Mental Health, WHO, Geneva) ; the upcoming 1995 conference will be presided by Herbert Y. Meltzer (Cleveland, USA). As the name « interface » suggests, these conferences aim at exploring the area where biology and clinical psychiatry affect each other or have links with each other. « Interfacing » has now been made a catch-word by the development of computing and electronics. We believe that the exploration of other interfaces is also necessary in the field of psychiatry. The major psychoses have been accurately described in all their clinical facets by masters such as Kraepelin ; however, the validation of these diagnostic concepts and the need to devise more affective treatments make it necessary to explore the molecular, biological, and chemical foundations of these illnesses.

Family, we would like to acknowledge the help of many friends and collaborators ; among the people to whom we are the most indebted are Sandra Schouler and Sylvie Mann for the painstaking work of preparing the manuscripts for publication.

J.-P. Macher, M.-A. Crocq, J.-F. Nedelec
Rouffach, September 1995

Bio-clinical psychiatry
[from chapter 1 to chapter 17]

Mapping brain function
[from chapter 18 to chapter 60]

1

Molecular genetic studies of bipolar illness

W.H. BERRETTINI [1], T.N. FERRARO [1], H. CHOI [1], L.R. GOLDIN [5], S.D. DETERA-WADLEIGH [5], D. MUNIEC [5], W-T. HSIEH [3], M. HOEHE [4], J. GUROFF [5], D. KAZUBA [5], J.I. NURNBERGER Jr., E.S. GERSHON [5]

[1] Department of psychiatry and Human Behavior, Jefferson Medical College, Thomas Jefferson University, 1025 Walnut Street, 312 College, Philadelphia, PA, 19107, USA.
[2] Institute for Psychiatric Research, University of Indiana, Indianapolis, IN, 46202, USA.
[3] Abbott Laboratory Department 9RF, Building R1V, 5th Floor, 14th Street and Sheridan Road, North Chicago, IL, 60064, USA.
[4] Harvard Medical School, Department of Genetics, Church Lab 25 Shattuck Street, Boston, MA, 02115, USA.
[5] Clinical Neurogenetics Branch, National Institute of Mental Health, 9000 Rockville Pike, Building 10, Room 3N218, Bethesda, MD, 20892, USA.

Twenty-one bipolar (BP) pedigrees were studied for linkage to chromosomes 1, 6, 8, 10q, 11q, 12, 13, 15, 17 and 18. These pedigrees include 365 informative persons, 159 of whom have BPI, schizoaffective, BPII with major depression or recurrent unipolar diagnoses. Using an autosomal dominant disease model with 85% or 50% age-dependent penetrance, two and three-point linkage analyses were performed under broad and narrow affection status models. None of these analyses provided minimal support (lod score > 3.7) for linkage. A lod score of 2.6 was observed at D18S32 in a three-point heterogeneity analysis (including D18S45) when an autosomal dominant, 50% penetrance model was used, with 30% of families linked. Simulations indicate that a score of this magnitude would be expected if only 30% of families were linked to a given marker. These results indicate that a gene for a common form of BP disease is unlikely to be found within the chromosomal regions covered by the DNA markers used. However, the region of 18p11 deserves further study.

Twin, family and adoption studies of bipolar (BP) disease are consistent with complex inheritance [1]. Rice *et al.* [2] reported that a single locus was not favored over a mixed model of transmission, a result non-Mendelian illnesses are difficult because of reduced penetrance, unknown mode of transmission, phenocopies (individuals with the syndrome from non-genetic causes) and non-allelic genetic heterogeneity [3-5]. Despite these obstacles, confirmed linkages have been reported for osteoarthritis [6-8], Alzheimer's disease [9-13] and breast cancer [14].

Previous linkage studies of BP disease are controversial. Linkage to 11p15 markers [15] has been weakened by absence of positive lod scores in numerous other pedigrees [16-19], and by evaluation of newly ascertained individuals in the original by several investigators [24-27], and some of the original evidence for linkage to color blindness and G6PD deficiency in one report[23] was not confirmed by genotyping with relevant Xq28 DNA markers [28]. Thus, there are no confirmed linkage studies in BP disease.

Preliminary results regarding genomic screening for a subset of these 21 BP pedigrees [29] have been published for most regions of chromosome 5 [30] and chromosomes 1, 10q, 11q, 13, 15 and 17 [31]. Gejman *et al.* [32] reported negative lod scores for 57 markers in a variable subset of these families. More recent results are provided here.

Methods

The 21 BP families have been described previously [29]; (*see* Tables I, IIA and IIB for descriptions and simulations regarding the poser to detect linkage). 20 pedigrees were studied with each marker (mean +/- 2). 328 individuals were genotyped at each marker (+/- 27). Mean marker heterozygosity is 64% (+/- 16). Table IV lists probes and loci studied. Laboratory and genotyping methods were as described previously [31].

Table I. Descriptive summary of twenty-one bipolar pedigrees.

	Informative persons	Ill Persons*
Total for 21 pedigrees	365 (50%) +	159 (40%)
Mean (+/-SD) per pedigree	17 +/- 7	7.6 +/- 2.3

Informative persons are defined as affected or as a parent, adult child (older than 24) or adult sibling of an affected person. Genotypes can be determined on 98% of the informative persons and 98% of the ill persons from the available DNA samples, given a sufficiently polymorphic marker (so that alleles for some deceased persons can be deduced from the genotypes of their spouses and children).
Adapted from Berrettini *et al* [29].
* under affection status model two (see Table III).
+ percent males given in parentheses.

Table IIA. Simulations assuming linkage and heterogeneity for 20 bipolar families.

Alpha*	Theta^	Mean maximum lod scores for 200 replicates	
		Homogeneity	Heterogeneity
0.25	0.01	2.37 (0.32) #	4.26 (0.52) **
0.25	0.05	1.70 (0.18)	2.95 (0.30)
0.50	0.01	7.59 (0.86)	10.5 (0.94)
0.50	0.05	5.91 (0.76)	7.50 (0.86)^

* Alpha is percent of families linked to the locus under study.
^ Theta is the recombination fraction.
\# The number in parentheses indicates the percent of replicates for which the lod score exceeded 3.0.
** The number in parentheses indicates the percent of replicates for which the lod score exceeded 3.7.

Using 20 BP pedigrees described in Berrettini et al. [29], 200 replicates (assuming linkage) were calculated for those persons whose genotypes can be determined from available cell lines. A dominant 90% penetrance disease model was employed, with a disease gene frequency of 0.5% for alpha=0.5, and 0.25% for alpha=0.25. Marker heterozygosity = 70%. Affection status model two (Table III) was used to define the illness.

Table IIB. Average simulated lod scores with a single marker locus.

Family	Informative # Persons	Affected* Persons	Recombination fraction	
			0.01	0.05
16	15	4	.90	.69
48	34	8	2.92	2.39
65	11	5	.88	.75
68	15	8	1.63	1.34
92	15	7	1.27	.96
137	14	5	.89	.68
278	20	6	1.21	.99
441	11	8	1.37	.99
488	9	5	.85	.73
643	23	7	2.24	1.64
1 442	18	12	2.20	1.64
1 482	29	11	3.13	2.33
1 483	8	5	.57	.51
1 484	26	6	1.87	1.44
1 505	19	9	1.65	1.14
1 412	14	6	1.11	.90
1 516	23	12	2.48	2.07
1 520	20	12	1.81	1.47
1 532	8	6	.68	.56
1 536	15	7	1.18	.93
9 002	18	9	1.49	1.20
Mean	**17 +/-7**	**7.6 +/- 2.3**	**1.54**	**1.21**

Lod scores for 21 BP pedigrees were calculated using the SIMLINK program [41], assuming a linked marker with a 70% heterozygosity, a dominant 90% penetrance disease model and a disease gene frequency of 1%. Only those persons whose genotypes can be determined are included in these simulations. Adapted from Berrettini et al. [29].
\# Informative person refers to an affected individual, or the adult (older than 24) child, sibling or parent of an affected subject.
* Affected person refers to model two in Table III: schizoaffective, BPI, BPII with major depression or recurrent UP diagnoses.

Linkage analyses were conducted with the LINKAGE package (version 5.03). Age-dependent penetrance (maximum 85% or 50% at age 50) was assumed in an autosomal dominant model with a disease gene frequency of 1.5%. Penetrance of the normal genotype was set at 0.1% to allow for a small number of phenocopies. Affection status models one and two (Table III) were used. As a check on published map distances, marker-marker recombination was calculated for many intervals. A few loci, localized cytogenetically, were placed on maps using data from these 22 families.

Table III. Affection status models.

Model 1 :	Bipolar I, Bipolar II with major depression and schizoaffective
Model 2 :	Model 1 + recurrent unipolar
Model 3 :	Model 2 + unipolar (single episode), cyclothymic personality, bipolar II with minor depression, unspecified functional psychosis, suicide, hypomania, eating disorders, other psychiatric disorder (hospitalized) and schizophrenia

Diagnoses are arranged in three affection status models for linkage analysis (see text for details).

Lod scores for individual families were reviewed to detect evidence for heterogeneity. Linkage analyses were done under heterogeneity, using the admixture test [33], for regions in which four or more families yielded lod scores consistent with linkage (Table IIB). A modified version of LINKMAP was used to estimate the fraction of families linked.

Results

Three-point analyses, assuming homogeneity, for affection status model two (and an 85% penetrance, dominant model) are shown for chromosomes 1, 6, 8, 10q, 11q, 12, 13, 15, 17 and 18 (Figure 1). Overlapping points are not shown (for visual clarity). The more negative of the two values is shown to reflect the negative influence of the loci adjacent to those in any given three-point analysis. The 50% penetrance lod scores are less negative, but provide no strong evidence for linkage to any region (data not shown).

Visual inspection of lod scores for individual families did not reveal any substantial evidence for heterogeneity. Admixture analyses (in a three-point calculation with D18S32 and D18S45) revealed a maximum lod score of 2.6 at D18S32 (assuming an autosomal dominant inheritance with 50% penetrance and a 1% disease gene frequency) with 30% of the families linked. Six of the families appeared linked by visual inspection, and their three-point lod scores are shown in Table V for the interval between D18S32 and D18S45 of D18S40.

Table V. Lod scores in 6 bipolar pedigrees for chromosome 18p11 markers.

Pedigree	Observed lod score*
0065	0.85
0278	1.18
1442	1.47
1483	0.81
1516	1.86
1536	0.84

* Observed lod score is the highest lod score observed in a three point analysis using D18S32 and D18S40 or D18S32 and D18S45 markers, calculated with an autosomal dominant, 50% penetrance analysis, using affection status model 2. Penetrance of the normal genotype was set at .001 (to allow for a small number of phenocopies) ; a BP disease gene frequency of 1% was employed.

Discussion

A single gene for a common heritable form of BP disease does not originate from the chromosomal regions studied. Weak evidence for linkage and heterogeneity was observed in 18p11 at the D18S32, D18S45 and D18S40 loci. A receptor-like protein tyrosine phosphatase gene has been described in this region [34]. Phosphorylation and dephosphorylation is a mechanism of receptor activation/deactivation, and these enzymes can be considered candidate genes for BP illness.

Lithium interacts with GTP binding proteins [35], and genes for GTP binding subunits are candidate genes for BP disease. A gene for an alpha subunit (GNAL) of a GTP-binding protein [36] has been localized to this interval [37]. This alpha subunit, Golf, may be expressed only in olfactory neurons found in the nasal epithelium, as no message was detected in a northern hybridization experiment using rat brain from which the olfactory bulbs were removed [36]. Human brain studies have not been reported.

In a conservative analysis (assuming only BPI and SA [manic] to be affected) with low penetrance, the power to detect linkage in these pedigrees would be greatly reduced. Exclusion of linkage should involve a conservative analysis. Additional BP families should be studied for these regions, so that power to detect linkage will be greater with combined results in a conservative meta-analysis.

Data were analyzed in an autosomal dominant model (assuming either 85 % or 50 % penetrance). Although the families were selected for unilineal transmission of illness [29], this selection criterion does not eliminate the possibility of recessive transmission. However, multiple analyses can spuriously elevate lod scores [38, 39], resulting in false claims of linkage. Because recessive illness was considered unlikely (by virtue of the structure of these families, a recessive analysis was not calculated). However, Clerget-Darpoux et al. [40] found that misspecifying the mode of inheritance as dominant (when it is actually recessive) markedly reduces power to detect linkage.

Linkage to a common form of BP illness in these families has been excluded (with the limitations noted above) for approximately 50% of the autosomal genome. Because genetic heterogeneity is likely in BP disease, the entire genome must be examined with large series of pedigrees to exclude linkages which may be valid for a small fraction of BP families.

Table IV. DNA probes for the linkage study of bipolar pedigrees.

Chromosome 1		Chromosome 6		Chromosome 8	
Probe	Locus	Probe	Locus	Probe	Locus
pMCT118	D1S80	PCR	F13A1	PCR	D8S264
pMCT58	D1S77	PCR	D6S202	PCR	D8S277
pCMM12.1	D1S76	PCR	D6S89	PCR	LPL
CRI-L336	D1S47	PCR	D6S109	PCR	D8S136
CRI-L1039	D1S71	PCR	D6S105	hNF-L	NEFL
pB8	FGR	pCH6	D6S10	PCR	D8S87
pYNZ2	D1S57	pH2.3	HSPA	pMS502	D8S162*
VC85	D1S85	pHHH157	D6S29	PCR	D8S166
p1-11B	D1S15	CRI-L171	D6S19	H25-3.8	CA2
p5-34	D1S21	PCR	TCTE	PCR	D8S164
p3-18	D1S17	PCR	D6S223	PCR	D8S88
p4-03	D1S19	CRI-R368	D6S23	PCR	D8S85
pL1.22	D1S2	PCR	D6S251	PCR	D8S198
CRI-S182	D1S38	CRI-L322	D6S26	CRI-L413	D8S32
pEFZ13	D1S64	PCR	D6S252	p380-8A	MYC
p6-02	D1S14	p3B10	D6S32	pHT 0.98	TG
pEFD53.2	D1S73	PCR	D6S87	CRI-L186	D8S34
p1-04	D1S9	PCR	D6S255	pH11F3b	CYP11B1*
HHH106	D1S67	pHmNSOD4	SOD2	pMCT128.2	D8S39
PUM24P	MUC1	CEB4	D6S133		
PCR	APOA2	pJCZ30	D6S37		
OS-6	D1S75	pMCOB12	D6S48		
pMLAJ1	D1S61	pYNZ132	D6S44		
pLamB2	LAMB2	CRI-L1065	D6S21		
EKH7.4	D1S65	CEB3	D6S132		
Ren2	REN	pTHH5	D6S39		
pYNZ23	D1S58				
DAF-H	DAF				
pTHH33	D1S81				
cYNA13	D1S74				
PCR	D1S102				
CRI-L1199	D1S68				

Chromosome 10		Chromosome 11		Chromosome 12	
Probe	Locus	Probe	Locus	Probe	Locus
pMCK2	D10S15	p3c7	D11S285	PCR	VWF
phage 10	D10S5	pMCMP1	PYGM	pPRPII2.2	PRB
PTB10.163	D10S22	pHB159	D11S146	pHLA2M.1	A2M
CDC2	CDC2	pSS6	INT2	PCR	D12S62
pCMM17.1	D10S16	PCR	D11S534	PCR	D12S61
pTHHS4	D10S14	PCR	D11S527	WEAV214	COL2A1
PCR	D10S109	pCJ52.99M2	D11S89	p9F11	D12S4
5-1	D10S1	PHI 6-2	D11S85	p11-1-7	D12S6
PCR	D10S109	p2-7-1D6	D11S84	EDF33.2	D12S14
pHHH105	D10S13	STMY	STMY	PCR	D12S43
PCR	D10S91	CJ52.208M2	D11S351	PCR	D12S64
p1-101	D10S4	PCR	D11S29	pDL32B	D12S7
OS-2	D10S20	PCR	CD3	PCR	D12S58
HPa2GEN	a2C10	PNE	PBGD	PCR	PLA2
PCR	D10S173	PCR	D11S490	PCR	D12S60
CRI-L368	D10S12	HBI18P2	D11S147	cMS623	D12S42*
HOAT-1	HOAT	PCR	D11S836	Chd TC-15	D12S65*
pMCT122.2	D10S36	PHI 2.25	D11S83	CMS618	D12S41*
EFD75	D10S25	PCR	D11S874		
		PCR	D11S127		
		CRI-L605			

Table IV (continued).

Chromosome 13		Chromosome 15		Chromosome 17	
Probe	Locus	Probe	Locus	Probe	Locus
PCR	D13S115	PCR	D15S97	p144D6	D17S34
pG2E3.1	D13S11	CRI-L146	D14S46	pYNZ22.1	D17S30
cMS604	D13S70*	pCMW-1	D15S24	pYNH37.3	D17S28
pHV10	D13S6	PCR	ACTC	pHY12-1	D17S1
pCR1359	D13S33	pTHH1142	D15S25	p10-5	MYH2
p7F12	D13S1	PCR	CYP	PCR	D17S520*
pTH162	D13S37	pMSI-14	D15S1	pEW301	D17S58
p68RS2.0	RB1	CRI-L442	D15S48	PHHH202	D17S33
pCR1324	D13S31	pDP151	D15S2	pUC10-41	D17S71
WC25	D13S39	pEFZ33	D15S45	PCR	D17S740
p9D11	D13S2	pEKD49.3	D15S29	pEW206	D17S57
p1E8	D13S4	pEKD49.2	D15S38	pEW207	D17S73
PCR	D13S122	pEKZ104.1	D15S30	PCR	THRA1
pCR1318	D13S32	pVNM18.1	D15S35	pHHH152	D17S32
PCR	D13S64	pKKA25		pE51	NGFR
p9A7	D13S3	PCR	D15S111	PCR	D17S579*
pCR1323	D13S35	pTHH55	D15S27	pCMM86	D17S74
CEB5	D13S107	pEFD85.7	D15S37	pEW101	D17S40
		cMS620	D15S86	PCR	D17S515
		pJU201	D15S3	pHtk9	TK1
				pTHH59	D17S4
				cEFD52	D17S26
				pRMU3	D17S24
				pKKA35	D17S75

Chromosome 18	
Probe	Locus
p74	D18S3
PCR	D18S59
PCR	D18S62
pHHH163	D18S21
PCR	D18S53*
PCR	D18S40
pMS615	D18S32*
PCR	D18S45
PCR	D18S47
L2.7	D18S6
pS71BH3	SSAV1
PCR	D18S35
pB12	GRP*
PCR	D18S42
pMS1-3	D18S19
OS-4	D18S5
EcoG	MBP
pAC404	D18S27
CRI-L159	D18S17
cMS440	D18S31

The probes and loci studied for linkage to BP disease are listed in the order in which they appear (pter-qter) on linkage maps in Figure 1. For marker linkage map references see Legend to Figure 1. Those loci marked with an asterisk have been placed on the linkage map using data from these pedigrees. In every case, the marker-marker linkage data from these pedigrees were in agreement with linkage maps, cytogenetic localization and/or personal communications (listed in the legend to Figure 1) regarding the locus.

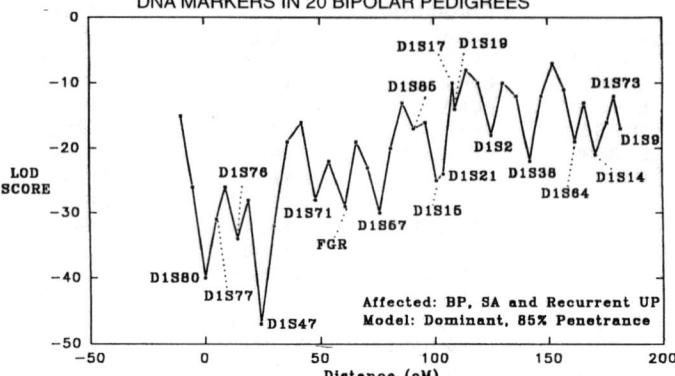

Figure 1A. THREE-POINT LINKAGE ANALYSIS OF CHROMOSOME 1p DNA MARKERS IN 20 BIPOLAR PEDIGREES

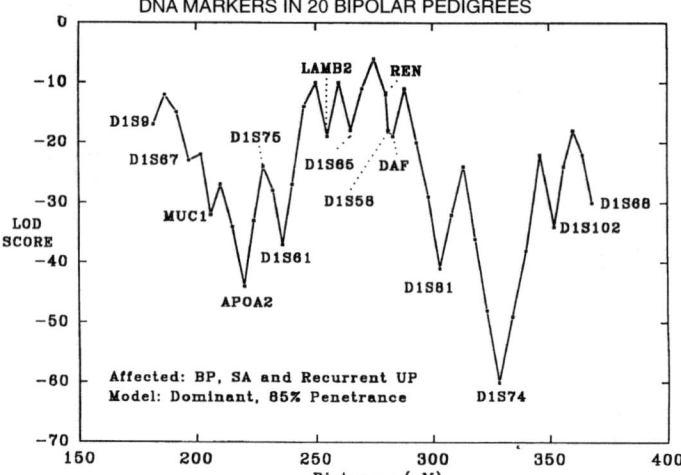

Figure 1B. THREE-POINT LINKAGE ANALYSIS OF CHROMOSOME 1q DNA MARKERS IN 20 BIPOLAR PEDIGREES

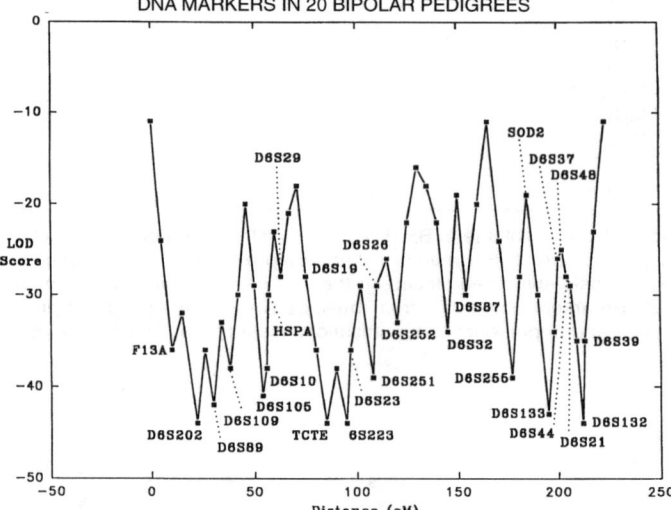

Figure 1C. THREE-POINT LINKAGE ANALYSIS OF CHROMOSOME 6 DNA MARKERS IN 20 BIPOLAR PEDIGREES

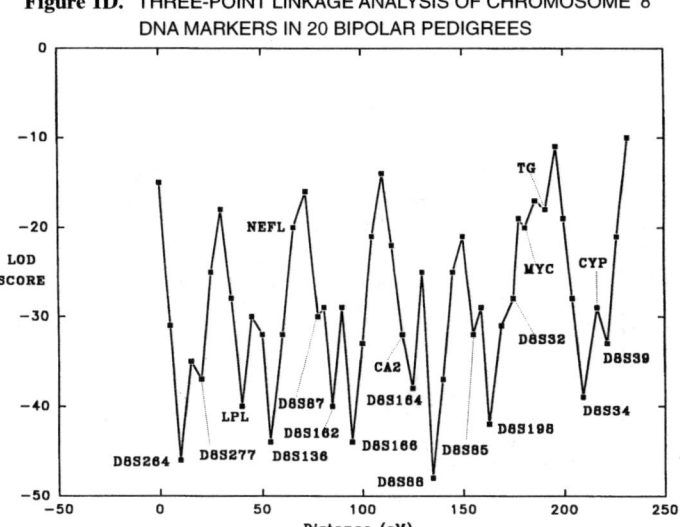

Figure 1D. THREE-POINT LINKAGE ANALYSIS OF CHROMOSOME 8 DNA MARKERS IN 20 BIPOLAR PEDIGREES

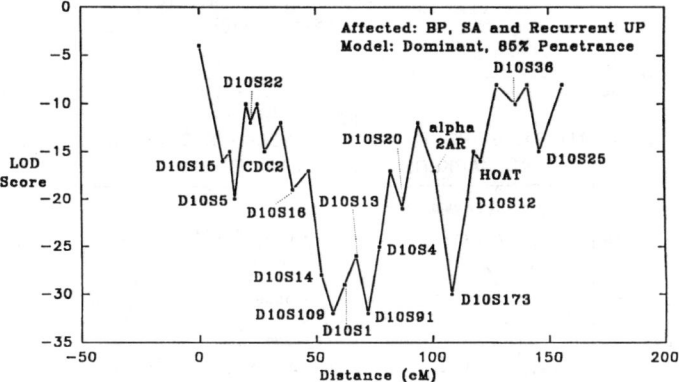

Figure 1E. THREE-POINT LINKAGE ANALYSIS OF CHROMOSOME 10q DNA MARKERS IN 20 BIPOLAR PEDIGREES

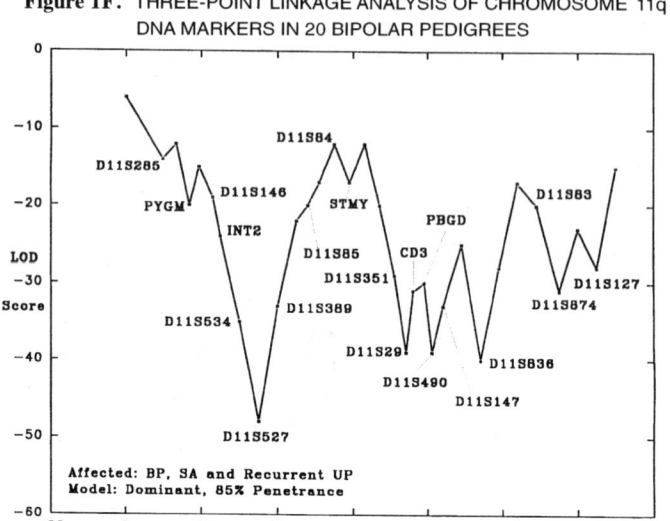

Figure 1F. THREE-POINT LINKAGE ANALYSIS OF CHROMOSOME 11q DNA MARKERS IN 20 BIPOLAR PEDIGREES

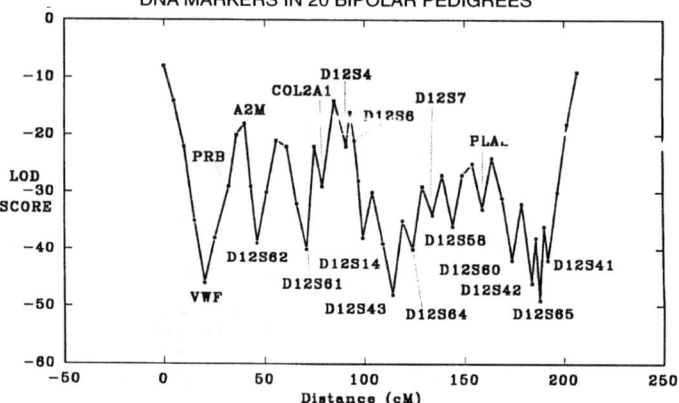

Figure 1G. THREE-POINT LINKAGE ANALYSIS OF CHROMOSOME 12 DNA MARKERS IN 20 BIPOLAR PEDIGREES

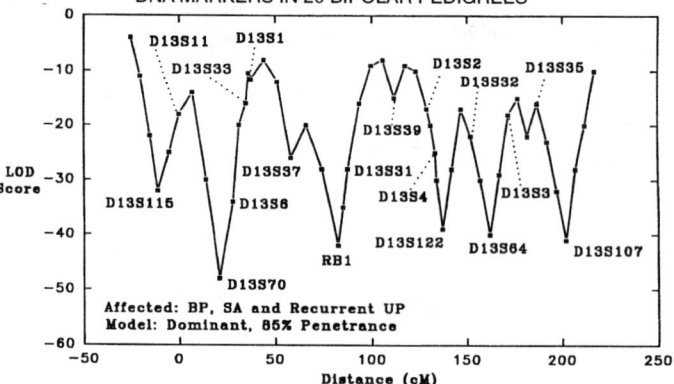

Figure 1H. THREE-POINT LINKAGE ANALYSIS OF CHROMOSOME 13 DNA MARKERS IN 20 BIPOLAR PEDIGREES

MOLECULAR GENETIC STUDIES OF BIPOLAR ILLNESS

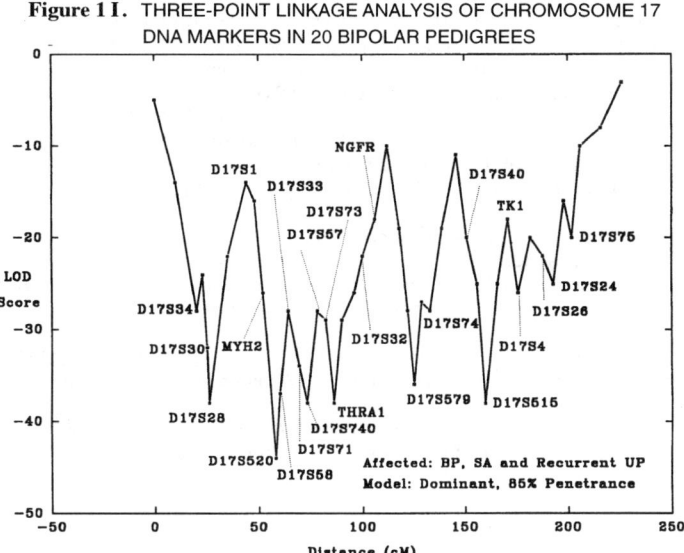

Figure 1 I. THREE-POINT LINKAGE ANALYSIS OF CHROMOSOME 17 DNA MARKERS IN 20 BIPOLAR PEDIGREES

Figure 1 J. THREE-POINT LINKAGE ANALYSIS OF CHROMOSOME 18 DNA MARKERS IN 20 BIPOLAR PEDIGREES

Legend to Figure 1 :
Three-point linkage analysis of the identified loci was conducted (under homogeneity) as described in the text, assuming an autosomal dominant, 85% penetrance disease model, disease gene frequency of 1%, with schizoaffective, bipolar I, bipolar II with major depression and recurrent unipolar considered as affected (affection status model two in Table III). Penetrance of the normal genotype was set at 0.1%. Lod scores for at least one point midway between any two adjacent markers were always calculated. These midpoint lod scores are not always shown on the maps if the markers are separated by less than 5% recombination, for reasons of visual clarity. The overlapping lod scores for adjacent pairs of markers are not shown for reasons of clarity. Rather, the most negative lod score of the two values is shown, so that the negative influence of the unincluded adjacent markers is approximated in each map. Distances between markers are congruous with the references given below. Where two or more maps disagreed on the distance, the actual distance used was that most closely reflected by our own data, in two-point analysis from these 22 families.

Map references :
Nearly all markers listed in Table IV (and shown in Figure 1) are on the linkage map published by the NIH/CEPH Collaborative Mapping Group [42]. D8S264, D8S277 and D18S53 are mapped in Weissenbach et al. [43]. Map locations of some markers were obtained from the Genome Data Base at Johns Hopkins University. Additional references are as follows.
Chromosome 1 :   Dracopli et al. [44]; Buetow et al. [45] (for D1S75).
Chromosome 6 :   Hoehe et al. [46]; Blanche et al. [47]; Nguyen et al. [48]; Wilkie et al. [49]; Bowcock et al. [50], personal communication for D6S202 from Huda Zoghbi.
Chromosome 8 :   Tomfohrde et al. [51]; Arnour et al. [52] (for D8S162); Weissenbach et al. [42] (for D8S264 and D8S277).
Chromosome 10 :   White et al. [53]; Decker et al. [54].
Chromosome 11 :   Julier et al. [55]; McConville et al. [56]; Hauge et al. [57].
Chromosome 12 :   O'Connel et al. [58]; Wang et al. [59]; Armour et al. [52] (for D12S41 and D12S42).
Chromosome 13 :   Bowcock et al. [60]; Armour et al. [52] (for D13S70); Vergnaud et al. [61] (for D13S107).
Chromosome 15 :   Bowcock et al. [62]; Nakamura et al. [63]; Vergnaud et al. [61] (for D15S86).
Chromosome 17 :   Nakamura et al. [64]; Wright et al. [65]; Haines et al. [66]; Fain et al.l [67]; O'Connel et al. [68].
Chromosome 18 :   Armour et al. [52] (for D18S32 and D18S31); Straub et al. [69]; O'Connel et al. [70]; Le Beau et al. [71]; personal communication from Ivan Balaazs for D18S27.

Acknowledgements

This work was supported by a grant to WHB by the National Association for Research in Schizophrenia and Depression (NARSAD). We thank Anita Roe for a grant to the Foundation for Advanced Education in the Sciences.

Ray White's Laboratory has provided more than 75 probes, for which we are very grateful. We thank James Weber and Joan Overhauser for providing unpublished data on numerous microsatellites. We acknowledge the following individuals for providing probes: Ingrid Caras (DAF), Sandra Gendler (MUC1), Nicholas Dracopoli (D1S9, D1S13, D1S14, D1S15, and FGR), M. Goossens (PBGD), S.K. Karathanasis (APOA1), Clive Dickson and G. Peters (INT-2), N.D. Spurr (STMY and CDC2), E. Dietzsch (D11S29), Brian Kobilka and Robert Lefkowitz (alpha 2 C10), V. Ramesh (HOAT-1), Professor C.H.C.M. Buys (D13S11, D13S12 and D13S22), T. Dryja (RB), W. Cavenee (D13S39 and D13S41), A.E. Bale (D13S31, D13S32 and D13S35), D. Barker (D17S58, D17S58, D17S57 and D17S73), M.V. Chao (NGFR), K.K. Kidd (TK1), John Armour (D18S32, D18S31, D13S70, D8S162, D12S41, D12S42 and D15S86), Gilles Vergnaud (D13S107), Jean-Louis Mandel (D18S3), Uta Francke (SSAV1), Jean-Pierre Julien (NEFL), Eliot Spindel (GRP), Stanley Prusiner (MBP), Ivan Balazs (D18S27), Perrin White (CYP11B1) and Carlo Croce (MYC). We wish to thank the many investigators who made their probes available to us through the American Type Culture Collection. D12S65 was kindly provided to us through the Japanese Cancer Research Resources Bank. We gratefully acknowledge the technical assistance of Nina Harris, Chris Ballas, Amy Wagner, David Heydt, Joan Barrick, Teresa Collela, Eric Goldstein, Mia Norlin, David Garth and Charles Cappellari.

References

1. Nurnberger J.I. Jr., Goldin L.R. and Gershon E.S., Genetics of psychiatric disorders. In : Winokur G., Clayton P., eds., *The Medical Basis of Psychiatry*, New York: Sunders WB Co., 1986; 486.
2. Rice J.P., Reich T., Andreasen N.C., Endicott J., Van Eerdewegh M., Fisherman R., Hirschfield R.M.A., Klerman G.L., *Arch. Gen. Psychiatry*, 1987; 44: 441.
3. Risch N., Genet. *Epidemiol.*, 1990; 7: 3.
4. Ott J., *Am. J. Hum. Genet.*, 1990; 46: 219.
5. Martinez M.M., Goldin L.R., *Genet. Epidemiol.*, 1990; 7: 219.
6. Palotie A., Veisanen P., Ott J., Ryhanen L., Elima K., Vikkula M., Cheah K., Vuorio E., Peltonen L., *Lancet* i, 1990; 924.
7. Knowlton R.G., Katzenstien P.L., Moskowitz R.W., Weaver E.J., Malemud C.J., Pathria N., Jimenez S.A., Prockop D.J., *New Eng. J. Med.*, 1990; 322: 526.
8. Ala-Kokko L., Baldin C.T., Moskowitz R.W., Prockop DJ, *Proc. Nat. Acad. Sci.*, 1990; 87: 6565.
9. St. George-Hyslop P.H., Tanzi R.E., Polinsky R.J., Haines J.I., Nee L., Watkins P.C., Myers R.H., Feldman R.G., Pollen D., Drachman D., Growdon J., Brunni A., Froncin J-F., Salmon D., Frommett P., Amaducci L., Sorbi S., Piacentini S., Stewart G.D., Hobbs W.J., Conneally P.M., Gusella J.F., *Science*, 1987; 235: 885.
10. Van Broeckhoven C., Van Hul W., Backhovens H., Van Camp G., Wehnert A., Stinissen P., Raeymaekers P., De Winter G., Gheuens J., Martinand J.J., Vandenberghs A., *Am. Hum J. Genet.*, 1988; 43: a205.
11. Goate A.M., Haynes A.R., M.J., Owen MJ, *Lancet*, 1989; i, 352.
12. Pericak-Vance M.A., Bebout J.L., Gaskell P.C. Jr, Yamaoka L.H., Hung W-Y, Alberts M.J., Walker A.P., Bartlett R.J., Haynes C.A., Weish K.A., Earl N.L., Heyman A., Clark C.M., Roses A.D., *Am. J. Hum. Genet.*, 1991; 48: 1034.
13. Schellenberg G.D., Bird T.D., Wijsman E.M., Orr H.T., Anderson L., Nemens E., White J.A., Bonnycastle L., Weber J.L., Alonso M.E., Potter H., Heston L.L., Martin G.M., *Science*, 1992; 258:668.
14. Hall J.M., Lee M.K., Newman B., Morrow J.E., Anderson L.E., Huey B., King M-C., *Science*, 1990; 250: 1684.
15. Egeland J.A., Gerhard D.S., Pauls D.L., Sussex J.N., Kidd K.K., Allen C.R., Hostetter A.M., Housman D.E., *Nature*, 1987; 325: 783.
16. Detera-Wadleigh S.D., Berrettini W.H., Goldin L.R., Boorman D., Anderson S., Gershon E.S., *Nature*, 1987; 325: 806.
17. Hodgkinson S., Sherrington R., Gurling H.M.D., Marchbanks R.M., Reeders S.T., Mallet J., Peturson H., Brunjolfsson J., *Nature*, 1987; 325: 805.
18. Gill M., McKeon P., Humphries P., *Med J. Genet.*, 1988; 25: 634.
19. Mitchell P., Waters B., Morrison N., Shine J., Donald J., Eissman J., *J. Aff Disorders*, 1991; 20: 23.
20. Kelsoe J.R., Ginns E.I., Egeland J.A., Gerhard D.S., Goldstein A.M., Bale S.J., Pauls D.L., Long R.T., Kidd K.K., Conte G., Housman D.E., Paul S.M., *Nature*, 1989; 342: 238.
21. Winokur G., Clayton P.J., Reich T., eds., *Manic-depressive Illness*. St Louis, C.V. Mosby Co., 1969; 112.
22. Mendlewicz J., Fleiss J.L., Biol. *Psychiatry*, 1974; 9: 261.
23. Baron M., Risch N., Hamburger R., Mandel B., Kushner S., Newman M., Drumer D., Belmaker R.H., *Nature*, 1987; 326: 289.
24. Gershon E.S., Targum S.D., Matthysse S., Bunney W.E. Jr., *Arch. Gen. Psychiatry*, 1979; 36: 1423.

25. Berrettini W.H., Goldin L.R., Gelernter J., Gejman, Gershon E.S., Detera-Wadleigh S., *Arch. Gen. Psychiatry*, 1990; 47: 336.
26. Del Zompo M., Bocchetta A., Ruiu S., Goldin L.R., Berrettini W.H., Association and Linkage studies of affective disorders. In : Racagni G., Brunello N., Fukuda T., eds. *Biological Psychiatry* (vol 2). New York, Elsevier Science Pub Co, Inc, 1991; 446.
27. Van Broeckhoven C., De Bruyn A., Raeymaekers P., Sandkuijl L., Mendelbaum K., Delvenne V., Mendlewicz J., *Proc. 8th Intl. Cong. Hum. Genet.*, 1991; 49: 362.
28. Baron M., Freimer N.F., Risch N., Lerer B., Alexander J.R., Straub R.E., Asokan S., Das K., Peterson A., Amos J., Endicott J., Ott J., Gilliam C., *Nature Genet.*, 1993; 3: 49.
29. Berrettini W.H., Goldin L.R., Martinez M.M., Maxwell T., Smith A.L., Guroff J.J., Kazuba D.M., Nurnberger J.I. Jr., Hamovit J., Simmons-Alling S., Robb A.S., Gershon E.S., *Psychiat. Genet.*, 1991; 2: 125.
30. Detera-Wadleigh S.D., Berrettini W.H., Goldin L.R., Martinez M., Hsieh W-T., Hoehe M., Coffman D., Rollins D.Y., Muniec D., Choi H., Wiesch D., Guroff J., Gershon E.S., *Neuropsychopharmacology*, 1992; 6: 219.
31. Berrettini W.H., Detera-Wadleigh S.D., Goldin L.R., Martinez M., Hsieh W-T., Hoehe M., Choi H., Muniec D., Ferraro T.N., Guroff J.J., Kazuba D., Harris N., Kron E., Nurnberger J.I. Jr., Alexander R.D., Gershon E.S., *Psychiat. Genet.*, 1991a; 2: 191.
32. Gejman P.V., Martinez M., Qiuhe C., Friedman E., Berrettini W.H., Goldin L.R., Koroulakis P., Ames C., Lerman M.A., Gershon E.S., *Neuropsychopharmacology* (in press).
33. Smith G.A.B., *Ann. Hum. Genet.*, 1963; 27: 175.
34. Gebbinck M.F.B.G., van Etten I., Hateboer G., Suijkerbuijk R., Beijersbergen R.L., van Kessel A.D., Moolenaar W.H., *FEBS Letters*, 1991; 290: 123.
35. Manji H.K., *Am. J. Psychiatry*, 1992; 149: 746.
36. Jones D.T. and Reed R.R., *Science*, 1989; 244.
37. Overhauser J., Mewar R., Rojas K., Lia K., Kline A.D., Silverman G.A., *Genomics*, 1993; 15: 387.
38. Weeks D.E., Lehner T., Squires-Wheeler E., Kaufman C., Ott J., *Genet. Epidemiol.*, 1990; 7: 237.
39. Clerget-Darpoux F., Babron M.C., Bonaiti-Pellie C., *Genet. Epidemiol.*, 1990; 7: 245.
40. Clerget-Darpoux F., Bonaiti-Pellie C., Hochez J., *Biometrics*, 1986; 42: 245.
41. Boehnke M., *Am. J. Hum. Genet.*, 1986; 39: 513.
42. NIH/CEPH Collaborative Mapping Group, *Science*, 1992; 258: 67.
43. Weissenbach J., Gyapay G., Dib C., Vignai A., Morissette J., Millasseau P., Vaysseix G., Lathrop M., *Nature*, 1992; 359: 794.
44. Dracopoli, O'Connell P., Elsner T.I., Lalouel J-M., White R.L., Buetow N.H., Nishimura D.Y., Murray J.C., Helms C., Mishra S.K., Donis-Keller H., Hall J.M., Lee M.K., King M.C., Attwood J., Morton N.E., Robson E.B., Mahtani M., Willard H.F., Royle N., Patel I., Jeffreys A.J., Verga V., Jenkins T., Weber J.L., Mitchell A.L., Bale A.E., *Genomics*, 1991; 9: 686.
45. Buetow K.H., Nishimura D., Green P., Nakamura Y., Jiang O., Murray J.C., *Genomics*, 1990; 8: 13.
46. Hoehe M.R., Leppert M., Lalouel J-M., Hsieh W-T., Stauffer D., Holik J., Berretttini W.H., Byerley W.F., Gershon E.S., *Genomics* (in press).
47. Blanche H., Zoghbi H.Y., Jabs E.W., De Gouyon B., Zunec R., Dausset J., Cann H.M., *Genomics*, 1991; 9: 420.
48. Nguyen J., Charmley P., Grody W.W., Cederbaum S.D., King M-C., Gatti R.A., *Cytogenetc. Cell Genet.*, 1990; 54: 95.
49. Wilkie P.J., Polymeropoulos M.H., Trent J.M., Small K.W., Weber J.L., *Genomics*, 1993; 15: 225.
50. Bowcock A.M., Azuma T., Barnes R.I., Wu S-H., Bell G.I., Taggart T., *Genomics*, 1992; 13: 398.
51. Tomfohrde J., Wood S., Chertzer M., Wagner M.J., Wells D.E., Parrish J., Sadler L.A., Blanton S.H., Daiger S.P., Wang Z., Wilkie P., Weber J.L., *Genomics*, 1992; 14: 144.

52. Armour J.A.L., Povey S., Jeremiah S. and Jeffreys A.M., *Genomics*, 1990; 8: 501.
53. White R., Lalouel J-M., Nakamura Y., Donis-Keller H., Green P., Bowden D.L., Mathew C.G.P., Easton D.R., Robson E.B., Morton N.E., Gusella J.F., Haines J.L., Retief A.E., Kidd K.K., Murray J.C., Lathrop G.M., Cann H.M., *Genomics*, 1990; 6: 393.
54. Decker R.A., Moore J., Ponder B., Weber J.L., *Genomics*, 1992; 12: 604.
55. Julier C., Nakamura Y., Lathrop M., O'Connel P., Leppert M., Litt M., Mohandas T., Lalouel J-M., White R., *Genomics*, 1990; 7: 335.
56. McConville C.M., Formstone C.J., Hernandez D., Thik J., Taylor A.M.R., *Nucl. Acids Res.*, 1990; 18: 4335.
57. Hauge X., Browne D., Litt M., Abstracts: Genome Maping and Sequencing. Cold Spring Harbor Laboratory, May 6-10, 1992.
58. O'Connell P., Lathrop G.M., Law M., Leppert M., Nakamura Y., Hoff M., Kumlin E., Thomas W., Elsner T., Ballard L., Goodman P., Azen E., Sadler J.E., Cai G.Y., Lalouel J-M., White R., *Genomics*, 1987; 1: 93.
59. Wangand Z., Weber J.L., *Genomics*, 1992; 13: 532.
60. Bowcock A., Osborne-Lawrence S., Barnes R., Chakravarti A., Washington S., Dunn C., *Genomics*, 1993; 15: 376.
61. Vergnaud G., Mariat D., Apiou F., Aurias A., Lathrop M., Lauthier V., *Genomics*, 1991; 11: 135.
62. Bowcock A.M., Barnes R.I., White R.L., Kruse T.A., Tsipouras P., Sarfarazi M., Jenkins T., Vilioen C., Litt M., Kramer P.L., Murray J.C., Vergnaud G., *Genomics*, 1992a; 14: 833.
63. Nakamura Y., Lathrop M., O'Connell P., Leppert M., Barker D., Wright E., Skolnikc M., Kondoleon S., Litt M., Lalouel J-M., White R., *Genomics*, 1988; 2: 302.
64. Nakamura Y., Lathrop M., O'Connell P., Leppert M., Lalouel J-M., Whit R., *Genomics*, 1988a; 3: 342.
65. Wright E.S., Goldgar D.E., Fain P.R., Barker D.F., Skolnick M.H., *Genomics*, 1990; 7: 103.
66. Haines J.L., Ozelius L.J., McFarlane H., Menon A., Tzall S., Martiniuk F., Hirschorn R., Gusella J.F., *Genomics*, 1990; 8: 1.
67. Fain P.R., Goldgar D.E., Wallace M.R., Collins F.S., Wright E., Hguyen K., Barker D.F., *Am. J. Hum. Genet.*, 1989; 45: 721.
68. O'Connell P., Plaetke R., Norisade M., Odelberg S., Jorde L., Chance P., Leppert M., Lalouel J-M., White R., *Genomics*, 1993; 15: 38.
69. Straub R.E., Speer M.C., Luo Y., Rojas K., Overhauser J., Ott J., Gilliam T.C., *Genomics*, 1993; 15: 48.
70. O'Connell P., Lathrop G.M., Leppert M., Nakamura Y., Muller U., Lalouel M-M., White R., *Genomics*, 1988; 3: 367.
71. Le Beau M.M., Overhauser J., Straub R.E., Silverman G., Gilliam T.C., Ott J., O'Connell P., Francke U., Geurts van Kessel A., *Cytogenet. Cell Genet.* 1991 (in press).

2

The question of a «nuclear depressive syndrome»

O. DOERR-ZEGERS

Psiquiatria y Psicoterapia Luis Thayer, OJEDA n° 0115 of 502, CL Santiago de Chile (Chili)

The author reviews the series of difficulties inherent to the diagnosis of the depressive illness, as well as the different attempts to determine something like a «nuclear depressive syndrome». Then he refers to a previous paper in which he also made a similar attempt. Unlike to what occurs in DSM-III and ICD 10, among other modern diagnostic systems, the symptoms appeared linked among them and with the underlying process by essential relationships and not only by contiguity. The problem of the operational systems and of their known lack of specificity lies in the fact that they do not distinguish between symptom and phenomenon. The first is only the visible element of a chain of links which conceals itself. The phenomenon, on the contrary, is «what shows itself by itself» (Heidegger) and encompasses both the symptom and the underlying process. As a contribution to phenomenological diagnosis of depression, the author attempts to make an analysis of corporality of a depressive patient, finding that its most striking feature is «chrematization» (from greek word «chrema», that means a useless thing) or «cadaverization». This phenomenon would be always present in a real depression, only that it would be more or less evident according to its severity. This feature discovered through phenomenological intuition permits the comprehension if both, the diversity of particular symptoms of depression as well as the form in which they tend to cluster in the concrete cases.

Any approach to the subject of depression has to face first of all the question of its definition. If, following the tradition, we take mood disturbance as the fundamental symptom, we immediately find ourselves with the problem that in many other morbid conditions the mood appears as being affected. Thus, there are schizophrenic patients who occasionally present a depressive mood, and the same is valid for epileptics, organics, and above all, for neurotics. The limits between depression and obsessive-compulsive neurosis, agoraphobia or the now called «generalised anxiety disorder» are extremely unprecise. But perhaps the greatest difficulty is the one stated by transitions towards normality. Too frequently we observe confusion between sentimental problems, work failures or normal mourning and a depressive illness. In our experience, psychiatrics overdiagnose depressive illness, whereas, on their side, internists and other specialists underdiagnose it.

The difficulty inherent to the diagnosis of depression led quite early to an attempt in establishing something like a nuclear depressive syndrome, that is to say, those symptoms which have to be always present to speak of depression. And thus, for Kraeplin, the fundamental symptoms are «difficulty in seizing stimuli and thinking, depressive or anxious dysthy and inhibition of the will». Beuler also distinguishes three fundamental symptoms: depressive dysthimia, slowing of the course of thought and retardation of centrifugal functions (decisions, acts, movements). Kurt Schneider, following Max Scheler, describes as the basic symptom involvement of «vital feelings», being the most specific those directly corporal, such as the case of precordial oppression and/or pain, globus melancholicus and pain in the nape of the neck. In 1966 Pichot describes five groups of symptoms which would always be present in an authentic depressive syndrome: one group surrounding depressive mood, another self-aggressiveness, another one slowing, another decrease in vitality, and finally, a group composed of somatic symptoms. In 1968 Pfeiffer, based on transcultural studies between Germany and Indonesia, concludes that «the only symptoms not determined by the type or degree of civilisation or culture, are a difficult to define» change in mood and the perturbation of vegetative functions such as sleep, appetite and libido.

Long before the appearance of the current diagnostic criteria for depressive illness, such as RDC (Research Diagnostic Criteria), the criteria of the Saint Louis School or DSM-III and DSM-III-R, at the end of the 60's we had also attempted to determine something like a nuclear depressive syndrome. In our study, carried out in the Psychiatric Hospital of Conception, Chile, we found three groups of symptoms which could be considered essential and directly deriving from the presupposed underlying process, namely:

1. Involvement of the «lived body» or corporality («Befindlichkeit» in German), in which mood disturbance appears only as one more expression of a very complex phenomenon which also includes lack of energy, anxiety, nauseas, feeling of cold and the «vital symptoms» of Schneider.

2. Involvement of those functions that Beuler designated «centrifugal», that is to say, those which connect us with the external world, among which psychic and motor retardation are the most characteristic manifestations. The difficulty in paying attention, in concentrating, in taking decisions, loss of strength of the voice and slowing down of body movements are other forms in which the same phenomenon reveals itself. The latter was also considered by Kraepelin as being essential in this illness.

3. Involvement of biological rhythmicity: all the vital rhythms are inverted, suspended or at least disturbed. And we talk of rhythmicity and not of rhythms because the disturbance is not referred only to particular rhythms such as sleep or digestion, but also to the way existence unfolds itself in time, so characteristically rhythmic and periodic. And thus, there is a daily rhythm, a monthly one, a seasonal one and a vital one, that is to say, of the whole life, and all of them appear altered.

Two other groups of independent symptoms can also be present, although not regularly: delusional ideas with the three typical depressive contents and self-aggressiveness, which includes suicidal ideation and attempts.

In that opportunity we also proposed the existence of a unique illness, which we would later call «melancholic depression». We also questioned the classic distinction between endogenous and reactive depression and -following Tellenbach- the endless number of other types of depression described throughout the century, as is the case of «basic depression» of Schneider, «vitalised reactive depression» of Weitbrecht, «exhaustion depression» of Kielholz or the «existential depression» of Haefner. The proposal of DSM-III (1980) of one only type of depression, namely, «major depression», as opposed to the 20 different types described in ICD 9 of the World Psychiatric Association (this would change in ICD 10), confirmed our point of view. The 9 criteria in DSM-III in opposition to the 21 in Hamilton's scale, are also close to what we found in Conception. The difference lies in the fact that DSM-III does not distinguish between symptom and phenomenon and that the first ones appear in a list where their only link is contiguity. Our proposition deals, in a certain way, with the same symptoms, but seen in their internal relationships and as deriving from wider phenomena (change in corporality or in rhythmicity, for example), which in turn would be rooted in something like a common denominator of depressiveness, probably the disturbance in temporality. Thus, symptoms 1, 2 and 6 of DSM-III-R (depressed mood, anhedonia and energy loss) correspond to the first group of symptoms of our list, those which surround change in corporality; symptoms 5 and 8 (psychomotor slowing and decrease in thought capacity) correspond to the second group, disturbance of the «body in action» or involvement of centrifugal functions, whereas symptoms 3 and 4 (weight increase or loss, insomnia or hypersomnia) correspond to the group of involvement of biological rhythmicity. Finally, symptoms 7 and 9 of DSM-III (uselessness or guilt ideas) correspond to the fourth set of symptoms described by us, that of depressive delusional ideas.

We believe that diagnostic criteria such as DSM-III, ICD 10 or RDC, by remaining in the sphere of symptoms, commit two fundamental mistakes: first, the lists will be necessarily incomplete. Two examples: first, when in symptom Nr. 6 DSM-III speaks of «energy loss», why not also mention languor or heaviness of the limbs?; or why not mention such important symptoms as anxiety, the vital symptoms of Schneider or feeling of cold ? and second, it overlooks essential relationships between particular symptoms, such as the one between insomnia and appetite loss (both rhythmic alterations) or between decrease in thought capacity and the general slowing down (both derived from the complex phenomenon of psychomotor retardation).

The distinction between symptom and phenomenon goes back to the book «Being and Time» by Heidegger and has great importance in the development of anthropological-phenomenological psychiatry (Hofer, Tellenbach, Haefner, Blankenburg, Tatossian, Doerr-Zegers). In his book the german philosopher made, in a certain way, a definitive analysis of the problem. For him the symptoms or manifestations only announce a disturbance which is not evident in itself. The phenomenon, in turn, is «what shows itself by itself», and it includes at the same time the symptom which announces it and the disturbance which underlies it. Somatic medicine is fundamentally concerned with the recognition and management of symptoms. If symptom is defined as «the visible element of a functional complex» (Haefner) and a previous knowledge of the laws ruling the underlying patho-physiologic whole, or illness, is supposed, then the jump from the external manifestation to the illness as a whole will be legitimate, and that is diagnosis. In psychiatry, on the contrary, this procedure is not possible, since the assumptions founding the diagnostic process of somatic medicine are not given, at least in what refers to the so called endogenous psychoses. If in spite of this, one insists on the merely symptomatologic sphere, e.g. discouragement, fatigue, weight loss, guilt ideas, etc. one unavoidably falls into confusions and tautologies. Müller-Suur demonstrated that in schizophrenia diagnosis is almost always done on the basis of the «schizophrenic» character of the symptoms, that is to say, a tautology. A psychiatry exclusively oriented to the external manifestations or symptoms is not qualified to answer what «schizophrenic» means, which in a tacit way is allowing diagnosis and consensus.

Attempt at a phenomenology of depressive corporality

In a further experience with affective disorders structured in the framework of the new admissions unit of the Psychiatric University Clinic in Santiago, Chile, the following clinical features became evident: First, we proved what we had stated in 1971, in the sense that the distinction between endogenous and reactive depression lacked justification and that depressions as such were all «endoreactive» and appeared in that characteristic personality described by Tellenbach as «typus melancholicus» (1961). This last one was later empirically demonstrated by von Zerssen and collaborators in Germany and more recently by Anneliese Doerr and Sandra Viani in Chile. Second, we gradually became sure of the need, already suggested in 1971, to distinguish between melancholic and non melancholic depressivity, e.g. the depressive symptom appearing in other pathologies such as schizophrenia, epilepsy and neurosis, and in normal people. Third, we became convinced that the substantial element of the phenotypic difference between one depressive picture and another was the intensity, and what appears as so different, for example, a simple vital depression and a depressive stupor were fundamentally one and the same phenomenon, only in different degrees. The last version of ICD, Nr. 10, agrees with us by defining one only depressive episode (F 31), but distinguishing four different intensities: mild, moderate, severe without psychotic symptoms and severe with psychotic symptoms. Fourth, something like an atmospheric emanation directly emerging from melancholic depressions became increasingly evident:; we called it «Melancholie-Gefühl» (sensation of what is melancholic), parodying Rümke with his classic «Praecox-Gefühl» (sensation of what is schizophrenic). This intuitive knowledge, susceptible of being also learned by younger colleagues, was demonstrated as fundamental in distinguishing melancholic depressions (which more or less correspond to the major depressive episode of DSM-III) from non-melancholic ones. Our atmospheric experience of melancholic depressivity has a certain relationship with expressions found in Tellenbach's «Geschmack und Atmosphäre» (Taste and Atmosphere) (1968), when he speaks of the «loss of vital freshness» of the depressive.

Blankenburg demands of the phenomenological experience that it be «decidedly more open to all the modalities of being of that which faces us, that is to say, it has to be capable of being more natural than natural experience itself», but at the same time it has to be «more scientific than scientific experience, insofar it is not limited to one only transcendental project, but it rather transforms all the ways of being in general in its central theme». Following Blankenburg's recommendations, we will elaborate a phenomenology of this atmospheric experience in the encounter with an extreme case of melancholic depression: a depressive stupor. For such analysis the attitude of the researcher would resemble as much as possible that of a person without psychiatric experience, somebody still able of a complete naiveté. For such an observer the immobility of the patient will not be «psychomotor retardation», and her silence will not be «stuporous mutism», etc., but simply the different aspects of the being with whom the observer comes across in that moment and which affect him in such or such a way. Because of the limited space we will omit the patient's clinical report. Following, we will present the phenomenological analysis :

The patient remains in front of us silent and motionless. Her glance is gloomy and dull, it does not transmit any message, there is in it no sign of interior life. Her skin is pale, yellowish and dry. We do not feel her persistent silence as denying a dialogue, but rather as not being present. In a certain way she is not there, since that natural polarised tension occurring in interpersonal encounters, called «antikry» by the Greeks, does not appear between me and her. Among the fundamental characteristics of the interhuman encounter, as they were first described by von Baeyer and then by Tellenbach, stands out vis-a-vis, or being one in front of the other in a permanent exchange of gestures, emotions and words. Behaviour with respect to the other in an encounter is always frontal. Only in this manner is it possible to understand the seriousness of the gesture of «turning one's back» or of «avoiding to look». The patient remains insensible to all my attempts to bring her to something like a contraposition, to make her oppose me as an other, and curiously, the feeling she begins to provoke in us is increasingly further from sorrow or compassion. There is something in her disagreeably alien, almost sinister. This impression of what is disagreeable and alien is rather the result of the experience of a vacuum, there where one was prepared to meet a living and different spirit more or less communicative, familiar, open, sympathetic, interesting, etc.

Let us try to go deeper into this feeling of disagreeable strangeness provoked in us by the patient. The first thing which comes to us is a very corporal sensation that floods us, difficult to express in words, although close to the nausea of Sartre. We experience similar sensations, for example, before a corpse in the autopsy table. Suddenly we realise that the opacity of her glance, that her motionlessness and silence have in common something cadaverous. In her whole being there is something like a thing, we could almost say material, preventing a reciprocity to arise between her existence and mine. There is no coming and going of a personal flow, there is no exchange between her glance and mine, between her happening and mine. Instead of an authentic interpersonal encounter, what has occurred between us is hardly colliding myself with her, encountering something and not encountering with. This character of «thing» irradiating the almost purely material presence of the patient is also made evident through her availability. She is not seated or standing in front of me, but only put there, and I feel that I could dispose of her at my will as of an utensil. In fact, I submit her to a neurologic examination and she offers no resistance, as well as no help, and I return to the original impression of examining a corpse, although less rigid.

If we wanted to express this form of her being or presenting herself in front of others with the richness of the greek language, we would have to say that her antikry (her way of facing) is not enantiotic, that is to say, reciprocal, but chrematic. For the Greeks, «chrema» is an object with which I can have only a utilitarian treatment, but which is useless to me. In a certain way «chrema» is the opposite of «physis». We find again an analogous contraposition in Gabriel Marcel in his polarity between the «body I have» and the «body I am». I have my eyes and my glance. The body I have is always on the way towards the thing, towards the corpse; on the contrary, the body I am is always gesture, meaning and transcendence, that is to say, spirit.

Undoubtlessly, the stuporous and chrematic body of our patient is nearer to the body I have than to the body I am. What she has lost is precisely her capacity to open herself to the other, to signify, to face, or said in greek, to be enantiotic. Her glance has lost not only its brightness, but it has sunk behind the eyes, being impossible for her to know the world, process so accurately defined by Sartre with the words: «connaître c'est manger des yeux» (to know is to eat with the eyes). In a certain way the total loss of appetite experienced by our patient has also involved the eyes, namely, the appetite of the spirit.

But stupor is not the only form depression in which the body of the depressive acquires the described chrematic transformation. Stupor only represents the final stage of a body process in becoming a thing, or chrema, which is already announced in the slight initial languor, in the vital symptoms such as precordial oppression, feeling of cold, heaviness of the limbs, but also in the so common fact that depressive patients tend to excessively worry about their body and they do not have any other subject but their somatized anguish or their obstructed digestion or their lack of appetite or their pertinacious insomnia. Every true depressive, every melancholic depression in our terminology, shows us a certain degree of chrematization and this would be a specific phenomenon, whose adequate grasping could be transformed into a fundamental weapon for an unequivocal diagnosis of depressive illness.

And now we return to the initial point, namely to the problem of the strict definition of depression as such and the need of an adequate order of its manifestations that goes beyond the mere addition of symptoms linked only by contiguity. From the three fundamental phenomena described by us characteristic of melancholic depression and around which its concrete manifestations are grouped, two of them can be directly perceived by the examinator: the group surrounding vital dysthimia and the group surrounding psychomotor retardation, since they are different ways in which the phenomenon of chrematization shows itself. In that sense, what the patient lives as languor, discouragement, feeling of cold, etc. is seen in a concrete way by the physician as paleness, opacity of the glance, frontal wrinkle in omega, greater or lesser motionlessness, etc. In the same way, what the patient lives as difficulty in concentrating, in taking decisions or as rumination of thoughts, is perceived by the examiner as slowing of movements, lack of direction of the glance, in-decision in the gestures, latency in the answers, etc. The third group, which is the expression of involvement of biological rhythmicity, cannot be perceived in phenomenological intuition, but being a subjective symptom, it is as the same time easy to objectify: even with instruments, and the same is valid for decrease in appetite and in weight or for slowness or acceleration of digestion. But the important thing is that this alteration of rhythms can also be conceived as an expression of the process of chrematization occurring in the depressive body. Life is movement from the past towards the future and this movement is always given in the form of rhythms and periods in consonance with cosmic rhythms, as has been stated by Tellenbach in his concept of endogenous psychoses as «endocosmogenic» illnessess. The phenomenon of suspension, inversion or at least alteration of biological fundamental rhythms that we observe in all melancholic depressions represents another form of expressing this process of chrematization, since it means a loss of consonance with the world and of the temporal condition of existence.

«Chrematization» process and endogenity

What we have called chrematization and conceived as a fundamental phenomenon of depressivity, from which its three groups of constituent symptoms can be inferred: alteration of the lived body (dysthimia), of the body in action (psychomotor retardation) and of the body in time (involvement of vital rhythms), has a very close relationship with one of the essential contribution made by phenomenological psychiatry to the understanding of depressive illness: Tellenbach's concept of endogenity. This author, following Goethe, conceives endogenity as an animated nature, as an originary form which shows itself in its development through certain somatic and psychic characteristics. «Imprinted form that by living develops itself», says Goethe in the poem dedicated to the primordial orphic words. And Tellenbach specifies, «The way of being of the endon is transubjective and consequently metapsychologic, but at the same time transobjective and consequently metasomatologic». This means that the endon is previous to the division between psyche and soma and it determines both of them, but at the same time it is subsequent, because in the relationship of consonance with the world, this one can also determine and shape the «endon» in the way the world and others teach us. Nobody has expressed in a better way this wonderful interaction than Goethe, when he says in his Theory of Colors: «The eye owes its existence to light. Among varios rudimentary and indifferent organs, light chooses an organ which resembles it, and thus it forms the eye from the light and for the light, so that the interior light goes out to meet the exterior one». Let us think, for example, in the phenomenon of language and how in it we need both the learning capacity originated from what is endogenous and the presence of the mother, whose language the boy slowly learns to imitate, until he comes to own the «mother tongue».

For Tellenbach this endon which reveals itself through maturative phenomena can also become spoiled in its development and those failures would come to be endogenous psychoses and in particular depression. In this last one, as in no other illness, all the manifestations of what is endogenous appear deformed, from rhythmycity up to the different talents or capacities, which vanish in that typical phenomenon of «not being able» considered by Binswanger as a central feature of melancholia.

There is no doubt that Tellenbach's concept of endogenity represents a sort of resurrection of the ancient greek concept of «physis». The noun «physis» comes from the verb «phyo», which means to grow or increase, that is to say, the same meaning of endon as «imprinted form that by living develops itself». The Greeks used this word to designate both nature in general as well as human nature, conceiving this last one as a «small nature», which in a way contains the whole «great» one. According to Heidegger (1953) the word physis meant for the classic Greek «both the sky and the earth, both the stones and the plants, the animals and the human being; but also the history of the human being as work of men and gods, and finally, or above all, the gods themselves under the sign of destiny. Physis is emerging which is made evident from what is hidden...». That is to say, physis «is the being itself by means of which the entity can come to remain and be then observed». The meaning of «nature» for the latin world is much more limited: it means to be born and birth, but also temperament and character. With this the greek concept of physis is lost and one could state that the reductionist and dichotomic character showed by the natural sciences in the history of the West -at least in what is referred to the study of the human being- is related with that reducing transformation carried out by Rome by translating the word «physis» to «nature». In philosophy after Aristotle the concept of «psyché», what is psychic, has been opposed to «physis», and thus we speak today of «psycho-physical unity», attempt of union which is precisely alluding to how separated these two forms of revealing itself the human nature have become. However, in its original meaning «psyché» was contained in «physis», it was a possible manifestation of it. What was certainly outside of «physis» was « nomos », that is to say, what is ethic, and «techné», technique in the sense of knowing how to dispose, install or modify what is given. «Nomos» and «techné» have in common their association with liberty. Both imply deciding between one option or another and the creativity implicit in technical action is based in that called liberty. «Physis» is, on the other hand, what is given, in some way, that escaping self-availity.

Now, what is really opposed to «physis» is «chrema ». « Chrema » means the loss of creative potentiality, motionlessness and whole availability. What is chrematic is what is referred to things in their most privative, material and devitalized sense, that is to say, the contrary not only of «physis», but also of «endon». We saw that in phenomenological analysis the chrematization of the being of the depressive person appeared as what is substantial in depressivity. From this process of loss of the physical condition, in the sense of «physis», one is able to understand the discouragement, the lack of strength, the anhedonia, the multiple pains and the somatized anxiety which imprisons the subject in its body, but also the «not being able» of psychomotor retardation and the suspension of the rhythmic condition of existence. Because, if «physis» is the transcended nature, «chrema» is the inanimated nature and the chrematization process suffered by the depressive person is only a progressive loss of the capacity of transcending the body towards the world and towards action, but without losing its anchorage in the order of the cosmos through its rhythms and periods. When we say that «physis» is transcended nature, we mean that it contains both, all that is involuntary, determined, outside self-availability, proper of what Heidegger calls «Geworfenheit» or «state of being ejected» or of being thrown into the world (1927, 1963) -and which is expressed in the physical structure, abilities and rhythms -as well as an opening towards the spirit. In the other words, «physis» is not only what is «geworfen», but also «das Entwerfen», not only what is ejected, but also the project, or better said, the capacity of projecting and being projected. A return to the chrematic condition is therefore a path towards death in the most literal sense. When there are no projects there is no future, when there is no future there is no time, when there is no time there is no movement. Many depressive patients report, when recovering from the episode, that they felt «dead in life». Heidegger, without having ever seen a depressive patient, only from his deep knowledge of human nature and his brilliant intuitions, came to say in «Being and Time»: «Die Gedrücktheit zwingt das Dasein auf seine Geworfenheit zurück, aber so, daß diese gerade verschlossen wird» (Gloominess forces existence back into its state of being ejected, but in such a way that it closes itself). It is difficult to find a deeper description of what occurs with the existence of a depressive person: he is pushed towards his feasibility, towards his condition of mere determined nature, and even further, towards inanimated nature, through the described chrematization process, but without even having the possibility of knowing that he is sheltered and protected in and by it, as we feel when sleeping, the clearest and most familiar example of our periodic return to what is endogenous.

In summary, depression would not only be conceived as a failure of endogenity, but also a retracting of that long road covered by the human being from «chrema» up to «physis» or, in other words, a sort of return of the spirit to its material condition.

References

1. American Psychiatric Association. *Diagnostic and Statistical Manual of Mental Disorders*. 3rd. Edition Revised (DSM III R). Washington, D.C. : APA (1987).
2. Baeyer, W, von. « Der Begriff der Begegnung in der Psychiatrie». *Der Nervenarzt* 1955 ; 26: 369-376.
3. Binswanger L. *Melancholie und Manie*. Pfullingen: Neske Verlag, 1964.
4. Blankenburg W., «Aus dem phänomenologischen Erfhrungsfeld innerhalb der Psychiatrie». *Schweiz. Arch. Psychiat. Neurol.* 1962 ; 90: 412-421.
5. Bleuler E. and Bleuler M. *Handbuch der Psychiatrie*. Berlin-Göttingen-Heidelberg: Springer Verlag, 10. Auflage 1966, Pag. 408.
6. Dörr-Alamos A. and Viani S. *Personalidad premorbida en los distintos cuadros efectivos*. Thesis to be a candidate for the title of Licenciate in Psychology. Santiago : Universad Diego Portales 1991.
7. Dörr-Zegers O. *et al.* «Del analisis clinico-estadistico del sindrome depresivo a una comprension del fenomeno de la depresividad en su concepto patogenetico». *Rev. Chil. Neuropsiquiat.* 1971 ; 10: 17-39.

8. Dörr-Zegers O. Analisis fenomenelogico de la depresividad en la melancolia y en la epilepsia. *Actas Luso-Espanolas Neurol. Psiquiat. y Cs. Afines*, 7 (2° Etapa): 1979 ; 291-304.
9. Dörr-Zegers O. and Tellenbach H. Differentialphänomenologie des depressiven Syndroms. *Der Nervenarzt* 1980 ; 15: 113-118.
10. Dörr-Zegers O. Dimensiones de la depresion. *Apuntes de Medecina Clinica* 1988 ; 27: 11-21.
11. Goethe W. von. Farbenlehre. In: *Naturwissenschaftliche Schriften*. Band I. Zürich-Stuttgart: Artemis Verlag 1966.
12. Goethe W. von. Orphische Grundworte. In: *Naturwissenschaftliche Schriften*. Band II. Zurich-Stuttgart: *Artemis Verlag 1966*.
13. Haefner H. Die existentielle Depression. *Arch. Psychiat. Nervenkr.* 1954 ; 191: 351-364.
14. Haefner H. «Symptom und Diagnose». In: Arzt im Raum des Erlebens. Hrgs. v. H. Stolze. München: *Lehmann-Verlage* 1959.
15. Heidegger M., *Sein und Zeit* 1927. Tübingen: Niemayer Verlag, 10. *Auflage* 1963.
16. Hofer G., «Phänomen und Symptom». *Der Nervenarzt* 1954 ; 25: 342-344.
17. Kielholz, P., «Diagnostik und Therapie der depressiven Zustandsbilder». *Schweiz. Med. Wochenschr.* 1957 ; 87: 107.
18. Kraepelin E., Einführung in die Psychiatrie. Leipzig: Barth *Verlag* 1916.; pag. 359.
19. Marcel G., *Être et avoir*. Paris: Montaigne 1955.
20. Müller-Suur H., «Die schizophrenen Symptome und der Eindruck des Schizophrenen». *Fortschr. Neurol. Psychiat.* 1958 ; 26: 140.
21. Pfeiffer W.M., «Die Symptomatik der Depression in transkulturelle Sicht». In: *Das depressive Syndrom*. München-Berlin-Wien: Urban & Schwarzenberg 1969. S. 151-168.
22. Pfeiffer W.M., *Transkulturelle Psychiatrie*. Stuttgart: Thieme Verlag 1971.
23. Pichot P., «Les dimensions des dépressions». *L'Evolution psychiatrique* 1969 ; 34: 297-312.
24. Rümke H., «Das Kernsymptom der Schizphrenie und das 'Praecoxgefühl'». *Zentral Gesamte Neurol Psychiatrie* 1942 ; 102: 168-169.
25. Sartre J.P., *L'Être et le Néant*. Paris : Gallimard 1943.
26. Scheler M., «Wesen und Formen der Sympathie». Frankfurt: Schulte Verlag 1948.
27. Schneider K., «Pathopsychologie der Gefühle und Triebe». Leipzig: Georg Thieme 1935.
28. Schneider K., «Klinische Psychopathologie. Stuttgart: «Thieme Verlag» 1959.
29. Tatossian A. *Phénoménologie des psychoses*. Paris-New York-Barcelona-Milan: Masson 1979.
30. Tellenbach H., «Annäherung an die Daseinanalyse.Phänomenologische Erfahrungsweise in Abgrenzung von der psychiatrischen une analytischen». Almanach für Neurologie u. *Psychiatrie* 1961.
31. Tellenbach H. Melancholie. Problemgeschichte, Endogenität, Typologie, Pathogenese, Klinik 1961. Berlin-Heidelberg-New York-Tokyo: Springer-Verlag, *4. Auflage* 1983.
32. Tellenbach H. *Geschmack une Atmosphäre*. Salzburg: Otto Müller Verlag 1968.
33. Tellenbach H., «Zur Psychopathologie der Zyklothymie». *Der Nervenarzt* 1977 ; 48: 335-341.
34. Weitbrecht H.J., «Zur Typologie depressiver Psychosen». *Fortschr. Neurol. Psychiat.* 1952 ; 20: 247.
35. Weitbrecht H.J., «Psicopatologia comparada de los estados depresivos». *Actas Luso-Espanolas de Neurol. Psiquiat.* 1968 ; 27: 407-415.
36. World Health Organization, International Classification of Diseases (ICD 10). Geneva 1987.
37. Zerssen D. von. Objektivierende Untersuchungen zur prämorbiden Persönlichkeit endogen Depressiver. In: Hippius, Selbach éds. *Das depressive Syndrom*. München-Berlin-Wien: Urban & Schwarzenberg 1969.
38. Zerssen D. von, «Personality and Affective Disorders». In: Paykel, E.S. *Handbook of Affective Disorders*. New York: Churchill Livingstone 1982 ; 213-228.

3

The nuclear depressive syndrome seen from a phenomenology of the corporality

O. DOERR-ZEGERS

Psiquiatria y Psicoterapia Luis Thayer, OJEDA n° 0115 of 502, CL, Santiago de Chile, Chili.

The problem of the delimitation of the syndrome

Any approach to the theme of depression has to face first of all the question of its definition. If following tradition, we take the mood compromise as fundamental symptom, we immediately find ourselves with the problem of the transitions toward normality, as well as with the fact that in many other morbid conditions the mood appears being affected, not being always easy distinguish among them. So, there are schizophrenic patients who occasionally present a depressive mood, and the same is valid for epileptics, organics, and above all, for neurotics. The limits between depression and obsessive-compulsive neurosis, agoraphobia or the now called «generalised anxiety disorder» are extremely unprecise. But perhaps the greater difficulty is the one stated by the transitions towards normality. With too much frequency we see the confusion between sentimental problems, work failures or normal mournings and a depressive illness. We also see the negative consequences brought by the administration of some strong antidepressant in these cases: multiple subjective discomforts, in addition to the impression they give in their family and social environment of being «strange» or «drugged». In our experience, psychiatrists over diagnose the depressive illness, whereas, on their side, internists and physicians of other specialities sub diagnose it. They do not think about this diagnosis in front of isolated somatic symptoms or diffuse discomforts without organic substrate, and the patients are submitted to innumerable examinations resulting all of them negative, being then disqualified as «functional» sick persons and declared cured after prescription of benzodiazepines. With it, the underlying depressive picture not only does not improve, but even more, the patient feels intellectually more impaired, and with no scarce frequency he acquires a serious dependence on this type of medicines.

The difficulty inherent to the diagnosis of depression early led to an attempt to stablish something like a nuclear depressive syndrome which were the direct expression of a disturbance in the underlying physiological process. So, Kraepelin states that the fundamental symptoms would be «difficulty for seizing stimuli and for thinking, depressive or anxious dysthimia and inhibition of the will». Bleuer also distinguishes three fundamental symptoms: depressive dysthimia, the inhibition of the course of thought and the inhibition of the centrifugal functions (decisions, acts, movements). Kurt Schneider, following Max Scheler, describes as fundamental symptom the compromise of the vital feelings, being among them the most specific those directly corporal, such as the case of precordial oppression and/or pain, globus melancholicus and pain in the nape of the neck. Pichot described in 1966 five groups of symptoms which would be always given with greater or lesser intensity in the depressive syndrome: one group around the depressive mood, another one around the self-aggressiveness, another one around the slowliness, another one around the vitality decrease, and finally, a group composed by the somatic symptoms. Pfeiffer, in 1968, and based on transcultural studies between Germany and Indonesia, comes to the conclusion that the fundamental symptoms, which are not determined by the type or degree of civilization or culture, are a «difficult to define» change in the frame of mind, and the perturbation of vegetative functions such a sleep, appetite and libido. Both inhibition and motoric agitation, hypocondriac and guilt ideas, and suicide ideas or attempts would be culturally determined symptoms, so that they would not belong to the nuclear depressive syndrome.

Quite before the appearance of the now current diagnostic criteria for the depressive illness, such as RDC (Research Diagnostic Criteria), the criteria of Saint Louis School or DSM-III and DSM-III-R, at the end of the 60's we already attempted to determine something like a nuclear depressive syndrome. With this objective we carried out clinical-statistical study about the theme in the Psychiatric Hospital of Concepcion, Chile. This institution offered the following advantages: 1st. it was the only psychiatric hospital of the zone and attended a population of about one million inhabitants; 2nd. thanks to the tradition imposed by Professor Auersperg, the filling cards were typed and kept with an uniform criterion, which included, besides the usual date referring to near and remote anamnesis, from a chapter of hereditary backgrounds to a meticulous psychopathological description of the patients, passing by a description of the premorbid and of the circumstances probably precipitating the illness. We review the filing cards of all the patients hospitalized during the five years previous to our arrival to that hospital. Now, we limited the study to the 55 cases of unipolar depression. The intention was to determine which symptoms or phenomena were always present in those pictures in which the tradition, taking in account their form of presentation and evolution, had spoken of «endogenous depression». That is the way we found three groups of symptoms or symptomatic complexes which were always present (to see enclosed picture):

1st. The compromise of the lived body or corporality (Befindlichkeit), in which the lack of vitality appeared as another expression of a very much complex phenomenon which also included anguish, nauseas, sensation of cold and the vital symptoms of Schneider.

2nd. The compromise of the functions called by Beuler «centrifugal», that is to say, those which connect us with the external world, among which the psychic and motor inhibition is the most characteristic manifestation. The difficulty in paying attention, in concentrating, in taking decisions, the loss of strength of the voice and the motoric slowness are other forms in which the same phenomenon reveals itself. This phenomenon was also considered by Kaepelin as being essential in this illness.

3rd. The compromise of the biological rhythmicity: all the vital rhythms are inverted, suspended or at least disturbed. And we talk of rythmicity and not of rhythms because the disturbance is not referred only to particular rhythms as sleep or digestion, but also to the way of unfolding the existence in time, so characteristically rhythmic and periodic. And thus, there is a daily rhythm, a monthly one, a seasonal one and a vital one, that is to say, of the whole life, and all of them appear altered in some extent.

These three phenomena-through some one of their respective particular symptoms- appeared in 100% of these depressive patients admitted to the Psychiatric Hospital of Concepcion between January 1st., 1962 and December 31st., 1966. But there were two other groups of symptoms which can not be reduced to the previous ones: the delusional ideas, which appeared in about 60% of the cases (which means that in general they were serious cases), and the symptomatic complex of self-aggressiveness, which includes the suicidal ideas and acts, present in 20% of them.

Sympton and phenomenon

We published this work in 1971. 20 years have gone by and we have had the opportunity of seeing and treating innumerable cases of depression, and we must confess that experience has come to widely corroborate what we found in that groups of ill persons on Concepcion. In that opportunity we also stated the existence of an unique illness, which we would call later «melancholic depression». We also questioned the clasic distinction between endogenous and reactive depression and -following Tellenbach- the endless number of other types of depression described throughout the century, as it is the case of the «basic depression» of Schneider, the «vitalized reactive depression» of Weitbrecht, the «depression by exhaustion» of Kielholz or the «existential depression» of Haefner. The proposition of DSM-III of 1980 of one only type of depression a such, «major depression», as opposed to the 20 different types described in ICD 9 of the World Association (this would change in ICD 10), gave us the reason. The 9 criteria of DSM-III in opposition to the 21 of the Hamilton's scale, are also near enough to what we found in Concepcion. The difference lies on the fact that DSM-III does not distinguish between symptom and phenomenon and that the first ones appear in a list where the only thing uniting them is a contiguity relationship. In our proposition it deals, in certain way, with the same symptoms, but seen in their internal relationships and as deriving from wider phenomena (change of the corporality or of the rhythmicity, for example), which in turn would be rooted in something like a common denominator of depressiveness and which is the disturbance of temporality. Thus, symptoms 1, 2 and 6 of DSM-III-R (depressed mood, anhedonia an energy loss) correspond to the first group of symptoms of our order, the change of corporality; symptoms 5 and 8 (psychomotor slowness and decrease of the thought capacity) correspond to the second group, the one of the alteration of the «body in action» or compromise of the centrifugal functions, whereas symptoms 3 and 4 (weight increase or loss, insomnia or hypersomnia) correspond to the group of the compromise of biological rhythmicity. Finally, symptoms 7 and 9 of DSM-III (uselessness or guilt ideas) correspond to the fourth set of symptoms described by us, which is accessory, because it is not always present, the one of the depressive delusional ideas.

We think that this type of diagnostic criteria such as the ones of DSM-III, of ICD 10 or of RDC, by staying in the sphere of symptoms, fall in two fundamental mistakes: first, the lists will be necessarily incomplete (when in symptom Nr. 6 of DSM-III they talk of «energy loss», why not to mention also the decay or the limbs heaviness?; or why not to mention such important symptoms as anguish, as vital symptoms of Schneider or the sensation of cold?); and second, they overlook essential relations between particular symptoms, such as the one existing between insomnia and appetite and weight loss (both rhythmic alterations) or between the decrease of the thought capacity and the slowness (both are forms derived of the complex phenomenon of inhibition).

The distinction between symptom and phenomenon goes back to the work Being and Time by Heidegger (1927) and has had a great importance in the development of anthropological-phenomenological psychiatry (Hofer, 1954; Tellenbach, 1956, 1961; Haefner, 1959; Blankenburg, 1962; Tatossian, 1979; Doerr-Zegers, 1980). There the great german philosopher made an in certain way definitive analysis of the problem, which after more than 60 years has not lost its validity. For him the symptoms or manifestations only announce a distubanced which is not showed in itself. The phenomenon, in turn, is «what is showed in itself», and it includes at the same time the symptom which announces it and the disturbance which underlies it. Somatic medicine is fundamentally worried about recognition and management of symptoms. If symptom is defined as «the visible element of a functional complex» (Haefner), and a previous knowledge of the laws ruling the hidden parts of that pathophysiologic wholeness which is the illness is supposed, then the jump from external manifestation or symptom to the illness as wholeness will be legitimate, and that is diagnosis. In psychiatry, in turn, this procedure is not adequate, since the assumptions legitimating the diagnostic process of somatic medicine are not given in it, at least in what refers to the so called endogenous psychoses: both the anatomic substrate and the pathogenic mechanisms are unknown in it. If in spite of it one insists on the merely symptomatologic sphere, e.g. discouragement, fatigue, weight loss, guilt ideas, etc. one will unavoidably fall in confusions and tautologies. Müller-Suur (1958) demonstrated that in schizophrenia diagnosis is almost always done on the base of the «schizophrenic» character of each one of its symptoms, that is to say, it is a tautology. A psychiatry exclusively oriented to the external manifestations or symptoms is not qualified to answer what does this «schizophrenic», which in a tacit way is allowing diagnosis and consensus, mean.

Diagnoses based on additions of symptoms, such as the case of the majority of the present systems of diagnostic criteria in fashion, do not even reach this level of tautology, which at least employs -although not deepening in it- that «schizophrenic» or that «depressive» which in any way contains in itself what is essential in these mysterious illenesses.

Towards a phenomenology of the corporality of the depressive

Between 1970 and 1976 we worked in the Psychiatric Clinic of University of Chile, filling the function of Chief of Policlinic during almost the half of that period. In a daily meeting, at the end of the morning, we reviewed together with younger collaborators all the new cases who had consulted. Very soon one of the more urgent tasks posed to the team was the one of realizing a conceptual clarification, a syndromatic definition and the establishment of clear differential criteria in the framework of the diversity of psychopathologic pictures with depressive symptoms in everyday practice. The usual shortage of beds obliged in most of the cases to carry out an ambulatory treatment, which allowed us to observe ourselves the spontaneous evolution of the evolution under tymoleptics, as well as the dissimilar therapeutic response of the different clinical and evolutive forms of depression.

During this experience in common the following clinical evidences began being imposed to us: in the first place, we proved what we stated in the paper of 1971, in the sense that the distinction between endogenous and reactive depression lacked justification and that depressions as such were all «endoreactive» and they appear in that characteristic personality described by Tellenbach as typus melancholicus (1961). This last one was later empirically demonstrated by von Zerssen and collaborators in Germany and more recently by Anneliese Dörr and Sandra Viani in Chile. In the second place, we made ourselves secure of the idea, already suggested in 1971, of the need of distinguishing between melancholic and non melancholic depressivity, e.g. the depressive symptoms appearing in other pathologies such as schizophrenia, epilepsy and neurosis, or also in normal people. In the third place, we became convinced that the substantive element of the phenotypic difference between one depressive picture and another was the intensity, and that what appears as so different, for example, a simple vital depression and a depressive stupor were fundamentally one and the same phenomenon, only that in different degrees. (We will see later which is the element that in the phenomenological analysis is imposed as the most central of melancholic depression and whose transformation can offer different intensity degrees.) The last version of ICD, Nr. 10, agrees with us by defining one only depressive episode (F 31), but distinguishing intensities: mild, moderate severity, serious severity without psychotic symptoms and serious severity with psychotic symptoms. In the fourth place, something like an atmospheric emanation directly emerging from the melancholic depressions began being imposed to us each time more; we called it «melancholie-Gefühl» (sensation of what is melancholic), parodying Rümke with his classic

«Praecox-Gefühl» (sensation of what is schizophrenic). This intuitive knowledge, susceptible of being also learned by the younger colleagues, was demonstrated as fundamental for distinguishing melancholic depressions (which more or less correspond to the major depressive episode of DSM-III) from the non-melancholic ones. Out atmospheric experience of melancholic depressivity has a certain relationship with expressions found in the book by Tellenbach, «Geschmak and Atmosphäre» (Taste and Atmosphere) (1968), when he speaks of the «loss of the vital freshness» of the depressive.

Blankenburg (1962) demands of the phenomenological experience that it be «decidedly more open to all the modalities of being of that facting us, that is to say, it has to be able of being of that facting us, that is to say, it has to be able of being more natural that the natural experience itself», but at the same time it has to be «more scientific than the scientific experience, in the measure that it is not limited to one only transcendental project, but it rather transforms in its central theme all the ways of being in general». Following the recommendations of Blankenburg, we attempted, some years ago, to make a phenomenology of this atmospheric experience with respect to the encounter with an extreme case of melancholic depression: a depressive stupor. For such analysis the attitude of the researcher will have to resemble as much as possible to the one of person without psychiatric experience, somebody still able of a complete naiveté. For such an observer the immobility of the patient will not be an «inhibition», and her silence will not be a «stuporous mutism», etc., but simply the different aspects of the being with whom the observer comes across in that moment and which affect him in such or such way. We will summarise here the results of that research:

The patient stays in front of us silent and motionless. Her glance is gloomy, without brightness, it dones not transmit any message, there is in it no sign of inferior life. Her skin is pale, yellowish and dry. We do not feel her persistent silence as denying a dialogue, but rather as not being present. In a certain way she is not in front of us, since that natural polarised tension occurring in the interpersonal encounters and called «antikry» by the Greeks is not produced between her and me. Among the fundamental characteristics of the interhuman encounter, as they were described first von Beayer (1955) and then by Tellenbach (1961, it stands out vis-a-vis, being one in front of the other in a permanent interchange of gestures, emotions and words. The behaviour with respect to the other in the encounter is always frontal. Only there it is understood the seriousness that can have the gesture of «turning one's back» or of «avoiding to look». The patient remains insensible to all my attempts to bring her to something like a contraposition, to make that she opposes me as an other, and it is curious, but the feeling she begins to provoke us more and more with draws from sorrow or compassion. There is something in her disagreeably alien, almost sinister, but not as in the cases of paranoids, who are strange to us by their excess of meaningfulness and of possible references which overwhelm us and surpass us. This impression of what is disagreeable and alien is rather the results of the experience of a vacuum there where one was prepared to meet a person, an alive and different spirit more or less communicative, familiar, open, sympathetic, interesting or whatever it be.

Let us to go more deeply into this feeling or disagreeable strangeness provoked in us by the patient. The first thing which is imposed to us is a very corporal sensation inundating us, difficult to express in words, although close to the Nausea of Sartre (1943). We experience similar sensations, for example, before a corpse in the autopsy table. Suddenly we realise that the opacity of her glance, that her immobility and her silence have in common something cadaverous. In her whole being there is something like a thing, we almost would say material, preventing the arising of a reciprocity between her existence and mine. There is no come and go of the personal flow, there is no exchange between her glance and my glance, between her happening and mine.

Instead of an authentic interpersonal encounter, what has occurred between us is hardly colliding myself with her, encountering something and not encountering-with. This character of thing irradiating the almost purely material presence of the patient is also made evident in its availability. She is not seated or standing in front of me, but only put there, and I feel that I could dispose of her as of an utensil at my service. In fact, I submit her to a neurologic examination and she offers no resistance, as well as no help, and I come back to the original impression of examining a corpse, although less rigid.

If you would like to express this form of her being or presenting in front of the other with her richness of the greek language, we should have to say that her antikry (her way of facing) is not enantiotic, that is to say, reciprocal, but chrematic. For the Greeks, «chrema» is an object with which I can have only an utilitarian treatment, but which is of not use for me, that is to say, an unuseful object. In a certain way «chrema» is the opposite to «physis». We find again an analogous contraposition in Gabriel Marcel (1955) with his polarity between the «body I have» and the «body I am». I have my eyes and I am my glance. The body I have is always on the way towards the thing, towards the corpse; on the contrary, the body I am is always gesture, signification and transcendence, that is to say, spirit.

There is no doubt, the stuporous and chrematic body of our patient is nearer the body I have than the body I am. What she has lost is precisely her capacity to confide to the other, to signify, to face, or said in greek, to be enantiotic. Her glance has lost not only its brightness, but it has sunk behind the eyes, being impossible for her to know the world, process so accurately defined by Sartre (1943) with the words: «connaître c'est manger des yeux» (to know is eating with the eyes). In a certain way the total loss of appetite experienced by our patient has also involved the eyes, namely, the appetite of the spirit.

But stupor is not the unique form of depression in which the body of the depressive acquires the described chrematic transformation. Stupor only represent the end of a body process to become thing and chrema which is already announced in the slight initial decay, in the vital symptoms as precordial oppression, in cold, in the heaviness of the limbs, but also in the so common fact that the depressives tend to excessively worry about their body and they do not have any other theme but the somatized anguish or the obstructed digestion or that lack of appetite or that pertinacious insomnia. Every true depressive, every melancholic depression in our terminology, shows us certain degree of chrematization and this indeed would be a specific phenomenon, whose adequate apprehension could be transformed in a fundamental weapon for an unequivocal diagnosis of depressive illness.

And now we return to the initial point, namely the problem of the strict definition of depression as such and of the need of an adequate order of its manifestations surpassing the mere addition of symptoms whose unique nexus among them is contiguity. From the three fundamental phenomena described by us as characteristic of melancholic depression and around which are grouped their concrete manifestations, reviving at the same time from them, two, the group around vital dysthimia and the group around inhibition can be directly perceived by the examiner, since they are different ways in which the phenomenon of chrematization shows itself: what the patient lives as decay, discouragement, sensation of cold, etc., is seen in a concrete way by the physician as paleness, opacity of the glance, frontal wrinkle in omega, greater or lesser immobility, etc. In the same way, what the patient lives as difficulty of concentration, of decision or as rumination of thoughts, is perceived by the examiner in the slowness of movements, the lack of strength of the voice, the lack of direction of the glance, the indecision of the gestures, the latency in the answers, etc. The third group of symptoms, which is the expression of the compromise of biological rhythmicity, can not be perceived in the phenomenological intuition, but being a subjective symptom, it is at the same time easy to objectify: the sleep alteration can be measured, even with apparats, and the same is valid for the decrease of the appetite and of the weight or for the slowness or acceleration of digestion. But the important is that this alteration of the rhythms can also be conceived as expression of the process of chrematization occurring in the depressive body. Life is movement from the past towards the future and this movement is always given in the form of rhythms and periods and in consonance with the cosmic rhythms, as it has been developed by Tellenbach (1975) in his concept of endogenous psychoses as endocosmegenic illnesses. The phenomenon of suspension, inversion or at least the alteration of the biological fundamental rhythms that we observe in all the melancholic depressions represents another form of expressing this process of chrematization, since it means a loss of the consonance with the world and of the temporal condition of the existence.

What we have called chrematization and conceived as the fundamental phenomenon of depressivity, from which its three groups of constituent symptoms would be inferred: the alteration of the lived body (dysthimia), of the body in action (inhibition) and of the body in time (compromise of the vital rhythms), has very intimate relationships with this essential contribution made by phenomenological psychiatry to the understanding of the depressive illness: the concept of endogenity of Tellenbach (1961). This author, following Goethe, conceives endogenity as an animated nature, as an originary form which is showed in its development through certain somatic and psychic characteristics. «Locked up form that living is developed», says Goethe in the poetry dedicated to the primordial orphic words. And Tellenbach specifies, «The way of being of the endon is transubjective and consequently metapsychologic, but at the same time transobjective and consequently metasomatologic». This means that the endon is previous to the division between psyche and soma and it determines both of them, but at the same time it is subsequent, because in the relationship of consonance with the world this can also determine and shape the «endon» in the way like the world and the others teach us. Nobody has expressed better this wonderful interaction than Goethe, when he says in his Theory of the Colors: «The eye owes its existence to the light. Among various rudimentary and indifferent organs, the light chooses an organ which resembles it, and thus it forms the eye from the light and for the light, so that the interior light goes out to meet the exterior one». Let us think, for example, in the phenomenon of the language and how in it both that learning capacity originated from what is endogenous and of the presence of the mother, whose language is the boy slowly learns to imitate, until arriving to own the «mother tongue» are needed.

Now, this endon which reveals itself very specially through the maturative phenomena can also become spoiled in its development and those failures would end up by being the endogenous psychoses and in particular depression for Tellenbach (1975). In this last one, as in no other illness, all the manifestations of what is endogenous appear deformed, from the rhythmicity up to the different talents or capacities, which vanish in that typical phenomenon of «not being able» considered by Binswanger (1960) as the most central fact of melancholy.

There is no doubt that Tellenbachs concept of endogenity (1961, 1967, 1975) represents a sort of resurrection of the ancient greek concept of «physis». The noun «physis» comes from the verb «phyo», which means to grow or increase, that is to say, the same meaning of endon as «living form developing itself». The Greeks used this word to designate both nature in general an human nature, thinking this last one as a «little nature», which in a way contains the whole «great» one. According to Heidegger (1953) the word physis meant for the classic Greek «both the sky and the earth, both the stones and the plants, the animals and the human being; but also the history of the human being as work of men and gods, and finally, or before everything, the gods themselves under the sign of destiny. Physis is emerging which is made evident from what is hidden...» That is to say, physis «is the being itself by means of which the entity can get to remain and be then observed». The meaning of «nature» for the latin world is much limited: it means to be born and birth, but also temperament and character. With this greek concept of physis gets losts and one could state that the reductionist and dichotomic character showed by the natural sciences in the history of the West -at least in what is referred to the study of the human being- is related with that reducing transformation done by Rome by traducing the word «physis» by «nature». In philosophy after Aristotle the concept of «psyché», what is psychic, has been opposed to «physis», and thus we speak today of «psychophysic unity», attempt of union which is precisely alluding to how separated have been these two forms of revealing itself the human nature. However, in its original meaning «psyché» was contained in «physis», it was a possible manifestation of it. What was certainly out of «physis» was the «Nomos», that is to say, what is ethic, and the «techné», the technic in the sense of knowing to dispose, to install or to modify what is given. «Nomos» and «techné» have in common its association with liberty. Both deciding between one option or another and the creativity implicit in the technical action are based in that called liberty. «Physis» is, on the other hand, what comes given from behind, in some way that escaping selfavaibility, in the last place, the «endon».

Now, what is really opposed to «physis» is «chrema». «Chrema» means the loss of the creative potentiality, immobility, whole availability. What is chrematic is what is referred to things in its most privative, material and devitalized sense, that is to say, the contrary not only to «physis», but of «endon». We saw before that in the phenomenological analysis the chrematization of the being of the depressive appeared as what is substantive of depressivity. From this process of loss of the physical condition, in the sense of «physis», one is able to understand the discouragement, the lack of strengths, the anhedonia, the pains and the somatized anguish which imprisons the subject in its body, but also the «not being able» of the inhibition and the suspension of the rhythmic condition of the existence. Because, if «physis» is the transcended nature, «chrema» is the inanimated nature and the chrematization process suffered by the depressive is only a progressive loss of the capacity of transcending the body towards the world (not feeling the body as assumption of health) and towards action, but without losing its anchorage in the order of cosmos through its rhythms and periods. When we say that «physis» is transcended nature, we want to mean that it contains both all that is involuntary, determined, outside the selfavailability, proper of what Heidegger calls «Geworfenheit» or «state of thrown» or of being thrown to the world -and which is expressed in the physical structure, but also in the abilities and in the rhythms- as well as an opening towards the spirit. In the other words, «physis» is not only what is «geworfen», but also «das Entwerfen», not only what is thrown, but also the project, or better expressed, the capacity of projecting and being projected. The return to the chrematic condition is therefore a way towards death. When there are no projects there is no future, when there is no future there is no time, when there is no time there is no movement. Many depressive patients report when going out of the episode that they felt «dead in life». Heidegger, without having ever seen a depressive patient, only from his deep knowledge of human nature and his brilliant intuitions, got to say in «Being and Time»: «Die Gedrücktheit zwingt das Dasein auf seine Geworfenheit zurück, aber so, daB diese gerade verschlossen wird» (Gloominess forces the existence back into its state of thrown, but in such a way that this itself is closed). It is difficult to find a deeper description of what occurs with the existence of the depressive: he is pushed towards his feasibility, towards his condition of mere determined nature, and even farther, towards the inanimated nature, and even farther, towards the inanimated nature, through the described chrematization process, but without even having the possibility of knowing that he is sheltered and protected in and by it, as we feel when sleeping, the clearest and quotidianest example of our periodic return to what is endogenous.

In summary, depression would not be a failure of endogenity, but also a retracing of that long road done by the human being from «chrema» up to «physis» or, said with other words, it is a sort of return of the spirit to its material condition.

4

A role for CRF in the pathophysiology of affective and anxiety disorders? Laboratory and clinical studies

M.J. OWENS, C.B. NEMEROFF

Laboratory of Neuropsychopharmacology
Department of Psychiatry and Behavioral Sciences
Emory University School of Medicine
Atlanta, Georgia, USA

«I saw Kazak out of the corner of my right eye. His eyes were pinwheels. His teeth were white daggers. His slobber was cyanide. His blood was nitroglycerine. He was floating toward me like a zeppelin, hanging lazily in the air.
My eyes told my mind about him. My mind sent a message to my hypothalamus, told it to release the hormone CRF into the short vessels connecting my hypothalamus to my pituitary gland. The CRF inspired my pituitary gland to dump the hormone ACTH into my bloodstream. My pituitary had been making and storing ACTH for just such an occasion. And nearer and nearer the zeppelin came.
And some of the ACTH in my bloodstream reached the outer shell of my adrenal gland, which had been making and storing glucocorticoids to my bloodstream. They went all over my body, changing glycogen to glucose. Glucose was muscle food. It would help me fight like a wildcat or run like a deer».

Kurt Vonnegut, Jr.
Breakfast of Champions

Although its existence has been postulated since the 1950's and its physiological actions accurately depicted in fiction by Vonnegut in 1973, CRF was only isolated and characterized a little more than 10 years ago (Vale *et al.* 1981). Simply stated, CRF is the major physiological regulator of the pituitary-adrenal axis and, therefore, of the endocrine stress response.

However, in the past 5 years, overwhelming evidence has accumulated that is concordant with the hypothesis that in addition to its hypophysiotropic role, CRF functions as a neurotransmitter within the central nervous system (CNS). It appears that

CRF and its naturally occurring homologs have been utilized by organisms throughout the evolutionary tree to play a preeminent role in mediating the stress response. Although these compounds may have originally functioned simply to mobilize sources of energy to help flee predators or other life threatening conditions, as animals developed evolutionarily, CRF appears to have taken on a more complex role in integrating not only the endocrine but also the autonomic, immunological, and behavioral responses of an organism to stress (Owens and Nemeroff 1991). Moreover, alterations in the activity of one or another CRF neuronal system may occur in a number of the major neuropsychiatric disorders including depression, certain anxiety disorders, anorexia nervosa, and Alzheimer's disease.

Because the literature clearly suggests that CRF-containing neurons in the CNS, apart from, but in concert with, those that regulate pituitary-adrenal axis activity, also mediate the autonomic and behavioral responses to stress, it is of paramount importance to study the function and regulation of these nonendocrine CRF neurons. Moreover, because a considerable clinical literature (*vide infra*) indicates that CRF neuronal circuits are pathophysiologically involved in certain psychiatric illnesses, study of CRF neuronal systems may lead to the development of novel treatment strategies.

Our group and others have attempted to localize the anatomical site of action for the behavioral effects of CRF. Because CRF is known to directly influence noradrenergic cell firing in the locus coeruleus (Valentino *et al.* 1983), and because of the well-established hypothesis linking noradrenergic neurotransmission with stress, anxiety, and depressive disorders (Bloom 1979, Redmond 1987), we examined the behavioral effects of microinfusion of CRF into the locus coeruleus (Butler *et al.* 1990). Anxiogenic activity was assessed in rats placed in a novel open field containing a small, darkened compartment that was nonthreatening to the rats. Bilateral infusion of CRF (1 to 100 ng) into the locus coeruleus produced a dose-dependant increase in the time spent in the darkened compartment and decreased the amount of time spent exploring outside the compartment or venturing into the inner squares of the open field, all indices of anxiogenic behavior. In addition, significant increases in the concentration of the norepinephrine metabolite, 3,4-dihydroxyphenglycol, was observed in forebrain NE projection areas after intra-locus coeruleus CRF injection. These data suggest that CRF produces its anxiogenic effects, at least in part, by increasing the activity of locus coeruleus noradrenergic neurons. The source(s) of this CRF innervation is not clearly understood. However, Koegler-Muly *et al.* (1993) reported that electrolytic lesions of the central nucleus of the amygdala (CeA), a source of CRF perikarya, result in significant decreases in significant decreases in CRF concentrations within the locus coeruleus, suggesting that one source of CRF innervation of the locus coeruleus may be the CeA.

Our group has reported that both acute immobilization stress and chronic exposure to a series of unpredictable stressors alter the concentration of CRF immunireactivity in various microdissected rat brain regions (Chappell *et al.* 1986). Of particular interest is the finding that both acute and chronic stress resulted in a 2-fold increase in the concentrations of CRF in the locus coeruleus, an area known to be electrophysiologically responsive to applied CRF. In addition, chronic stress decreased CRF concentrations in the dorsal vagal complex, which also contains a number of nuclei that are CRF responsive. These cells are believed to be involved in the regulation of autonomic function.

In view of these findings, we sought to determine whether clinically efficacious anxiolytic and antidepressant drugs alter CRF function in the locus coeruleus. Acute administration of the triazolobenzodiazepine, alprazolam, decreases CRF concentrations in the locus coeruleus (Owens et al. 1989, 1991). The time course of these acute effects were investigated; the decrease in CRF concentrations in the locus coeruleus produced by a single dose of alprazolam persisted for 3 hours. This time course corresponds very closely with the bioavailability and metabolism of alprazolam in the rat. Moreover, CRF concentrations in the locus coeruleus remained decreased during the course of 13 days of continuous administration, which indicates a lack of tolerance to this neurochemichal effect of the anxiolytic. In addition, CRF concentrations in the dorsal vagal complex were decreased 24 hours following abrupt alprazolam with drawal. These latter changes are, not surprisingly, similar to those observed following stress.

It is certainly of interest to test the hypothesis that the effects of clinically efficacious anxyolitics act, in part, by their effects on CRF neurons, because this is an effect opposite to that observed following exposure to stress. As noted previously, CRF has been shown to increase the firing rate of noradrenergic locus coeruleus neurons. Thus, CRF may intrinsically modulate the activity of the major CNS noradrenergic cell body population, a circuit that has long been implicated in the pathophysiology of stress, anxiety and depression. It is unclear at present whether classical benzodiazepines (diazepam, lorazepam, etc.) or anxiolytic partial agonists alter regional brain CRF immunoreactivity or whether treatment with anxiolytics or antidepressants abolishes stress-induced alterations in CRF neuronal activity. However, preliminary data suggests that diazepam and lorazepam also decrease CRF concentrations in the locus coeruleus, the differences between drugs apparently dependent only upon dose and pharmacokinetic properties (Owens and Nemeroff 1993).

For many of the same reasons that we study the effects of benzodiazepines on CRF neurons, we have recently examined the acute and chronic effects of the putative antidepressant nefazodone on CRF neurons (Owens et al. 1993). Neither acute nor chronic (28 day) administration of nefazodone altered regional brain CRF concentrations, but chronic administration resulted in a significant up-regulation of CRF binding sites in the frontal cortex, an effect opposite to that observed in suicide victims (*vide infra*). Like many other antidepressant agents, chronic nefazodone decreased the density of cortical ß-adrenergic and 5-HT2 receptor binding. Because of the inability at present to directly measure CRF release in extrahypothalamic brain regions, experiments aimed at measuring CRF concentrations and CRF mRNA expression, and CRF receptor binding kinetics and CRF receptor mRNA expression in the basal state and after exposure to stress or in animal models of anxiety or depression are the next logical steps in determining whether CRF plays a role in the mechanism of action of these drugs.

Preclinical studies clearly support a preeminent role for CRF neurons of both hypothalamic and extrahypothalamic origin in orchestrating an organism's response to stress. Moreover, stress has been implicated in precipitating depressive episodes and suicidality in genetically vulnerable individuals (Anisman and Zacharko 1982, Wilde *et al.* 1992). We have recently hypothesized that early life stressors may contribute to this vulnerability in later life. Indeed, Nemeroff *et al.* (1993) have recently observed that separation of rat pups from their mothers at either day 9 or 12 results in alterations in pituitary and brain CRF receptors. Preliminary findings suggest that these changes may persist into adulthood (Owens and Nemeroff, unpublished observations).

The concentrations of preclinical findings raises the possibility that CRF neuronal dysregulation could contribute to human illness. Many of the effects of centrally administered CRF closely resemble certain of the signs and symptoms of major depression. With this in mind, one of the most reproducible findings in biological psychiatry is the hyperactivity of the hypothalamic-pituitary-adrenal (HPA) axis in patients with major depression as evidenced by hypercortisolemia, cortisol non-suppression to dexamethasone and other measures of activity of this axis. A number of investigators have studied the mechanism(s) that result in these HPA axis abnormalities. Although there is evidence for adrenal gland alterations in depression (i.e., enhanced cortisol responses to exogenously administered ACTH and adrenal gland enlargement), most evidence points to a primary alteration in the CNS that leads to hyperactivity of the HPA axis, with CRF neuronal hyperactivity the most plausible candidate.

The most widely studied method to scrutinize the pathophysiology of the HPA axis is measurement of the neuroendocrine response to exogenously administered CRF. In a standardized CRF stimulation test, both rat/human CRF and ovine CRF produce robust ACTH, β-endorphin, β-lipotrophin, and cortisol responses following intravenous or subcutaneous administration in normal subjects (Hermus *et al.* 1984; Watson *et al.* 1986). A number of investigators have observed a blunted ACTH or β-endorphin response with a normal cortisol response in patients with major depression compared with controls (Holsboer *et al.* 1984; Gold *et al.* 1986; Amsterdam *et al.* 1987; Kathol *et al.* 1989; Young *et al.* 1990; Krishnan *et al.* 1993). In contrast, Rupprecht *et al.* (1989) observed blunted ACTH, but normal β-endorphin, responses in depressed individuals. A recent study by Amsterdam *et al.* (1988) found that depressed patients exhibited a normal ACTH response to CRF following clinical recovery suggesting that the blunted ACTH response, like dexamethasone non-suppression, may be a «state» marker for depression.

Several hypotheses have been introduced to explain the mechanism of this blunted ACTH response to administered CRF. One hypothesis is that the blunted ACTH responses result primarily pituitary responsiveness to CRF in the face of long term hypersecretion of CRF from the median eminence and the resultant down-regulation of pituitary CRF receptors. The data, when scrutinized, support this hypothesis more strongly than an alternative hypothesis suggesting altered sensitivity of the pituitary to glucocorticoid negative feedback, though this may play some role. This has not yet been tested directly by measurement of anterior pituitary CRF receptor density of CRF mRNA in the PVN in post-mortem tissue from depressed patients. In fact, two groups (von Bardeleben and Holsboer 1989; Krishnan *et al.* 1992; Carroll, Ritchie and Nemeroff, unpublished observations) have found that following dexamethasone pretreatment, depressed patients exhibit greater increases in plasma ACTH and cortisol concentrations than normals following CRF administration (*i.e.*, depressed patients escape from dexamethasone suppression). These results further suggest that the blunted

ACTH responses to exogenously administered CRF observed in depressed patients are not solely or even primarily due to hypercortisolemic negative feedback. In addition, a recent landmark study (Schlaghecke et al. 1992) reported that long term glucocorticoid therapy exerted a very variable effect on the ACTH response to CRF. Although most studies in depression are concordant, differences exist and are likely the result of differences in the patient population under study (depression severity, misdiagnosis, comorbidity, etc.) and/or ACTH assay methodological differences. In any case, further studies are needed. However, no matter the number of studies, these neuroendocrine studies purported to be a «window to the brain» will always represent an indirect, secondary measure of CNS activity. It is also important to recognize the fact that pituitary ACTH responses likely reflect hypothalamic CRF neuronal activity; CRF neurons in limbic and cerebrocortical areas are likely involved in the pathophysiology of depression.

In order to directly test the hypothesis that the synaptic availability of CRF is increased in patients with depression, and possibly those with other psychiatric illnesses, we and others have measured the concentration of the peptide in cerebrospinal fluid (CSF). Pst et al. (1982) have comprehensively reviewed the fact that for neuropeptides found in both CSF and plasma, there is marked CSF-plasma dissociation indicating that neuropeptides are secreted directly into CSF from brain tissue, and that CSF neuropeptide concentrations are not derived from the systemic circulation. Thus, CSF CRF concentrations likely reflect the concentrations of CRF in extracellular fluid contiguous with extrahypothalamic CRF neurons.

Evidence that CSF CRF concentrations are derived from non-hypophysiotropic CRF have been provided from studies in which CSF CRF concentrations were repeatedly measured over the course of the day. Garrick et al. (1987) reported that CSF CRF concentrations were not positively correlated to CSF cortisol concentrations in rhesus monkeys, which directly reflect plasma cortisol concentrations. In fact, CSF CRF concentrations reach their peak approximately 12-14 hours prior to the peack for CSF cortisol; CRF is similarly dysynchronous with plasma ACTH concentrations. Kalin et al. (1987) also reported that CSF CRF concentrations in rhesus monkeys are not entrained with pituitary-adrenal activity. It is evident that CSF CRF concentrations are not merely a reflection of median eminence CRF release. Although the source of CSF CRF remains unknown, CRF neurons in cortical, limbic, and brainstem regions are all in close proximity to the ventricular system and likely contribute to CSF CRF. Relevant to these findings is our recent report (Owens et al. 1990) that there are circadian alterations in regional brain CRF concentrations.

In a developmental study of pediatric patients, we found that CSF CRF concentrations were highest in the immediate postnatal period (Hedner et al. 1989). CSF CRF concentrations decrease significantly during the first postnatal year compared to the immediate postnatal period and by one year of age are similar to that observed in adults.

We have shown in a series of studies that CRF concentrations are significantly elevated in the CSF of drug-free patients with major depression (Nemeroff et al. 1984, Arato et al. 1986,

Banki et al. 1987, France et al. 1988, Widerlöv et al. 1988) or following suicide (Arato et al. 1989). In our first study, we measured the CSF concentration of CRF in 10 normal controls, 23 depressed patients, 11 schizophrenics, and 29 demented patients. The CSF concentration of CRF was elevated in the depressed patients compared to all of the groups; 11 of the 23 depressed patients had CSF CRF concentrations higher than the highest normal controls (Nemeroff et al. 1984). In our second study we measured the CSF concentration of CRF in 54 depressed patients, 138 neurological controls, 23 schizophrenic patients, and 6 manic patients. The depressed patients exhibited a marked, two-fold elevation in CSF CRF concentrations (Banki et al. 1987). In a third study we reported that patients with major depression had higher CSF CRF concentrations than patients with chronic pain (France et al. 1988). Our fourth study, conducted in Budapest, also found increased CSF CRF concentrations in depressed patients (Arato et al. 1986). Finally, a fifth study was conducted in which we measured CSF CRF concentrations collected post-mortem from the cisternal space in depressed suicide victims and sudden death controls. Again, CSF CRF concentrations were elevated in the depressed group (Arato et al. 1989). Although as a total group, Roy et al. (1987) did not find any difference between depressed patients and controls, those patients who were dexamethasone nonsuppressors exhibited higher concentrations of CSF CRF than depressed DST suppressors. Recently, Risch et al. (1991) have confirmed our findings of elevated CSF CRF concentrations in depressed patients.

In order to determine whether elevated CSF CRF concentrations in depression represent a state or trait marker, Nemeroff et al. (1991) measured CSF CRF concentrations in depressed patients before and after a course of electroconvulsive therapy (ECT). Before ECT, depressed patients exhibited elevated CSF CRF concentrations compared to controls. Twenty-four hours after their final ECT treatment, a significant decrease in CSF CRF concentrations was observed. This finding indicates that CSF CRF concentrations, like hypercortisolemia, represent a state, rather than a trait, marker of depression.

Because depression is a major determinant of suicide (Van Praag 1985) and more than 50% of suicides are accomplished by patients with major depression, we hypothesized that if CRF is chronically hypersecreted in major depression, a reduced (down-regulated) number of CRF receptors may be present in the brain tissue of suicide victims. To test this hypothesis, we measured the number and affinity of CRF receptors in the frontal cortex of 26 suicide victims and 28 control subjects (Nemeroff et al. 1988). The suicide group exhibited a 23% reduction in the number of CRF binding sites compared with controls. We have recently confirmed this findings in Broadman's area 12 of the frontal pole in a second group of suicide/depressed victims (unpublished observations). This findings further suggests that CRF is hypersecreted within the CNS of patients with major depression. Clearly, further studies in which CRF receptors, CRF receptor mRNA, and CRF mRNA is measured in other brain regions are of great interest.

Because both CRF and ACTH possess trophic properties, we hypothesized that hypersecretion of CRF might result in pituitary and adrenal gland alterations in depression. In brief, we have found that depressed patients exhibit pituitary gland enlargement as assessed by magnetic resonance imaging (MRI) (Krishnan et al. 1991) and adrenal gland hypertrophy as assessed by computed tomography (CT) scanning (Nemeroff et al. 1992) likely due to CRF and ACTH hypersecretion, respectively.

Clearly, one of the most exciting areas of research is the possibility of the development of a CRF antagonist for the treatment of depression and/or anxiety. Although computer-aided drug design of such a large peptide is difficult, the recent cloning of the CRF-binding protein and the CRF receptor will greatly aid in the elucidation of the active portion of the peptide or the active site on the receptor. These discoveries may lead to the rational design of lipophilic peptidomimetics which may possess clinical utility. Alternatively, we are investigating whether antisense knockdown strategies aimed at the CRF receptor might provide a novel form of pharmacotherapy.

Considering that CRF was first isolated barely 10 year ago, one marvels at the wealth of knowledge that has been gathered to date. We believe that in the next decade a plethora of more detailed information regarding the basic neurobiology of CRF will be forthcoming. Even more exciting to us are the possibilities that pharmacological agents based upon neuropeptides in general, and CRF in particular, may find utility in the treatment of neuropsychiatric disorders.

Acknowledgements

Supported by NIMH MH-42088 and the John D. and Catherine T. MacArthur Foundation Network on Depression.

References

1. Amsterdam J.D., Maislin G., Winokur A., Kling M., Gold P. Pituitary and adrenocortical responses to the ovine corticotropin releasing hormone in depressed patients and healthy volunteers. *Arch Gen Psychiatry* 1987 ; 44:775-781.
2. Amsterdam J.D., Maislin G., Winokur A., Berwish N., Kling M., Gold P. The oCRH stimulation test before and after clinical recovery from depression. *J Affect Dis* 1988 ; 14:213-222.
3. Anisman H., Zacharko R.M. Depression: the predisposing influence of stress. *Behav Brain Sci* 1982 ; 5:89-137.
4. Arato M., Banki C.M., Nemeroff C.B., Bissette G. Hypothalamic-pituitary-adrenal axis and suicide. In: Mann J.J., Stanley M., eds. *Psychobiology of Suicidal Behavior*. New York: Academy of Science, New York, 1986; 263-270.
5. Arato M., Banki C.M., Bissette G., Nemeroff C.B. Elevated CSF CRF in suicide victims. *Biol Psychiatry* 1989 ; 25:355-359.
6. Banki C.M., Bissette G., Arato M., O'Connor L., Nemeroff C.B. CSF corticotropin-releasing factor-like immunoreactivity in depression and schizophrenia. *Am J Psychiatry* 1987; 144:873-877.
7. Bloom F.E. Norepinephrine mediated synaptic transmission and hypotheses of psychiatric disorders. In: Meyer E., Brady J., eds. *Research in the Psychobiology of Human Behavior*. The Johns Hopkins University Press, Baltimore, 1979 ; 1-11.
8. Butler P.D., Weiss J.M., Stout J.C., Nemeroff C.B. Corticotropin-releasing factor produces fear-enhancing and behavioral activating effects following infusion into the locus coeruleus. *J Neurosci* 1990 ; 10:176-183.

9. Chappell P.B., Smith M.A., Kilts C.D. et al. Alterations in corticotropin-releasing factor-like immunoreactivity in discrete rat brain regions after acute and chronic stress. *J Neurisci* 1986; 6:2908-2914.
10. France R.D., Urban B., Krishnan K.R.R. et al. CSF corticotropin-releasing factor-like immunoreactivity in chronic pain patients with and without major depression. *Biol Psychiatry* 1988; 23: 86-88.
11. Garrick N.A., Hill J.L., Szele F.G., Tomai T.P., Gold P.W., Murphy D.L. Corticotropin-releasing factor: a marked circadian rhythm in primate cerebrospinal fluid peaks in the evening and is inversely related to the cortisol circadian rhythm. *Endocrinology* 1987; 121:1329-334.
12. Gold P.W., Loriaux D.L., Roy A. et al. Responses to corticotropin-releasing hormone in the hypercortisolism of depression and cushing's disease. *New Eng J Med* 1986; 314:1329-1334.
13. Hedner J., Hedner T., Lundell K.H., Bissette G., O'Connor L., Nemeroff C.B. Cerebrospinal fluid concentrations of neurotensin and corticotropin-releasing factor in pediatric. *Biol Neonate* 1989; 55:260-267.
14. Hermus A.R.M.M., Pieters G.F.F.M., Pesman G.J. et al., Differential effects of ovine and human corticotropin-releasing factor in human subjects. *Clin Endocrinol* 1984; 21: 589-595.
15. Holsboer F., Von Bardellelben U., Gerken A., Stalla G.K., Muller O.A. Blunted corticotropin and normal cortisol response to human corticotropin-releasing factor in depression. *New Eng J Med* 1984; 311:1127-1137.
16. Kalin N.H., Shelton S.E., Barksdale C.M., Brownfield M.S. A diurnal rhythm in cerebrospinal fluid corticotrophin-releasing hormone different from the rhythm of pituitary-adrenal activity. *Brain Res* 1987; 426:385-391.
17. Kathol R.G., Jaeckle R.S., Lopez J.F., Meller W.H. Consistent reduction of ACTH responses to stimulation with CRH, vasopressin and hypoglycemia in patients with major depression. *Br J Psychiatry* 1989; 155:468-478.
18. Koegler-Muly S., Owens M.J., Kilts C.D., Ervin G.E., Bissette G., Nemeroff C.B. Potential corticotropin-releasing factor pathways in the rat brain as determined by bilateral electrolytic lesions of the paraventricular nucleus and the central amygdaloid nucleus. *J Neuroendocrinol* 1993; 5:95-98.
19. Krishnan K.R.R., Doraiswamy P.M., Lurie S.N. et al. Pituitary size in depression. *J Clin Endocrinol Metab* 1991; 72:256-259.
20. Krishnan K.R.R., Rayasam K., Reed D. et al., The corticotropin-releasing factor stimulation test in patients with major depression: relationship to dexamethasone suppression test results. *Depression* 1993; 1:133-136.
21. Nemeroff C.B., Widerlov E., Bissette G. et al. Elevated concentration of CSF corticotropin-releasing factor-like immunoreactivity in depressed patients. *Science* 1984; 226:1342-1344.
22. Nemeroff C.B., Owens M.J., Bissette G., Andorn A.C., Stanley M. Reduced corticotropin-releasing factor binding sites in the frontal cortex of suicide victims. *Arch Gen Psychiatry* 1988; 45:577-579.
23. Nemeroff C.B., Bissette G., Akil H., Fink M. Neuropeptide concentrations in the cerebrospinal fluid of depressed patients treated with electroconvulsive therapy: corticotropin-releasing factor, β-endorphin and somatostatin. *Br J Psychiatry* 1991; 158:59-63.
24. Nemeroff C.B., Krishnan K.R.R., Reed D., Leder R., Beam C., Dunnick N.R. Adrenal gland enlargment in major depression: a computed tomography study. *Arch Gen Psychiat* 1992; 49:384-387.
25. Nemeroff C.B., Owens M.J., Plott S.J., Levine S. Increased density of regional brain CRF binding sites after maternal deprivation. *Soc Neurosci Abstr* 1993; 6.2.
26. Owens M.J., Bissette G., Nemeroff C.B. Acute effects of alpralozam and adinazolam on the concentrations of corticotropin-releasing factor in the rat brain. *Synapse* 1989; 4:196-202.

27. Owens M.J., Bartolome J., Schanberg S.M., Nemeroff C.B. Corticotropin-releasing factor concentrations exhibit a diurnal rhythm in hypothalamic and extrahypothalamic brain regions: differential sensitivity to corticosterone. *Neuroendocrinology* 1990; 52:626-631.
28. Owens M.J., Nemeroff C.B. The physiology and pharmacology of corticotropin-releasing factor. *Pharmacol Rev* 1991; 43:425-473.
29. Owens M.J., Vargas M.A., Knight D.L., Nemeroff C.B. The effects alprazolam on corticotropin-releasing factor neurons in the rat brain: acute time course, chronic treatment and abrupt withdrawal. *J Pharmacol Exp Ther* 1991; 258:349-356.
30. Owens M.J., Nemeroff C.B. Acute effects of benzodiazepines on regional brain CRF concentrations: comparison of alprazolam, diazepam and lorazepam. *Soc Neurosci* 1993; (Abstr) 763.2.
31. Owens M.J., Dole K.C., Knight D.L. Nemeroff C.B., Preclinical evaluation of the putative antidepressant nefazodone. *Depression* (submitted) 1993.
32. Post R.M., Gold P., Rubinow D.R., Ballenger J.C., Bunney W.E., Goodwin F.K. Peptides in cerebrospinal fluid of neuropsychiatric patients: an approach to central nervous system peptides function. *Life Sci* 1982; 31:1-15.
33. Redmond D.E. Jr. Studies of the nucleus locus coeruleus in monkeys and hypotheses for neuropsychopharmacology In: Meltzer H.Y. (ed.) *Psychopharmacology: The Third Generation of Progress.* Raven Press, New York 1987; 967-976.
34. Risch S.C., Lewine R.J., Jewart R.D. et al., Relationship between cerebrospinal fluid peptides and neurotransmitters in depression In: Risch S.C. (ed.) *Central Nervous System Peptide Mechanisms in Stress and Depression.* American Psychiatric Press, Inc., Washington 1991; 93-103.
35. Roy A., Pickar D., Paul S., Doran A., Chrousos G.P., Gold P.W. CSF corticotropin-releasing hormone in depressed patients and normal control subjects. *Am J Psychiatry* 1987; 144:641-645.
36. Rupprecht R., Lesch K.P., Muller U., Beck G., Beckmann H., Schulte H.M. Blunted adrenocorticotropin but normal β-endorphin release after human corticotropin-releasing hormone administration in depression. *J Clin Endocrinol Metab* 1989; 69:600-603.
37. Schlaghecke R., Kornely E., Santen R.T., Ridderkamp P. The effect of long-term glucocorticoid therapy on pituitary-adrenal responses to exogenous corticotropin-releasing hormone. *New Eng J Med* 1992; 226:226-230.
38. Vale W., Spiess J., Rivier C., Rivier J. Characterization of a 41-residue ovine hypothalamic peptide that stimulates secretion of corticotropin and β-endorphin. *Science* 1981; 213:1394-1397.
39. Valentino R.J., Foote S.L., Aston-Jones G. Corticotropin-releasing factor activates noradrenergic neurons of the locus coeruleus. *Brain Res* 1983; 270:363-367.
40. Van Praag H.M. Biological suicidal research: outcome and limitations *Biol Psychiatry* 1985; 21:1305-1323.
41. Von Bardeleben J., Holsboer F. Cortisol response to a combined dexamethasone-human corticotropin-releasing hormone challenge in patients with depression. *J Neuroendocrinol* 1989; 1:485-488.
42. Vonnegut Jr., K. *Breakfast of Champions.* Delacorte Press, 7th edition, New York 1973.
43. Watson S.J., Lopez J.F., Young E.A., Vale W., Rivier J., Akil H. Effects of low dose ovine corticotropin-releasing hormone in humans: endocrine relationship and β-endorphin/β-lipotropin responses. *J Clin Endocrinol Metab* 1986; 66:10-15.
44. Widerlov E., Bissette G., Nemeroff C.B. Monoamine metabolites, corticotropin-releasing factor and somatostatin as CSF markers in depressed patients. *J Affect Dis* 1988; 14:99-107.
45. Wilde E.J., Kienhorst I.C.W.M., Diekstra R.F.W., Wolters W.H.G. The relationships between adolescent suicidal behavior and life events in childhood and adolescence. *Amer J Psychiat* 1992; 149:45-51.
46. Young E.A., Watson S.J., Kotun J. et al. β-lipotropin-β-endorphin response to low-dose ovine corticotropin releasing factor in endogenous depression. *Arch Gen Psychiatry* 1990; 47:449-457.

5

Evaluation of anxiety, depression and management of psychotic anxiety in schizophrenic patients

O. BLIN[1], J.M. AZORIN[2]

[1]*Pharmacologie Clinique, CHU Timone, 13385 Marseille Cedex 5, France.*
[2]*Clinique de Psychiatrie et Psychologie Médicale, CHU Timone, 13385 Marseille Cedex 5, France.*

None of the widely used, validated anxiety and depression scales could be used to specifically assess anxiety or depression in schizophrenic patients. However, it seems important to correctly assess depression and anxiety in psychotic patients before classifying and subtyping them. Therefore we proposed two rating scales: the «Psychotic Anxiety Scale» and the «Psychotic Depression Scale». In the manuscript, we also reviewed the different drugs that could be used in the management of psychotic anxiety.

Anxiety and depression in psychotic patients

Psychotic anxiety is a well known symptom. Its frequency and severity in psychotic patients contrast with the scarcity of the literature on this subject. Even the DSM-III-R [1] does not mention it and psychotic anxiety never appears as a diagnostic criteria. However, the existence and severity of psychotic anxiety in a given patient is one of the factors that may intervene in the choice of the treatment by the clinician. Several pharmacological approaches are possible.

There has been some controversy about the nature of the relationship between depression and psychosis. Some authors label «psychotic depression» depressive states with mood congruent features such as delusions or hallucinations (DSM-III-R). Others have emphasised the occurrence of depression in schizophrenic or delusional patients. Whatever the case, it could be sometimes difficult to differentiate some psychotic symptoms from depressive features. Recently Carpenter *et al* [2], for example, have noticed that negative symptoms such as restricted affect, diminished emotional range, poverty of speech, diminished sense of purpose and diminished mind drive might be, in some cases, due to depression or anxiety. Therefore, it seems important to correctly assess depression and anxiety in psychotic patients before classifying and subtyping them, particularly when one deals with the positive-negative distinction.

Evaluation of psychotic depression

None of the widely used, validated depression scales (MADRS, HAM-D) could be used to specifically evaluate psychotic depression. Depression only appeared in BPRS and PANSS as a sole item. However, the principal component analysis of the PANSS revealed a distinct affective component [3]. Therefore we recently developed the Psychotic Depression Scale, the scale designed for evaluating anxiety in psychotic patients (Appendice I). Our approach consisted of first determining the clinical elements underlying the evaluation of depression. In accordance with clinical interviews with psychotic patients, 32 items were chosen from the PANSS, the CPRS, CIDI, SANS and ERD (Widlöcher). Items were classified according to 3 groups: Psychotic items, Mood items and Behavioral items. This list of items has been tested in more than 100 schizophrenic patients and factor analysis will be published.

Evaluation of psychotic anxiety

Few studies have focused on psychotic anxiety. This aspect of schizophrenia did not receive much attention from clinicians, researchers or pharmacologists. One possible explanation of that fact is that up to a recent past, none of the validated anxiety scales could be used to specifically evaluate psychotic anxiety. Anxiety only appeared in BPRS and PANSS as a sole item. However, the principal component analysis of the PANSS, as previously mentioned, revealed a distinct affective component, including anxiety. Thus, psychotic anxiety could be considered as a important dimension in schizophrenic patients. Therefore we recently developed and validated the Psychotic Anxiety Scale, the first scale designed for evaluating anxiety in psychotic patients (Appendice II).

Our approach consisted of first determining the clinical elements underlying the evaluation of anxiety. In the course of clinical interviews with psychotic patients, 18 items were chosen. The list of these items was tested in schizophrenic patients. A principal component factorial analysis revealed that 4 factors accounted for respectively 32%, 14.7%, 14% and 7% of the variance. The first factor may be considered as representative of general severity and of exteriorisation of anxiety, while the second assesses patient inhibition. The third factor is interpreted as characterising the patient's dimension of self aggressiveness, and the fourth represents the changes in anxiety over time. Since no valid reference scale currently exists, the validity of the PAS was shown by calculating the correlation between the total PAS score and the clinician's overall evaluation of anxiety (R=0.663, p<0.001), and determining the correlation of each separate item with the clinician assessment of anxiety (p<0.05 for 11 items). We also validated the inter-rater reliability of the PAS [4-5]. Furthermore, a recent study performed by others showed that the PAS score was inversely correlated with the hydroxy-haloperidol/haloperidol ratio in treated schizophrenic patient [6].

Drug management of psychotic anxiety

Neuroleptics and psychotic anxiety

In the choice of a treatment, it would be usefull to know if a drug is anxiolytic or not. Let's consider the chronological management of psychotic anxiety and first, the neuroleptics. Different classifications have been proposed. First the clinical classification of Lambert and Revol. In this classification, levomepromazine which is mainly characterised by sedative neuroleptic activity and which is assumed by french psychiatrists to be anxiolytic, is opposed to the standard neuroleptic drug, haloperidol, which controls the positive symptoms of schizophrenia and which is assumed to be devoid of anxiolytic properties. One consequence is that french psychiatrists usually prescribe a combinaison of these 2 drugs. Other clinical classifications have been proposed (Delay and Denicker, 1961; Bobon *et al.*, 1972; Deniker and Ginestet, 1973, for a review see [7]). However, the anxiolytic properties of neuroleptics were not used as a classifying item until the classification of Kampsambelis *et al.* [8] who pointed out 3 clinical actions which should be selected in a present classification of neuroleptics: the anxiolytic effect, that is the specific antianxiety action upon psychotic anxiety; psychic reorganisation effect and thymoleptic effect. The biochemical classification is also important to consider. The antidopaminergic activity is the common point of neuroleptics and to a certain extent, it is possible to establish a link between the therapeutic activity and the dopaminolytic activity of these compounds. However, neuroleptics often exhibit other pharmacological properties: mainly adrenolytic, histaminergic and cholinergic blocking properties.

More recently, the development of different classes of neuroleptics have provided some interesting information.

For the benzamides and particularly amisulpride or remoxipride, a medline search did not provide any references on the anxiolytic activity of these drugs in schizophrenic patients. However, it can be noted that a benzamide such as sulpiride has been claimed to demonstrate anxiolytic properties at least in neurotic patients.

Zupenthixol, a thioxanthene, demonstrates sedative properties and has been shown to be effective on anxiety as assessed on VAS in mania and schizophrenic patient (10-40 mg). Its efficiency on the cluster anxiety-depression of the BPRS has been shown in open as well as in double-blind studies [9].

Clozapine, an atypical neuroleptic and a tricyclic dibenzodiazepine derivative, is moderately active on the dopaminergic pathways, blocking D1 and D2 receptors and also has adrenergic alpha 1, histamine H1, and muscarinic blocking activity. The drug is a serotonin 5HT2 antagonist and interestingly, this compound has been demonstrated to be effective on anxiety and tension in schizophrenic patients (see for example the studies published by Gerlach, Ekblom, Lapierre, Singer, for a review see [10]).

Benzodiazepines and psychotic anxiety

Since the 60', another therapeutic approach has been the benzodiazepines. Taking into account the double-blind trials, recent reviews show that response is highly variable, about one-third to one-half of patients improve, benzodiazepines are potentially most useful as adjuncts to neuroleptics in the acute management of psychotic agitation, relatively high doses of benzodiazepines may be associated with better response, and therapeutic effects, when seen, develop rapidly but diminish after several weeks in some patients. Features that predict response, amenable schizophrenic symptoms to benzodiazepines, role of benzodiazepines in maintenance therapy remain to be determined.

Serotonergic drugs and psychotic anxiety

Pilot studies have been conducted with serotonergic antagonists in schizophrenia. Cyproheptadine, a non-specific 5 HT antagonist, has some effects on negative symptoms of schizophrenia. 5 HT 3 blockers such as ondansetron display some efficiency in generalised anxiety. Two open, uncontrolled multicenter studies have tested various doses. In these studies ondansetron demonstrated an antipsychotic activity, but the efficacy was inversely related to the dose [11]. A double-blind study on 114 patients did not confirm these results.

5 HT2 lockers may improve schizophrenic patients. Ritanserin, a highly specific 5 HT2 antagonist can be described as a thymosthenic agent which restores energy and mood, reduces inhibition and anxiety. In schizophrenic patients, at an average dose of 20 mg daily, associated with classical neuroleptic therapy, Ritanserin was reported to improve both positive and negative symptoms [12].

New antipsychotic and psychotic anxiety

Since both dopaminergic and serotonergic receptor blocking properties are related to antipsychotic activity, the idea raised to develop a compound which demonstrates both pharmacological properties. Recently, the anxiolytic profiles of different kinds of neuroleptics, levomepromazine, haloperidol and risperidone, a drug with combined 5HT2 and dopamine-D2 receptor blocking properties, have been compared in the treatment of acute exacerbation of schizophrenia accompanied by symptoms of psychotic anxiety. 62 schizophrenic patients were included in a 4-week, randomised, double-blind, individual dose titration and parallel-group trial. The effects of the medications were assessed by means on the PANSS, the Psychotic Anxiety Scale (PAS), and the Clinical Global Impression (CGI). Safety evaluations were also performed. The results showed that risperidone, a potent 5 HT2 and D2 antagonist was more effective than both haloperidol and levomepromazine in reducing psychotic anxiety, the latter two drugs being comparable. Furthermore, risperidone caused less extrapyramidal symptoms than haloperidol [13-15].

Conclusion

The literature points out the need to specifically assess the effects of neuroleptics on both anxiety and depression in psychotic patients. In order to fulfil these requirements, we recently demonstrated the validity and the sensitivity to change of the PAS, the first scale intended to evaluate anxiety in psychotic patients. We propose here a new scale intended to evaluate depression in schizophrenic patients.

Acknowledgements

The authors wish to thank Dr Ph Bouhours for his helpful criticism and suggestions in the preparation of this work.

Psychotic Anxiety Scale ©
(Blin o. & Azorin J.M., 1992).

INSTRUCTIONS:
This scale is designed to assess a patient's psychotic anxiety over the past week. Check the appropriate rating for each item. Refer to the Manual for item definitions and description of anchoring points.

	0		2		4		6
1. Unconsciousness of the affliction	❑	❑	❑	❑	❑	❑	❑
2. Derealization	❑	❑	❑	❑	❑	❑	❑
3. Physical depersonalisation	❑	❑	❑	❑	❑	❑	❑
4. Psychic depersonalisation	❑	❑	❑	❑	❑	❑	❑
5. Ineffable depth of anxiety	❑	❑	❑	❑	❑	❑	❑
6. Inhibition of thought	❑	❑	❑	❑	❑	❑	❑
7. Perplexity	❑	❑	❑	❑	❑	❑	❑
8. Transmission of the anxiety to the examiner	❑	❑	❑	❑	❑	❑	❑
9. Reactivity to the surroundings	❑	❑	❑	❑	❑	❑	❑
10. Progression mode within the past week	❑	❑	❑	❑	❑	❑	❑
11. Motor inhibition	❑	❑	❑	❑	❑	❑	❑
12. Painful character of the affect felt	❑	❑	❑	❑	❑	❑	❑
13. Self-aggressiveness	❑	❑	❑	❑	❑	❑	❑
14. Lack of control of anxiety by the patient	❑	❑	❑	❑	❑	❑	❑
15. Hetero-aggressiveness	❑	❑	❑	❑	❑	❑	❑
16. Agitation	❑	❑	❑	❑	❑	❑	❑
17. Genuineness of experienced anxiety	❑	❑	❑	❑	❑	❑	❑
18. Global evaluation of anxiety by the examiner	❑	❑	❑	❑	❑	❑	❑

Psychotic Depression Scale ©
(Azorin J.M., Blin O., 1992).

1. PSYCHOTIC ITEMS	0		2(slight)		4(important)		6(extreme)
Autistic preoccupations	☐	☐	☐	☐	☐	☐	☐
Guilt feelings	☐	☐	☐	☐	☐	☐	☐
Guilty ideas of reference	☐	☐	☐	☐	☐	☐	☐
Ideas of persecution	☐	☐	☐	☐	☐	☐	☐
2. MOOD ITEMS							
Depression	☐	☐	☐	☐	☐	☐	☐
Somatic concern	☐	☐	☐	☐	☐	☐	☐
Sadness	☐	☐	☐	☐	☐	☐	☐
Inability to feel	☐	☐	☐	☐	☐	☐	☐
Pessimistic thoughts	☐	☐	☐	☐	☐	☐	☐
Suicidal thoughts	☐	☐	☐	☐	☐	☐	☐
Indecision	☐	☐	☐	☐	☐	☐	☐
Hopelessness	☐	☐	☐	☐	☐	☐	☐
Self depreciation	☐	☐	☐	☐	☐	☐	☐
Lack of self confidence	☐	☐	☐	☐	☐	☐	☐
Loss of interest/pleasure	☐	☐	☐	☐	☐	☐	☐
Brooding	☐	☐	☐	☐	☐	☐	☐
Discouragement	☐	☐	☐	☐	☐	☐	☐
3. BEHAVIOR ITEMS							
Concentration difficulties	☐	☐	☐	☐	☐	☐	☐
Failing memory	☐	☐	☐	☐	☐	☐	☐
Lack of appropriate emotion	☐	☐	☐	☐	☐	☐	☐
Withdrawal	☐	☐	☐	☐	☐	☐	☐
Early wakening	☐	☐	☐	☐	☐	☐	☐
Loss of appetite	☐	☐	☐	☐	☐	☐	☐
Increase in appetite	☐	☐	☐	☐	☐	☐	☐
Loss of weight	☐	☐	☐	☐	☐	☐	☐
Increase in weight	☐	☐	☐	☐	☐	☐	☐
Loss of interest/pleasure/work	☐	☐	☐	☐	☐	☐	☐
Lassitude, tiredness, lack of energy	☐	☐	☐	☐	☐	☐	☐
Fatiguability	☐	☐	☐	☐	☐	☐	☐
Psychomotor agitation	☐	☐	☐	☐	☐	☐	☐
Psychomotor retardation	☐	☐	☐	☐	☐	☐	☐
Slowness and underactivity	☐	☐	☐	☐	☐	☐	☐

References

1. American Psychiatric Association. *DSM-III-R*, Masson, Paris.
2. Carpenter W.T. Jr, Heinrichs D.W., Wagman A.M.I. *Am J Psychiatry* 1988; 145 578.
3. Kay S.R. (ed.) *Positive and negative syndromes in schizophrenia, Clinical and experimental psychiatry monograph n°5*. Brunner/Mazel, New York, 1991.
4. Blin O., Lecrubier Y., Azorin J.M., Souche A., Fondarai J. *Psychiatr and Psychobiol.* 3 1988; 255.
5. Blin O., Azorin J.M., Lecrubier Y., Souche A., Fondarai J. *Encéphale XV* 1989; 543.
6. Vaiva G. *PhD thesis*, Lille, 1992.
7. Deniker P., Ginestet D. *Encycl Med Chir* 1973; 37860 b 20, 2.

8. Kapsambelis V., Gekiere Cl., Ginestet D. *Encéphale XVI* 1990; 63.
9. Heikkilä L., Eliander H., Vartiainen H., Turunen M., Pedersen V. *Current Med Res Opinion* 12 1992; 594.
10. Péré J.J., Castaigne J.P. *Actualités Psychiatriques* Sept 1991; 28.
11. Meltzer H.Y. International Congress Series 968, *Biol Psychiatr* 2 1991; 891.
12. Gelders Y.G. *Br J Psychiatr* 155 (suppl 5) 1989; 33.
13. Blin O., Azorin J.M., Bouhours Ph. *Biol Psychiatr* 29 1991; 328S.
14. Blin O., Azorin J.M., Bouhours Ph. *Clin Pharmacol Ther* 51 1992.
15. Blin O., Azorin J.M., Bouhours Ph, Fondarai J. *Clin Neuropharm* 15 1992; 169B.

6

Endogenous opioids and their putative role in disturbances of social behavior, in particular autism

J.K. BUITELAAR

Department of Child and Adolescent Psychiatry, P.O. Box 85500, 3508 GA Utrecht, The Netherlands.

Data from animal studies support the involvement of opioids derived from the pro-opiomelanocortin system in the neuroregulation of social behavior. In general, low dosages of beta-endorphin appear to increase approach behavior, whereas high dosages tend to decrease social interaction. The neuropeptide ORG 2766, a synthetic adrenocorticotrophic hormone (4-9) analog, was shown to modulate disturbances in social behavior elicited by environmental manipulations. Possible opioid hypotheses of infantile autism are discussed, and empirical evidence is briefly reviewed.

Autism is a chronic persisting psychiatric disorder that is characterized by specific deficits in social interaction. In addition, the disorder is characterized by repetitive stereotyped behavior patterns and a deviant development of cognitive, language and communicative functions. Deficits in the area of social behavior and communication include impairments in the pragmatics of nonverbal communication as the use of eye contact and gestures [1]. The neurobiological basis of the autistic symptomatology is unknown. In this paper we examine to what extent neuropeptides of the pro-opiomelanocortin system (POMC) are involved in the neuroregulation of the autistic syndrome. First, a survey is presented of animal studies, which were concerned with the part played by POMC peptides in the neuroregulation of social behavior. Subsequently, a review is presented of research on the POMC system in autistic children. Finally, we will give an overview of the data from two controlled clinical trials designed to evaluate the efficacy of ORG 2766, a synthetic adrenocorticotrophic hormone (4-9) analog, in modulating the social behavior deficits of autistic patients.

The pro-opiomelanocortin (POMC) system

The POMC system is one of the three known opioid systems in the brain, along with the pro-dynorphin and the pro-enkephalin system. Most POMC containing neurons in the brain are found in the arcuate nucleus of the ventral hypothalamus. From here these neurons project to numerous brain structures, e.g. red nucleus of the stria terminalis, septum, amygdala, preoptic area, several hypothalamic nuclei, the periaquaductal grey matter, the nucleus ambiguous and the nucleus tractus solitarius. POMC is also synthesized in the pituitary gland, in the rat in the intermediate as well as in the anterior lobe. The anterior pituitary endocrine cells process the POMC is also synthesized in the pituitary endocrine cells process the POMC to ACTH, beta-lipotropine (beta-LPH) and beta-endorphin. The intermediate lobe and the neuronal structures process the precursor further to synthesize alpha-melanocyte stimulating hormone (alpha-MSH), beta-endorphin and smaller fragments. It should be stressed that due to differences in the degree of post-translational processing various modified forms of alpha-MSH and beta-endorphin exist also in the brain and in the pituitary, resulting in tissue specific sets of end products with distinct biological properties [2,3].

Peptides and social behavior in animals

Attachment behavior

Most research into the neuroregulation of attachment behavior has been done by Panksepp and collaborators [4,5]. Attachment behavior was investigated by studying the reaction to separation. The separation reaction, and particularly separation distress constitutes an index of the nature and quality of the existing attachment. As an easily operationalized measure, identical in different animal species, the socalled distress-vocalization (DV) is used, i.e. in animals various forms of squeaking and yelping. (A limitation of this research paradigm is that DV is only one of the manifestations of limitation of this research paradigm is that DV is only one of the manifestations of separation distress, and that pharmacological influences of endorphins and neuropeptides on other manifestations - dysphoria, motor phenomena - have not been investigated.) In the first instance this research was carried out in puppies, young guinea-pigs and chickens. Administration of morphine, either centrally or peripherally, supresses the DV to a dose-dependent degree. This effect can be blocked by naloxone, an opioid antagonist. Administration of naloxone alone causes increase of the DV. Many endorphins have morphine-like effects, the effect of beta-endorphin being by far the strongest.

The effects of endorphins on DV exhibit specificity in the behavioral and brain-localizatory senses [4]: (1) a behavior-specific effect, i.e. the effect is not produced via changes of the sedation level or of motor behaviors; and (2) brain-localization-specific effects, i.e. influence on the DV can only be brought about by electric stimulation of the central nervous system in specified areas (region near the anterior commissure, the dorsomedial thalamus, the amygdala and the mesencephalic periventricular grey matter) where endogenous opioid systems are localized. DVs provoked by such electric stimulation can be reduced by administration of morphine and aggravated by naloxone.

It was initially believed that these endorphin effects on DV were neurochemically specific as well. This was qualified somewhat by subsequent research [6-8]. Beside all opiates and endorphins, alpha-2-noradrenergic agonists (clonidine), glutamate receptor agonists, somatostatin, oxytocin and vasotocin also prove capable of greatly reducing DVs. Some reduction of DVs is also accomplished with tricyclic antidepressants (imipramine). An increase of DVs is brought about by opioid antagonists (naloxone, naltrexone) but also by, dextro- and levo-amphetamine, atropine, arginine vasopressin, alpha-MSH and ACTH (1-24). The last-mentioned two peptides cause biphasic effects, low doses increasing the DV and high doses reducing it.

These finding points to a distinct involvement of endogenous opioids in the regulation of separation distress reactions. However, other receptor systems also play a part in the regulation of separation distress: glutamate and noradrenergic receptors, serotoninergic and cholinergic systems. Panksepp [4] interpreted the findings as supporting his hypothesis that hyperfunction of endogenous opioid systems block the entering into social relationships. They alleged that a hyperactive endogenous opioid system reduced social interest. Results from other experimental designs, however, confound the picture and fail to support this simple and straightforward interpretation.

Approach behavior

In this experiments, use is often made of preceding social isolation of animals. The functioning of endogenous opioid systems is affected by previous brief or protracted social isolation, presumably through changing the number or sensitivity of the opioid receptors [4,9,10].

Low doses of morphine in rats reduce approach behavior. This effect of morphine is attenuated by previous social isolation. Naloxone in this experimental design had contradictory effects. The question whether naloxone antagonizes the morphine effect has not been investigated [11]. In young guinea-pigs, low doses of morphine lead to less approach behavior toward the mother. Naloxone has no effect in this design. Previous social isolation cancels the morphine effect [12].

Niesink and Van Ree used the dyadic interaction model to study social behavior in rats [13,14]. After brief social isolation of rats, an increased frequency of social behaviors was seen, whereas after adjustement to low intensity of light, social behaviors were seen to decrease under high-intensity illumination. Great importance attaches to the finding that ORG 2766 can 'normalize' these experimentally induced changes in social behavior [13]. Changes in motor behavior induced by environmental manipulations are also counteracted by ORG 2766 [15]. These normalizing effects of ORG 2766 prove to be naltrexone-reversible, which implies that these behavior-modulating effects of ORG 2766 are brought about via endogenous opioid systems.

Conversely, ACTH (4-10) and ACTH (1-24) enhance in a number of designs the effect of environmental manipulations on social and motor behavior.

Further research findings suggest that these normalizing and stabilizing effects of ORG 2766 originate in the amygdala by influencing the integration of sensory stimuli [16]. Data from binding studies and social interaction experiments also support the hypothesis that endogenous opioid systems in the amygdala are particularly important for social behavior [17,18].

Beta-endorphin in isolated rats mainly increase social contact [19]. Moreover, beta-endorphin in low doses has a positive, i.e. stimulating effect on the frequency of social interactions in non-isolated rats [14,19,20]. Higher doses of beta-endorphin caused a reduction of social behavior in rats [21].

In the non-isolated rat, gamma-MSH unlike beta-endorphin decreases contact behavior in particular [14], while ACTH (4-10) reduces all social interactions [22]. Accordingly, there appears to exist a functional antagonism between gamma-MSH and ACTH (4-10) on the one hand, and beta-endorphin on the other where social behavior is concerned [14].

Other social behaviors

The influence of endogenous opioid systems on numerous other aspects of social behavior has also been studied in animal experiments. Morphine reinforces the contact comfort (the tendency of young chickens to fall asleep in the hands of a human experimenter), naloxone weakens it [23,24]. Both morphine and naloxone inhibit imprinting in chickens [4,23].

Morphine causes an increase of playing ('pinning') behavior in rats, while naloxone inhibits it [25-28]. After brief social isolation, pinning behavior and social grooming increase in young rats. This increase is weakened by naltrexone, while opioids (morphine and beta-endorphin) enhance it. Apart from opioid systems, dopaminergic systems also pay a part in the regulation of these behaviors [29].

Endogenous opioids influence social, friendly behavior in dogs, such as face licking and tail wagging [30]. According to Panksepp, the importance of social rewards decreases under the influence of morphine, which leads to persistence of learnt behavior patterns. Naloxone, on the other hand, hastens the extinction of social learning behavior [31]. Opioids in rats influence dominance hierarchy in groups [28] and determine the balance between agonistic-aggressive and defensive-submissive behavior in mice [32]. Endogenous opioid systems are also involved in the regulation of social behavior of squirrel monkeys in groups. After naltrexone, the subordinate monkeys take more social initiatives and display more marking behavior. Naltrexone does not affect the dominant monkeys. Finally, social conflicts in mice leads to violent and protracted changes in the functioning of endogenous opioid systems [33-35].

Summary: POMC and social behavior

These data indicate that opioid systems in the brain are involved with a certain chemical specificity in the neuroregulation of the intensity of emotions and of distress reactions that occur after social isolation. POMC peptides also play a neurobiological part in various other types of social behavior. It has however not been demonstrated that opioid systems constitute a necessary and/or sufficient biological condition for these social behaviors.

The effects of manipulations of the POMC depend on the test design selected. Making a priori predictions on the direction of the effect is difficult. This may mean that, in dependence on the test design, only certain parts of the opioid system, certain receptors or receptors types play a part.

The effect of both morphine and beta-endorphin on social behavior and playing behavior is biphasic: in low doses they stimulate social contact, in higher doses they inhibit it. This suggests that the main influence of POMC peptides on social behavior is a stabilizing and modulating one. A normalizing and stabilizing effect has been demonstrated most clearly for ORG 2766.

The activity of the POMC system influences social behavior. However, the inverse is true as well: social experiences (social isolation, social conflicts) exert a distinct influence on the activity of the endogenous opioid systems.

In a number of test designs a functional antagonism is demonstrable between beta-endorphin on the one hand and ACTH related peptides (gamma-MSH and alpha-MSH) on the other. All these compounds, both beta-endorphin and the ACTH related peptides gamma-MSH and alpha-MSH derive from the same precursor molecule POMC.

These effects of POMC peptides on social behavior can theoretically be explained in various ways, namely via a) coping with the stress accompanying pleasure in social contact, c) reduction of aversion, e.g. decrease of (social) fear, d) influence on the general activity level, e) change of the information processing of social stimuli, or f) a combination of these possibilities. It should be noted that in experimental paradigms these possibilities are difficult to distinguish from another. Asking for an explanation also implies asking how specific this effect of POMC peptides on social behavior is. Up to now, empirical support has been found for possibilities c) reduction of aversion and e) change in information processing.

POMC hypotheses on autism

Panksepp has advanced the hypothesis of a hyperfunctioning endogenous opioid system in autism [36]. This might explain numerous symptoms in the domains of social behavior, information processing, stereotypies and brain maturation. However, the biphasic effects on different types of social behavior and the finding that the direction of the effect often depends on the experimental conditions give rise to problems of interpretation within the framework of this hypothesis. Also, there are equally good grounds to postulate hypofunctionality of ACTH/MSH peptidergic systems.

An alternative, soberer hypothesis is that which postulates imbalance and dysfunctioning of the endogenous opioid system and of other peptides originating from the POMC system. This may involve hyper- as well as hypoactivity of parts of this system, and also changes in number and sensitivity of subpopulations of opioid receptors.

Another possibility is a disturbance of the functional antagonism between beta-endorphin and the ACTH/MSH peptides, e.g. due to disturbances in the formation and splitting of the various POMC derivatives. This hypothesis is supported by growing evidence that opioids and ACTH/MSH peptides constitute a balanced system modulating numerous brain functions [2,3]. As a rule, opioids and ACTH/MSH peptides influence these brain functions in opposite ways, although identical effects have also been described. ACTH/MSH peptides and endorphins probably are acting by their own receptor system, but exert effects also by a pharmacological or functional, mutual agonism and/or antagonism.

Because post-translational bioprocessing of the POMC-peptides is subject to various enzymatical and biochemical factors, disturbances may easily result in different mixtures of peptides with concomitant neurobehavioral effects. Moreover, also other regulatory sites of the POMC-system itself, gene expression and transcription, translation, biodegradation, and receptorstructure and -sensitivity may be influenced by environmental and/or congenital factors. More detailed but speculative models of the possible involvement of endogenous opioid systems in the pathogenesis of the autistic symptomatology can be found in Sandman and Kastin [37] and in Chamberlain and Herman [38].

The POMC system in autism

To what extent are POMC hypotheses on autism supported by results of empirical studies in autistic children? We will briefly discuss two lines of evidence: measurements of levels of endorphins and other neuropeptides in the body fluids of autistic patients, and results from intervention studies in the POMC system in autism.

Measurement of endorphins and neuropeptides in autism

There are several reports on endorphin plasma levels in autism. Weizman *et al.* report a study in which the blood humoral-endorphin concentration was measured in 10 autistic children [39]. The endorphin level in autistic children was significantly lower than in a group of control children (N=11). The same researchers reported later plasma immunoreactive beta-endorphin to be significantly lower in 22 autistic patients as compared with 22 schizophrenic patients and 22 controls [40]. In an Italian study in 12 autistic children two different patterns of plasma beta-endorphin levels were observed, the first one characterized by very high levels and the second one by very low levels, compared to mentally retarded controls [41]. There was no correlation between the clinical characteristics of the subjects and endorphin levels [42]. Another report on 4 autistic subjects fund elevated plasma beta-endorphin levels in 3 subjects, and normal levels in one child [43]. In an adult autistic sample (N=8, mean age 26 years) plasma beta-endorphin levels were reported to be lower compared to healthy controls but not significantly different from mentally retarded controls [44]. In a larger sample of mentally retarded adults with self-injurious behavior (SIB) and/or stereotypy, plasma beta-endorphin was lower than in mentally retarded controls [45]. Unfortunately, this report does not indicate whether and to which extent these self-injurious subjects were also autistic.

There are three reports available on CSF endorphin levels. In the first study raised levels of endorphin-fraction II were found in the CSF in autistic children (N=20). The major opioid in fraction II was met-enkephalin, and not beta-endorphin [46]. Ross *et al.* [47] measured a significantly elevated CSF beta-endorphin level in 8 autistic children; there was however no correlation between the reduction of beta-endorphin levels with fenfluramine and the clinical response. Conversely, in a group of 31 autistic children, and 8 children with Rett syndrome, CSF beta-endorphin levels were significantly lower compared to healthy adult controls [48]. The Rett syndrome is characterized by symptoms of autistic-like behavior, progressive loss of motor, cognitive and language skills, and the development of a very restricted repertory of stereotyped hand movements, which seem to develop only in girls. In the other studies, elevated CSF beta-endorphin-like immunoreactivity had been reported in girls with the Rett syndrome [49-51].

Taken together, there are many inconsistencies in the data on plasma and CSF beta-endorphin levels in autism. These inconsistencies may relate to discrepancies in assay techniques, clinical and etiological heterogeneity within the autistic syndrome, and failures to account for co-existing abnormalities in other neurotransmitter or neuromodulator systems.

Interventions in the POMC system in autism: opioid antagonists

Four studies have examined the effects of naltrexone in a placebo-controlled acute-dosage design. In two pilot studies by Herman *et al.* it was found that naltrexone did not favorably affect social behavior, but reduced measures of hyperactivity and stereotypy in small samples of autistic subjects [52,53]. In two other studies some beneficial effects of naltrexone on social behavior were reported: the first one indicated a combination of tranquilizing and socially stimulating effects in 10 autistic children [54], and the second one described an improvement of eye-contact and smiling along with a decrease of hyperactivity and automutilation in 2 subjects [55].

At this stage, there are three reports available on subchronic placebo-controlled naltrexone treatment in autism. In the first one, positive behavioral effects could be substantiated only on a global clinical consensus rating, but not on detailed formal rating scales in a parallel-design in 18 subjects [56]. In the second one, 1.0 mg/kg naltrexone every 48 hours produced a significant reduction in autistic symptomatology in 12 autistic children in a crossover design; 7 individuals turned out to be a drug-responder [42]. The third study included 4 subjects in a crossover design; 3 subjects were considered to be drug-responders. The group statistics however were flawed by excluding the non responding subject from the analysis [43]. All three responders had elevated baseline plasma beta-endorphin levels which normalized after naltrexone treatment; however, beta-endorphin levels also normalized after dosages of naltrexone which did not exert clinical effects. Finally, positive effects of naltrexone on social behavior of autistic subjects have been found in an open-label treatment [57].

In sum, naltrexone appears to be use in the treatment of some autistic children; however, it is not clear whether the main effect is on social behavior in particular, or on more general measures of overactivity and behavioral disorganization. Further controlled treatment studies are warranted.

Interventions in the POMC system in autism: ORG 2766

ORG 2766 was chosen for a pharmacological intervention in autism for several reasons. It was shown to counteract changes in social behavior elicited by environmental manipulations in rats [13]. Furthermore, ORG 2766 exerted a positively valued influence on the structure of social behavior in animal experiments. ORG 2766 was reported also to exert some beneficial effects on social behavior in elderly people. ORG 2766 has no substantial steroidogenic activity and is active on oral administration. We will present an overview of the data from two controlled clinical trials designed to evaluate the efficacy of ORG 2766 in modulating the social behavior deficits of autistic patients.

Subjects were outpatient children with a diagnosis of autistic disorder according to DSM-III-R criteria. The diagnosis was made independently by two child psychiatrists on the basis of all available clinical records. The ages of the subjects ranged from 5 to 15 years, IQ scores ranged from 22 to 99. In both trials a double-blind and placebo-controlled crossover design was employed. After a 2-week baseline period the children were randomly assigned to their treatment sequence, ORG 2766 - placebo or placebo - ORG 2766. Treatmentorder groups were matched by IQ and age. Both trials differed with respect to the length of the period of active treatment and the dosage of ORG 2766 administered. Active treatment was in the first and second trial respectively 20 mg ORG 2766/day per child during 4 weeks, and 40 mg ORG 2766/day per child during 8 weeks.

Treatment effects were evaluated by means of an ethologically analyzed playroom observation and by means of behavior checklist ratings. Behavior elements of child and experimenter were monitored by an event-recorder in a semi-structured playroom session which lasted 20 minutes. The analysis was focused on changes in frequencies of behavior elements as well as on shifts in the structure of behavior. Particularly the degree of interactional dependency of the child's behavior on the behavior of the experimenter was expressed in information-statistical measures, which served as an index of the social interaction between child and experimenter [58].

Behavior ratings were completed independently by the parents and the teachers on the Aberrant Behavior Checklist, and by the investigators on the Clinical Global

Impressions Scale. At the end of the study the parents rated double-blind their treatment preference by specifying their period of choice («period 1», «period 2» or «no preference»).

Fourteen autistic children were enrolled in the first trial [58,59]. All children completed the study, no side effects were observed. In the playroom session ORG 2766 treatment was associated with an increase of changing toys, talk behavior and locomotion, and a decrease of stereotyped behaviors. The analysis of the structure of behavior revealed, after ORG 2766 treatment, an increased amount as well as an improved quality of the social interaction between child and experimenter. In particular, after ORG 2766 gaze and smile behaviors of child and experimenter showed stronger temporal contingencies. However, in the overall analysis of the checklist ratings completed by parents and teachers no significant ORG 2766 effects were found. The investigators identified 8 children as an individual drug-responder. Treatment effects became apparent after the use of ORG 2766 during 4 weeks and not after 2 weeks. Hence, and because effects were found in the playroom condition only, a second clinical trial was conducted with a higher dosage of ORG 2766 (40 mg/day per child) during a longer treatment period (8 weeks).

Twenty-one autistic children participated in the second trial [60]. Again no physical side-effects were reported by parents or teachers, nor did we observe physical side-effects. ORG 2766 treatment was associated with significantly more play behavior in the playroom session. In regard of the structure of behavior only after ORG 2766 connections were found between «play» and child's gaze behaviors. This reflects an improved communicative quality of the play. The analysis of the information-statistical measure indicated an increased social interaction between child and experimenter after ORG 2766.

This time significant drug effects appeared in the analysis of the checklist ratings, namely on the ABC-parents sum score and social withdrawal subscale and on the CGI severity and improvement ratings. All drug effects were in the intended direction with ameliorated ratings in the ORG 2766 condition. Parents double-blind treatment preferences completed after the finish of the trial favored ORG 2766 treatment more than placebo. According to an algorithm of the checklist ratings 9 subjects were ascertained as an individual responder.

In these two clinical trials ORG 2766 exerted an activating and social interaction stimulating influence on the behavior of autistic children. In the second trial these effects were substantiated not only in the playroom observation, but also on the checklist ratings. It is of interest to note that ORG 2766 was able to induce shifts in temporal contingencies of behavior elements, affecting in particular those aspects (attunement of eye-contact and gestures) in which autistic children were deficient compared to nonautistic retarded controls [1, 61].

Since the social behavior modulating effects of ORG 2766 in the dyade interaction model could be demonstrated to be naltrexone reversible, which indicates that ORG 2766 exerts this effect via an interaction with endogenous opioid systems [13,16], the behavioral effects induced by ORG 2766 in these autistic children may be mediated by endogenous opioid systems also.

Concluding remarks

So far, the empirical, evidence for opioid hypotheses on disturbed social behavior, and in particular on autism is inconclusive. Treatment studies suggest that agents like naltrexone and ORG 2766, which have an impact on endogenous opioids systems, do benefit some autistic children. To find further evidence supporting the neuroendocrine hypotheses mentioned, useful research strategies may be more intensive direct measurement of neuro-endocrine parameters in autistic children during pharmacological challenges. Another promising strategy could be neuro-imaging studies which visualize opioid receptor systems in the brain by means of specific tracers. These tracers are in the process of being developed and tested in various research centers. However, a disadvantage of both strategies may be that merely static information is provided on the POMC system, i.e. on the functioning in autistic children at the time of study. In theory it is possible that during the development of the (autistic) child disorders in neuroendocrine functions have occurred which subsequently can no longer be objectified as such. These disturbances have, as it were, left no 'endocrine fingerprints'.

Finally, some relativation is in due place. Opioids, endorphins and neuropeptides have been ascribed neuroregulatory roles in virtually all classes of psychiatric disorders. Further research has to clarify whether the implication of the POMC-system in autism is of a nonspecifical nature, or is based upon more specific associations with pathophysiological mechanisms underlying autism.

References

1. Buitelaar JK, Van England H, De Kogel CH, De Vries H, Van Hooff JARAM. *J Child Psychol Psychiat* 1991; 32:995-1015.
2. O'Donohue TL, Dorsa DM. *Peptides* 1982 ; 3:353-395.
3. De Wied D, Jolles J. *Physiological Reviews* 1982 ; 62:976-1059.
4. Panksepp J, Herman BH, Vilberg T, Bishop P, DeEskinazi FG. *Neuroscience and Biobehavioral Reviews* 1980 ; 4:473-487.
5. Sahley TL, Panksepp J. *J Autism Dev Disord* 1987; 17:210-216.
6. Panksepp J, Siviy S, Normansall L. *The Psychobiology of Attachment and Separation* (eds.) Reite M, Fields T. Orlando : Academic Press 1985, 3-50.
7. Panksepp J, Normansell L, Herman BH, Bishop P, Crepeau L. *The Physiological Control of Mammalian Vocalizations* (ed.) Newman JD. New York: Plenum Press 1988, 263-300.
8. Panksepp J, Lensing P. *Proceedings of the International Conference on The Experimental Biology of the Autistic Syndromes* (March 29-31, Durham UK) 1989.
9. Geller EB, Braberman S, Biunno I, Harakal C, Adler MW. *Federation of the Proceedings of Science* 1977; 36:993.
10. Schenk S, Britt MD, Atalay D, Charleson S. *Pharmacol Bioch Beh* 1982; 16:841-842.
11. Herman BH, Panksepp J. *Pharmacol Bioch Beh* 1978 ; 9:213-220.
12. Panksepp J, Najam N, Soares F. *Pharmacol Bioch Beh* 1979; 11:131-134.
13. Niesink RJM, Van Ree JM. *Science* 1983 ; 221:960-962.
14. Niesink RJM, Van Ree JM. *Neuropeptides* 1984 ; 4:483-496.

15. Wolterink G, Van Ree JM. *Brain Research* 1987; 421:41-47.
16. Wolterink G, Van Ree JM. *Neuropeptides* 1989; 14:129-136.
17. Panksepp J, Bishop P. *Brain Res Bull* 1981 ; 7:405-410.
18. File SE, Rodgers RJ. *Pharmacol Bioch Beh* 1979 ; 11:313-318.
19. Niesink RJM. Social Behavior of Rats. Thesis, Utrecht: University of Utrecht, 1983.
20. Van Ree JM, Niesink RJM. *Life Sciences 33* (suppl. I): 1983; 611-614.
21. Meyerson B. *Eur J Pharmacol* 1981 ; 69:453-463.
22. File SE. *Peptides* 1981 ; 2:255-260.
23. Panksepp J, Bean NJ, Bishop P, Vilberg T, Sahley TL. *Pharmacology, Biochemistry and Behavior* 1980 ; 13:673-683.
24. Vilberg TR, Bean N, Bishop P, Porada K., Panksepp J. Society of Neuroscience Abstracts 1977; 3:975.
25. Panksepp J, Beatty WW. *Behavioral and Neural Biology* 1980 ; 30:197-206.
26. Beatty WW, Costello KB. *Pharmacology Biochemistry and Behavior* 1982; 17:905-907.
27. Panksepp J, Siviy S, Normansall L. *Neurosciences and Biobehavioral Reviews* 1984 ; 11:131-134.
28. Panksepp J, Jalowiec J, De Eskanazi FG, Bishop P. *Behavior and Neurosciences* 1985 ; 99:441-453.
29. Niesink RJM, Van Ree JM. *Neuropharmacology* 1989 ; 28:411-418.
30. Panksepp J, Herman BH, Vilberg T, Bishop P, DeEskanazi FG. *Neurosciences and Biobehavioral Reviews* 1978 ; 4:473-487.
31. DeEskanazi FG, Panksepp J. Society of Neuroscience Abstracts 1979 ; 5:1037.
32. Benton D, Brain PF. *Endorphins, Opiates and Behavioural Processes* (eds.) Rodgers RJ and Cooper SJ. New York: Wiley and Sons, 1988, 215-235.
33. Miczek KA, Thompson ML, Shuster L. *Science* 1982 ; 215:1520-1522.
34. Miczek KA, Thompson ML, Shuster L. *Annals of the New York Academy of Science* 1986 ; 467:14-29.
35. Teskey GC, Kavaliers M, Hirst M. *Life Sciences* 1984; 35:303-315.
36. Panksepp J. *Trends in Neuroscience* 1979; 2:174-177.
37. Sandman CA, Kastin AJ. *Applications of Basic Neuroscience to Child Psychiatry* (eds.) Deutsch S I, Weizman A and Weizman R. New-York: Plenum Press, 1990; 101-124.
38. Chamberlain RS, Herman BH. *Biol Psychiatry* 1990; 28:773-793.
39. Weizman R, Weizman A, Tyano A, Szekely B, Weissman BA, Sarne Y. *Psychopharmacology* 1984 ; 82:368-370.
40. Weizman R, Gil-ad I, Dick J, Tyano S, Szekely GA, Laron ZJ. *Am Acad Child Adolesc Psychiatry* 1988 ; 27:430-433.
41. Marchetti B, Scifo R, Batticane N, Scapagnini U. *Brain Dysfunct* 1990 ; 3:346-354.
42. Scifo R, Batticane N, Quattropani MC, Spoto G, Marchetti B. *Proceedings of OASI Conference*, Sicily, October 1991.
43. Leboyer M, Bouvard MP, Launay J-M, et al. *J Autism Dev Disord* 1992; 22:309-319.
44. Sandman CA, Barron JL, Chicz-DeMet A, DeMet EM. *J Autism Dev Disord* 1991 ; 21:83-87.
45. Sandman CA, Barron JL, Chiicz DeMet A, DeMet EM. *Am J Ment Retard* 1990 ; 95:84-92.
46. Gillberg C, Terenius L, Lonnerholm G. *Arch Gen Psychiat* 1985; 42:780-783.
47. Ross DL, Klykylo WM, Hitzemann R. *Pediatric Neurology* 1987; 3:83-86.
48. Gillberg C, Terenius L, Hagberg B, Witt-Engerstrom I, Eriksonn I. *Brain Dev* 1990 ; 12:88-92.
49. Zappella M, Genazzini A, Facchinetti F, Hayek G. *Brain Dev* 1990 ; 12:221-225.
50. Brase DA, Myer EC, Dewey WL. *Life Sciences* 1989; 45:359-366.
51. Budden SS, Myer EC, Butler IJ. *Brain Dev* 1990 ; 12:81-84.
52. Herman BH, Hammock MK, Arthur-Smith A, et al. Society for Neuroscience Abstracts 1986 ; 12:1172.

53. Herman BH, Asleson GS, Borghese IF, *et al. Proceedings of the 38th Annual Meeting of the American Academy of Child and Adolescent Psychiatry*, San Fransisco: AACAP, 1991.
54. Campbell M, Overall JE, Small AM, *et al. J Am Acad Child Adolesc Psychiatry* 1989; 28:200-206.
55. Leboyer M, Bouvard MP, Dugas M. *Lancet* 1988; 1:715.
56. Campbell M, Anderson LT, Small AM, Locasio JL, Lynch NS, Choroco MC. *Psychopharmacol Bull* 1990 ; 26:130-135.
57. Leboyer M, Bouvard MP, Lensing P, *et al. Brain Dysfunct* 1990; 3:285-298.
58. Buitelaar JK, Van Engeland H, De Kogel CH, De Vries H, Van Hooff JARAM and Van Ree JM. *Biol Psychiatry* 1992 ; 31:1119-1129.
59. Buitelaar JK, Engeland H, Van Ree JM, De Wied D. *J Autism Dev Disord* 1990 ; 20:467-478.
60. Buitelaar JK, Van Engeland H, De Kogel CH, De Vries H, Van Hooff JARAM and Van Ree JM. *J Am Acad Child Adolesc Psychiatry* 1992; 31:1149-1156.
61. Buitelaar JK, Van Engeland H, De Kogel CH, De Vries H, Van Hooff JARAM and Van Ree JM. *Experientia* 1992; 48:391-394.

7

The D₃ dopamine receptor as a target for antipsychotics

D. LEVESQUE[1], P. SOKOLOFF[1], J. DIAZ[1], M.P. MARTRES[1], C. PILON[1], J.C. SCHWARTZ[1,2]

[1]Unité de Neurobiologie et Pharmacologie, Centre Paul-Broca de l'INSERM, 2ter, rue d'Alésia, 75014 Paris, France
[2]Laboratoire de Physiologie, Faculté de Pharmacie, Université René-Descartes, 75006 Paris, France.

The dopamine receptor family

During the past few decades the idea the brain dopamine (DA) receptors are involved in the antipsychotic action of neuroleptics has widely been accepted among scientific community. This was supported by the fact that most neuroleptics share, among others, the common property to interact with DA receptors. Based on their opposite effect on adenylate cyclase activity and on their pharmacological profile, two DA receptor subtypes, termed D_1 and D_2, were proposed to mediate the various actions of DA [1]. Advances in molecular biology have completely modified this somewhat simplistic view, in regard to what we know now, of the dopaminergic neurotransmission. This approach led to the identification and the cloning of the genes corresponding, not only to D_1 and D_2 receptor subtypes [2-5], but also to additional and less expected ones termed D_3 [6], D_4 [7], and D_5 [8,9]. Some important characterisitics of the DA receptor family are shown in Table 1.

The amino acid sequences, as deduced by the established nucleotide sequences of corresponding complementary DNAs, reveal that they belong to a larger superfamily, that of receptors with seven transmembrane domains and coupled to their intracellular transduction system by a GTP binding regulatory protein (G protein) [10]. All G protein-coupled receptors comprise a parttern of seven streches of 20-25 hydrophobic amino acid residues postulated to form transmembranes α-helices, connected by alterning extracellular and cytoplasmic loops composed of hydrophilic residues [10]. The DA receptor family can be divided in two groups according to their gene organisation : "D_1-like" with intronless genes, i.e. those of the D_1 and D_5 receptors, in which the coding nucleotide sequence is continuous, and "D_2-like" or intron containing genes which possed discontinuous DNA fragments (exons), interspersed among sequence (introns) that do not form a part of the mature messenger RNA (mRNA). This is observed with D_2, D_3 and D_4 receptors subtypes (Figure 1). This latter gene organisation may also lead, via a mechanism of alternative splicing, to the biosynthesis of several distinct proteins encoded by a unique gene (see Figure 1 and [11-13]).

Table I. Synopsis of the domapine receptor family.

	D_1-like receptors		D_2-like receptors		
	D_1	D_5	D_2	D_3	D_4
Coding sequence :	446 a.a.	477 a.a.	D_{2A} : 443 a.a. D_{2B} : 414 a.a.	400 a.a.	387 a.a.
Chromosome localisation	5 q31-q34	4 p 16.3	11 q22-q23	3 q13.3	11 p
Highest brain densities :	Neostriatum	Hypothal. Hippocamp.	Neostriatum	Isl. Calleja Nucleus accumbens	Medulla Frontal cortex
Pituitary :	No	No	Yes	No	Yes
DA affinity :	µM	µM	Sub-µM	nM	Sub-µM
Characteristic agonists :	SKF 38393	SKF 38393	Bromocriptine	7-OH-DPAT	?
Characteristic antagonists :	SCH 23390	SCH 23390	Haloperidol	UH 232	Clozapine
Adenylate cyclase	Stimulates	Stimulates	Inhibits	?	?

a.a. amino acid, Hypothal. : Hypothalamus, Isl. : Islands, Hippocam. : Hippocampus, 7-OH-DPAT : 7-hydroxy-N,N' dipropyl aminotetralin.

This definition of two subfamilies of DA receptors based on genetic informations is also consistent at the level of their pharmacology. Indeed, D_1-like subtypes possess a high, subnanomolar affinity for compounds like SCH 23390 and SKF 38393, previously classified as D_1 receptor selective agents, whereas D_2-like receptor subtypes have only micromolar affinity for these drugs (see Table II). The opposite feature is observed with (-) sulpiride, for example. More generally, D_2-like receptor subtypes also have a better affinity for neuroleptics than D_1-like receptor subtypes. Among new members of the DA receptor family the D_3 receptor has interesting properties ; it possesses a good affinity for most neuroleptics (Table II and ref. [6]), and its brain localisation is restricted to the ventral part of the striatal complex [6,14], which is associated with the limbic system, controlling cognitive functions and emotional behaviour. Both properties suggest that the blockade of the D_3 receptor may participate in the antipsychotic activity of neuroleptic drugs.

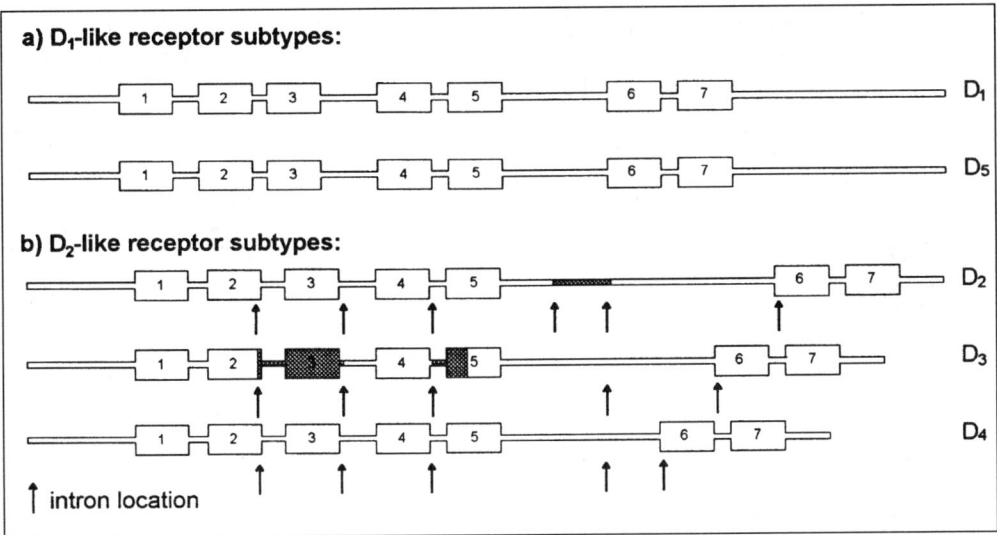

Figure 1. DA receptor gene organisation. Boxes represent transmembrane domains along the coding sequence. Arrows indicate position of introns and shaded areas correspond to alternatively spliced exons. Note that the second spliced exon in the D₃ receptor mRNA sequence uses an internal acceptor site present in transmembrane domain 5.

Focus on the D₃ receptor sybtype

The open reading frame of the D₃ receptor correspond to a sequence of 446 amino acid residues in the rat, but only 400 residues in humans, the main difference residing at the level of the third putative intracytoplasmique loop (i3) [6,15]. Since i3 loop is mainly responsible for specific interaction with G protein [10], it is likely that this difference may lead to distinct coupling of the D₃ receptor in both species. However, D₃ receptor has yet unidentified signal transduction pathway. The amino acid sequence of the human D₃ receptor displays 46% overall homology with that of the D₂ receptor, a value increasing to 78% when only the putative transmembrane domains, which are though to form the binding pocket for DA and dopaminergic drugs [10], are considered. For the D₂ receptor, alternative splicing has been shown to produce two receptor isoforms that differ by a stretch of 29 amino acids in i3 loop (Figure 1). Although they display similar pharmacology, they have different patterns of expression among cerebral areas [11,12]. Moreover, treatment with haloperidol predominantly enhances the abundance of the smaller isoform in brain [11], and pituitary [12]. On the other hand, there is no clear evidence that both isoforms are functionally distinct. For D₃ receptor, two truncated forms have been detected in rat [13] and human [15]. These truncated mRNA lead to the formation of the protein of 109 (the splicing introduces a frameshift leading to a premature stop codon) or 428 amino acids. However, when spliced variant of the rat D₃ receptor mRNA are expressed in transfect cell lines they do not show any DA specific binding [15]. Hence, the functional signifiance of the process of alternative splicing remain elusive. We may speculate that this processing mechanism represents a way to control the abundance of a specific functional transcript. It cannot be exclude that defects in alternative splicing mechanisms, leading to the formation of inactive receptors, may occur during psychiatric disorders.

Table II. Pharmacology of dopamine receptor subtypes*.

	D_1-like receptors		D_2-like receptors		
	D_1	D_5	D_2	D_3	D_4
Dopamine[a]	2000	250	2000	30	540
7-OH-DPAT	5300	-	60	0,7	650
Apomorphine	700	400	70	70	4[b]
Bromocriptine	700	500	5	7	300
Pergolide	1400	900	20	2	-
Quinpirole	14,000	-	1400	40	50
SKF 38393	150	100	10,000	5000	10,000
Antogonists					
Haloperidol	30	40	0,6	3	5
Pimozide	-	-	10	11	40
Thioproperazine	-	-	0,5	1	50
(-) Sulpiride	40,000	80,000	10	20	50
UH 232	-	-	40	10	-
Clozapine	140	250	70	500	9
SCH 23390	0,3	0,3	1000	1000	3500

* Values shown are inhibition constants exprimed in nM, and were obtained with cell lines expressing respective DA receptor subtypes from human [7,8,16], except for values of 7-OH-DPAT which are from rat [17].
[a]Value in presence of guanyl nucleotide.
[b]High affinity component.

The distribution of the D_3 receptor gene transcript (mRNA) in rat brain areas, as established by *in situ* hybridization histochemistry markedly differs from those of the D_1 or D_2 receptor gene transcript [14]. For instance, only a week D_3 receptor hybridization signal was detected in restricted parts of the striatum, whereas the whole striatum contains the highest densities of DA axons and D_2 receptor mRNA [14]. By contrast, D_3 receptor mRNA is highly expressed in areas of the ventral striatum. These areas include the olfactory tubercle-island of Calleja complex, and the anterior and the shell part of the nucleus accumbens (Figure 2 and ref. [14]). There is also a weak D_3 receptor signal in the substantia nigra and the ventral tegmental area [6,14] and after unilateral 6-hydroxy-DA injection, degeneration of DA neurons was followed by an ipsilateral reduction of the D_3 receptor mRNA in these regions [6]. These data suggest that D_3 receptor are also expressed by DA neurons and may play autoreceptor functions. This is consistent with its pharmacological profile, where many DA autoreceptor selective-agents (like 7-OH-DPAT, quinpirole or TL 99, for example) show a better affinity at the D_3 receptor than non-autoreceptor selective-agents [6].

Autoradiography of the D_3 receptor protein recently performed with the first selective D_3 receptor ligand [^{3}H]7-hydroxy-N,N' dipropyl aminotetralin ([^{3}H]7-OH-DPAT) [17] shows that the pattern of expression of the D_3 receptor protein overlaps almost exactly the distribution of its mRNA (Figure 2). This suggests that the D_3

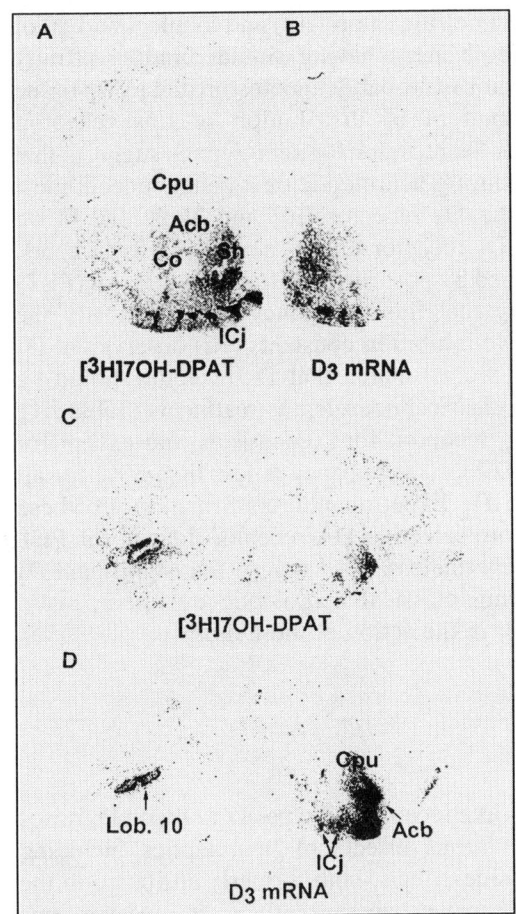

Figure 2. Comparison of autoradiographic localization of [³H]7-OH-DPAT specific binding to rat brain section (A and C) with the distribution of D_3 receptor mRNA measured by *in situ* hybridization (B and D). Frontal (A and B) and sagittal (C and D) sections at approximately similar levels were either incubated with [³H]7-OH-DPAT (0,5 nM) or hybridized with a ³²P-labelled complementary RNA probe. Acb, Accumbens ; Co, core of the nucleus accumbens ; Sh, shell part of the nucleus accumbens ; Cpu, Caude-putamen ; Lob. 10 lobule 10 of the cerebellum ; Icj, island of Calleja.

receptor is expressed on dendrites, perikarya or short axons rather than on axons of distant neurons. Using ([³H]7-OH-DPAT for labelling the D_3 receptor in the brain, we also confirmed two importants characteristics of the D_3 receptor ; its high affinity for DA (Ki-8nM in olfactory tubercle) and the low modulatory effect of guanyl nucleotides on its binding (KI-9 nM in presence of a guanyl nucleotide analogue) [17]. Both properties, which indicate a peculiar mode of interaction with the neurotransmitter in a subset of dopaminoceptive neurons, suggest that DA might act through D_3 receptors at some distance from the terminals that release it and/or occupy the D_3 receptor for a longer period of time than in the case of other DA receptor subtypes. Such quasi-hormonal mode of action is consistent with the high expression of the D_3 receptor in the core of the island of Calleja, whereas DA axons surround these islands making only few contacts with granule cells [18], and since the background DA concentration in the extracellular space in the striatum is 5-20 nM [19] D_3 receptor should be subjected to a tonic stimulation. The level of D_3 receptor binding site expression is about 2 orders of magnitude lower than the expression of the D_2 receptor in the brain : the highest level being observed in the olfactory tubercle (17 fmol/mg of protein) and lobule 9 and 10 of the cerebellum (11 fmol/mg of protein), both areas having similar binding affinity (0,7 nM). In fact, the density of the D_3 receptor is probably underestimated using tissue homogenates because of the restricted pattern of distribution of this receptor.

On the other hand, the high affinity of the D_3 receptor for neuroleptics suggests that this receptor may be significantly occupied during neuroleptic treatments. Indeed, most neuroleptics possess a good affinity for the D_3 receptor ([6] and Table II). If we calculate the theoretical occupancy of the D_3 receptor during neuroleptic treatments, based on DA receptor occupancy data obtained by positron emission tomography (PET) scan using [^{11}C] raclopride [] (considering that this occupancy reflects mostly the occupancy at the D_2 receptor), and respective inhibition constants (Ki) observed at D_2 and D_3 receptors *in vitro* for these drugs, we estimated that D_3 receptor should be occupied, *in vivo*, between 5 to 75% during classical neuroleptic treatments (Table III). We also estimated the occupancy at the D_4 receptor, for comparison, and except for clozapine (for which D_4 is occupied over 90%), its occupancy is less than 50% for all the drugs subjected to the test (Table III). Experimental confirmation of these speculations are however needed, using more selective DA receptor ligands for PET scan studies in similar *in vivo* paradigms. Nevertheless, this suggests that significant D_3 receptor occupancy could be reached during classical neuroleptic treatment, again arguing for a participation of the D_3 receptor in the action of these drugs.

Conclusion

The identification of three distinct DA D_2-like receptor subtypes D_2, D_3 and D_4 raises the important question of assigning the various effects of neuroleptics including beneficial therapeutic effects and undesired side-effects, both formerly attributed to the blockade of a single D_2 receptor entity. These answers are currently under investigations and constitute and exciting and promising field of research in neuro-sciences.

Table III. *In vivo* DA receptor occupancy.

	Receptor occupancy (%)		
	D_2*	D_3	D_4
Haloperidol (3mg)	87	58	44
Pimozine (4 mg)	77	75	43
Chlorpromazine (100 mg)	80	61	20
Sulpiride (400 mg)	74	59	27
Raclopride (4 mg)	72	57	2
Clozapine (300 mg)	65	21	93

* Data from PET scan usiing [^{11}C] raclopride [20].

At this stage of our knowledge much caution is needed, but two clues point to the D_3 receptor as a key receptor as a key receptor in the antipsychotic effect ; its recognition by neuroleptics and its selective expression in phylogenetically old part of the brain, known as the limbic system. Defects in limbic functions are likely to be involved in mood, emotion and behavior disturbances. The D_4 receptor is also blocked by some antipsychotics, such as clozapine, but it cannot be recognized as the common target for antipsychotics since several highly potent compounds are poorly recognized by this receptor. On the other hand, the D_2 receptor shares the criterion of being well recognized by neuroleptics, but its ubiquitous and high level of expression in the dopaminergic areas, especially the neostriatum and pituitary, suggest that its blockade is also responsible for the important motor and endocrine side-effects elicited by classical neuroleptics. However, its participation in the antipsychotic action of neuroleptics cannot be ruled out.

The next step will be the development of more selective DAergic drugs (preferably antagonists). Performances in this field have markedly increased in using cell lines transfected with specific receptor subtypes. In this regard, 7-OH-DPAT is the first representative of this new generation of selective agent that have been screened using this system, and story is far from over.

References

1. Kebabian JW, Calne DB, *Nature* 1979 ; 277 ; 93.
2. BunzowJR, Van Tol HHM, Grandy DK, Albert P, Salon J, McCrisite D, Machida CA, Neve KA, Civelli O, *Nature* 1988 ; 336 : 783.
3. Zhou QZ, Grandy DK, Thambi L, KushnerJA, Van TolHHM, Cone R, Pribnow D, Salon J, Bunzow JR, Civelli O, *Nature* 1990 ; 347 : 76.
4. Dearry A, Gingrich JA, Falardeau P, Fremeau RT, Bates MD, Caron MG, *Nature* 1990 ; 347 : 72.
5. Sunahara RK, Niznik HB, Weiner DM, Stormann TM, Brann MR, Kennedy JL, Gelernter LE, Rozmahel R, Yang Y, Israel Y, Seeman P, O'Dowd BF, *Nature* 1990 ; 347 : 80.
6. Sokoloff P, Giros B, Martes MP, Bouthenet ML, Shwartz JC, *Nature* 1990 ; 347 : 146.
7. Van Tol HHM, Bunzow JR, Guan HC, Sunahara RK, Seeman P, Niznik HB, Civelli O, *Nature* 1991 ; 350 : 610.
8. Sunahara RK, Guan HC, O'Dowd BF, Seeman P, Laurier LG, Ng G, George SR, Torchia J, Van Tol HHM, Niznik HB, *Nature* 1991 ; 350 : 614.
9. Tiberi M, Jarvie KR, Silvia C, Falardeau P, Gingrich JA, Godinot N, Bertrand L, Yang-Feng TL, Fremeau RT, J, Caron MG, *Proc Natl Acad Sci USA* 1991 ; 88 : 7491.
10. Dohlman HG, Thorner J, Caron MG, Lefkowitz RJ. *Annu Rev Biochem* 1991 ; 60 : 653.
11. Giros B, Sokoloff P, Martres MP, Riou JF, Emorine LJ, Schwartz JC, *Nature* 1989 ; 342 : 923.
12. Monsma FJ, Mc Vittie LD, Gerfen CR, Mahan LC, Sibley DR, *Nature* 1989 ; 342 : 926.
13. Giros B, Martres MP, Pilon C, Sokoloff P, Schwartz JC, *Biochem Biophys Res Commun* 1991 ; 176 : 1584.
14. Bouthenet ML, Souil E, Martres MP, Sokoloff P, Giros B, Schwartz JC, *Brain Res* 1991 ; 564 203.
15. Giros B, Martres MP, Sokoloff P, Schwartz JC, CR *Acad Sci Paris III* 1990 ; 311 501.
16. Sokoloff P, Andrieux M, Besançon R, Pilon C, Martres MP, Giros B, Schwartz JC, *Eur J Pharmacol Mol Biol* 1992 ; 225 : 331.
17. Lévesque D, Diaz J, Pilon C, Martres MP, Giros B, Souil E, Schott D, Morgat JL, Schwartz JC, Sokoloff P. *Proc Natl Acad Sci USA* 1992 ; 89 : 8155.
18. Fallon JH, Loughlin SE, Ribak CE, *J Comp Neurol* 1983 ; 218 : 91.
19. Zetterström T, Sherp T, Marsden CA, Ungerstedt U, *J Neurochem* 1983 ; 41 : 1769.
20. Farde L, Wiesel FA, Nordström AL, Sedvall G. *Psychopharmacology* 1989 ; 99 : S28.

8

Multihormonal responses to a series of neuroendocrine challenges in psychiatry: a multivariate approach

F. DUVAL, M.-C. MOKRANI, M.-A. CROCQ, M. JAUTZ, P. BAILEY, T. S. DIEP, E. E. DE ANDRADE, A. DE ANDRADE, J.-P. MACHER

From the Research Center for Applied Neuroscience in Psychiatry (FORENAP), Rouffach, France.

This study used a multivariate neuroendocrine approach to attempt to find external validators for the classification of inpatients meeting proposed DSM-IV criteria for major depressive episode, schizophrenia, or schizoaffective disorder. We wanted to know whether it was possible to identify patterns of hormonal response abnormalities specific for these clinical entities, thus defined, and for some of their clinical subtypes. We examined multihormonal responses to a neuroendocrine test battery including the apomorphine test, the protirelin test, and the dexamethasone suppression test (DST).

Apomorphine is a short-acting dopamine receptor agonist which decreases prolactin (PRL) secretion [1], and stimulates secretion of growth hormone (GH) [2], adrenocorticotropic hormone (ACTH) and cortisol [3]. The hormone response to apomorphine has been widely used to evaluate dopaminergic function in psychiatric patients [4]. In schizophrenia, GH and PRL responses differ from study to study: unchanged [5,6], decreased [7], or showing greater variability [8,9] when compared with normal controls. In major depression it is generally accepted, but not universally [10], that GH and PRL response to apomorphine is unaltered [4,11]. To our knowledge, no previous published study has examined the ACTH and/or cortisol response to apomorphine in psychiatric patients.

The protirelin test and the DST have been reported in many investigations to be state-dependent markers of major depression. The protirelin test, which assesses thyroid axis function, is blunted in approximately 30% of depressed patients [12]. We recently reported that the difference between evening and morning thyrotropin response to protirelin (ΔΔthyrotropin) [13] improves the diagnostic value of the protirelin test since about 75% of major depressed patients have a blunted ΔΔthyrotropin [14]. The picture is less clear concerning the PRL response to protirelin: exaggerated [15], blunted [16,17], or unchanged [18,19] responses have been found in depression. Post-DST cortisol nonsuppression, corresponding to disinhibition of the hypothalamic-pituitary-adrenal axis [20], is noted in 40%-50% of depressed patients; in very severe depression the sensitivity is higher (60%-70%) [21]. However, abnormal results of the DST and protirelin test have also been reported in other psychiatric disorders including alcoholism [22-24], mania [25-27], dementia [28,29], and schizoaffective disorder [30,31]. In schizophrenia abnormal results have rarely been found [32-36].

Thus, we investigated a combined approach of hormone responses to apomorphine (PRL, GH, ACTH and cortisol), 8 AM and 11 PM protirelin (thyrotropin and PRL), and dexamethasone (cortisol) in a large population of hospitalized and unmedicated subjects (n=104). Moreover, to demonstrate overall hormonal differences between the clinical groups we chose to perform a factorial correspondence analysis [37]. This type of multivariate analysis is performed on a contingency table recording the frequency of normal and abnormal responses to each neuroendocrine test in each diagnostic group or subgroup.

This approach was selected in order to fulfil at least three functions: (1) external validation of pre-existing clinical diagnostic criteria; (2) indication of possible underlying pathophysiological processes; (3) identification of appropriate psychopharmacological treatments [38].

Study methods

Subjects

Patients were recruited from the inpatient service of Sector VIII of the Centre Hospitalier of Rouffach (France). The population consisted of 86 inpatients and 18 hospitalized control subjects without psychiaric disorder (Table I). All subjects gave their informed consent to participate in this study and they underwent both a standard clinical interview and a structured interview—Schedule for Affective Disorders and Schizophrenia-Lifetime Version [39]. This research was approved by the local ethical committee.

Patients were classified according to DSM-IV criteria by consensus of two psychiatrists and a psychologist, without knowing the results of endocrine investigations. The patients were separated into 3 groups: 46 major depressives, 26 schizophrenics and 14 schizoaffectives. Among the depressed patients, 9 met the criteria for the melancholic subtype, and the remaining 37 were nonmelancholic; 7 had a history of bipolarity (bipolar I disorder), all the others had a history of recurrent major depression; all met the criteria for a severe major depressed episode without psychotic features. Sixteen schizophrenic patients met criteria for paranoid type and ten met criteria for disorganized type; all had a chronic course with acute exacerbation. All schizoaffective patients had a history of bipolarity and were depressed at the time of the

Table I. Demographic and clinical features of patients and healthy controls.

DSM-IV Diagnosis	No.	M/F	Age, y (mean±SD)	Total score (mean ±SD) HRSD	BPRS
Major Depression	46	27/19	35.6±10.5	27.4±6.4†	41.9±7.6
With Melancholia	9	3/6	41.3±9.3	34.8±3.0	49.1±7.0
Without Melancholia	37	24/13	34.2±10.4	25.6±5.8	40.2±6.7
Bipolar I Type	7	3/4	43.8±6.6	28.6±5.4	41.0±5.0
Recurrent Type	39	24/15	35.2±10.5	27.2±6.7	42.1±8.0
Schizophrenia	26	20/6	32.9±10.7	19.8±10.3	58.4±17.7‡
Paranoid Type	16	11/5	35.0±11.5	21.0±11.5	55.8±17.5
Disorganized Type	10	9/1	29.5±9.7	17.8±8.4	46.5±9.1
SAD	14	9/5	34.9±8.8	22.4±9.8	60.3±14.8
Control	18	9/9	33.9±6.7	...	.

SAD indicates schizoaffective disorder, M/F Male/Female, HRSD Hamilton Rating Scale for Depression (17-item), BPRS Brief Psychiatric Rating Scale. †$P<0.001$ vs. SCZ, ‡$P<.00001$ vs. MDE with the Bonferroni corrected two-tailed test.

study. The intensity of clinical symptoms was evaluated with the Brief Psychiatric Rating Scale (BPRS) [40] and the severity of depression with the 17-item Hamilton Rating Scale for Depression (HRSD) [41].

The control group consisted of 18 hospitalized normal volunteers. All were free of concomitant psychiatric and medical illness. None had a personal or family history of major psychiatric illness.

All patients had been drug-free for a minimum of 10 days; this wash-out was supervised in hospital. All subjects were within 15% of ideal body weight. Subjects with history of endocrine diseases; major medical illness (including organic brain syndrome); alcoholism or drug abuse; recent pronounced weight change; previous treatment with lithium salts, carbamazepine, long-acting neuroleptics, carbamates, MAOIs or ECT; and women taking oral contraceptives were excluded. No benzodiazepine was taken during the washout period.

All subjects were on a caffeine-restricted diet for at least three days before testing and their environment was synchronized, with diurnal activity from 8 AM to 11 PM, and nocturnal rest (sleep).

Procedures

On day 1, the first protirelin stimulation test was carried out at 8 AM. Subjects were in bed, non-smoking and fasting from 7 PM on the previous day. An indwelling cannula was inserted at 7 AM into a forearm vein and kept open with an isotonic saline infusion. Two hundred micrograms of protirelin (Protiréline Roche®, Produits Roche, Neuilly-sur-Seine, France) was injected intravenously over two minutes at 8 AM. Blood was drawn for assay of plasma thyrotropin and PRL at the following times: 15 minutes before protirelin injection (t-15), immediately before protirelin injection (t0), and 15, 30 and 60 minutes after TRH injection (t15, t30, t60). The challenge was repeated at 11 PM on the same day, with the injection of a further 200 µg of protirelin I.V. and the same sampling intervals. Subjects were awake before and during the evening sampling and kept without food from 6 PM.

A dexamethasone suppression test was started at midnight, with oral ingestion of 1 mg of dexamethasone (Dectancyl, Laboratoires Roussel, Paris, France) followed by the assay of plasma cortisol at 8 AM, 4 PM, and 11 PM on the next day [42].

On day 7, an apomorphine test (Apomorphine Méram, Melun, France) was carried out at 9 AM. After an overnight fast, subjects were awoken at 7 AM, and a cannula was inserted into a forearm vein and kept open with an isotonic saline infusion. Three baseline blood samples were drawn before subcutaneous injection of 0.75 mg apomorphine hydrochloride (at -30, -15, and 0 minutes) and further samples for the assay of PRL, GH, ACTH, and cortisol were collected at 15, 30, 60, 90, 120, and 150 minutes.

Assays

Blood samples were immediately centrifuged at 1 500 g and 4°C, plasma samples were then stored at -20°C until assay. Hormone concentrations were determined by immunoassay techniques based on enhanced luminescence (thyrotropin, PRL, cortisol) or radioimmunoassay techniques (GH, ACTH). Average intra-assay and inter-assay coefficients of variation were respectively: thyrotropin: 5.1 % - 7 %, sensitivity < 0.04 µU/ml (Amerlite TSH-60 Assay, Amersham International plc, Amersham, UK); PRL: 5.5 % - 6 %, sensitivity < 1.3 ng/ml (Amerlite Prolactin Assay, Amersham International plc, Amersham, UK); cortisol: 6.2 % - 8.9 %, sensitivity < 3 nmol/l (Amerlite Cortisol Assay, Amersham International plc, Amersham, UK); ACTH: 5 % - 6.3 %, sensitivity < 10 pg/ml (ACTHK-PR, CIS® Oris industrie, Gif-sur-Yvette, France); GH: 2.8 % - 4.5 %, sensitivity < 0.1 ng/ml (hGH «Coatria», BioMérieux, Marcy-l'Etoile, France).

Statistical analysis

Baseline thyrotropin (TSHB) and PRL (PRLB) values were defined as the mean of the two samples before protirelin injection (t-15 and t0). Δthyrotropin and ΔPRL were defined as the maximum increment above the baseline values after protirelin injection. $\Delta\Delta$thyrotropin was defined as the difference between 11 PM-Δthyrotropin and 8 AM-Δthyrotropin. $\Delta\Delta$PRL was defined as the difference between 11 PM-ΔPRL and 8 AM-ΔPRL.

The highest post-DST plasma cortisol value in any blood sample obtained at 8 AM, 4 PM, and 11 PM on day 2 was used to evaluate the cortisol response to DST.

The parameters analyzed during the apomorphine test were as follows: baseline GH (GH_B) value, defined as the mean of the three samples before apomorphine injection (at -30, -15, and 0 minutes); baseline PRL (PRL_B), ACTH ($ACTH_B$), and cortisol ($cortisol_B$) values, defined as the level at time 0 (34). This was chosen rather than the mean of the three samples before apomorphine injection since the values of these hormones declined sharply in the morning owing to the circadian rhythm [43,44]. To be included in the study subjects had to have GH_B value <2 ng/ml and PRL_B <20 ng/ml in men and <25 ng/ml in women.

The basal PRL area under the cuve ($PRL_{B\ AUC}$) was calculated as follows: PRL_B x 150 minutes. The PRL suppression area ($PRL_{S\ AUC}$), defined as the difference between $PRL_{B\ AUC}$ and PRL_{AUC} after apomorphine was highly correlated with PRL_B ($\rho=0.92$, n=104; P<.0001); to avoid this source of bias the PRL response to apomorphine was expressed as a percentage of change from baseline according to the formula: ($PRL_{S\ AUC}/PRL_{B\ AUC}$)x100 [6]. PRL suppression thus defined was unrelated to PRL_B ($\rho=0.15$). The GH, ACTH, and cortisol responses to apomorphine were expressed as the maximum increments above baseline values (ΔGH, $\Delta ACTH$ and $\Delta cortisol$ respectively).

Between-group differences were tested for significance by analysis of variance, and where significant, by two-tailed Student's t test. Bonferroni's adjustment was used for multiple comparisons. Within-subject differences were evaluated for significance with two-tailed paired t test. When the data precluded the use of parametric statistical tests, the following non-parametric methods were used: Kurskal-Wallis H test (one-way analysis of variance), Mann-Whitney two-tailed U test (comparison of two groups), Wilcoxon two-tailed signed-rank T test (differences for paired data). Correlations between quantitative variables were estimated by means of the Spearman rank coefficient (ρ). Categorical data were analyzed by χ^2 or Fisher's Exact test (two-tailed). The level of statistical significance was set P=.05.

The form of multivariate analysis chosen was a factorial correspondence analysis (FCA) [37]. This analysis is based on categorical data recorded in a contingency table, i.e normal and abnormal responses to each endocrine test (column) in each diagnostic group or subgroup (row). The thresholds of abnormal test results were determined using a receiver operating characteristic (ROC) analysis [45]. FCA may be regarded informally as a form of principal component analysis in which the contribution of each element in a row (or column) of the contingency table is weighted according to the contribution of the row (or column) to the total variance of the table. This form of analysis is thus particulary suited to summarizing the results of a number of tests performed on a number of predefined groups, since tests (or groups) which do not contribute much to the total variance will receive relatively low weighting.

Results and discussion

Patients and controls were not significantly different on age and sex. Table II displays the results of the protirelin, dexamethasone and apomorphine tests.

Protirelin test

Thyrotropin responses
There was no significant difference between control, schizophrenic, schizoaffective and depressed groups in TSH_B both at 8 AM and at 11 PM. In patients and controls

Δthyrotropin obtained with our procedure exhibited a diurnal variation: at 11 PM responses were significantly higher than at 8 AM (all P <.001 by paired t test). At 11 PM—but not at 8 AM—depressed patients had lower 11 PM-Δthyrotropin than schizophrenic patients. In our sample the sensitivity of the protirelin test in depression was low in the morning (11% [5/46], defining thyrotropin blunted criterion as Δthyrotropin < 3.5 μU/ml); in the evening the sensitivity was increased (30% [14/46], defining thyrotropin blunted criterion as Δthyrotropin < 6 μU/ml).

The percentage of blunted responses in the other groups, for the morning and evening protirelin test, was respectively: 5% and 0% in control subjects, 15% and 15% in schizophrenic patients, and 0% and 21% in schizoaffective patients.

ΔΔthyrotropin values were lower in the depressed group than in the control and schizophrenic groups. Defining blunted ΔΔthyrotropin as less than 2.5 μU/ml, 76% (35/46) of the depressed and 57% (8/14) of the schizoaffective patients showed the abnormality. The specificity was 95% in controls and 85% in schizophrenic patients. Thus the ΔΔthyrotropin, which reflects a chronobiologic dysregulation of the hypothalamic-pituitary-thyroid axis (HPT), does not seem specific for major depression. It can be suggested that the reduced ΔΔthyrotropin is more probably linked to depressed mood rather than to major depression as defined by the DSM-IV criteria.

No significant sex or age effects were found for thyrotropin parameters (i.e. baselines and responses to protirelin). Despite a trend towards a positive correlation between ΔΔthyrotropin values and total HRSD scores in the depressed group (ρ=-.31; n=46; P<.04), no significant differences were observed for the thyrotropin parameters among the depressed subgroups (i.e with or without melancholic features, recurrent vs. bipolar types). In the schizophrenic group, disorganized patients had a trend towards lower Δthyrotropin values both at 8 AM (t=2.13; df=24; P=.04)and at 11 PM (t=2.12; df=24; P=.04) than paranoid patients.

PRL responses

There was no difference in 8 AM- and 11 PM-PRL_B between patients and controls. PRL responses to protirelin (ΔPRL) – which correlated positively with thyrotropin responses – were higher in the evening than in the morning in both groups (all P <.001 by T test) except for the schizoaffective group. ΔPRL were lower in men than in women both at 8 AM (mean ΔPRL, 23.8±19.4ng/ml [n=65] and 45.9±29.1ng/ml [n=39] respectively; P <.00001 by U test) and 11 PM (mean ΔPRL, 31.7±21.1 ng/ml and 58.6±32.7 ng/ml respectively; P <.00001 by U test). However, there were no significant differences in ΔPRL values between groups when comparing men and women separately. PRL parameters (baselines and responses to protirelin) were independent of age and severity of the symptoms as evaluated by means of HRSD and BPRS scores. No significant differences were found for these parameters among the subtypes of depressed or schizophrenic patients.

ΔΔPRL values – which were unrelated to sex and age – were significantly blunted in schizoaffective patients. Defining blunted ΔΔPRL as less than 0 ng/ml,17% (8/46) of the depressed and 29% (4/14) of the schizoaffective patients showed the abnormality. Despite its modest sensitivity, this result gives evidence for the nocturnal

Table II. Basal hormone values and hormonal responses to neuroendocrine challenge tests in patients and healthy controls (mean±SD).

	MDE (n=46)	SCZ (n=26)	SAD (n=14)	HC (n=18)	ANOVA	MDE vs. SCZ	MDE vs. SAD	MDE vs. HC	SCZ vs. SAD	SCZ vs. HC	SAD vs. HC
8 AM Protirelin test											
Basal Thyrotropin, µU/ml	1.21±0.56	1.42±0.80	1.38±0.49	1.23±0.49	...	...	...	...	...	...	...
ΔThyrotropin, µU/ml	6.88±2.94	7.60±4.04	7.06±3.82	8.90±4.72	...	...	...	...	...	...	...
Basal Prolactin, ng/ml	10.2±5.3	10.8±4.5	11.2±7.4	11.9±4.9	...	...	...	...	...	...	...
ΔProlactin, ng/ml	33.2±26.0	28.1±17.4	31.5±41.4	35.4±20.6	...	...	...	...	...	...	...
11PM Protirelin test											
Basal Thyrotropin, µU/ml	0.96±0.36	1.46±0.78	1.17±0.51	1.32±0.75	.0055	$P<.005$	...	...	...	...	...
ΔThyrotropin, µU/ml	8.45±3.51	11.54±5.29	9.06±4.02	12.92±5.38	.0011	$P<.03$	...	$P<.001$	...	...	...
Basal Prolactin, ng/ml	6.8±4.4	7.3±4.5	10.1±8.5	8.5 ±5.0	...	...	...	...	...	...	...
Δ Prolactin, ng/ml	41.4±28.2	38.6±23.8	33.0±28.8	54.3±35.9	...	...	...	...	...	...	...
ΔΔThyrotropin, µU/ml	1.58±1.76	4.28±2.46	2.00±1.75	4.02±1.22	.00001	$P<.00001$	...	$P<.00001$	$P<.03$	...	$P<.003$
ΔΔProlactin, ng/ml	8.1±10.7	10.4±10.9	1.65±14.3	18.9±20.2	.0170	...	...	...	...	...	$P<.03$
Post-dexamethasone cortisol level, nmol/l	79±96	89±130	144±189	44±56	...	...	...	...	...	...	...
Apomorphine test											
Basal growth hormone, ng/ml	0.3±0.2	0.6±0.5	1.0±1.0	0.4±0.3	...	...	...	...	...	...	...
ΔGrowth hormone, ng/ml	12.5±7.6	13.4±17.2	10.9±10.9	14.3±11.4	...	...	...	...	...	...	...
Basal prolactin, ng/ml	7.3±3.9	7.3±4.3	9.1±6.2	9.6±5.4	...	...	...	...	...	...	...
Prolactin suppression, %	37±18	30±25	27±15	37±17	...	...	...	...	...	...	...
Basal ACTH, pg/ml	27.4±16.7	23.5±14.0	30.0±18.5	20.9±15.8	...	...	...	...	...	...	...
ΔACTH, pg/ml	42.9±57.9	33.4±70.0	12.8±37.6	32.5±53.4	...	...	...	...	...	...	...
Basal cortisol, nmol/ml	302±110	328±147	358±116	291±107	...	...	$P<.03$	...	...	...	...
ΔCortisol, nmol/ml	105±131	97±133	-3±77	182±205	.0073	...	...	...	...	...	$P<.02$

MDE indicates major depressive episode, SCZ schizophrenia, SAD schizoaffective disorder, HC healthy controls ; and ANOVA, analysis of varianc. P values are adjusted using Bonferroni's correction to compensate for the number of post hoc comparisons.

hyposensitivity of the pituitary TRH receptors in some depressed and schizoaffective patients.

Dexamethasone suppression test

The cortisol levels had skewed distributions so we analyzed logarithmic transformed data. Post-DST cortisol values were not significantly related to age or sex. Although control, schizophrenic, schizoaffective and depressed groups did not differ significantly in post-DST cortisol values, the subgroup of depressed patients with melancholic features had higher values than controls (t=3.47; df=25; P <.002), disorganized schizophrenics (t=3.61; df=17; P <.003), and depressed patients without melancholic features (t=2.53; df=44; P=.01). No correlation between post-DST cortisol values and HRSD and BPRS scores was found.

Defining DST nonsuppression as a plasma cortisol level in excess of 120 nmol/l in any of the three samples (8 AM, 4 PM, or 11 PM): 33% (3/9) of the melancholic, 28% (4/14) of the schizoaffective and 31% (5/16) of the paranoid patients were DST nonsuppressors. These results cast doubt on the utility of the DST, used alone, as a biological marker of depression.

Apomorphine test

Effects on GH concentration

GH_B levels did not differ between patients and controls and were unrelated to age or sex. ΔGH values correlated negatively with age in the overall population (ρ=-.43; n=104; P <.00001), in controls (ρ=-.74; n=18; P=.002), in the depressed patients (ρ= .47; n=46; P <.002), and in the schizophrenic patients (ρ=-.61; n=26; P <.003), but not in the schizoaffective patients (ρ=-.11). However, patients and controls did not differ significantly in ΔGH values (H=2.8; n=104; P>.40).

Athough there was no significant difference between the groups for the mean GH responses, there were more blunted ΔGH values (i.e. < 4 ng/ml) in the schizophrenic (42% [11/26]) and schizoaffective (36% [5/14]) groups in than in other groups (χ^2=11.39; df=3; P=.009).

It is believed that the localization of the dopamine receptors which stimulate the secretion of GH is in the hypothalamus. Our results suggest a blunted sensitivity of the dopamine receptors at this level in some schizophrenic and schizoaffective patients. However, the effect of apomorphine on GH requires the participation of acetylcholine and GH releasing factor neurons, and other neurotransmitters such as GABA, norepinephrine, and cholecystokinin are probably involved in the GH response to apomorphine. Moreover, age diminishes the apomorphine-induced GH stimulation. These confounding factors limit the value of the GH response to apomorphine in the investigation of dopaminergic function in psychiatry.

Effects on PRL concentration

Analysis of the PRL_B levels showed that these were unrelated to age but tended to be lower in male than in female subjects (F=2.28; df=1,98; P <.04). After adjustment for sex there was no statistical difference in the PRL_B levels between patients and controls. The extent of inhibition of PRL secretion by apomorphine correlated negatively with age ($\rho= -.29$; n=104; P=.003) but was unrelated to sex. However, no difference was found between patients and controls for PRL suppression. In the depressed group, bipolar patients were slightly older than recurrent (unipolar) patients (mean, 43.8±6.6 years [n=7], and 35.2±10.7 years, respectively [n=39]) (t=2.09; P <.05). However, after adjustment for age, PRL suppression was lower in patients with bipolar type (mean,12±12%) than in patients with recurrent depressive episode (mean, 41±16%) (F=14.67; df=1,43; P=.0004).

Defining blunted PRL suppression as less than 15%, 71% (5/7) of the bipolar depressed patients vs. 5% (2/39) of the recurrent depressed patients showed the abnormality as did 11% of controls, 23% in schizophrenic patients, and 21% in schizoaffective patients.

Apomorphine stimulates the dopamine D_2 receptors on the lactotrophs and inhibits PRL secretion. The baseline PRL levels were comparable across the groups suggesting no residual effects of neuroleptics in the schizophrenic and schizoaffective groups. The blunted PRL suppression in the bipolar depressives might suggest a hyposensitivity of the pituitary D_2 receptors in this diagnosic category.

Effects on ACTH concentration

There was no age or sex effect for $ACTH_B$ and $\Delta ACTH$ values. These parameters were not significantly different between the schizophrenic, schizoaffective, depressed, and control groups. However, in further analyses of subgroups of patients we found that paranoid and schizoaffective patients had lower $\Delta ACTH$ values than depressed (both P<.01 by U test) and disorganized patients (both P <.02 by U test). In the schizophrenic group only, there was a negative relationship between the total BPRS scores and $\Delta ACTH$ values ($\rho=-.46$; n=26; P=.02).

The mechanisms underlying the ACTH stimulation by apomorphine are not completely understood. It has been recently suggested that the D_3 receptors are probably involved in the regulation of corticotropin releasing hormone (CRH) and therefore of ACTH release. Our findings may be in accordance with the hypothesis that dopaminergic mechanisms are involved in some aspects of psychosis but not all; this emphasizes the difference between schizoaffectives and paranoid schizophrenics, on the one hand, and disorganized schizophrenics, on the other. Thus, hyposensitivity of dopaminergic receptors – and may be more specifically of D_3 receptors – can be suggested downstream of the hypothalamic level in paranoid and schizoaffective patients.

Effects on cortisol concentration

$Cortisol_B$ values tended to be positively correlated with age ($\rho=.22$; n=104; P <.03), but were unrelated to sex. No significant difference was observed among $cortisol_B$ of patients and controls. $\Delta cortisol$ values – which were unrelated to sex or age, but strongly correlated with $\Delta ACTH$ values ($\rho=.74$; n=104; P<.00001) – were lower in the schizoaffective group than in the control and depressed groups. No significant difference was found for the cortisol parameters (baseline, and response to apomorphine) among the subtypes of depressed or schizophrenic patients. Moreover, these parameters were correlated neither with HRSD nor with BPRS scores.

When defining blunted Δcortisol as a response below 0 nmol/l, 64% (9/14) of the schizoaffective patients and 31% (5/16) of the paranoid schizophrenics showed the abnormality. Consequently, apomorphine-induced cortisol release is blunted in schizoaffectives and to a lesser degree in paranoid schizophrenics.

In summary, the lower responsiveness of ACTH and cortisol to apomorphine may be of greater interest as a diagnostic marker (or index) in paranoid schizophrenic and schizoaffective states; lower responsiveness of GH to apomorphine – which probably involves different pathways from those mediating ACTH (and cortisol) responses – is seen in the schizoaffective patients and in a wider range of schizophrenic patients. The diminished apomorphine-induced prolactin suppression – which is not correlated with ACTH, cortisol, or GH responses – seems to be found preferentially in the bipolar I depressed patients. Concentrating briefly on the other tests, the protirelin test is more frequently blunted in depression and in some schizoaffective patients, and the DST does not appear specific for depression.

Factorial correspondence analysis

Given the apparent inconsistencies when analysing single tests one may wonder whether it is possible to identify neuroendocrine profiles specific to clinical entities. Multivariate statistical techniques represent the most satisfactory approach to this problem. Thus, we chose to perform a factorial correspondence analysis.

The axes of the analysis shown in Figure 1 can be interpreted in terms of links between biological parameters and clinical categories.

The parameters that most contributed to the first component (C1) were the blunting of ΔΔthyrotropin and ΔΔPRL, and also normal ΔΔthyrotropin. The second component (C2) was defined primarily by blunting of cortisol and GH to apomorphine. The diagnostic categories that most contributed to the first component were the control and depressed groups. In the second component, the schizoaffective group contributed the most.

Thus, the first axis shows a link between depression and the chronobiological dysregulation of the TRH test, and the second axis shows a link between dopaminergic dysregulation and productive psychotic symptoms. Therefore, it is possible to determine specific abnormality profiles among the four groups:

- major depressed patients are characterized by blunted 11 PM-Δthyrotropin and ΔΔthyrotropin, and normal hormonal responses to apomorphine.

- schizophrenics are characterized by blunted GH, cortisol and prolactin responses to apomorphine and normal 11 PM-Δthyrotropin and ΔΔthyrotropin test.

- schizoaffectives are more difficult to characterize because they associate abnormalities found both in schizophrenics such as blunted GH, cortisol and PRL responses to apomorphine, and in depressives such as DST non-suppression and blunted ΔΔPRL.

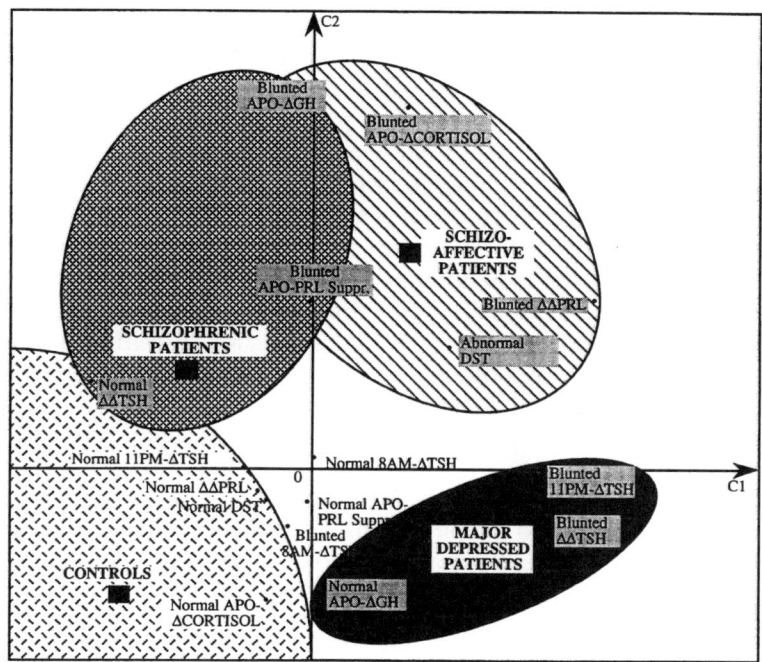

Figure 1. Simultaneous representation of the four diagnostic categories and the test response modalities, namely: normal or abnormal.

Two additional factorial correspondence analyses were performed focusing on 6 diagnostic subcategories and neuroendocrine test response modalities. The first analysis concerned 2 diagnostic subtypes of depressives: with or without melancholic features, and 2 schizophrenic subtypes: paranoid or disorganized, vs. control and schizoaffective groups. This analysis yielded similar results: the same neuroendocrine parameters contributed to the construction of the axes. Melancholics remained close to nonmelancholic depressives. On the contrary paranoids were distinct from disorganized schizophrenics and were characterized by coexistence of a blunted GH response to apomorphine and normal thyrotropin responses to protirelin. The second additional analysis was based on the depressed types: bipolar or recurrent vs. paranoid and disorganized schizophrenic, schizoaffective and control groups. This analysis showed that the profiles were different: bipolars were characterized by blunted 8 AM-Δthyrotropin and PRL suppression to apomorphine.

Conclusion

Our study clearly shows that results of endocrine tests vary according to diagnosis, and therefore could be useful in the classification of subjects. Moreover, this multihormonal approach provides important information on pathophysiology such as chronobiological dysregulation of the HPT axis in depression and dysregulated dopaminergic function in productive psychotic symptomatology. This is of great interest in devising an appropriate therapeutic strategy.

Nevertheless, it remains difficult to find pathognomonic «biological markers» of clinical psychiatric diagnoses, even if these latter are operationnally defined, since we lack detailed knowledge of the relationship between these diagnoses and their biological correlates. The problem has been formulated by Zimmermann et al [46]: «How does one validate a biologic marker for endogenous depression when a valid clinical definition does not exist?» A number of studies, including this present one, have shown the biological heterogeneity of current psychiatric diagnoses; this would suggest the incorporation of biological criteria in future research classification systems [47]. Classifications taking account of clinical, biological, and therapeutic data would establish a better foundation for psychiatric nosology.

Acknowledgements

The authors express their gratitude to Mrs Gabrielle Wagner in providing the test kits for hormonal determination, to the physicians, the nurses and the psychologists of the Sector VIII, Centre Hospitalier Rouffach, and to Mrs Geetha Savarimouttou-Toussaint for her contribution to the translation of this article.

References

1. Lal S. de la Vega CE, Soures TL, Friesen HG. Effect of apomorphine on growth hormone, prolactin, luteinizing hormone and follicle-stimulating hormone levels in human serum. *J Clin Endocr Metab* 1973 ; 37:719-724.
2. Lal S. de la Vega CE, Soures TL, Friesen HG. Effect of apomorphine on human growth hormone secretion. *Lancet* 1972; ii:661.
3. Jezova D, Vigas M. Apomorphine injection stimulates b-endorphin, adrenocorticotropin, and cortisol release in healthy man. *Psychoneuro-enocrinology* 1988 ; 13:479-485.
4. Lal S. Apomorphine in the evaluation of dopaminergic function in man. *Prog Neuropsychopharmacol Biol Psychiatry* 1988 ; 12:117-164.
5. Meltzer HY, Goode DJ, Fang VS, Schyve P, Young M. Dopamine and schizophrenia. *Lancet* 1976;2:1142.
6. Meltzer HY, Kolakowska T, Fang VS, Fogg L, Robertson A, Lewine R, Strahilevtz M, Bush D. Growth hormone and prolactin response to apomorphine in schizophrenia and the major affective disorders. *Arch Gen Psychiatry* 1984 ; 41:512-519.
7. Tamminga CA, Smith RC, Pandey G, Frohman LA, Davis JM. A neuroendocrine study of supersensitivity in tardive dyskinesia. *Arch Gen Psychiatry* 1977 ; 36;1199-1203.
8. Rostrosen J, Angrist BM, Paquin J, Halperin FS, Sachar EJ. Neuroendocrine studies with dopamine agonists in schizophrenia. *Psychopharmacol Bull* 1978 ; 14:14-17.
9. Lieberman JA, Jody D, Alvir JM, Ashtari M, Levy DL, Bogerts B, Degreef G, Mayerhoff DI, Cooper T. Brain morphology, dopamine, and eye-tracking abnormalities in first-episode schizophrenia. *Arch Gen Psychiatry* 1993 ; 50:357-368.

10. Ansseau M, Von Frenckell R, Cerfontaine JL, Papart P, Franck G, Timsit-Berthier M, Geenen V, Legros JJ. Blunted response of growth hormone to clonidine and apomorphine in endogenous depression. *Br J Psychiatry* 1988 ; 153:65-71.
11. Jimerson DC, Cutler NR, Post RM, Rey A, Gold PW, Brown GM, Bunney WE. Neuroendocrine responses to apomorphine in depressed patients and healthy subjects. *Psychiat Res* 1984 ; 13:1-12.
12. Duval F, Macher JP, Mokrani MC. Difference between evening and morning thyrotropin responses to protirelin in major depressive episode. *Arch Gen Psychiatry* 1990 ; 47:443-448.
13. Loosen PT, Prange AJ. Serum thyrotropin response to thyrotropin-releasing hormone in psychiatric patients: a review. *Am J Psychiatry* 1982 ; 139:405-416.
14. Duval F, Mokrani MC, Oliveira Castro J, Crocq MA, de Andrade EE, Macher JP. Circadian effects on the TSH response to TRH in depressed patients. *Clin Neuropharm* 1992 ; 15:384-385A.
15. Baumgartner A, Gräf KJ, Kürten I. Prolactin in patients with major depressive disorder and healthy subjects. I: cross sectional study of basal and post-TRH and postdexamethasone prolactin levels. *Biol Psychiatry* 1988 ; 24:249-267.
16. Witschy J, Schlesser M, Fulton C, Orsulak P, Giles D, Fairchild C, Crowley G, Rush J. TRH-induced prolactin release is blunted in females with endogenous unipolar major depression. *Psychat Res* 1984 ; 12:321-331.
17. Brambilla F, Semeraldi E, Sachetti E, Negri F, Cocchi D, Muller EF. Deranged anterior pituitary responsiveness to hypothalamic hormones in depressed patients. *Arch Gen Psychiatry* 1978 ; 35:1231-1238.
18. Roy A, Pickar D. TRH-induced prolactin release in unipolar depressed patients and controls. *J Psychiat Res.* 1988 ; 22:221-225.
19. Duval F, Mokrani MC, Crocq MA, Rosenberg S, Oliveira Castro J, Valdivieso S, Macher JP. Circadian variations in response to protirelin test in major depressive episode. *Eur Psychiatry* 1991 ; 6:79-88.
20. Kathol RG, Jaeckle RS, Lopez JF, Meller WH. Pathophysiology of HPA axis abnormalities in major depression: an update. *Am J Psychiatry* 1989 ; 146:311-317.
21. APA Task Force on Laboratory Tests in Psychiatry. The dexamethasone suppression test: an overview of its current status in psychiatry. *Am J Psychiatry* 1987 ; 144:1253-1262.
22. Loosen PT, Prange AJ, Wilson IC. TRH (protirelin) in depressed alcoholic men: behavioral changes and endocrine responses. *Arch Gen Psychiatry* 1979 ; 36:540-547.
23. Dackis CA, Bailey J, Pottash ALC, Stuckey RF, Extein IL. Specificity of the DST and the TRH test for major depression in alcoholics. *Am J Psychiatry* 1984 ; 141:680-683.
24. Banki CM, Arato M, Papp Z. Thyroid stimulation test in healthy subjects and psychiatric patients. *Acta Psychiatr Scand* 1984 ; 70:295-303.
25. Extein IRL, Pottash ALC, Gold MS, Cowdry RW. Using the protirelin test to distinguish mania from schizophrenia. *Arch Gen Psychiatry* 1982 ; 39:77-81.
26. Targum SD. Neuroendocrine challenge in clinical psychiatry. *Psychiatr Ann* 1983 ; 13:385-507.
27. Godwin CD, Greenberg LB, Shukla S. Consistant dexamethasone suppression test results with mania and depression in bipolar illness. *Am J Psychiatry* 1984 ; 141:1263-1265.
28. Raskind M, Peskind E, Rivard MF, Veith R, Barnes R. Dexamethasone suppression test and cortisol circadian rhythm in primary degenerative dementia. *Am J Psychiatry* 1982 ; 139:1468-1471.
29. Molchan SE, Lawlor B, Hill JL, Mellow AM, Davis CL, Martinez R, Sunderland T. The TRH stimulation test in Alzheimer's disease and major depression: relationship to clinical and CSF measures. *Biol Psychiatry* 1991 ; 30:567-576.

30. Sauer H, Koehler KG, Sass H, Hornstein C, Minne HW. The dexamethasone suppression test and thyroid stimulating hormone response to TRH in RDC Schizoaffective patients. *Eur Arch Psychiatr Neurol Sci* 1984 ; 2 34:264-267.
31. Kiriike N, Izumiya Y, Nishiwaki S, Maeda Y, Nagata T, Kawakita Y. TRH test and DST in schizoaffective mania, and schizophrenia. *Biol Psychiatry* 1988 ; 2 4:415-422.
32. Langer G, Ashauer H, Koinig G, Resch F, Schonbeck G. The TSH response to TRH: a possible predictor of outcome to antidepressant and neuroleptic treatment. *Prog Neuropsychopharmacol Biol Psychiatr* 1983 ; 7:335-342.
33. Wolkin A, Peselow ED, Smith M, Lautin A, KahnI, Rostosen J. TRH test abnormalities in psychiatric disorders. *J Affective Disord* 1984 ; 6:273-281.
34. Carroll BJ. Dexamethasone suppression test: a review of contemporary confusion. *J Clin Psychiatry* 1985 ; 46:13-24.
35. Kaneko M, Murata S, Hoshino Y, Takahagi K, Yokoyama F, Watanabe M, Kumashiro H. Dexamethasone suppression test in schizophrenia: its relation to monoamine metabolism in hypothalamic-pituitary-adrenal axis. *Neuropsychobiol* 1990-91 ; 24:12-16.
36. Duval F, Mokrani MC, Crocq MA, Weber N, Rosenberg S, Castro Oliveira J, Valdivieso S, Macher JP. Multihormonal responses to neuroendocrine tests in psychiatric patients. In: Macher JP, Crocq MA, eds. New prospects in psychiatry: the bio-clinical interface I. Amsterdam, NL:*Elsevier* 1992 : 192-205.
37. Benzecri JP. L'analyse des données. Vol 1: La Taxinomie, Vol 2: Correspondances. Paris, France: *Dunod* 1973.
38. Duval F, Mokrani MC, Jautz M, Crocq MA, de Andrade EE, de Andrade A, Diep TS, Macher JP. Predictive bio-clinical profiles of antidepressant responses in major depression. *Psychol Med.* 1993 ; 13:1325-1328.
39. Spitzer RL, Endicott J. Schedule for Affective Disorders and Schizophrenia–Lifetime Version. Bethesda, Md: National *Institute of Mental Health* 1977.
40. Overall JE, Gorman DR. Brief Psychiatric Rating Scale. In: Guy W (ed) ECDEU Assessment Manuel for Psychopharmacology, rev. ed., Rockville, Maryland, pp 157-169.
41. Hamilton MA. A rating scale for depression. *J Neurol Neurosurg Psychiatry* 1960 ; 23:56-62.
42. Carroll BJ, Feinberg M, Greden JF, Tarika J, Albala AA, Hasket RF, James NM, Kronfol Z, Lohr N, Steiner M, de Vigne JP, Young E. A specific laboratory test for the diagnosis of melancholia: standardisation, validation, and clinical utility. *Arch Gen Psychiatry* 1981 ; 38:15-22.
43. Reinberg A, Touitou Y, Guillemant, Levy F, Lagoguey M. Rythmes circadiens et circannuels des résultats d'épreuves fonctionnelles en endocrinologie. Ann Endocrinol (Paris). 1982;43:309-335.
44. van Cauter E, Refetoff S. Multifactorial control of the 24-hour secretory profiles of pituitary hormones. *J Endocrinol Invest* 1985 ; 8:381-391.
45. Metz CE. Basic principles of ROC analysis. *Semin Nucl Med* 1978 ; 8:283-298.
46. Zimmerman M, Coryell W, Pfohl B. The validity of the dexamethasone suppression test as a marker for endogenous depression. *Arch Gen Psychiatry* 1986 ; 43:347-355.
47. Carroll BJ. Diagnostic validity and laboratoriy studies: rules of the game. In: The validity of psychiatric diagnosis , Robins LN and Barrett JE (eds). Raven Press, Ldt, *New York* 1989 ; pp229-245.

9

Composite diagnostic evaluation system at the major psychiatric disorders

P. GASZNER, T.A. BAN

National Institute of Psychiatry and Neurology, Budapest, Hungary.
Vanderbilt University, Department of Psychiatry, Nashville, USA.

The Composite Diagnostic Evaluation (CODE) System is a polydiagnostic nosologic method in psychiatry. At the affective disorders the CODE-DD (Depressive Disorders) and the CODE-HD (Hyperthymic - manic, hypomanic and euphoric - Disorders), at the schizophrenic area the CODE-SD (Schizophrenic Disorders) are the good systems to use. This systems include the rating scales (symptoms), the glossary, the severity subscales, the semi-structured interview and the «decision trees» (for the diagnoses). This diagnostic tool good for the psychiatric research, first of all for the clinical psychopharmacology.

CODE is the Composite Diagnostic Evaluation: and the CODE-System is a methodology in psychiatric polydiagnostic nosology. It renders nosologic concepts accessible for validation and allows for the comparison of different systems of diagnostic classifications.

Two of the Composite Diagnostic Evaluation Systems from the area of affective psychosis are the Composite Diagnostic Evaluation of Depressive Disorders (CODE-DD) [3] and the Composite Diagnostic Evaluation of Hyperthymic Disorders (CODE-HD) [/7]. At he schizophrenic psychosis it is used the Composite Diagnostic Evaluation of Schizophrenic Disorders (CODE-SD) [4].

CODE-DD

The differential therapeutic responsiveness to antidepressants has focused attention on the heterogeneity of patient populations within depressive illness. To break the created impasse in therapeutic progress, there is a need for a shift in emphasis in clinical psychopharmacological research from the demonstration of therapeutic efficacy to the identification of treatment responsive populations. The purpose of the Composite Diagnostic Evaluation of Depressive Disorders (CODE-DD) is to facilitate this development.

In CODE-DD, a diagnostic assessment scale is presented (Rating Scale for Depressive Diagnoses - RSDD) with a severity subscale (Rating Scale for the Assessment of Severity in Depressive Disorders) (RSASDD). One of the unique properties of the RSDD is that, by employing a specially devised algorithm, it can provide diagnoses within 25 systems of diagnostic classifications of depressive disorders simultaneously. The classifications were selected on the basis of their relevance to the conceptual development of the different forms and subforms of depressive illness.

There is increasing evidence that a valid nosology is an essential prerequisite for a meaningful interpretation of contributions from the neurosciences with possible relevance to depressive illness. Because of this, CODE might contribute to bridging the widening gap between neuropharmacological research and its clinical psychopharmacological applications. From a practical point of view, however, probably the most important is that CODE-DD might also be a suitable instrument for the identification of treatment responsive, nosologically meaningful populations, within depressive illness.

CODE-DD is one of the Composite Diagnostic Evaluations based on the principles outlined in the Prolegomenon to the Clinical Prerequisite [2].

CODE-DD was developed for the differentiation of subforms within unipolar depressive disorder and not for the differentiation of unipolar depression from other psychiatric disorders. Therefore, CODE-DD should be used only in preselected patients with depressive illness.

To achieve its objective, CODE-DD had to be set out in a systematic and detailed manner. Accordingly, chapter one deals with symptoms, chapter two with the elicitation of these symptoms and chapter three with the organisation of these symptoms into distinct depressive illnesses.

The CODE for the bipolar disorders is not ready today.

CODE-HD

As in CODE-DD, CODE-HD utilises a diagnostic assessment scale; Rating Scale for Hyperthymic Diagnoses (RSHD), and a severity subscale: Rating Scale for the Assessment of Severity in Hyperthymic Disorders (RSASHD).The RSHD is based on 95 variables characteristic of hyperthymic illness, each of which is assessed in terms of «present» or «absent». This 95 variables - 90 at CODE-DD and 127 at CODE-SD -are presented in the order of the «dynamic totality» of psychiatric disease.

The RSASHD, a subscale of the RSHD, consists of 40 items. Its structure is very similar to the Rating Scale for the Assessment of Depressive Disorders from CODE-DD. This 40 items are grouped under 10 headings, each representing a different affected area of mental functioning in hyperthymic illness. Each fur items under each of the 10 «functional areas» are presented in hierarchical order with each item assigned a score from one to four. In the ultimate analysis, however, the RSASHD provides one interpretable score only. This total score is based on the sum total of 10 component scores; one score - the highest - from each of the functional areas.

The Glossary of Variables in Hyperthymic Disorders (GVHD) consist of 95 items presented in the order of the RSHD. To facilitate the reliable use of the RSHD, the glossary definitions were adopted - mainly - from the English edition of the AMDP and AGP Systems [6,7]. Each variable of the RSHD is perceived as a «code» responsible for a distinct form of clinical expression. It is assumed that it is this «code» which provided for the components of the «determining structure» of hyperthymic/manic, hypomanic and euphoric/diseases, reflected in hyperthymic illness.

In Chapter Two: to obtain the information necessary for completing the RSHD, a Semi-Structured Interview for Hyperthymic Disorders (SSIH) was devised. It consists of 95 sets of questions, identified by Roman numerals: each set corresponding with one specific RSHD variable, identified by an Arabic numeral. Regardless of the number of questions - identified by the letters of the alphabet - included in any single set, there is only one single response to each set (RSHD variable).

It should be noted that it is difficult, if not impossible, to construct a structured or semi-structured interview which is equally suitable across populations with different socio-cultural background and educational level. There will always be questions which some patients will not understand. The interviewer will be expected to interpret all these questions (including technical terms) for the patient and ascertain that relevant answers are obtained.

The SSIHD consists almost exclusively of «suggestive questions» which need to be answered with a «yes» or «no».

In the SSIHD all responses are dichotomous, i.e., «present» or «absent», and refer to the presence (RSHD Pres) or absence (RSHD Abs) of the RSHD variable regardless of the answer to any single SSIHD question. Furthermore, with few exceptions - which are explicit through the nature of the variable or the sentence structure of the question - all the responses are based on the presence or absence of the variable during the interview period.

In the third part of CODE-HD, the «decision tress» based on the 18 classifications, consist of from five to 227 variables, from three to 174 decision clusters and from three to 236 diagnoses. 17 original classifications consist seven German (two E. Kraepelin's, one-one K. Schneider's, E.Bleuler's, Jaspers', Leonhard's and Vienna's), three European (CATEGO, ICD-9 AND ICD-10), five American (St Luis, Taylor and Abrams', RDC, DSM-III and DSM-III-R) and two «mania rating scale» (Beigel and

Murphy's, Leff, Fisher and Bertelsen's). The last classification is our original system, the Composite Diagnostic Classification (CDC) of Hyperthymic Disorders.

When using CODE-HD one must not be forgotten diagnoses are based on the RSHD variables, the meaning of which, even at best, can only approximate the meaning of the variables on which the different diagnostic systems are based. It is probably even more important to understand that the diagnostic criteria in the majority of systems - including those diagnoses which are based on statistical treatments of rating scales - had to be generated from their own descriptive data.

Although the theory behind CODE-HD and the CODE-DD remains the same, in the preparation of CODE-HD we have made an attempt to overcome some of the shortcomings of CODE-DD. For example: we tightened the correspondence between the glossary and the questions of the semi-structured interview; decreased the number of the «neutral» questions of the introduction, i.e., information collected over and above the information covered by the SSIDD: and eliminated the possibility of direct overruling in the response to the RSDD variable the answers given by patients. By these changes we hope CODE-HD will be an even more reliable instrument and in keeping with the theory on which the CODE - System is based.

CODE-SD

CODE-SD stand for Composite Diagnostic Evaluation of Schizophrenic Disorders; and in CODE-SD the CODE method is employed in the polydiagnostic evaluation of patients subsumed under the different forms and subforms of schizophrenic disorders. Similar to the other CODEs, such as, for example, the prototype CODE-DD, CODE-SD has the unique capability of providing multiple diagnoses on the basis of a single interview.

Of the five classifications included in CODE-SD, three, i.e., Bleuler's (1911), Schneider's (1950) and Leonhard's (1957) are conceptually derived, whereas two, i.e., DSM-III-R and ICD-10, are consensus-based; and of the three conceptually derived classifications two, i.e., Bleuler's and Schneider's are derived by the application of a psychopathologic (analytic) approach and one, i.e., Leonhard's, by the application of a nosologic (holistic) approach. Accordingly, in Bleuler's and Schneider's classifications, diagnosis represents the sum, of symptoms and signs present, whereas in Leonhard's classification, diagnosis represents a distinctive form or subform, which - in keeping with the principles of polytethic taxonomy - can be constructed in many ways and from a number of different constituents.

To ascertain that all the necessary information is available for all diagnostic decisions, a Rating Scale for Schizophrenic Diagnoses (RSSD) was constructed. It consists of 127 items (variables) of schizophrenic illness, each of which is assessed in terms of «present» or «absent». And to assist in the elicitation of the necessary information, a Semi-structured Interview for Schizophrenic Disorders (SSISD) was prepared with a series of (optional) questions addressed to the patient and a series of (optional) questions addressed to the interviewer.

Scoring of the RSSD, regardless of whether on the basis of an open-ended or a semi-structured interview, yields five diagnoses, i.e., one diagnosis in each diagnostic system; and information on how each of the five diagnostic decisions was reached.

CODE-SD consists of 127 variables with each variable representing a symptom or sign relevant to the diagnosis of schizophrenia in one or more of the five diagnostic classifications of schizophrenia included in CODE-SD. By assessing the presence or absence of each of the 127 variables presented in alphabetic order in the Rating Scale for Schizophrenic Disorders (RSSD), all the relevant information for a diagnosis within each of the five systems of diagnostic classifications (Table I).

To improve the reliability of diagnosis, the RSSD is supplemented by a glossary, in which each of the 127 variables is given a descriptive definition, with primary consideration to the source, i.e., to the description or definition used for the variable in the diagnostic system(s) from which the variable was derived (Table II). To prevent confusion by conflicting definitions in different diagnostic systems, for symptoms and/or signs encountered in more than one diagnostic system, the method referred to as «splitting of the concept» was used. By employing this method, nominally similar symptoms and signs in different diagnostic systems were entered into the glossary under two or more names, each with a distinctive definition.

In the preparation of the glossary of definitions, the sources consulted included the AGP System [7] : the AMDP System [6] : the Composite Diagnostic Evaluation of Depressive Disorders [3] : the DCR Budapest-Nashville [10] : the Diagnostic and Statistical Manual of Mental Disorders, Third Edition-Revised [1]: Fish's Clinical Psychopathology, Second Edition [8] : Landmark's Manual for the Assessment of Schizophrenia [9] the International Classification of Disease, Tenth revision [12] : and Taylor's Neuropsychiatric Mental Status Examination [11].

The «decision trees» are to create diagnosis (Table III).

The CODE System is a good psychiatrical language representing the valid nosological method at the research work. It is possible to use exact multicenter international study in the field of affective disorders and schizophrenia, as well as in clinical psychopharmacology.

Table I.

No.	Variable	Present	Absent
103	Rambling speech		
104	Recurrent thoughts of death		
105	Responding to inner experiences		
106	Restricted thinking		
107	Scenic hallucinations		
108	Self-absorbed attitude		
109	Self-reference hallucinosis		
110	Slow replies		

Table II.

| P | A |

Automatic obedience

The following of commands to perform actions regardless of the consequences (FISH). It is also referred to as «command automatism».

| P | A |

Bizarre delusions

False beliefs with content that cannot be encountered and cannot occur. It involves a belief that is regard as totally impossible by patient's culture (DSM-III-R).

| P | A |

Blunted affect

Observable decrease in emotional responsiveness, primarily in terms of intensity. It is characterized by «meager» feelings (AGP).

| P | A |

Bodily hallucinations

Unfounded somatic perceptions including touch, pain, vestibular, etc. Also referred to as «coenesthetic hallucinations» (AMDP).

| P | A |

Catatonic excitement

An extreme form of hyperactivity, without an identifiable motive, that is not in response to hallucinatory experiences (DSM-II-R).

| P | A |

Catatonic negativism

Motiveless resistance to all instructions or attempts to be moved. When passive, the patient resists any attempts to be moved; when active, patient does the opposite of what he/she is asked to do (DSM-II-R). In case of «Gegenhalten» patient resists being moved with the strength equal to that applied.

| P | A |

Catatonic posturing

Voluntary assumption of odd, unnatural, awkward and/or (DCR), bizarre postures (DSM-III-R) with all and/or parts of the body. In case of «catalepsy» patient maintains the assumed posture for an extended period.

Table III.

	A. Eugen Bleuler's criteria	
1.	Derailment	33/
	Desultory thinking	34/
	Driveling	37/
	Echolalia	38/
	Incoherence	65/
	Neologisms	81/
	Thought blocking	118/
	Verbigeration	125/
	Woolliness of thinking	127
2.	Autism	8/
	Autistic delusions	9/
	Empty autism	42/
	Hallucinatory rich autism	56
3.	Ambivalence	4
4.	Blunted affect	12/
	Emotional impoverishment	41/
	Flat affect	50/
	Inappropriate affect	64
All 4 present, stop		Definite Schizophrenia
3 present, stop		Probable Schizophrenia
2 present, stop		Possible Schizophrenia
Less than 2 present, stop		Other Psychiatric Dis.

References

1. American psychiatric Association. *Diagnostic and Statistical Manual of Mental Disorders*. Third Edition-Revised. Washington, 1987.
2. Ban T.A. *Prog, Neuropsychopharmacol, and Biol, Psychiat,* 1987 ; 11:527-580.
3. Ban, T.A. Composite Diagnostic Evaluation of Depressive Disorders. J.M. *Productions, Brentwood* 1989.
4. Ban, T.A. Composite Diagnostic Evaluation of Schizophrenic Disorders. In press.
5. Gaszner, P. and Ban, T.A. Composite Diagnostic Evaluation of Hyperthymic Disorders J.M. *Productions Brentwood* 1993.
6. Guy, W. and Ban, T.A. (edited and translated). *The AMDP System. Manual for the Assessment and Documentation of Psychopathology*. Springer, Berlin 1982.
7. Guy, W. and Ban, T.A. (edited and translated). *The AGP System. Manual for the Documentation of Psychopathology in Gerontopsychiatry*. Springer, Berlin 1985.
8. Hamilton, M. (ed.). *Fish's Clinical Psychopathology*. John Wright and Sons, Ltd., Bristol 1985.
9. Landmark, J. A Manual for the Assessment of Schizophrenia. *Acta Psychiatrica Scandinavica* 65. Supplementum 1982 ; 298.
10. Petho, B. and Ban, T.A. in collaboration with Kelemen, A., Ungvari, G., Karczag, I., Bitter, I., Tolna, J. (Budapest), Fjetland, O. (Nashville, TN). *Psychopathology* 1988. ; 21:153-239.
11. Taylor, M.A. *The Neuropsychiatric Mental Status Examination*. Pergamon Press, New York,1986. 12.
12. World Health Organization. International Classification of Diseases. 1990. Revision. World Health Organization, Geneva 1990.

10

Predictive bio-clinical profiles of antidepressant responses in major depression

F. DUVAL, M.-C. MOKRANI, M.-A. CROCQ, M. JAUTZ, P. BAILEY, T. S. DIEP, E. E. DE ANDRADE, A. DE ANDRADE, J.-P. MACHER

From the Research Center for Applied Neuroscience in Psychiatry (FORENAP), Rouffach, France.

The aims of this study were two-fold:
- Firstly, using clinical, psychological and biological variables, to derive profiles predictive of short-term response to antidepressants in depressed adults;
- Secondly, to explore the connection between clinical response and changes in biological indicators.

A number of previous studies with similar goals have been performed [1], but to our knowledge this is the first to examine a wide range of neuroendocrine and psychological variables in a population of this size.

Study methods

Subjects

We studied 57 inpatients meeting DSM-III-R criteria for major depression [2]. There were 23 males and 34 females, age (mean ± standard deviation) 40.1 ± 12.4; all were unipolar and severely depressed (17-item Hamilton Depression Scale Score 28.2 ± 6.2 [3]; 11 met criteria for melancholic type and 7 had mood-congruent psychotic features.

Nineteen had concomitant symptoms of anxiety, with a score greater than 15 on the Hamilton Anxiety Scale [4].

Evaluation of personality

A psychodynamic assessment of each patient was made by our Department of Psychology. Using psychometric tests (D48 or PM38, Binois-Pichot, Benton, Figure de Rey, WAIS) and personality tests (Rorschach, TAT, MMPI), psychological criteria [5,6] were applied to classify the mode of functioning of the personality. Seventeen were found to have a neurotic mode of functioning but without meeting DSM-III-R criteria for any personality disorder. These may be regarded as "neurotic-normals" [6]. Twenty-one had a borderline mode of functioning, which includes the DSM-III-R categories borderline (n=11), narcissistic (n=3), dependent (n=3) and self-defeating (n=4). Six had a psychotic mode of functioning without however showing any signs of psychotic decompensation; these correspond to the DSM-III-R category schizoid personality disorder. Finally, 13 patients could not be classified because their depressive disorder was too severe.

Neuroendocrine investigations

Patients were maintained free from any psychotropic medication, under medical and nursing observation, for at least 10 days. After this wash-out period two challenge tests with TRH (200 µg iv) were performed on the same day at 8am and 11pm; plasma TSH was measured 15 minutes before, just before, and 15, 30 and 60 minutes after TRH injection. This strategy was adopted because we had already shown that the TSH response to TRH is increased in the evening compared with the morning [7]. Following this, dexamethasone 1mg was given orally at midnight and plasma cortisol was measured the following day at 8am, 4pm and 11pm [8]. Patients were excluded if they had a history of physical illness, medical treatment or drug abuse which could affect the neuroendocrine tests.

The patients were compared with 30 healthy controls, hospitalised under comparable conditions (notably timing of meals and sleep), in order to provide norms for the neuroendocrine tests. The control group was comparable to the patients in age (36.0 ± 10.2) and sex (13 males, 17 females).

After one month of inpatient antidepressant treatment the same neuroendocrine tests were repeated in all the patients.

Plasma hormone levels were determined using highly sensitive luminescence-coupled immunoenzymatic methods (sensitivity: TSH < 0.04 µU/ml, cortisol < 3 nmol/ml).

Antidepressant treatment

Antidepressant treatment was given in an open-label manner and chosen according to clinical presentation, history of the disorder and, where applicable, response to previous treatment and side-effects. In this way it was hoped to optimize the response to treatment.

Three different antidepressants of three different types were used:
- Selective serotonin reuptake inhibitors: fluoxetine in 23 patients, daily dose 43.5 ± 11.5 mg, range 20-60mg;
- Tricyclics: amitriptyline in 18 patients, daily dose 203 ± 47 mg, range 150-300 mg;
- Reversible inhibitors of monoamine oxidase type A: toloxatone in 16 patients, daily dose 1 190 ± 50 mg, range 1 000-1 200 mg.

Antidepressants were given under supervision on the ward, at doses known to be effective (1). Changes in dose were made according to clinical response.

The criteria of clinical response were defined in terms of the Hamilton Depression Scale (HAM-D). Although the use of this particular scale to quantify change in depressed mood is open to question, it was chosen because of its ease of use and its general acceptance in the Anglo-Saxon literature. We followed Frank *et al* [9] in defining response in terms of absolute rather than relative scores: good response was defined as a final HAM-D score less than 8, poor response as a final score greater than 14, and a partial response as a final score between these limits.

Results and discussion

After one month's treatment, 46% of the patients were classified as responders, 21% as partial responders and 33% as nonresponders (Table I). This response rate is comparable with that generally reported in the literature [10]. The proportion of males and females is similar across the three response groups; the partial responders however are younger. The intensity of symptoms at baseline - estimated using the HAM-D - does not differ between the three groups; furthermore the efficacy of the different antidepressant drugs is comparable.

Table I. Demographic characteristics of groups defined by antidepressant treatment response.

	Responders	Partial responders	Non-responders
Number (%)	26 (46%)	12 (21%)	19 (33%)
Sex (M/F)	9/14	8/4	8/13
Age (y)*	40±12	34±11**	43±12
HAM-D score (Day 1)	27±5	27±5	31±6
HAM-D score (Day 28)	5±1	11±1	23±6
Fluoxetine	14	3	6
Amitriptyline	7	4	7
Toloxatone	5	5	6

* mean ± SD
** p < 0.05 Comparing partial responders with nonresponders (Student's t-test, two-tailed).

Table II shows the results of the neuroendocrine tests performed before and after treatment.

Pretreatment 8am ΔTSH, a measure of the stimulation of TSH by TRH, is on average lower in the nonresponders. In other words the nonresponders show hyposensitivity of pituitary receptors to TRH stimulation, perhaps owing to hypersecretion of endogenous TRH [11]. 8am ΔTSH values do not change with treatment even in the responder group.

For chronobiological reasons, the TSH response is greater at 11pm than at 8pm. The 11pm test is performed close to the peak of circadian secretion of TSH, when the target receptors are most sensitive to stimulation; thus hyposensitivity is easier to demonstrate at 11pm than at 8am. The pretreatment 11pm ΔTSH is reduced in nonresponders and partial responders, showing hyposensitivity to TRH; on the other hand, responders are comparable to controls. After treatment, 11pm ΔTSH does not change in nonresponders or in partial responders; it rises significantly in responders.

The difference between 11pm response and 8am response, which we refer to as ΔΔTSH, is a more refined measure of thyroid axis activity since, as we have recently shown, it takes account of the feedback effect of the thyroid hormones (Duval et al. 1993). Pretreatment ΔΔTSH is reduced in all three groups irrespective of response to treatment, though the reduction is greater in nonresponders. This would be expected from the preceding results since ΔΔTSH is correlated with 8am ΔTSH ($r=0.37$, $n=57$, $p<0.01$) and 11pm ΔTSH ($r=0.73$, $n=57$, $p<0.00001$).

Table II. Results of neuroendocrine tests performed in 30 controls and in 57 depressed patients before and after antidepressant treatment.

	Controls n=30	Responders n=26	Partial Responders n=12	Non-responders n=19
8 am-ΔTSH				
Day 1	7,80±3,77	6,28±3,96	5,67±2,29	3,66±1,93**
Day 28		7,28±3,49	5,72±2,09	4,22±2,16
11 pm-ΔTSH				
Day 1	11,53±4,38	9,52±4,37	6,97±2,94*	4,99±2,72***
Day 28		11,40 ±4,28††	7,09±2,34	5,77±3,33
ΔΔTSH				
Day 1	3,75±1,29	2,45±1,98*	1,30±1,07***	1,26±1,42***
Day 28		3,93±1,66†††	1,37±1,36	1,55±1,67
DST				
Day 1	45,2±45,3	87,1±94,1	101,5±99,3*	122,9±33,8*
Day 28		32,8±15,8†	51,8±40,3†	135,5±168,0

* $p < 0.01$, ** $p < 0.001$, *** $p < 0.00001$: Comparison vs. controls (two-tailed Student's t-test).
† $p < 0.05$, †† $p < 0.01$, ††† $p < 0.001$: Intra-group comparison before and after treatment (two-tailed Student's t-test for paired data). ΔTSH : Maximent increment in plasma TSH level above baseline. ΔΔTSH : Difference between 11 pm- and 8 am- ΔTSH. DST : Highest post-dexamethasone suppression test cortisol value (statistical test performed after logarithmic transformation of data). Mean±SD.

After antidepressant treatment, ΔΔTSH increases significantly only in the responders; it does not change in nonresponders or partial responders. This suggests that antidepressant treatment response is associated with restitution of normal thyroid axis activity, which does not occur in partial or nonresponders. This confirms results which we have published previously [13].

The pretreatment dexamethasone test results show adrenocortical axis hyperactivity in partial and nonresponders. Responders also show some degree of cortisol nonsuppression but the mean does not differ significantly from that of the controls. After antidepressant treatment the hypercortisolemia is reduced, except in the nonresponders. These results are also consistent with the published literature [14].

Thresholds defining normal and abnormal responses can be defined by Receiver Operating Characteristic (ROC) analysis [15]; such an analysis shows that the biological markers that we studied during the acute depressive phase are also indicators of change in the clinical state (Figure 1).

Defining an abnormal 8am TRH test response as $\Delta TSH < 3.5$ µU/ml, 31% of the depressed patients had an abnormal (blunted) test prior to treatment. The relative lack of sensitivity of this test in depression has already been described [11]. However, if only the nonresponders are considered, the proportion showing blunting of 8am TRH response rises to 50%. Antidepressant treatment does not significantly increase 8am TRH response.

The 11pm TRH test is considered abnormal if ΔTSH is below 6µU/ml. At baseline 46% of the patients had an abnormal result. This test tends to normalize with treatment. Once again it is the nonresponders who are more likely to show this abnormality at baseline (almost three-quarters) and after treatment.

The criterion for a blunted ΔΔTSH is a value below 2.5µU/ml. Almost three-quarters of the depressed patients have a blunted response prior to treatment. Normalization occurs only in the responder group; blunting persists in partial and nonresponders. Thus ΔΔTSH appears to be a chronobiological marker of thyroid axis dysregulation in hospitalized depressed patients and its normalization accompanies good clinical response to treatment.

Cortisol nonsuppression after dexamethasone seems on the other hand to be a marker of severity of depression. In this study 26% of the patients had a pre-test cortisol greater than 140nmol/l (DST positive) and their mean HAM-D score was 31.6 ± 5.7, significantly higher ($p<0.01$, two-tailed t-test) than the score of the DST-negative patients (HAM-D 26.9 ± 5.9). However the percentages of DST-positive patients in the three response groups are virtually the same. After treatment the intra-group change in post-DST cortisol reached statistical significance only in the responder group, which shows that, in these patients, adrenocortical axis activity returned to normal.

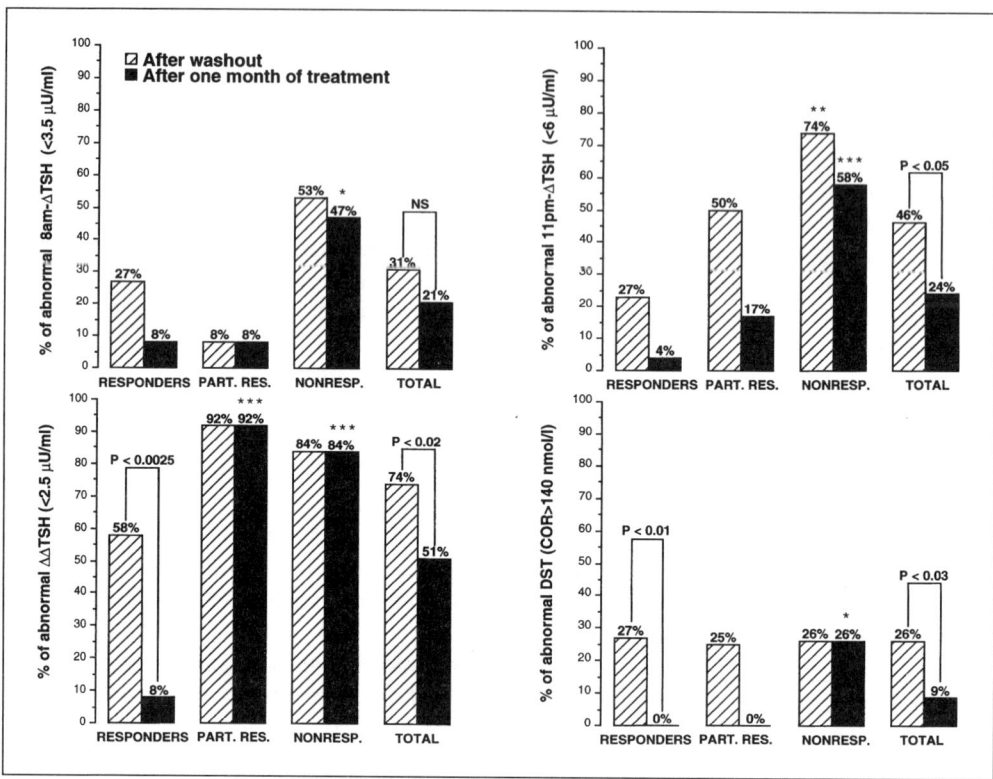

Figure 1. Endocrine tests in 57 depressed patients before and after one month of antidepressant treatment. * p<0.01, ** p<0.001, *** p<0.0001: compared with responders (Fisher's exact test, two-tailed).

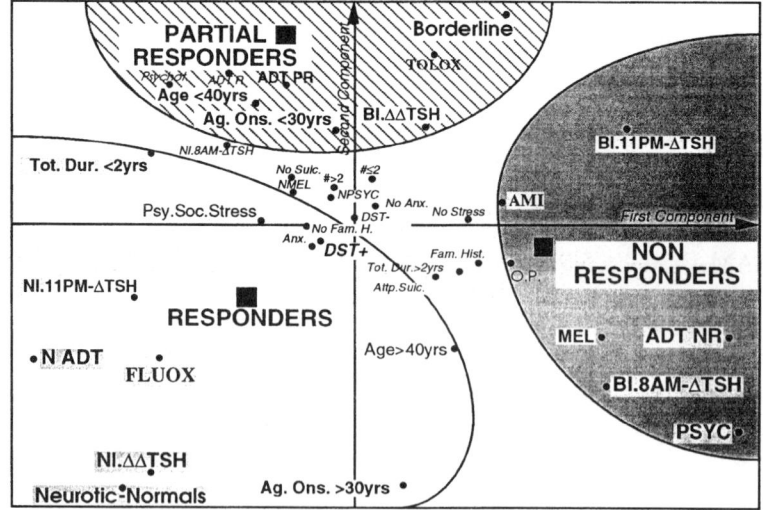

Figure 2. Graphical presentation of factorial correspondence analysis. The analysis contrasts three groups defined by response to one month's antidepressant treatment (responders, partial responders and nonresponders) in term of pretreatment clinical, psychological and biological characteristics.

Distribution of certain clinical characteristics did not differ significantly across the three response groups (Table III) when each characteristic was considered separately, with one exception: previous medication. All except one of the nonresponders had had previous antidepressant treatment, whilst 35% of the responders had never received an antidepressant.

Table III. Clinical and psychological characteristics of groups defined by antidepressant treatment response.

	Responders n=26	Partial responders n=12	Non-responders n=19
Age ≤ 40 years	13 (50%)	9 (75%)	7 (37%)
Melancholic features	4 (15%)	1 (8%)	6 (32%)
Psychotic features	2 (7%)	0 (0%)	4 (21%)
Anxiety symptoms	10 (38%)	4 (33%)	6 (31%)
Stressful event	16 (61%)	7 (58%)	8 (42%)
> 2 episodes	15 (58%)	6 (50%)	10 (53%)
Total duration of disorder < 2 yrs	10 (38%)	6 (50%)	3 (16%)
Age at onset of disorder ≤ 30 yrs	12 (46%)	8 (67%)	9 (47%)
Previous suicide attempt	11 (42%)	4 (33%)	10 (53%)
Previous antidepressant treatment	17 (65%)	10 (83%)	18 (94%)*
Family history of depression	4 (15%)	1 (8%)	4 (21%)
Personality :			
neurotic-normal	13 (50%)	1 (8%)	3 (16%)
borderline	5 (19%)	7 (58%)	9 (47%)
psychotic	3 (12%)	2 (17%)	1 (5%)
not defined	5 (19%)	2 (17%)	6 (32%)

* $p < 0.05$ Comparison responders vs. nonresponders (Student's t-test, two-tailed).

Figure 2 is a graphical representation of the results of a factorial correspondence analysis (FCA) performed on the clinical, psychological and neurobiological data whose univariate analysis has just been described. FCA in principle «permits analysis of large amounts of numerical data by replacing a table which is difficult to understand with one which is easier to understand and is a good approximation» [16]. In the present study such an analysis can be used to describe the characteristics of the three groups defined by response to treatment (responders, partial responders or nonresponders).

The graphical presentation can be made completely using only two axes: the first accounts for 63% and the second for 37% of the total variance. The first axis contrasts responders with nonresponders and the second contrasts responders with partial responders.

The principles used to choose the main factors loading on each axis (response groups and variables) can be summarized as follows:
- Each factor must have a high relative contribution to the total variation explained by the axis, in other words it must play an important part in accounting for the deviation of an element from the mean. The minimum relative contribution is generally set at 100/n; in this study n=57, thus the lower limit is 1.75.

- The factors with relative contributions above this minimum are selected in descending order of magnitude until the cumulative sum of the relative contributions accounts for 70 to 80% of the variance explained by the axis.

- The cosine squared of the angle between the factor and the axis must be greater than 0.80.

- The co-ordinates of these factors on the axes are then inspected to see if they lie on the same side or on opposing sides of the axis.

The three groups are well separated in the FCA and their biological and clinical characteristics can be defined:

- The **nonresponders** are characterised mainly by a blunted 8am ΔTSH, by mood-congruent psychotic features and by a history of poor response to antidepressants. They differ from responders in having a blunted 11pm ΔTSH, melancholic features, and a lack of response to tricyclics such as amitriptyline. This does not of course imply that amitriptyline is an inefficacious antidepressant; rather it appears that, in this patient group, it is not the treatment of choice.

- The **responders** are characterized mainly by a normal $\Delta\Delta$TSH. They respond to treatment with selective serotonin reuptake inhibitors, especially if they have not previously been treated with an antidepressant. Finally, they show neurotic («neurotic-normal») functioning in personality tests. There are further characteristics which distinguish responders from non-responders: history of psychosocial stress in the preceding year, total duration of disorder less than two years, normal 11pm ΔTSH. When compared with partial responders the full responders are older, with a later age of onset (after age 30) and a positive DST.

- The **partial responders** do not have a well-defined profile and cannot be clearly separated from the nonresponders. On the other hand there are certain characteristics which distinguish them from the responders: borderline personality functioning, blunted $\Delta\Delta$TSH, lower age of onset both of the present episode and of the disorder. This group consists in fact of patients with markedly abnormal personalities associated with depressive features who, in our clinical experience, often develop chronic dysthymia.

Conclusions

The profiles of the three patient groups (responder, partial responder and nonresponder) are largely consistent with other published studies [1]. This confirms that the technique of factorial correspondence analysis, which has received little attention in the Anglo-Saxon literature, is indeed suitable for investigating biological correlates of clinical psychiatric phenomena (in this case, antidepressant treatment response). Despite some limitations in our methodology (e.g. treatment was not given double-blind) it sems that certain conclusions can be drawn regarding treatment strategies:

1. Selective serotonin reuptake inhibitors seem to be perfectly suitable as first-line treatment for depression, especially when there is no evidence for chronobiological dysfunction of the thyroid axis and when the disorder is of relatively recent onset (absence of chronicity). A positive DST would also point to this choice of treatment.

2. In cases of major depression associated with known abnormality of the personality in young patients with isolated ΔΔTSH blunting, antidepressant treatment alone will probably not suffice. This is consistent with a number of studies showing mediocre response to antidepressants in borderline patients [17, 18]. Because of this some authors have suggested giving low doses of neuroleptics [19, 20], or mood stabilisers such as lithium [21] or carbamazepine [22]; these treatments may sometimes be more effective than antidepressants. Others however have emphasized the importance of adding concomitant psychotherapy to psychotropic medication [23, 24]; this is an important aspect of our own clinical practice.

3. Finally, the nonresponders call for a different approach. This may include changing the antidepressant dose [25], changing to a different class of antidepressant [26], or - more controversially - the use of ECT [27]; or, as has also been suggested on an empirical basis, one may continue the antidepressant and add other treatments:

- mood stabilisers such as lithium [28,29] and carbamazepine [30];

- dopamine agonists such as bromocriptine [31];

- or, on the other hand, dopamine antagonists - neuroleptics - if psychotic symptoms are present [32];

- thyroid hormones: triiodothyronine (T3) seems to be more efficacious in this indication than thyroxine (T4) [33]. In our view, our results suggest that adding T3 to the existing treatment is indicated particularly if there is a blunting of TSH response to TRH, since this blunting could be secondary to hypersecretion of endogenous TRH. Now, as we have recently shown, thyroid hormones continue to exert feedback control in depressed patients. Thus it may be that treatment with exogenous thyroid hormone increases this negative feedback and in this way tends to correct the hypersecretion of endogenous TRH. Speculating further, the return to normal levels of TRH is perhaps part of the physiological normalisation which is associated with resolution of a depressive episode.

Whatever the endocrine basis of depression may be, our study shows clearly that the development of new and more effective antidepressants is necessary. Given what is known about the effects of antidepressants on gene expression, one of the most promising avenues of research may lie in the development of compounds acting on signal transduction proteins and on monoamine transport mechanisms in certain defined cerebral areas.

Acknowledgements

We should like to thank the nursing staff of Sector VIII; our colleagues in the Department of Psychology - Christine Rebourg, Carine Biessy, Nadine Carreras and Thérèse Addessa - for their help and support with this study; Roger Heymann for his advice concerning the interpretation of the factorial correspondence analysis; and Gabrielle Wagner, pharmacist, for performing the hormone analyses.

References

1. Agency for Health Care Policy and Research (AHCPR). *Depression in primary care.* Vol 2. *Treatment of major depression.*1993, Silver Spring, MD: AHCPR Publication, p 175.
2. American Psychiatric Association. *DSM-III-R: Diagnostic and Statistical Manual of Mental Disorders.* 3 rd edition rev American Psychiatric Press, Washington, DC, 1987.
3. Hamilton M. A rating scale for depression. *J Neurol Neurosurg Psychiat* 1960; 23:56-62.
4. Hamilton M. The assessment of anxiety state by rating. *Br J Med Psychol* 1959; 32:50-53.
5. Bergeret J. *La personnalité normale et pathologique.* 1974, Dunod, Paris.
6. Rossel F, Husain O, Merceron C. Reflexions critiques concernant l'utilisation des techniques projectives. *Bull Psychol* 1986; 39:721-728.
7. Duval F, Macher JP, Mokrani MC. Difference between evening and morning thyrotropin responses to protirelin in major depressive episode. *Arch Gen Psychiatry*, 1990; 47:443-48.
8. Carroll BJ, Feinberg M, Greden JF, Tarika J, Albala AA, Hasket RF, James NM, Kronfol Z, Lohr N, Steiner M, de Vigne JP, Young E. A specific laboratory test for the diagnosis of melancholia: standardization, validation, and clinical utility. *Arch Gen Psychiatry,* 1981; 38:15-22.
9. Frank E, Prien RF, Jarrett RB, Keller MB, Kupfer DJ, Lavori PW, Rush AJ, Weissman MM. Conceptualization and rationale for consensus definitions of terms in major depressive disorder. *Arch Gen Psychiatry* 1991; 48:851-855.
10. Klein DF, Gittelman R, Quitkin. *Diagnosis and drug treatment of psychiatric disorders: adults and children*, 2nd edition, Baltimore, Williams & Wilkins, 1980.
11. Loosen PT, Prange AJ. Serum thyrotropin response to thyrotropin-releasing hormone in psychiatric patients: a review. *Am J Psychiatry* 1981; 139:405-416.
12. Duval F, Mokrani MC, Crocq MA, Bailey P, Macher JP. Influence of thyroid hormones on morning and evening TSH response to TRH in major depression. *Biol Psychiatry* (in press).
13. Duval F, Mokrani MC, Oliveira Castro J, Crocq MA, Andrade EE, Macher JP. Ciracadian effects on the TSH response to TRH in depressed patients. *Clin Neuropharma* 1992;15 (Suppl 1):384-385A.
14. American Psychiatric Association task force on laboratory tests in psychiatry. The dexamethasone suppression test: an overview of its current status in psychiatry. *Am J Psychiatry* 1987; 144:1253-1262.
15. Metz CE. Basic principles of ROC analysis. *Sem Nucl Med* 1978; 8:283-298.
16. Benzecri JP. *L'analyse des données. Vol 1: La taxinomie, Vol 2: Correspondances.* 1973, Dunod, Paris.
17. Soloff PH, George A, Nathan RS, Schulz PM, Cornelius J. Patterns of response to amitriptyline and haloperidol among borderline patients. *Psychopharmacol Bull* 1988; 24:264-268.
18. Soloff PH, George A, Nathan RS, Schulz PM, Ulrich RF. Progress in pharmacotherapy of borderline disorders. *Arch Gen Psychiatry* 1986; 43:691-697.
19. Brinkely JR, Breitman BD, Friedel RO. Low-dose neuroleptic regimens in the treatment of borderline patients. *Arch Gen Psychiatry* 1979; 36:319-29.
20. Leone NF. Response of borderline patients to loxapine and chlorpromazine. *J Clin Psychiatry* 1982; 43:148-150.
21. Rifkin A, Quitkin F, Carrillo C, Blumberg AG, Klein DF, Oaks G. Lithium carbonate in emotionally unstable character disorder. *Arch Gen Psychiatry* 1972; 27:519-523.
22. Gardner DL, Cowdry RW. Positive efects of carbamazepine on behavioral dyscontrol in borderline personality disorder. *Am J Psychiatry* 1986; 143:519-522.
23. Blackburn IM, Bishop S, Glen AIM, Walley LJ, Christie JE. The efficacy of cognitive therapy and pharmacotherapy, each alone and in combination. *Br J Psychiatry* 1981; 139:181-189.

24. Mintz J, Mintz LI, Arruda MJ, Hwang SS. Treatment of depression and the functional capacity to work. *Arch Gen Psychiatry* 1992; 49:761-768.
25. Amsterdam J, Brunswick J, Mendels J. High dose desipramine, plasma drug levels and clinical response. *J Clin Psychiatry* 1979; 40:141-143.
26. Beasley CM, Sayler ME, Cunningham GE, Weiss AM, Masica DN. Fluoxetine in tricyclic refractory major depressive disorder. *J Aff Disorder* 1990; 20:193-200.
27. Electroconvulsive therapy. *Psychiatr Clin North Am* 1991; 14:793-1016.
28. Montigny C (de), Cournoyer G, Morissette R, Langlois R, Caile G. Lithium carbonate addition in tricyclic antidepressant drugs and lithium ion on the serotoninergic system. *Arch Gen Psychiatry* 1983; 40:1327-1334.
29. Price LH, Charney DS, Heninger GR. Efficacy of lithium-tranylcypromine treatment in refractory depression. *Amm J Psychiatry* 1985; 142:612-623.
30. Post RM, Uhde TW, Roy-Byrne PP, Joffe RT. Antidepressant effects of carbamazepine. *Am J Psychiatry* 1986; 143:29-34.
31. Waehrens J, Gerlach J. Bromocriptine and imipramine in endogenous depression. A double blind controlled trial in outpatients. *J Affective Disord* 1981; 3:193-202.
32. Charney DS, Nelson JC. Delusional and non delusional unipolar depression: further evidence for distinct subtypes. *Am J Psychiatry* 1981; 138:328-333.
33. Joffe RT, Singer W. Thyroid hormone use to enhance the effects of drugs. *Clin Neuropharma* 1992;15 (Suppl 1):389-390A.

11

Late auditory evoked potentials: contribution to diagnosis of schizophrenia and correlations with Andreasen's rating scales (SANS, SPAS)

M. SMETS [1], PH. GALLOIS [2], G. FORZY [2], P. HAUTECOEUR [2],
C.E. THOMAS III [1], J.M. HENNEBIQUE [1]

[1] CH Saint-Venant, 62350 Saint-Venant, France.
[2] CH Saint-Philibert, 59160 Lomme, France.

Schizophrenia remains one of the most complex and the most severe of the mental disorders. It seemed interesting to study information processing in schizophrenic patients [15]. In order to do this, we recorded auditory event-related brain potentials (ERPs) in patients who fulfilled the DSM-III-R diagnostic criteria for schizophrenia [1].

Materials and methods

Subjects

Two populations of schizophrenic patients (DSM-III-R) were compared with a sample of 30 control subjects (Table I).

Table I. Description of the three groups.

	N	mean age (years)	mean duration of illness (years)	patients on neuroleptic medication
group 1	17	34	10	16
group 2	20	29	3.5	20
controls	30	29		

Methods

Electrophysiological measures

Late auditory evoked potentials (AEPs) were studied in the three groups using an «odd-ball» paradigm: the subjects received bilateral stimuli through headphones: pure tones of 70 dB HL intensity and 20 ms duration. Frequent tones were of 750 Hz frequency and 85% probability, rare tones were of 2 000 Hz frequency and 15% probability. AEPs data were recorded from scalp needle electrodes situated in Pz and Fz (international 10-20 system) and referred to linked ears.

Subjects were instructed to raise their fingers as soon as they heard the target tone (2 000 Hz) and to ignore the frequent tones. We did two series of stimulations to verify reproducibility. Duration of recording session was about 30 minutes. We measured latency of N1, P2, N2 P3, N3 and amplitude of N1 and P3.

Clinical measures

In the second group, we also did clinical quantitative assessment of negative and positive symptoms of schizophrenia using Andreasen's rating scales (2, 3). We used the two complete scales for every patient and a time set covering the past month. Mean duration of investigation was about 70 minutes. All clinical measures were scored independently of the AEPs data.

Results

Clinical measures

In 5 patients, positive total score was greater than negative; in 11 patients, negative total score was greater than positive; in 4 patients, negative and positive total scores were equal.

Electrophysiological measures (Figure 1)

Figure 1 shows AEPs recorded in a normal control and a schizophrenic subject, elicited by infrequent and frequent tones in an «odd-ball» paradigm. In the first group (mean duration of illness: 10 years), we found anomalies in 13 patients (76.47 %). In the second group (mean duration of illness: 3.5 years), disturbances were found in 18 patients (90%).

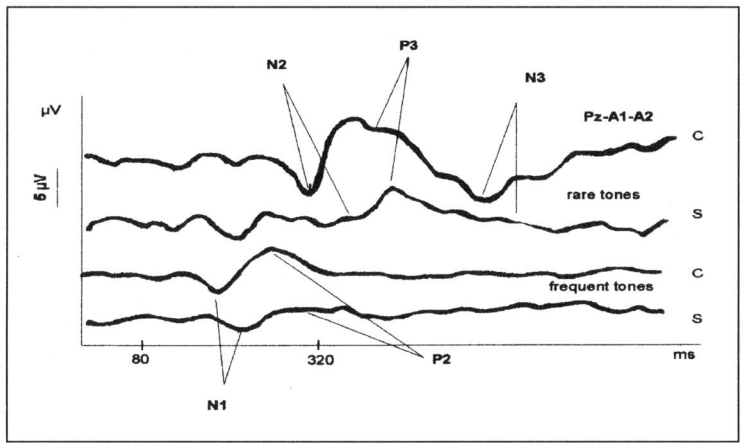

Figure 1. AEPs recorded in a normal control (C) and a schizophrenic subject (S).

Table II gives the statistically significant parameters (P < 0.01). We observed a lengthening of the latency of N1, N2, P3, N3 and a decreased amplitude of N1 and P3 in the two groups.

Table II. Statistically significant parameters (P < 0,01).

	latency (milliseconds)				amplitude (µvolts)	
	N1	N2	P3	N3	N1	P3
Controls	93.8±6.5	201.8±17.6	299.7±12.6	424.7±19.5	8±1.8	15.3±4.6
group 1	100.6±10.8	240.1±36.3	351.6±39.6	496.7±55.6	4.6±2.5	9.2±6.2
group 2	101.9±8.8	233.2±21.7	338.4±33.3	476±47.3	4.5±2.6	9.6±4.1

We also performed an analysis of correlation between clinical and AEPs data (Figure 2).

Discussion

This study allows three approaches.

Diagnosis

Although AEPs disturbances are not specific to schizophrenia, many studies showed anomalies [12,14]. These perturbations could be a vulnerability trait marker which is

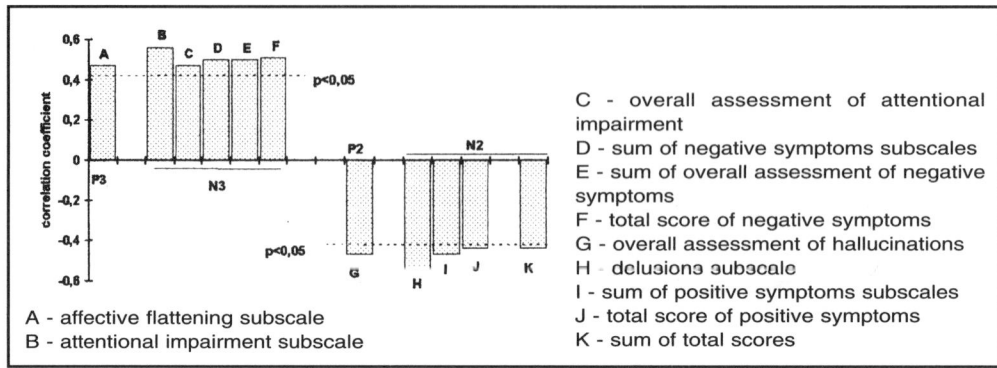

Figure 2. Statistically significant correlations between clinical and AEPs data.

stable over time [7, 9] or a symptomatic state [5,6]. This study found AEPs anomalies in the two groups: their existence in the early stages of illness (second group) would be in favour of the first hypothesis.

Etiopathogenetic hypothesis

At a functional level

Many authors observed impairments in the physiological processes underlying attention disorders in schizophrenics [13]. Our study confirmed these anomalies from first stages as indexed by N1, P2, N2, to later stages of categorization and decision making (P3, N3).

At a neuroanatomical level

The N1 modifications are pathophysiological indices of subcortical dementias [8, 10]. Various researchers, using brain imaging techniques (PET), have described anomalies located in the limbic structures [16]. Our results suggest an impairment of cerebral information processing, probably localized in the subcortical level.

Correlative analysis

Statistically significant correlations were observed between anomalies of the last stages of information processing (P3, N3) and negative symptoms, especially affective flattening and attentional impairment. The disturbances of the first stages of information processing (P2) and of automatic information processing (N2) were related to positive symptoms, notably hallucinations and delusions. The anomalies of N2 were also related to the sum of the total scores for negative and positive symptoms: an attentional impairment could be a main factor in the pathogenesis of schizophrenia [4, 11].

Conclusion

AEPs are disturbed in schizophrenia and might contribute to diagnosis of illness. This work shows that these disturbances are significantly correlated with clinical parameters.

References

1. American Psychiatric Association DSM III R. *Diagnostic and statistical manual of mental disorders*. Third edition, revised. American Psychiatric Association, Washington, DC, 1987.
2. Andreasen N.C. *Scale for the Assessment of Negative Symptoms* (SANS). Iowa City, Department of Psychiatry, University of Iowa. College of Medicine, 1981.
3. Andreasen N.C. *Scale for the Assessment of Positive Symptoms* (SAPS). Iowa City, Department of Psychiatry, University of Iowa. College of Medicine, 1984.
4. Barrett K., Mc Callum W.C., Pocock P.V. Brain Indicators of Altered Attention and Information Processing in Schizophrenic Patients. *Br. J. Psychiatry* 1986; 148: 414-120.
5. Duncan C.C. Current issues in the application of P300 to research in schizophrenia. In : *Schizophrenia concepts, vulnerability and intervention*. Straube E.R., Hahlwed K., Eds, 1990; 117-134.
6. Erlenmeyer-Kimling L., Cornblatt B. High-risk research in schizophrania a summary of what has been learned. *J. Psychiat. Res.*, 1987; 21, 4: 401-411.
7. Friedman D, Cornblatt B, Vaughan HJr, Erlenmeyer-Kimling L. Auditory event-related potentials in children at risk for schizophrenia: the complete initial sample. *Psychiatry Res.*, 1988; 26: 203-221.
8. Goodin DS. Aminoff MJ. Electrophysiological differences between subtypes of dementia. *Brain*, 1986; 109: 1103-1113.
9. Grebb JA, Weinberger DR, Morihisa JM. Electroencephalogram and evoked potential studies of schizophrenia. In : Nasrallah HA, Weinberger DE (eds). *Handbook of schizophrenia.* Vol.1. *The neurology of schizophrenia*. Elsevier, 1986; 121-140.
10. Hautecoeur P, Gallois Ph, Forzy G, Chatelet P, Choteau Ph, Dereux JF. Potentiels évoqués auditifs tardifs dans les affections cognitives sous-corticales. *Rev Neurol* 1991; 147, 4: 293-299.
11. Hemsley DR. Information processing and schizophrenia. In : Straube ER, Hahlweg K (eds). *Schizophrenia concepts, vulnerability and intervention*. 1990; 59-76.
12. Romani A, Merello S, Cozzoli L, Zerbi F, Grassi M, Cosi V. P300 and GT scan in patients with chronic schizophrenia. *Br. J. Psychiatry*, 1987; 151: 506-513.
13. Roth WT, Duncan CC, Pfefferbaum A, Timsit-Berthier M. *Applications of cognitive ERPs in psychiatric patients. Cerebral Psychophysiol.* Studies in event-related potentials, 1986; Suppl. 38: 419-38.
14. Saint-Clair D, Blackwood D, Muir W. P300 abnormality in schizophrenic subtypes. *J. Psychiat. Res.*, 1989; 23, 1: 49-55.
15. Smets M. *Etude des potentiels évoqués sensoriels et cognitifs chez 18 patients schizophrènes*. Thèse pour le Doctorat en Médecine, Lille, 1989.
16. Zec RF, Weinberger DR. Brain areas implicated in schizophrenia a selective overview. In: Nasrallah HA, Weinberger DR (eds). *Handhook of schizophrenia*. Vol 1. *The neurology of schizophrenia*, Elsevier, 1986; 175-206.

12

First pharmaco-electroencephalographic approach of Euphytose®

R. LUTHRINGER[1], G. LEFRANÇOIS[2], D. ROD[2], J.P. MACHER[1]

[1]Forenap, CH, 68250 Rouffach, France.
[2]Soekami-Lefrancq Laboratoires, 69, Boulevard Victor-Hugo, 95585 Saint-Ouen Cedex, France.

Euphytose® is a complex mixture of plant extracts comprising mainly of passiflora incarnata, valeriana officialis and cola nitida. The extract also contains hawthorn (crataegus oxyacantha), guarana (paullinia cupana) and bullota foetida, but in much lower quantities. The product has been used in France, on an empirical basis, since 1927, for its anxiolytic properties. The traditional medicinal properties and the synergistic effects of components may provide the rationale for the use of the Euphytose® mixture in clinical practice, particularly now that benzodiazepine (BZD) treatments are subject to growing criticisms because of their deleterious side effects.

In man, Euphytose® is reported to have no side effects, and a recent double-blind randomized study in patients suffering from generalized anxiety has shown that this complex mixture is as active as the BZD, oxazepam, and can efficiently replace this standard treatment (Guibert and Cholet, 1990).

In order to elucidate the mechanisms of action of Euphytose®, a first *in vitro* binding study on the total mixture and its individual components has been performed on rat CNS receptors (Valli *et al.*, 1991). The results showed that the association of plant extracts, Euphytose®, interacts with central benzodiazepine (BZD) receptors, alpha-2 adrenoreceptors and muscarinic H1 receptors with respective IC50 values of 37.1, 3.6 and 30.0 µg/mL. In contrast, Euphytose® did not show any interaction with peripheral BZD, 5-HT1 and 5-HT2 serotoninergic, alpha-1 adrenergic, D1 and D2 dopaminergic and M2 muscarinic receptors. These *in vitro* binding data demonstrated clearly the different interactions of Euphytose® with various neurotransmitter binding sites in the central nervous system. This is of importance in order to elucidate the mechanism of action of the putative anxiolytic and/or antidepressant effect of this drug.

A further animal study, including the Vogel test, the four plates test and the clonidine test, showed the anxiolytic potency of Euphytose®, as well as, at higher doses, the antidepressant potential activities. During this study several formulations of Euphytose® have been used. Two of them [Euphytose® (containing six plant extracts) and RUSL 311 (containing four plant extracts)] have shown good anxiolytic properties.

All these encouraging results as well as the empirical findings of Euphytose® users, have now to be confirmed in a double-blind clinical trial in anxious patients.

Nevertheless, before starting this clinical trial, it seemed important to investigate, in man, the bioavailability of Euphytose® and RUSL 311.

Thus, it was decided to carry-out a pharmaco-EEG study. Indeed quantified pharmaco-EEG is now, a validated and accepted technique (Saletu, 1976; Saletu et al., 1987; Saletu, 1987; Sannita et al., 1981) for early psychopharmacological investigation of new psychotropic molecules allowing to determine cerebral kinetics, pharmaco-EEG profiles, to establish correlations with plasma concentrations (Laurian et al., 1983; Saletu et al., 1988) and also to underscore psychopharmacological properties which had not been detected by classical methods of pharmacological or biochemical investigation in animals (Itil et al. 1972).

The aim of the present double-blind, cross-over, placebo controlled study was first to compare the CNS (Central Nervous System) bioavailability of Euphytose® and RUSL 311, after single dose administration at 2 different doses (2 and 4 tablets), second to determine the pharmaco-EEG profile and effects on Event Related Potentials (ERPs) of this compound. In addition, psychomotor tests (Hindmarch, 1980), Osgood mood profile scale (Spiegel and Aebi, 1983) clinical and biological safety of Euphytose® were also assessed.

Material and methods

Design, subjects, drugs, recording methods, statistics

Twelve healthy caucasian volunteers aged between 23 and 36 years (mean 28.5 ± 3.98 years), ranging in height from 156 cm to 175 cm (mean 166.4 ± 6.5 cm), weighing from 48 kg to 80 kg (mean 60.9 ± 9.4 kg) participated in this double-blind, placebo-controlled, cross-over study. They took no psychoactive drugs for 1 month before or during the study. Subjects received at daily intervals, in random order as single oral doses: placebo, RUSL 311 (2 and 4 tablets) and Euphytose® (2 and 4 tablets). The study was performed in accordance with the rules and regulations for the conduct of clinical trials stated by the World Medical Assembly at Helsinki, Tokyo, Venice and Hong-Kong and by the french law. Informed written consent was obtained. RUSL 311, Euphytose® or placebo were administered at approximately 9 a.m. after a day of wash-out and an overnight fast. During recordings, four light standard meals were given.

They were identical for every volunteer and each dose level. The breakfast, lunch (2) and supper were served before, 2 hours, 4-5 hours and 10-11 hours respectively after each drug administration. EEG and ERP parameters were collected before drug administration and 0.5h ; 0.75h ; 1h ; 1.25h ; 1.5h ; 2h ; 3h ; 4h ; 5h ; 6h and 7h after administration. OSGOOD scale was filled in by the volunteers before drug administration and again 1h, 2h, 4h, 6h and 7h after administration. At the same periods as OSGOOD scale, psychomotor tests have also been recorded.

During data acquisition subjects reclined in a comfortable armchair with their eyes closed in a sound-proofed and electrically shielded room. Twenty-eight EEG leads were recorded using an ear linked reference as well as 4 artifact channels (detection of eye movement, muscle activity, EKG and other potential causes of artifacts). Electrode placement was derived from the 10-20 system (Jasper, 1958) and the additional electrodes were placed in the center of four standard electrodes.

Spontaneous EEGs were initially recorded under 3-minute vigilance controlled (VC) conditions and then under 3-minute resting (R) conditions. Filter settings were 1-90 Hz. (12 db/octave). Data from the 32 channels were digitalized with a sampling frequency of 256 points/second and stored on a hard disk. The VC condition was not analyzed here, but ensured the same basal conditions for the R condition recordings.

The standard auditory «odd-ball» paradigm was used for P300 elaboration. Subjects listened to a series of two-tones, with a frequency of 500 Hz for frequent tones and a frequency of 2 000 Hz for infrequent tones. Subjects were asked to count the infrequent tones. The tones were presented binaurally through earphones with a duration of 0.5 sec. and an intensity of 85 db. The intertrial interval was randomized between 0.8 and 1.3 sec., with frequent tones presented in 85% and infrequent tones in 15% of all trials in order to obtain 20 trials in which the subject was asked to count. Each trial was recorded with a sampling frequency of 250 Hz and then averaged to calculate 28 mean curves for either frequent or infrequent trials. Four artifact channels were recorded and an on-line rejection of EEG activities higher than 70 µV was used. The same montage and the same references were used for data acquisition as for spontaneous EEG recordings, with the following filter settings (0.5 Hz and 30 or 70 Hz according to the amount of EMG activity). The length of the curve was 508 ms with an interpoint time of 4 ms.

CNV was obtained with a warning auditory stimulus (1000 Hz, 0.5 sec., 85 db) generated binaurally by earphones and followed, 1 sec. later, by an imperative auditory stimulus (750 Hz, 5 sec., 85 db) which could be stopped by the subject with a pushbutton. The recording procedures were the same as for P300 acquisition, but with adapted filter settings (0.016 Hz and 70 or 30 Hz).

For spontaneous EEG recordings, the artifact removal procedure was performed by two technicians trained in the field of electroencephalography on elementary 2-second epochs (512 points) over each 3-minute period. Amplitude spectra were then calculated for every 2-second period over a frequency range of 0.5 to 32 Hz., using the Fast Fourier Transform algorithm (Cooley and Tuckey,1965), in order to obtain 32 mean amplitude spectra for each subject and for each time. Finally, group spectra (mean and variance) for the 12 subjects were calculated.

Absolute and relative energies for delta (0.5-3.5 Hz), theta (4-7.5 Hz), alpha (8-12.5 Hz) and beta (13-32 Hz) bands were analyzed. The alpha band was divided into alpha 1 (8-9.5 Hz) and alpha 2 (10-12.5 Hz) and the beta band was broken up into beta 1 (13-17.5 Hz), beta 2 (18-20.5 Hz) and beta 3 (21-32 Hz). All these parameters were analyzed by means of mapping techniques.

The parameters analyzed for P300 were both latency and amplitude of peak P3 (evaluated on Cz lead). In addition, mean amplitude maps of P3 component (mean amplitude between 260 and 420 ms) were also analyzed. For the CNV, post-warning stimulus (first 500 ms after warning stimulus) and pre-imperative stimulus (500 ms preceding the imperative stimulus) maps were estimated.

The EEG and ERP maps were obtained, using a methodology previously described by some of us (Soufflet et al.,1991).

The Dynamic Statistical Decision Tree (DSDT) (Dago et al.,1991) procedure was used for topographical (maps) statistical analysis. DSDT integrates, on the one hand the modified [implementation of paired comparisons and non-parametric tests (Wilcoxon t test)] Significance Probability Mapping (SPM) technique (Duffy et al.,1981) to allow a global spatial evaluation, and on the other hand multidimensional tests for predefined sets of leads belonging to specific scalp regions (i.e. frontal, temporal, central, parietal, occipital) allowing the construction of statistical kinetic curves.

Results

Double-blind placebo-controlled EEG brain mapping investigations showed that single oral doses (2 and 4 tablets) of Euphytose® and RUSL 311 induced electroencephalotropic and psychometric changes as compared to placebo and had no clinically significant effects on clinical and biological parameters.

For spontaneous EEG, these changes were more important in resting recording conditions as compared to vigilance-controlled conditions. In absolute energy, the effects were generally characterized, by an increase of the global EEG activity, the alpha activity (mostly the alpha 2 band) and, only for the RUSL 311 doses, the beta activities. Delta and theta activities were only slightly and not systematically modified by the four administered formulations. In relative energy, alpha activities were increased as compared to placebo, with the most important effects observed after Euphytose® (2 tablets). Again delta and theta activities were only slightly modified unlike beta bands which showed increased values, only after the two Euphytose® doses.

The effects of Euphytose® and RUSL 311 on the ERPs were for the P300, at time 0.5h, a trend towards increased latencies concomitant with a trend towards decreased amplitudes. These effects were more important for the two Euphytose® doses as compared to the two RUSL 311 doses. Towards the end of the recordings (time 6h) the P300 latency showed a trend of shortened latencies for the four doses. CNV, which was only recorded from time 1.5h on, showed at this time point decreased mean amplitudes after the 4 tablets dose of Euphytose® unlike the three other treatments which induced increased mean amplitudes.

Psychometric measurements were only slightly modified by the four treatments. Thus, for the psychomotor tests, the Critical Fliker Fusion test was never modified, unlike the Multiple Choice Reaction Time test which showed a significant decrease of the Recognition phase after the two doses of RUSL 311 at time 2h and after Euphytose® (2 tablets) at time 7h. The Motor phase of this test was never modified by active treatments. Finally, the Total reaction time was decreased at time 7h after 2 tablets of RUSL 311. Osgood scale was only modified by the RUSL 311 (2 tablets) formulation at time 2h where Vigilance was increased and Extraversion was decreased.

Discussion

The primary objective of this study was to compare the CNS bioavailability of 2 Euphytose® formulations [Euphytose® (with six plant extracts) and RUSL 311 (with four plant extracts)], after single dose administration at 2 different doses (2 and 4 tablets).

According to the results observed with the used EEG and psychometric techniques it can be stated that the four treatments have shown CNS bioavailabilities, after single doses administrations.

Nevertheless, some differences of CNS effects can be described between the four treatments as far as the vigilance, the cognitive and the psychometric dimensions are concerned.

For vigilance, the present electroencephalotropic findings indicate that the two drugs have no deleterious effects on vigilance, according to the fact that delta and theta bands are never modified. Furthermore, the ASI (Alpha Slow wave Index) increase and the global mean complexity decrease are also good arguments for the absence of light and infraclinical deleterious effects on vigilance of the investigated treatments. In counterpart, the absence of modifications or the improvement of vigilance dimension for the Osgood scale and the Recognition reaction time for the Multiple Choice Reaction Time test combined with the ASI increase are further arguments suggesting some overall beneficial vigilance effects after Euphytose® and RUSL 311 at these doses and after single dose administration.

Nevertheless, on a more dynamic level, as assessed by the ERPs methods which allow the investigation of vigilance, as far as arousal is concerned, but also some cognitive skills (McCarthy and Donchin, 1978; Squires *et al.*, 1977; Sutton *et al.*, 1965; Squires *et al.*, 1975; Rohrbaught and Gaillard, 1983; Tecce, 1972), the effects on P300 latency and amplitude at time 0.5h are in favour of some effects of the verum drugs on the time needed by the subjects for the stimulus evaluation. The CNV decrease in amplitude after 4 tablets of Euphytose® may also be interpreted as a decreased arousal level after Euphytose® as compared to placebo, if the distraction-arousal hypothesis proposed by Tecce is considered (Tecce, 1972).

As far as the time-course of the encephalotropic effects (i.e. EEG and ERPs) of Euphytose® and RUSL 311 is concerned, significant changes, as compared to placebo, were observed between time 30 minutes until the end of the kinetic (7h), with a maximum of differences being present during the first two hours. The maximum of ERPs effects was present at time 0.5h unlike the spontaneous EEG where the effects were maximum at time 1.5h and 2h. After time 4 hours some differences still could be evidenced but at a lesser degree. The pharmacodynamics of the four treatments are a short onset and maximum of CNS activity between 1.5h and 2h and some lighter effects until the end of the 7h recordings.

Dose-encephalotropic effects in the present study showed that all the four doses were significantly different from placebo, although there were less important differences between the doses themselves. Only for the two Euphytose® doses the differential effect on CNV can be interpreted as a dose-effect.

Drug-encephalotropic different effects could be described between Euphytose® and RUSL 311. These differences were mostly retrieved on the beta band which was increased in absolute values after RUSL 311 doses and in relative values after Euphytose® doses. The effects on the alpha band were relatively homogeneous and no real difference could be evidenced. Finally, some differential effects could also be described for the ERPs and psychometric tests. These drug-effects have to be ponderated by the fact that as far as the topography of the EEG and ERPs activities is concerned no major differences between Euphytose® and RUSL 311 can be described. Thus, the maximum of effects are always present over fronto-central scalp areas.

Finally, the absence of effects on the motor part of the psychomotor tests is in good agreement of the absence of any peripheral effect of Euphytose® or RUSL 311.

In spite of these drug-encephalotropic differences, the pharmaco-EEG profiles of the four treatments are comparable and are suggesting three possible, clinically relevant, indications of these drugs. These indications are anxiolytic, antidepressant and vigilance improving capacities.

Anxiolytic and sedative properties of the benzodiazepines have been related to two different EEG changes: anxiolysis to an increase in beta activity (absolute and relative energies) and sedation to a decrease in alpha activity (with a concomitant increase of theta and delta activity), two parameters which can exhibit a different evolution (Matejcek, 1979; Kurowski *et al.*, 1982). On the one hand, no significant change in the alpha (or theta-delta) band appeared after Euphytose® or RUSL 311 in this study, in good agreement with the absence of sedative effects experienced by the subjects. On the other hand, the increase in beta absolute energies after RUSL 311 and beta relative energies after Euphytose® are good arguments of some anxiolytic capacities of the two formulations. It has to be stressed on the fact that this absence of clinical sedative effects is only seen with few anxiolytics of the benzodiazepine type, but these latter having often some sedative effects as shown by pharmaco-EEG or psychometric techniques (Itil *et al.*, 1973; Fink *et al.*, 1976; Herrmann and McDonald, 1978; Saletu and Grünberger, 1979; Grünberger and Saletu, 1980; Saletu *et al.*; 1981).

As suggested by Saletu (Saletu *et al.*, 1987) there are at least two types of antidepressants pharmaco-EEG profiles, which are the thymeretic one and the thymoleptic one. The former is characterized by an augmentation of alpha activity, an increase in amplitude, and eventually by attenuation of slow and fast activities indicating activating properties. This pharmaco-EEG profile can be observed with antidepressants as for example desipramine (Saletu *et al.*, 1985), nomifensine (Saletu *et al.*, 1982), fluoxetine (Saletu and Grünberger, 1985), low doses of sertraline (Saletu *et al.*, 1986), zimelidine (Saletu *et al.*, 1986) and moclobemide (Minot *et al.*, 1993). The latter is characterized by a concomitant increase of slow and fast activities and a decrease in alpha activity suggesting sedative qualities. This pharmaco-EEG profile can be observed after imipramine (Saletu and Grünberger, 1988), amitriptyline (Coppola and Herrmann, 1987), maroxepine (Herrmann *et al.*, 1991) and levoprotiline (Herrmann *et al.*, 1991). In addition to the two pharmaco-EEG profiles of antidepressants it seems that an intermediate profile exists, characterized by a concomitant increase of alpha activity, theta and eventually beta activities in absolute energy. As a representative drug of this group, tianeptine can be given as an example (Luthringer *et al.*, 1989).

The present findings indicate and activating effect of Euphytose® or RUSL 311 which leads to a pharmaco-EEG profile close to the thymeritic one and an improvement in vigilance.

The vigilance improvement is objectified by the increase of the ASI. Furthermore, the decrease of the global complexity is an additional argument in favour of an increase of the alpha peak activity and thus in vigilance.

Conclusion

In conclusion, it can be stated that the two treatments as well as the two doses per treatment have encephalotropic effects.

Among the two formulations and for each, the two tested posologies (i.e. 2 and 4 tablets), a choice has to be done for future therapeutic use: the more important modifications of the reactivity threshold with the six plants formulation (*i.e.* Euphytose®) and the lack of cognitive alterations after two tablets leads us to the choice of the six plants formulation using two tablets.

This choice seems to be the most adapted, as far as the desired therapeutic indication is concerned.

References

1. Cooley JW, Tuckey JW. An algorithm for the machine calculation of complex Fourier series. *Math. Comp.*, 1965 ; 19: 297-301.
2. Coppola R, Herrmann W.M. Psychotropic Drug Profiles: Comparisons by topographic maps of absoulte power. *Neuropsychobiology.* 1987 ; 18:97-104.
3. Dago KT, Luthringer R, Lengelle R, Toussaint M, Minot R, Macher JP. A new tool for pharmaco-EEG and EPs mapping kinetics: the dynamic statistical decision tree (DSDT). *European Neuropsychopharmacology*, 1991 ; 1: 477-478.
4. Duffy FH, Barthels PH, Burchfield JL. Significance probability mapping: An aid in topographic analysis of the brain electrical activity. *Electroencephalo Clin Neurophysiol*, 1981 ; 51: 455-462.

5. Fink M, Irwin P, Weinfeld RE, Schwartz MA, Conney AH. Blood levels and electroencephalographic effects of diazepam and bromazepam. *Clin Pharmacol Ther* 1976 ; 20 : 184-191.
6. Grünberger J, Saletu B. Determination of pharmacodynamics of psychotropic drugs by psychometric analysis. *Prog Neuro-Psychopharmacol.* 1980 ; 4:417-434.
7. Guibert S, Cholet R. Euphytose dans l'anxiété généralisée; étude en double aveugle versus oxazepam. *La gazette médicale*, 1990 ; 97:3-7.
8. Herrmann WM, McDonald RJ. A multidimensional test approach for the description of the CNS activity of drugs in human pharmacology. *Pharmacopsychiatria* 1978 ; 11:247-265.
9. Herrmann WM, Schärer E, Wendt G, Delini-Stula A. Pharmaco-EEG profile of maroxepine: Third example to discuss the predictive value of pharmaco-electroencephalography in early human pharmacological evaluations of psychoactive drugs. *Pharmacopsychiatry.* 1991 ; 24:214-224.
10. Herrmann WM, Schärer E, Wendt G, Delini-Stula A. Pharmaco-EEG profile of levoprotiline: Second example to discuss the predictive value of pharmaco-electroencephalography in early human pharmacological evaluations of psychoactive drugs. *Pharmacopsychiatry.* 1991 ; 24:206-213.
11. Hindmarch I. Psychomotor function and psychoactive drugs. *Br J Clin Pharmac* 1980 ; 10:189-209.
12. Itil TM, Polvan M, Hsu W. Clinical and EEG effects of GB94-94 a tetracyclic antidepressant : EEG model in discovery of a new psychotropic drug. *Curr Ther Res*, 1972 ; 14:395-414.
13. Itil TM, Hsu W, Cig E. "Anxiolytic" profile and "bioavailability" of clorazepate dipotassium based on quantitative pharmaco-electroencephalography. *Agressologie* 1973 ; 14:203-212.
14. Jasper HH. The ten twenty electrode system of the Internatinal Federation. *Electroencephalo and Clin Neurophysiol* 1958 ; 10: 371-375.
15. Kurowski M, Ott H, Herrmann WM. Relationship between EEG dynamics and pharmacokinetics of the benzodiazepine lormetazepam. *Pharmacopsychiat* 1982 ; 15:77-83.
16. Laurian S, Gaillard JM, Le PK, Schöpf J. Topographic aspects of EEG profile of some psychotropic drugs. *Adv Biol Psychiatr* 1983 ; 13:165-171.
17. Luthringer R, Minot R, Toussaint M, Macher JP. EEG and EP mapping of a new 5 HT AD: Stablon. *Biol Psychiat* 1989 ; 25:159.
18. Matejcek M. Pharmaco-electroencephalography : the value of quantified EEG in psychopharmacology. *Pharmacopsychiat* 1979 ; 12:126-136.
19. McCarthy G, Donchin E. A metric for thought: a comparison between P3 latency and reaction time. *Science* 1981 ; 211:77-80.
20. Minot R, Luthringer R, Macher JP. Effect of moclobemide on the psychophysiology of sleep/wake cycles: a neuroelectrophysiological study of depressed patients administered with moclobemide. *International Clinical Psychopharmacology* 1993 ; 7:181-189.
21. Rohrbaugh JW, Gaillard AWK. Sensory and motor aspects of the contingent negative variation. In: Gaillard. *Ritter, Tutorials in ERP research: the endogenous components.* North-Holland, Amsterdam, 1983.
22. Saletu B. Psychopharmaka, Gehirntätigkeit und Schlaf. Munich; Karger, 1976.
23. Saletu B, Grünenberger J. Evaluation of pharmacodynamic properties of psychotropic drugs : Quantitative EEG, psychometric and blood level investigations in normals and patients. *Pharmacopsychiatria* 1979 ; 12:45-58.
24. Saletu B, Grünberger J, Amrein R, Skreta M. Assessment of pharmacodynamics of a new "controlled-release" form of diazepam (Valium® CR Roche) by quantitative EEG and psychometric analysis in neurotic subjects. *J Int Med Res* 1981 ; 9:408-433.

25. Saletu B, Grünberger J, Linzmayer L, Taeuber K. The pharmacokinetics of nominfensine. Comparison of pharmacokinetics and pharmacodynamics using computer pharmaco-EEG. *Int Pharmacopsychiat* 1982 ; 17:43-72 .
26. Saletu B, Grünberger J, Kinzmayer L. Is amezinium metilsulfate - a new antihypotensive drug psychoactive ? Comparative quantitative EEG and psychometric trials with desipramine and meth amphetamine. *Curr Ther Res,* 1985 ; 28:800-826.
27. Saletu B, Grünberger J. Classification and determination of cerebral bioavailability of fluoxetine: Pharmacokinetic, pharmaco-EEG and psychometric analyses. *J clin Psychiat* 1985 ; 46:45-52.
28. Saletu B, Grünberger J, Linzmayer L. On central effects of serotonine re-uptake inhibitors: Quantitative EEG and psychometric studies with sertraline and zimelidine. *J Neural Transm* 1986 ; 67: 241-266.
29. Saletu B, Anderer P, Kinsperger K, Grünberger J. Topographic Brain Mapping of EEG. In: *Neuropsychopharmacology* - Part II. Clinical Applications (Pharmaco EEG Imaging). *Meth and Find Exptl Clin Pharmacol,* 1987 ; 9:385-408.
30. Saletu B. The use of pharmaco-EEG in drug profiling. In: Hindmarch I, Stonier PD (eds). *Human Psychopharmacology. Measures and Methods.* Vol. 1. John Wiley and Sons, Chichester, New-York : 1987 ; 173-200.
31. Saletu B, Grünberger P. Drug profiling by computed electroencephalography and brain maps, with special considerations of sertraline and its psychometric effects. *J Clin Psychiatr* 1988 ; 49 suppl. ; 59-71.
32. Sannita WG, Cabri M, Montano VF, Rosadini G. Quantitative EEG and behavioral effects in volunteers of a new benzodiazepine in relation to drug plasma concentration. *Ther Drug Monit,* 1981 ; 3:341-349.
33. Soufflet L, Toussaint M, Luthringer R, Koudou DT, Gresser J, Minot R, Macher JP. A statistical evaluation of the main interpolation methods applied to three dimensional EEG mapping. *Electroencephalo Clin Neurophysiol,* 1991 ; 79: 393-402.
34. Spiegel R, Aebi HJ. *Method for recording subjective drug effects in psychopharmacology, an introduction.* Wiley and Sons, Chichester 1983.
35. Squires NK, Squires KG, Hillyard SA. Two varieties of long latency positive waves to unpredictable auditory stimuli. *Electroenceph Clin Neurophysiol* 1975 ; 38:387-401.
36. Squires KC, Petruchowski S, Wickens C, Donchin E. The effects of stimulus sequence on event-related potentials: a comparison of visual and auditory sequences. *Percept Psychophys* 1977 ; 22:31-40.
37. Sutton S, Braren M, Zubin. J. ER. Evoked potential correlates of stimuli uncertainty. *Science,* 1965 ; 150:1187-1188.
38. Tecce JJ. CNV and psychological processes in man. *Psychol Bull* 1972 ; 77: 73-108.
39. Valli M, Paubert-Braquet M, Picot S, Fabre R, Lefrançois G, Rod D. Euphytose®, an Association of plant extracts with anxiolytic activity : investigation of its mechanism of action by an In vitro binding study. *Phytotherapy Research* 1991 ; 5:241-244.

13

Therapeutic sleep deprivation in patients resistant to antidepressants

S. KASPER[1], S. RUHRMANN[1], RH. VAN DEN HOOFDACKER[2]

[1] *Department of Psychiatry, University Bon, Bonn, Germany.*
[2] *Department of Psychiatry, University of Groningen, The Netherlands.*

> In some cases sleep may do more harm than good,
> in that flegmatick, cold, and sluggish melancholy...
> (it) fils the head ful of gros humors ;
> causeth destillations, rheumes,
> great store of excrements in the brain.
> Robert Burton, *The Anatomy of Melancholy*, 1651, page 90.

Research on the antidepressant effects of sleep deprivation (SD) has been carried out since the first description of Shulte in 1966. However, the knowledge about the depressiogenic effect of sleep is known to doctors already at least as long as the description of Burton in 1651 (*see* quotation above). The antidepressant response to SD has been achieved with either total (TSD) or partial sleep deprivation (PSD) of the second half of the night. In TSD the patient is not allowed to sleep for the day previous to the night of SD, during the whole night of SD and during the next day (40 hours), whereas in PSD the patient is kept awake for the second part of the night and the following day (*see* Table I). The typical antidepressant response to SD is rapid and dramatic in about 60% of patients with major depression (Kuhs and Tölle, 1992 ; Wu and Bunny, 1990 ; Wehr, 1990 ; Leibenluft and Wehr, 1992 ; Kasper, 1990) but is often reversed by recovery sleep or even naps, especially in morning hours (Wiegand *et al.*, 1992). Among the dimensions of depressive symptomatology which change most dramatically are : depressed mood, deactivation, anxiety, vulnerability, tiredness, motor excitement, drowsiness, self-esteem (*see also* Table II). Whereas non-responder to SD do not show these changes and are by enlarge also not negatively affected, it is noteworthy that age-matched healthy controls feel deteriorated on the items which are improved by depressed patients (*see* Figure 1). The medication status, on medication or without medication, does not seem to play a role for the acute effect of SD (e.g. on the day after then night without sleep). However, there is some evidence that antidepressants can prevent the relaps after the recovery night, at least partially (Kasper, 1992 ; Elsenga and v.d. Hoofdakker, 1983, 1990), especially if they excert a serotonergic mechanism of action.

Table I. Types of therapeutic sleep deprivation (SD).

Total SD	The patients are awake on the day prior to SD, during the SD-night and on the day after the night of SD
Partial SD (Late)[1]	Patients are allowed to sleep until 1 : 00 a.m. and are awake during the remaining night and the whole day
Phase advance therapy[2]	Patients are shifted in their sleep-wake cycle for 6 hours and sleep from 6 p.m. until 1 a.m. after 14 days shift back in hourly intervals until normal schedule
REM - deprivation[2]	Selective deprivation of REM sleep by acoustic stimuli

[1] Partial sleep deprivation (early) in which patients are asked to stay up until 1 : 00 a.m. and sleep thereafter has not been shown to be therapeutic effective.
[2] Just for research settings because very labor intensive and no apparent advantage over the other settings.

Table II. Efficacy of therapeutic sleep deprivation (SD).

Single night	60% of patients with major depression exhibit good antidepressive response on the day after a night of SD, however worsening after recovery night which can be partially prevented by the simultaneous usage of antidepressants	
Repeated SD	good response if adjunctive to antidepressants (e.g. twice a week)	
Improvement in following items*		
	Depression	49%
	Deactivation	39%
	Anxiety	32%
	Vulnerability	20%
	Tiredness	19%
	Motor excitement	18%
	Drowsiness	15%
	Self-esteem	10%

* EWL-L items (Janke and Debus 1977). Data from 50 responders (53% of a sample of medication free patients with major depression) (Kasper, unpublished observation)

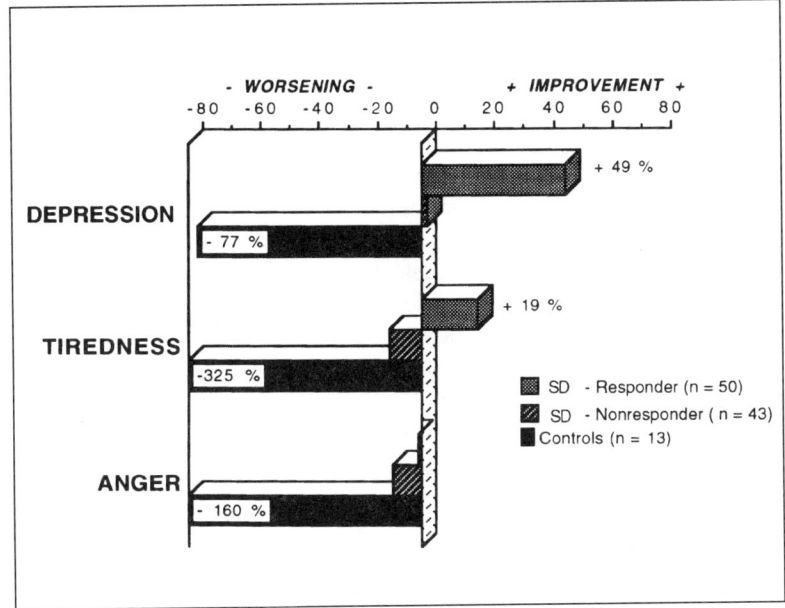

Figure 1. Efficacy of sleep deprivation (SD) in healthy controls, SD-Nonresponders and SD-responders.

As indicated in Table III there are several clinical indications for the usage of SD : it can be used for differential diagnosis of pseudodementia (Reynolds et al., 1987), prediction of subsequent antidepressant response (Kasper, 1992), and also, if used repetitively, as an adjunct to antidepressants in depressed patients which were considered as resistant to antidepressant alone.

Table III. Indications for therapeutic sleep deprivation (SD).

Therapeutic
Differential diagnosis to pseudodementia
Predication
+ Antidepressives : additive efficacy
Resistance to antidepressants

Non-response to antidepressants

Approximately 30% of patients of patients with major depression (or equivalent diagnosis and depressive symptomatology) do not respond to the first antidepressive treatment to which they are exposed at least for 4 weeks (Möller, 1991). Furthermore, there is an increasing number of patients refractory to antidepressants in inpatient services, at least in Germany. Different treatment strategies have therefore been developed to treat this patient group (Helmchen, 1990 ; Möller, 1991 ; Heimann 1974). These strategies include obligatory as well as facultative treatment steps. As a general rule antidepressants should be given for an adequate duration (4 weeks) and in an adequate dosage (equivalent to 150 mg amitriptyline). Furthermore, there is the need for the achievement of an adequate blood level, with the possibility to identify fast metabolizers. If patients do not respond to the first antidepressant to which they are exposed, which does not necessarily have to be a classical one, like the older tricyclic or tetracyclic compounds are often termed, there is the need for a switch to an antidepressant with a different mechanism of action (e.g. serotoninergic or noradrenergic). A next step can be the combination of an antidepressant with lithium and later also the addition of L-Tryptophane or L-Hydroxytryptophane (at present not available on the market). However, the combination with these compounds cannot be recommended for selective-serotonin-reuptake inhibitors (SSRIs). The addition of T_3 (25 - 50 ug/day) to antidepressant drugs may also be helpful (Joffe and Singer, 1990). A further step, if not already taken before, may be the application of a monoamine-oxidase-inhibitor (MAO-I) and finally electroconvulsive therapy (ECT) can be considered. However, it needs to be mentioned that ECT can also be the treatment of choice for a first intervention for a carefully selected group of patients.

Repetitive sleep deprivation (e.g. twice a week TSD or three times a week PSD) as well as light therapy (2500 lux, 2 hours each day, for at least 3 weeks) can be considered as an adjunctive therapy to antidepressants in every stage of the above mentioned treatment strategy. There are no data if repeated SD without antidepressants can be successfully used in patients which are considered as non-responders to antidepressants. Supportive psychotherapy has been shown to be helpful in patients with specific problem constellations and the addition of neuroleptics is necessary if depression is associated with a psychotic symptomatology.

Table IV. Adjunctive therapies to antidepressants in patients resistant to antidepressants alone.

Repeated sleep deprivation (partial or total)
Lithium (a level of 1.0 mmol/l should be reached)
Thyroid hormones (T_3, 25-50 mg/ day)
Light therapy (>2500 Lux for at least 3 weeks)

One of the shortcomings in the literature is the lack of operationalized criteria in the reports on treatment resistant depressions. A practical one would be (Kasper et al., 1992) : (1) non-response to at least three antidepressants with a different mechanism of action (one of them should preferably be a MAO-I), (2) duration of each medication for a least 4 weeks in a sufficiently high dosage - equivalent to 150 mg amitriptyline - and (3) at least one of the antidepressants was used in a combination therapy with another antidepressant.

Studies on the efficacy of SD in patients resistant to antidepressants

There are no studies available in the literature in which the antidepressant response of SD is described for patients resistant to antidepressants using operationalized criteria about nonresponsivenes to antidepressant medication. Furthermore, all of these studies have been carried out in a non-controlled fashion (for overview see Table V).

Pflug and Tölle (1971) and later Lit (1973) firstly mentioned that there is the same indication and efficacy for SD as for electroconvulsive therapy (ECT), but SD is the more physiological approach. Bhanji and Roy (1975) noticed that SD still can be beneficial even if patients do not respond to antidepressants as well as to ECT. Probably the most optimistic report is from van Scheyen (1997) who found that 60% of patients responded to SD if they were non responders to antidepressants and ECT. Table VI summarizes the studies which compared the efficacy of SD with ECT, but due to methodological shortcomings it is not possible to generalize these fidings.

Based on single case studies van den Hoofdakker et al. (1992) suggest that the addition of lithium to the combination of SD and antidepressants is capable to achieve an antidepressant response. Dessauer et al. (1985) performed a study in which SD was performed twice weekly additionally to tricyclic antidepressants (mostly amitriptyline). This group found a complete remission in 33% of their sample of patients which were considered as resistant to antidepressants.

Table V. Studies about the efficacy of sleep deprivation (SD) in patients resistant to antidepressants.

Authors	Design	Result
Pflug und Tölle, 1971	Discussion	Indication for SD = ECT
Lit, 1973	open (n = 10)	Indication for SD = ECT
Bhanji und Roy, 1975	open (n = 39)	Response to SD in AD-Nonresponse and/or ECT
van Scheyen, 1977	open (n = 19)	68% Response to SD 53% Response in Patients who are resistent to ECT and Antidepressants
Sack et al., 1985	open (n = 4)	"Phase - Advance Therapy"
Dessauer et al., 1985	open (n= 21)	Repeated SD (5x) 33% complete remission
v.d. Hoofdakker et al., 1992	open (n = 26)	Observation that the combination of AD + TSD + Lithium is successful
Kasper, 1990	open (n = 103)	Single TSD effective in AD-Nonresponders
Zimanova & Voijtechosky, 1974 Sidorowicz, 1976 Wasik und Puchalka, 1978 Manthey et al., 1983		Hint for Response to SD in AD-Nonresponse

SD = therapeutic sleep deprivation, TSD = total sleep deprivation, ECT = electroconvulsive therapy, AD = Antidepressants, AD-Nonresponse = patients considered as nonresponders to antidepressive medications

Table VI. Studies about the efficacy of sleep deprivation (SD) in relation to electroconvulsive therapy (ECT).

Authors	Design	Result
Pflug und Tölle, 1971	Discussion	Same Indication for SD as for ECT SD is a "physiological" therapy (in contrast to ECT).
SD is effective after ineffective ECT		
van Scheyen, 1977	open (n = 19)	53% Response In patients refectory to antidepressants and to ECT
ECT is effective after ineffective SD		
Larsen et al., 1976	open (n = 13)	ECT efficacious in patients which responded to SD or not
Kvist und Kirkegaard, 1980	open (n = 9)	ECT in only 2 of 9 patients effective who were non-responders to SD e.g. ; ECT and SD might have same mechanism of action

SD = therapeutic sleep deprivation, ECT = electroconvulsive therapy.

Based on theoretical considerations of the phase-advance (Wehr et al., 1979) of several biological rhythms in depression Sack et al. (1985) initiated a protocol in which patients (resistant to antidepressants) were advanced in their sleep-wake cycle. With this treatment approach patients were asked to go to bed at 6 pm and were woken up at 1 am. In the course of two weeks duration there was a nearly complete remission of depressive symptomatology, which also did not worsen, when patients were shifted back to a normal rhythm within 1 week (1 hour every day).

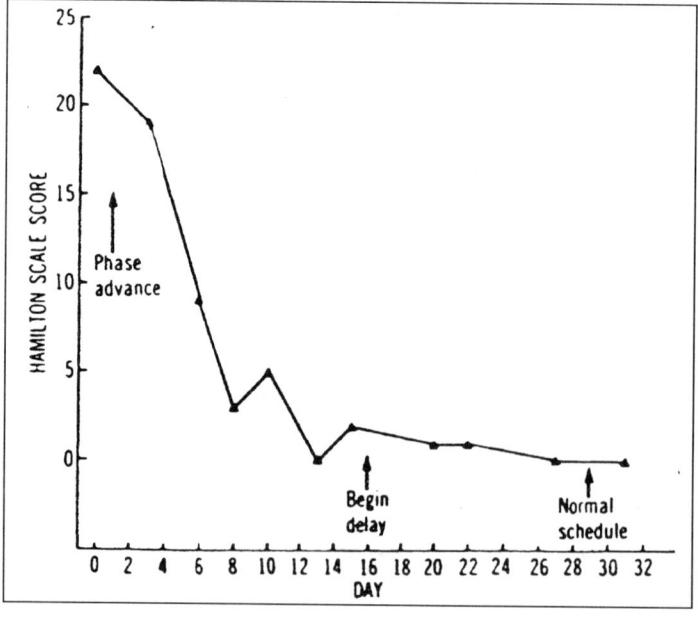

Figure 2. Phase-advance therapy in patients resistant to antidepressants (Sack et al., 1985).

In an approach to find out if a single night of TSD is effective in patients considered as resistant to antidepressants we studied the effect of TSD in 103 medication free (4 - 7 days) patients with major depression. Patients were predominantly unipolar (97 unipolar, 6 unipolar I) with a mean age (± SD) of 52 ± 13 years and 72% were female. TSD was carried out within different biologically oriented therapy protocols and there were no prospective operationalized criteria for antidepressant-nonreponse. However, we recorded very carefully the previous history, especially medication status of these patients. The knowledge of the previous history made it possible to compare patients with a high and low likelyhood for antidepressant-nonresponse. The duration of illness in our sample ranged between 14 and 386 days with a mean (±SD) of 107 ± 89 days. All patients were treated with antidepressants during their actual depressive phase previously to TSD. We defined the group of patients with duration of illness longer than 100 days as the potentially antidepressant-nonresponders (n = 52 ; mean ± SD duration of actual phase ; 174 ± 83 days) and compared the antidepressant effect of one single TSD in this group with the effect to TSD in a group of patients with a duration of illness shorter than 100 days (n = 51 ; mean ± SD duration of the actual phase ; 42± 22 days). Furthermore, we characterized extreme groups with a duration of illness between 14 and 30 days (n = 24) and a group with the duration of illness of 135 to 386 days (n = 24). As can be depicted from Figure 3 there was no difference in response to TSD between these groups. The mean daily difference scores (Kasper *et al.*, 1988) were 29% and 29% for the large groups and 25% and 29% for the extreme groups, respectively. These groups did also not differ in further clinical variables like age, gender, diagnosis, onset of illness or number of phases.

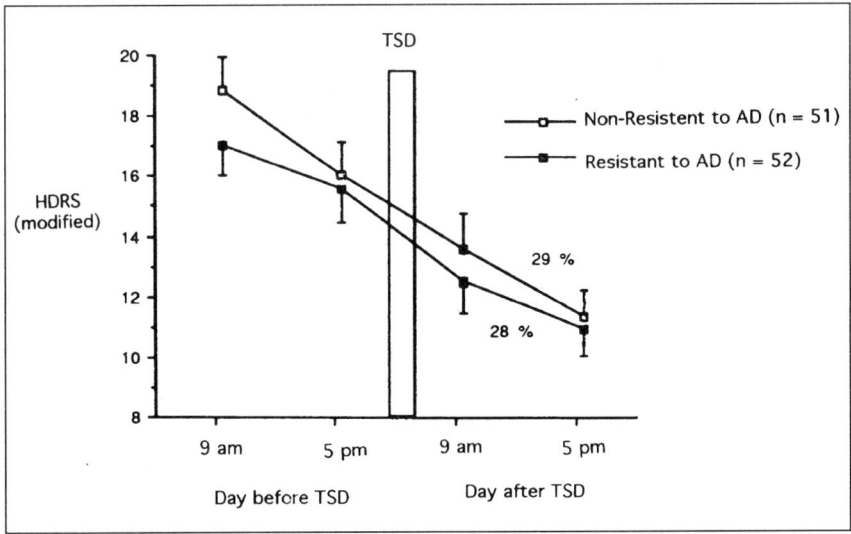

Figure 3. Efficacy of a single night of total sleep deprivation (TSD) in patients with and without resistance to antidepressants.

Sleep deprivation as a probe for the underlying biology in patients resistant to antidepressants

Since the antidepressant response to SD is rapid and not confounded by drug effects it can be serve as a model to study its underlying pathophysiology. Several approaches have been undertaken to explain the antidepressant effect of SD, nevertheless they are not conclusive as yet (Kuhs and Tölle, 1992) Changes of hypothalamus - pituitary - thyroid hormone - axis (HPT) have been discussed to be associated with the antidepressant response to SD (Baumgartner et al., 1986, Kasper et al., 1988). For the treatment of patients resistant to antidepressants changes in the HPT-axis seems to be specific interest since T_3 administration as an adjunct to antidepressants has been reported to be beneficial in over 20 studies (Kissling, 1990).

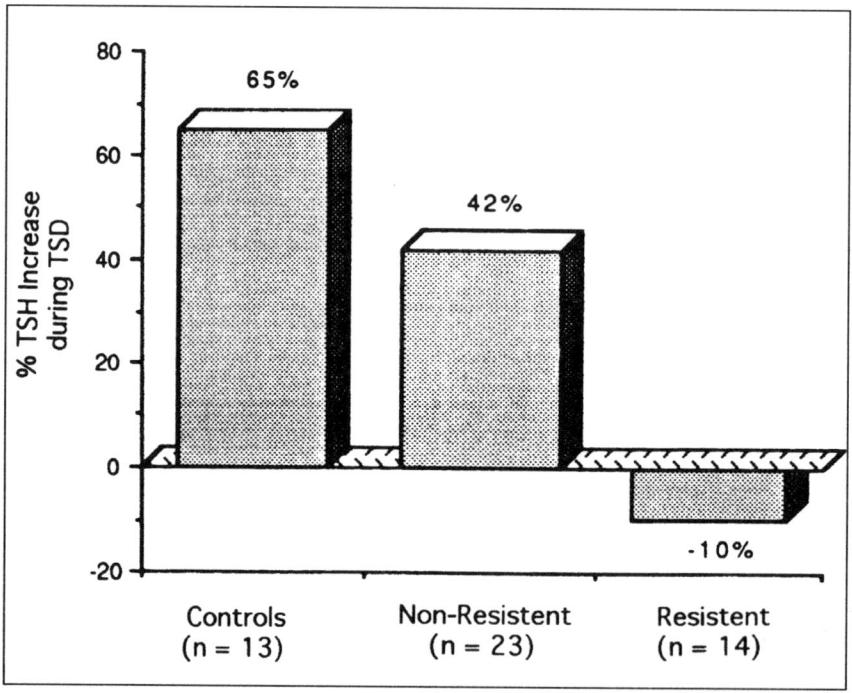

Figure 4. Delta night-time (2 a.m. values) thyreotropin (TSH) concentrations (night before SD in which patients and controls slept minus sleep derivation night) in patients with and without resistance to antidepressants and in healthy controls.

We therefore studied TSD-induced changes of thyroid hormones (free T_3 and T_4) as well as thyreotropin (TSH) in a subgroup of 37 patients of the above mentioned sample and also in 13 healthy controls. Since thyroid hormones as well as TSH peak at night time (Sack et al., 1987) we obtained 2 : 00 a.m. samples in the night before TSD in which patients and controls slept and also during the night of sleep deprivation.

Differences between these two values are expressed as delta values and outlined in Figure 4 for controls (n =13), depressed patients considered as resistant to antidepressants (n = 14) and depressed patients without this characteristic (n = 23). Whereas healthy controls had an increase of TSH values of 65%, there was just a 42% increase in depressed patients without AD nonresponse and no increase, even a 10% decline, in patients which were considered as resistant to antidepressants. Our finding might delineate the pathophysiological basis for the used clinical praxis to add thyroxine to depressed patients resistant to antidepressants (Joffe et al., 1990). A blunted reagibility to the physiological stimulation with TSD might indicate that the HPT-axis is hypofunctional. Since our group of patients also had higher $F-T_3$ levels (resistant to antidepressants : 2,1 pg/ml) nonresistant to antidepressants : 1,7 pg/ml) than healthy controls (1,3 pg/ml) this might be indicative that there are differences in energy consumption which might be linked to the antidepressant response to the therapeutic action of sleep deprivation.

Conclusion

There is some strong evidence that SD is of the use in the treatment of depressed patients refractory for antidepressants. Furthermore, it seems that the acute efficacy and probably also the efficacy of repeated SD is independent from the state of depression (e.g. acute versus chronic). Nevertheless, there are no controlled studies as yet published in the literature on this theme and in all studies there is a lack of prospective operationalized criteria for antidepressant-nonresponse. For practical treatment protocols we recommend repeated SD as an adjunct to antidepressants, but we are unable to recommend a specific class of antidepressants. A further exploration of the possibilities of the combination of SD and Lithium seems worthwhile since sudden and sustained improvements have been found in single case studies (van den Hofdakker et al., 1992). Since there is an cute antidepressant response to SD in at least 50% of patients characterized as therapy resistant depression and since this effect is not confounded by drug effects it can also serve as a tool for studying the underlying pathophysiology of this group of patients which has been seldomly being the subject of research in biologically oriented research protocols.

References

1. Baumgartner A, Meinhold H. Sleep deprivation and thyroid hormone concentrations. *Psychiatry Res.* 1986 ; 19 : 241-2.
2. Bhanji S, Roy G.A. The treatment of psychotic depression by sleep deprivation : A replication study. *Br J Psychiatry* 1975 ; 127 : 222-6.
3. Burton R. *The anatomy of melancholy* 1651 ; 90.
4. Dessauer M, Götze U, Tölle R. Periodic sleep deprivation in drug-refractory depression. *Neuropsychobiology* 1986 ; 13 : 111-6.

5. Elsenga S, Hoofdakker RH van den. Clinical effects of sleep deprivation and clomipramine in endogenous depression. *J Psychiatric Res* 1983 ; 17 : 361-74.
6. Elsenga S, Hoofdakker RH van den. Antidepressant medication and total sleep deprivation in depressives. In : Bunney, Hippius, Laakmann, Schmaub (Eds). *Neuropsychopharmacology* 1990 ; 639-51.
7. Helmchen H. Gestuftes Vorgehen bei Resistenz gegen Antidepressiva-Therapie. In : Möller (Hrsg) Therapieresistenz unter Antidepressiva-Behandlung. Springer, Berlin Heidelberg New York, 1990 ; 237-50.
8. Heimann H. Therapy-resistant depressions : symptoms and syndromes. *Pharmacopsychiatry* 1974 ; 7 : 139-44.
9. Hoofdakker RH van den, Gordijn MCM, Kasper S. On the contribution of sleep deprivation to the treatment of therapy-resistant depression (in preparation) 1992.
10. Janke W, Debus G. Die Eigenschaftswöterliste (EWL-L). Ein Verfahren zur Erfassung der Befindlichkeit. Hogreve, Göttingen 1977.
11. Joffe RT, Singer W. A comparison of triiodothyronime and thyroxine in the potentation of tricyclic antidepressants. *Psychiatry Res* 1990 ; 32 : 241-51.
12. Kasper S, Katzinski L, Lenare T, Richter P. Auditory evoked potentials and total sleep deprivation in depressed patients. *Psychiatry Res* 1988a ; 25 : 91-100.
13. Kasper S, Sack DA, Wehr TA, Kick H, Voll G, Vieira A. Nocturnal TSH and Prolactin secretion during sleep deprivation and prediction of antidepressant response in patients with major depression. *Biol Psychiatry* 1988b ; 24 : 631-41.
14. Kasper S. Schlafentzugstherapie - eine Chance bei Antidepressiva-Nonresponse. In : Möller HJ. (Ed) Therapieresistenz unter Antidepressiva-Behandlung. Springer, Berlin Heidelberg New york, 1990 ; 149-65.
15. Kasper S, Antidepressant medication and therapeutic sleep deprivation in depressed patients. In : Macher JP, Crocq MA (Eds) New york prospect in psychiatry. *The bioclinical interface I*. Elsevier Amsterdam London New York Tokyo, 1992 ; 215-22.
16. Kasper S, Höflich G, Ruhrmann S, Rao ML, Scholl HP, Möller HJ. Hormonelle Verlaufsparameter unter Electrokrampftherapie bei Patienten mit therapieresistenter Depression. In : Baumann P. (Ed) Biologische Psychiatrie der Gegenwart. Springer, Wien New york (im Drunck) 1992.
17. Kissling W. Antidepressiv wirksame Zusatzmedikation. In : Möller HJ (Ed) Therapieresistenz unter Antidepressiva-Behandlung. Springer, Berlin Heidelberg New York. 1990 ; 139-145.
18. Kuhs H, Tölle R. Sleep deprivation therapy. *Biol Psychiatry* 1991 ; 29 : 1129-48.
19. Kvist J, Kirkegaard C. Effects of repeated slepp deprivation on clinical symptoms and the TRH test in endogenous depression. *Acta Psychiatr Scand* 1980 ; 62 : 494-502.
20. Larsen JK, Lindberg ML, Skovgaard B. Sleep deprivation as treatment for endogenous depression. *Acta Psychiatr Scand* 1976 ; 54 : 167-73.
21. Leibenluft E, Wehr T.A. Is sleep deprivation useful in the treatment of depression ? *Am J Psychiatry* 1992 ; 149 : 159-68.
22. Lit A. Elektroschock en slaaponthouding. *Tijdschr Psychiatrie* 1973 ; 15 : 56-64.
23. Manthey I, Richter G, Richter J, Dreves B, Haiduk A. Untersuchungsansatz und erste Ergebnisse zur Wirking des Schlafentzugs beim depressiven Syndrom. Psychiatr. Neurol. *Med Psychol* 1983 ; 35 : 398-404.
24. Möller HJ. Therapieresistenz auf Antidepressiva : Risikofaktoren und Behandlungsmöglichkeiten. *Nervenarzt* 1991 ; 62 : 658-69.
25. Pflug B, Tölle R. Therapie endogener Depressionen durch Schlafentzug. *Nervenarzt* 1971 ; 42 : 117-24.

26. Reynolds CF. III, Kupfer DJ, Hoch CC, Stack JA, Houck PA, Berman SR. Sleep deprivation effects in older endogenous depressed patients. *Psychiatr Res* 1987 ; 21 : 95-109.
27. Sack DA, Nurnberger J, Rosenthal NE, Ashburn E, Wehr TA. Potentiation of antidepressant medication by phase advance of the sleep-wake cycle. *Am J Psychiatry* 1985 ; 142 : 606-8.
28. Sack DA, James SP, Rosenthal NE, Wehr TA. Deficient noctural surge of TSH secretion during sleep and sleep deprivation in rapid-cycling bipolar illness. *Psychiatry Res* 1987 ; 23 : 179-91.
29. Scheyen JD van. Slaapdeprivatie bij de behandling van unipolaire (endogene) vitale depressies. *Ned Tijdschr Geneeskd* 1977 ; 121 : 564-8.
30. Schulte W. Kombinierte Psycho-und Pharmakotherapie bei Melancholikern. In Kranz H. (Ed) Probleme Pharmakopsychiatrische Kombinations und Langzeitbehanddlungen. *Karger Basel* 1966 ; 150-69.
31. Sidorowicz W. Sleep deprivation in treatment of depression. *Psychiatr Pol* 1976 ; 10 : 503-7.
32. Wasik A, Puchalka G. Analysis of sleep deprivation as a treatment method in depressive states. *Psychiatr Pol* 1978 ; 12 : 463-8.
33. Wehr TA. Effects of wakefulness and sleep on depression and mania. In : Montpaisier I., Godbowt R. (eds.) Sleep and billogical rhythms. Basic mechanisms and application to psychiatry. Oxford Univ. Press, New York Oxford 1990 ; 42-86.
34. Wehr TA, Wirz-Justice A, Goodwin FK, Duncan W, Gillin JC. Phase advance of the circadian sleep-wake cycle as an antidepressant. *Science* 1979 ; 206 : 710-13.
35. Wiegand M, Riemann D, Berger M. Pathogenetic considerations on the antidepressant effect of sleep deprivation and the depressiogenic impact of daytime naps. In : Racagni G, Brunello N, Fukuda T. (Eds.) *Biological Psychiatry*, Vol. 1. *Excerpta Medica* 1922 ; 797-9.
36. Wu JC, Bunney WE. The biological basis of an antidepressant response to sleep deprivation and relapse : review and hypothesis. *Am J Psychiatry* 1990 ; 147 : 14-21.
37. Zimanova J, Vojtechowsky M. Sleep deprivation as a potentiation of antidepressive pharmacotherapy ? *Activ Nerv Sup* (Praha) 1974 ; 16 : 188-9.

14

Methodological difficulties in clinical trials in developing countries

D. MOUSSAOUI

University Psychiatric Center Ibn Rushd, Casablanca, Morocco.

Research in psychopharmacology is essential for developing countries, and encounters to a more or less extent, the same kind of difficulties than in industrialized countries. However, some of them are rather specific to developing countries. The first type concerns the investigators and their image. There is an almost complete absence of confidence of the pharmaceutical firms in clinical trials conducted in developing countries. They usually propose repetitive, confirmative, open trials to the psychiatrists of these countries, with almost no scientific value. On the other hand, it is true that the status of investigator is rather rare in developing countries, especially for nurses. As a matter of fact, therapeutic activities do not leave enough time to psychiatrists for research.

The second type of difficulties concerns the patients, generally illiterate, the patient and his family understand with difficulty the aim of a clinical trial, and very rarely accept to sign an informed consent. Ethical issues should be probably managed differently in a developing and in an industrialized country. On the other hand, demographic data collected from the patients and their families are not always accurate. Patients do have also a passive attitude toward the investigating team, and the prescriptions. The third kind of difficulty is clinical, concerning the unavailability of translated and validated rating scales and standardized interviews, not to mention cultural difficulties in the classification of mental disorders.

The proposed solutions need a multisectoral cooperation between the national associations of psychiatry, international NGOs, the WHO, and governmental regulatory agencies, in order to train psychiatrists from developing countries in methodology of psychopharmacological research. The pharmaceutical firms do have a responsibility as well, by monitoring rigorously good clinical trials conducted in developing countries.

It is obvious that there is no possible development of psychiatry in developing countries without progress in the field of psychopharmacology. As a matter of fact, the considerable pressure of demand of the community in mental health care is so heavy, mostly with severe psychotic patients, that the main therapeutic tool of psychiatrists in these countries remain psychotropic medications. Within the general situation characterized by lack of means, the budgets allocated to the purchase of medications is usually much below the real needs.

Therefore, psychiatrists from developing countries need to master the rules of psychopharmacology in an even better way than those of industrialised countries. S. Potkin, who worked in China for about two years, used to say: «It is too expensive for a developing country not to do research in psychopharmacology and biological psychiatry.» Among the most important aspects of the latters, clinical trials of psychotropic medications should be given a special attention [1].

In developing countries, universal difficulties are encountered when designing or conducting a clinical trial. As one can notice, there is a constant increase in the sophistication of the methodology of clinical trials, such as strict inclusion criteria for a better homogeneity of the studied group of patients, double-blind design, restriction of concomitant use of other medications, placebo control, wash-out periods, use of a fixed dose of a given medication, statistical methods.

Moreover, there are some specific methodologic difficulties in designing and conducting clinical trials in developing countries. These difficulties can be related to :
- the investigators ;
- the patient or ;
- the clinical domain.

Difficulties related to the investigators

Generally speaking, the investigators working in a developing country have a bad image, although sometimes, the same investigators might have good positions in research in an industrialised country. This bad image is due to many facts :
- There is hardly some training in research in the best departments of psychiatry in industrialised countries. In developing ones, unfortunately, it is clear that training in research is even less considered.
- Furthermore, there is no such training for, or a position as research nurse. Most of the time, residents or even psychiatrist, have to do the work of the nurses, in order to be sure that it is done correctly. It happens sometimes that research activities are perceived by the medical team as being a luxury in a developing country, or even detrimental to the patients.
- It is also obvious that for the vast majority of the health institutions, therapeutic activities lets little time for training and research. It is clear that, the less psychiatrists from developing countries conduct clinical trials, the less they will be able to do so, since methodology is evoluting very quickly.

All these reasons explain that pharmaceutical firms has little confidence in the clinical trials conducted in a developing country. That is why the kind of clinical trials usually proposed to the psychiatrists in developing countries are «me too» studies, or open trials with almost no scientific interest, and which real objective is to familiarize the clinician with the prescription of a considered psychotropic medication. Sometimes, suggestions are made to some clinicians to conduct clinical trials which are not completely ethical, for example due to insufficient toxicological data, or by including patients with possibly too high risk/benefit ratio. The solution for such problems is to submit all the clinical trials to local ethical committees.

Difficulties related to the patients

An important question is to know if ethical issues are universally applicable or not. For example, can informed consent be used the same way all over the world ? Our experience leads us to answer no to this question, because asking a patient to sign an informed consent in some developing countries, can be interpreted as a lack of confidence, and can threaten the doctor-patient relationship. This is probably why the positions of the good clinical practice of the World Health Organization (WHO) and the one of a European country like France, are slightly different on this matter [2,3].

On the other hand, data collection are most of the time difficult to realize with illiterate patients, compared to those having been educated. Patients coming from lower economic class, usually leaving in a traditional culture, tend also to be very passive in their relationship with the investigating team and toward the prescriptions. Their cooperation is therefore less than satisfactory. It is also important to stress that most of the patients are not used to verbalize their problems, and would rather express themselves through somatization.

Finally, the profile of the patients seen in many psychiatric institutions in developing countries are mainly severely psychotic patients in the public sector. Even academic institutions function sometimes as primary referral ones. Wash out periods for severely disturbed patients are not easy to respect. It is more difficult to recruit other kind of patients for various clinical trials in psychiatric institutions. Mildest cases of mental disorders can be found of course in the consultations of G.P.s, but they are even less prepared to participate to a study than psychiatrists.

Difficulties related to clinical aspects

From the clinical point of view, rating scales are seldom translated in the vernacular languages, and rarely validated. It is even more so for the semi-standardised interviews. On the other hand, there are still some unresolved issues concerning diagnosis and classification in psychiatry, both with DSM-III-R and ICD 10. So far, anthropological and cultural aspects have not been correctly addressed in these classifications.

What can be done ?

Psychiatrists and pharmacologists from developing countries should invest specially in improving their knowledge and their know-how in clinical trials and psychopharmacology. They should also be helped, for various reasons, to conduct better clinical trials :

- Helping psychiatrists and pharmacologists from developing countries is not only a matter of ethics, toward countries who suffer from many shortages. As a matter of fact, the kind of patients one can find in developing countries is difficult to find in industrialised ones. Never treated schizophrenics for example, are frequently found in developing countries, and can represent a unique field of research in psychopharmacology.

- The number of patients included in a clinical trial conducted in a developing country can be important, since catchment areas concern usually large populations. Instead of doing a multi-center, multi-national collaborative study with the methodologic difficulties related to such kind of research, a larger one can be conducted in a few centers from developing countries, which do have the technical know-how for a good clinical trial. This can save time and money for the pharmaceutical firm.

- Finally, transethnic-transcultural psychopharmacology is not only a fashionable trend of psychopharmacology, it is another way of making progress in the knowledge of psychobiology and psychopharmacology in general, for the best interest of the patients all over the world.

Who can do what ?

- In order to improve the situation of research in psychopharmacology in developing countries, pharmaceutical firms have some responsibility, as it has one in the continuing medical education. Organizing training seminars before a clinical trial, and monitoring it rigorously, are some of the tools which can improve the status of research in psychopharmacology in developing countries.

- Regulatory governmental agencies have also a responsibility. Depending on the available teams and their expertise, they should ask for a minimum of good studies in the country, before allowing the marketing of a new psychotropic medication.

- National societies of psychiatry and/or psychopharmacology do have a responsibility as well, by promoting the knowledge and the know-how in psychopharmacological research. International non governmental organizations (like the World Psychiatric Association - WPA, the Collegium Internationale Psychopharmacologicum-CINP, or the World Federation of Societies of Biological Psychiatry), as well as the WHO can also improve the research situation in psychopharmacology in developing countries. Both the WPA and the CINP have sections on education, the latter having a special programme of psychopharmacology directed toward developing countries. The WHO Network in Biological Psychiatry and Psychopharmacology has also, and since the mid 70's involved more and more centers from developing countries in these fields. It had, in particular, a special educational programme named «Travelling Seminar in Biological Psychiatry and Psychopharmacology». Finally, the WHO has recently sponsored a newsletter on transethnic and transcultural psychopharmacology, which is published in different languages.

These NGOs and the WHO can work more specifically on important issues like training for rating scales, and standardized interviews, as well as teaching good clinical practice.

In summary, the situation of research in psychopharmacology in developing countries is not at the level where it should be. There are obstacles due to the investigators themselves, to the patients and to the clinical domain in developing countries. The joint efforts of NGOs, the WHO, and the pharmaceutical firms, as well as regulatory agencies, can play an important role in order to improve the quality of research in psychopharmacology, especially concerning clinical trials, in developing countries.

References

1. Moussaoui D. Biological psychiatry in Arab countries. In: Shagass et al., eds *Biological Psychiatry 1985*, Elsevier 1986 ; 1531-1533.
2. World Health Organization. WHO guidelines for good clinical practice (GCP) for trials on pharmaceutical products. Division of Drug Management and Policies, Geneva, draft 8.9.1992, 20 p.
3. Ministère des Affaires Sociales et de l'Emploi - Ministère Chargé de la Santé et de la Famille - Bonnes Pratiques Cliniques, Paris, 1987, 21 p.

15

Value of computerized EEG and evoked potentials in the diagnosis of depressive pseudodementia

P. MORAULT[1,2], E. PALEM[1], M. BOURGEOIS[1], J. PATY[2,3]

[1] Unité d'Investigations Cliniques Approfondies, Hôpital Charles-Perrens, 121, rue de la Bêchade, 33076 Bordeaux, France.
[2] Service d'Explorations Fonctionnelles du Système Nerveux, Hôpital Pellegrin-Tripode, Place Amélie-Raba-Léon, 33076 Bordeaux, France.
[3] Laboratoire de Médecine Expérimentale, Université Bordeaux-II, rue Léo-Saignat, 33076, Bordeaux, France.

The accuracy of computerized EEG (cEEG) and evoked potentials (EP) in discriminating depressive pseudodementia from dementia was evaluated in 11 inpatients with recent cognitive impairment (all with DSM-III-R diagnosis of dementia). Recordings were performed during wash-out period, then all subjects underwent an ECT and/or antidepressant trial. After this trial, clinical improvement was significant in five patients, while the other six remained unimproved. The electrophysiological data of the two groups were retrospectively compared. Discriminant stepwise analysis showed that the combination of two cEEG parameters, symmetry of occipital alpha power and frontal alpha/theta ratio, was able to discriminate future responders from non-responders with a greater accuracy than clinical, classical EEG and EP parameters.

Severe cognitive and memory impairment often occurs during episodes of depression in the elderly. Sometimes, cognitive disturbances may dominate the clinical picture, but the diagnostic of depression (i.e. depressive pseudodementia) can be made because such disturbances respond favorably to antidepressant treatment (Azorin *et al.*, 1990). However, can a treatment have a nosographic specificity?

Running a therapeutic trial also poses methodological problems: treatment is empirical because only retrospective diagnosis is possible; what should the length of treatment be? When faced with a non-responder, practitioners must deal with a severe dilemma. On one hand, resistent depression is more frequent in the elderly. This provides a rationale for more aggressive treatment. On the other hand, antidepressant treatment and electroconvulsivotherapy (ECT) may have dangerous side effects in incipient dementia patients.

In such a context, practitioners emphasize the need for help in the difficult task of evaluating the potential reversibility of cognitive disturbances in patients with dementia-like symptoms. However, neither classical clinical examination, a specific list of pseudodementia criteria (Wells, 1979), or paraclinical date (dexamethasone suppression test, CT scan) have proved conclusive for diagnostic purposes (review in Azorin et al. 1990; Palem, 1991). Conventional EEG gives a slightly better performance in this difficult task. Abnormal EEGs are more frequent in demented versus pseudodemented patients (Nott and Fleminger, 1975; Ron et al 1979; Brenner et al. 1989). Yet all these studies require the contribution of trained clinical neurophysiologists whose subjectivity can be a prejudicial. Progress electroencephalography has provided new tools such as computerized electroencephalography (cEEG) and event-related potentials (ERP). Characteristic cEEG and ERP profiles have emerged for pure groups of major depressive and demented patients.

Given these considerations, the following questions are addressed in this paper: (1) Do clinically dementia-like patients whose cognitive disturbances will improve with an antidepressive trial exhibit characteristic cEEG and ERP profiles of depression? (2) Do patients whose cognitive disturbances will not improve with an antidepressive trial exhibit characteristic cEEG and ERP profiles of dementia? (3) If both are true, can the different cEEG and ERP profiles discriminate future responders from future non-responders?

The challenge of this longitudinal prospective study was to propose accurate but simple cEEG and ERP indexes of reversibility of cognitive disturbances in dementia-like patients.

Material and methods

Subjects

The experimental sample consisted of 11 inpatients aged from 62 to 88 (mean 75.33± 8 ; 4 men, 7 women) with recent cognitive impairment (less than one year). Patients were recruited from the adult psychiatric unit, the psychogeriatric unit at the «Centre Hospitalier Spécialisé Charles-Perrens», the neurological department and the geriatric unit at the «Centre Hospitalo Universitaire», Bordeaux. The study was explained to all subjects. However, given their cognitive disturbances, they were not considered to be competent to give informed consent, so this was obtained from family members.

Before participating in the study, all patients were required to meet specific psychiatric inclusion and exclusion criteria. Screening included a medical history and physical examination; laboratory tests, including thyroid function tests, serology, determination of folate and vitamine B12 levels; a dexamethasone suppression test (DST); an electrocardiogram and a chest X-ray film. They had cranial computed tomographic scans (CT scan) to rule out focal disease. All patients underwent a 1-week period free of alcohol and psychotropic drugs before beginning the study. They were considered to be medically stable but some required continuing medication for medical illnesses. Patients had independent diagnostic assessments performed by their attending practitioner and one of the authors (EP). They were included if they presented the A, B, C, D criteria of dementia according to DSM-III-R, and a Folstein Mini Mental State examination (MMSE) score of 24 or less (Folstein, 1975). The one DSM-III-R criterion not met was the circular exclusionary E criterion «cannot be accounted for by any nonorganic mental disorder, e.g., major depression accounting for cognitive impairment». In addition, they could not have any other concurrent psychiatric disorder, any neurologic disorder, or other cause of organic dementia (vascular dementia, Parkinson's disease, Huntington's disease, multiple sclerosis, HIV infection, normal pressure hydrocephalus, endocrine, toxic or traumatic dementia). Patients whose behavioral disturbances were incompatible for correct processing of EEG were excluded. Cognitive function was assessed with the Folstein MMSE, the Blessed A and B Scales (A=family information; B=patient examination) (Blessed, 1968). Severity of possible co-occurent depression was rated with the Montgomery and Asberg Depression Rating Scale (MADRS) (Montgomery and Asberg, 1976). The probability of belonging to a group (pseudodementia versus dementia) was assessed with the list of Wells' major clinical features differentiating pseudodementia from dementia (Wells, 1979). In the list, characteristic clinical symptom profiles are proposed for pseudodementia and for dementia in three categories: «clinical course and history», «complaints and clinical behavior», and «clinical features related to memory, cognitive and intellectual dysfunctions».

Procedure

Clinical evaluation and scale compilation, laboratory tests, DST, classical EEG and cEEG were performed during the first week (wash-out period). At the end of the week (D7), a second clinical and scale compilation was done (MMS, Blessed and MADRS) to exclude patients whose cognitive disturbances had improved with psychotropic drug withdrawal.

From D8, all subjects underwent a treatment trial that consisted of six or more ECT and/or antidepressant trials (clomipramine or fluvoxamine) for at least 6 weeks with adequate blood levels. Choice of treatment was done by the patients' attending practitioner, with one author's agreement (EP). If cognitive symptoms remained unimproved after the first trial (6 weeks of adequate antidepressant trial or up to 20 ECT sessions), a second trial with another of the three treatments was proposed, and eventually a third if disturbances were still persistent. These second and third trials were proposed earlier in cases of intolerance to one of them.

Clinical improvement was considered significant if MMSE and Blessed B scores increased 50% or more from the initial rating, according to Azorin's criteria (Azorin *et al.*, 1990). These patients were called «responders». Patients who remained unimproved were called «non-responders».

Clinical, laboratory and electrophysiological data were retrospectively compared between these two groups. Comparisons were made by using a non parametric test (Mann and Whitney). Comparisons of left versus right absolute power for each subject, for each frequency band, and for each scalp area were made by using a one-way analysis of variance (ANOVA) for pairwise comparisons. Pearson's correlations between mean dominant frequency in posterior area and clinical scores were calculated. A stepwise discriminant analysis was performed on clinical and electrophysiological data (P7M: BMDP Statistical Software, 1983).

Clinical and classical laboratory features

Of the 11 patients, 5 were responders and 6 non-responders. Neither clinical nor classical laboratory parameters could have anticipated the response to the antidepressant trial. Details of the clinical study have been presented elsewhere (Palem, 1991), and are summarized in Table I as means ± SDs.

Table I. Sample characteristics.

		Responders (n=5)	Non-Responders (n = 6)	P
Age (years)		74.1±6.6	76.5±9.8	-
MMSE	JØ	17.67±3.2	16.67±3.14	-
	J End	27.5±0.55	17.5±3.27	0.01
Blessed A	JØ	14.42±3.15	13.75±1.41	-
	J End	4.08±2.6	14.33±3.34	0.03
Blessed B	JØ	14.83±7.09	13.42±5.77	-
	J End	30.58±1.66	14.5±4.04	0.001
MADRS	JØ	25.5±11.83	21.5±8.98	-
	J End	5.17±1.17	9.5±5.24	-
Wells' criteria	Ps-D	12.67±1.03	9.17±3.25	0.04
	Dem.	9±1.41	12.67±3.56	-

- = no significant difference.

Conventional EEG and computerized EEG

Introduction

The aim of this study was to seek characteristic cEEG profiles similar to those described for pure groups of major depressive and demented patients. Depression is associated with power asymmetry (review in Timsit-Berthier, 1990). Dementia is associated with a decrease in mean dominant frequency, an increase in absolute and relative theta power, and a decrease in the alpha/theta ratio (Duffy *et al.*, 1984; Coben *et al.*, 1983, 1985; Pentilla *et al.*, 1985; Samson-Dollfus *et al.*, 1989; Gueguen *et al.*, 1987, 1991a-b).

EEG and cEEG recording protocols and data analysis

Silver/silver chloride electrodes were placed at Fp1, Fp2, F3, F4, F7, F8, T3, T4, T5, T6, C3, C4, P3, P4, O1, O2, and Fz, Pz. The reference electrode was passively linked ears. Electrode impedance were less that 3kW. Signals were recorded, amplified, the bandpass filtered from 0.16 to 30 Hz, and the analog record was printed with an 18-channel polygraph (EEG 1A97 Nicolet). Signals were digitized on a 10-bit A to D converter and stored (Pathfinder, Nicolet).

Subjects were seated in a quiet room. Recordings were made in three different conditions: eyes closed, eyes open and under light stimulation. All patients had complete 18-channel conventional EEGs performed before cEEG acquisition. Recordings included longitudinal, transverse bipolar and vertex referential montages. Visual analysis by two trained clinical neurophysiologists (PM and JP) eliminated artifact-contaminated EEG segments. Each selected epoch was analyzed using a fast Fourier transform (FFT) (Hjorth, 1975).

Conventional EEG scoring: Records were read blindly (just after recordings and before antidepressant trial) and independently by two clinical neurophysiologists, both with active practice (P.M. and J.P.). Criteria were: alpha frequency, abundance, topography and reactivity; slow activities were rated as rated as present or absent, focal or generalized. Records were classified as normal or abnormal. Comments were added by the interpreter as needed.

cEEG analysis: Data were analyzed only in the eyes closed situation. Absolute and relative power (power in frequency band/total power 0-30Hz) were calculated for the delta (0.5-3.5Hz), theta (4-7.5Hz), alpha (8-13Hz) and beta 1 (13.5-22Hz) frequency bands, for each electrode. The ratio of power alpha/theta and the mean dominant frequency for each frequency band and for the total frequency band (1-30Hz) were also calculated for each electrode. Values were averaged across 6 selected scalp areas to provide the final cEEG measures. These scalp areas were those proposed by Gueguen *et al.* (1991a), taking account of modifications in blood perfusion with SPECT analysis in dementia. They were: anterior right (F4-F8) and left (F3-F7); central right (C4) and left (C3); posterior right (T6-P4-O2) and left (T5-P3-O1).

Results

Conventional EEG scoring

All the EEGs were classified as normal in responders and abnormal in non-responders by at least one EEG interpreter. Four records were classified by both interpreters as normal in responders and five as abnormal in non-responders.

Generalized background slowings were noted by both interpreters in 5 non-responders and in 1 responder, and by 1 interpreter in 2 responders.

Computerized EEG results

Absolute and relative powers seemed to be lower in delta-theta bands and higher in alpha-beta 1 bands for future responders, but comparisons between the two groups exhibited few significant differences only in right anterior and left posterior areas.

Symmetry of activities: Comparison of left versus right absolute powers for each subject exhibited a significant asymmetry in alpha ($F(1,14)=10.61$, $P=0.006$) and in beta bands ($F(1,14)=4.99$, $P=0.042$) for future responders and no asymmetry for future non-responders. These significant differences were noted in central and posterior scalp areas. This asymmetry was always a left hypoactivity versus right. This led us to propose an alpha symmetry index (left/right alpha absolute power in posterior areas). The further from 1 the index, the more asymmetric the activities. Comparison showed a significant difference of this index between groups ($P=0.01$) (Figure 1).

Frequencies: The mean dominant frequencies for the total frequency band (1-30Hz) were slower for future non-responders, and significant in posterior areas (Figure 2). However, non difference was noted when analyzing the mean dominant frequency for each frequency band.

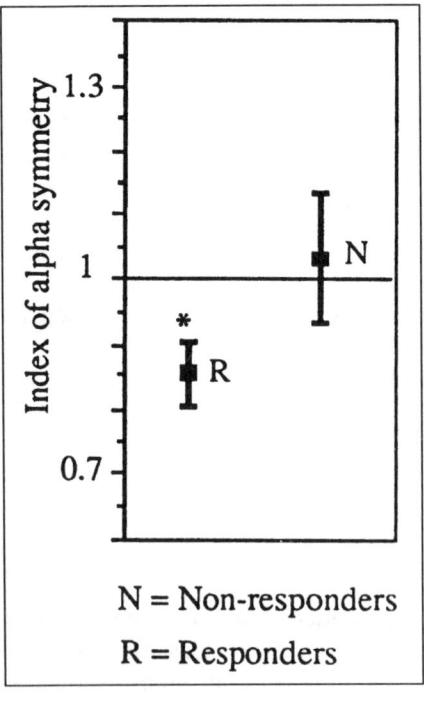

Figure 1. Index of symmetry of alpha activities (left/right) in responders and non-responders.
(* : $P \leq 0.05$).

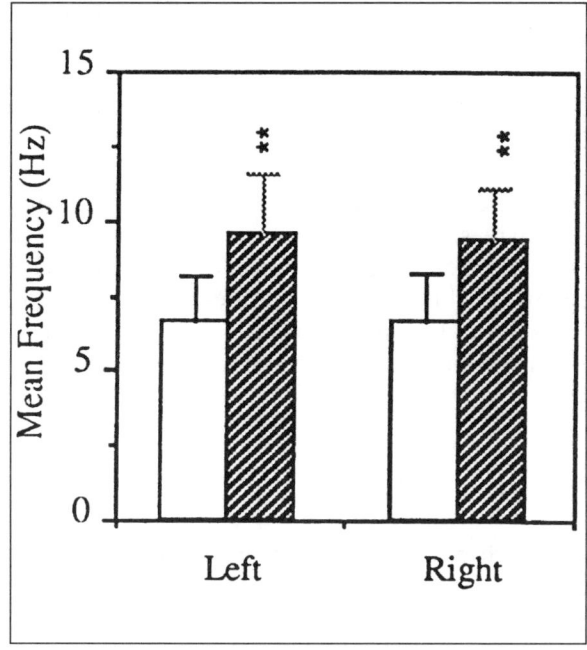

Figure 2. Histograms of mean posterior frequency for total frequency band (1-30 Hz) in responders and non-responders.
(**:P≤0.01).

Correlations between mean posterior frequency (MPF) and clinical parameters: There was no correlation between MPF and age, gender, A and B Blessed scales and MADRS scores, and Wells' pseudodementia features. There was a positive correlation with MMSE scores for the whole population (r=0.665; f=7.14; P=0.02) (Figure 3) and a negative correlation with Well's dementia features (r=0.633; P=0.03). Group analysis revealed a positive correlation between MPF and MMSE scores for future responders (r=0.901; f=12.873; P=0.03), but no relation for future non-responders. Furthermore, if a responder and a non-responder had the same MMSE scores, MPF was always lower for the latter. There was also a strong negative correlation between MPF and the index of alpha power symmetry (r=0.813; f=17.527; P=0.002). The higher the frequency, the more asymmetric the alpha powers.

Stepwise discriminant analysis

Discriminant analysis was proposed on clinical parameters rated at admission (age, gender, MMSE, A-B Blessed and MADRS scores, and Well's features), and on cEEG parameters measured on each area: mean dominant frequency in 1-30Hz band, absolute power of each frequency band, alpha/theta power ratio, index of alpha power symmetry and mean posterior frequency (MPF). A total of 46 parameters were included in this analysis.

Step 0 represents f values. The most pertinent parameters were: «index of alpha power symmetry in posterior areas» in rank 1, «alpha/theta power ratio in right anterior areas» in rank 2 and «MPF» in rank 3. The first clinical parameters were Well's features (pseudodementia features in rank 7 and dementia features in rank 9).

Stepwise analysis gave «index of alpha power symmetry» at step 1, «absolute theta power in left anterior areas» at step 2 and «MMSE scores» at step 3. The combination of the three parameters discriminated the two groups with a 100% sensitivity and a 100% specificity.

These three classical parameters are not of common clinical use because they require averaging of electrode values across scalp areas. In order to provide more direct cEEG measures, we sought the most pertinent electrodes for each area and evaluated the sensitivities and specificities of the measured values. These electrodes were O1-O2 for index of alpha symmetry and MPF, and F7 for alpha/theta power ratio. Cut-off values were 7.8Hz for MPF, 1 for index of alpha symmetry and 1 for alpha/theta power ratio.

A new cEEG index can be proposed:

$$\text{Index EEGq} = \frac{\text{alpha O1/O2}}{\text{alpha theta F7}}$$

With a cut-off value of 0.7, this ratio discriminates the 2 groups with a 100% sensitivity and a 100% specificity. All responders were below 0.6, all non-responders were above 0.8. Respective sensitivities and specificities are presented in Table II.

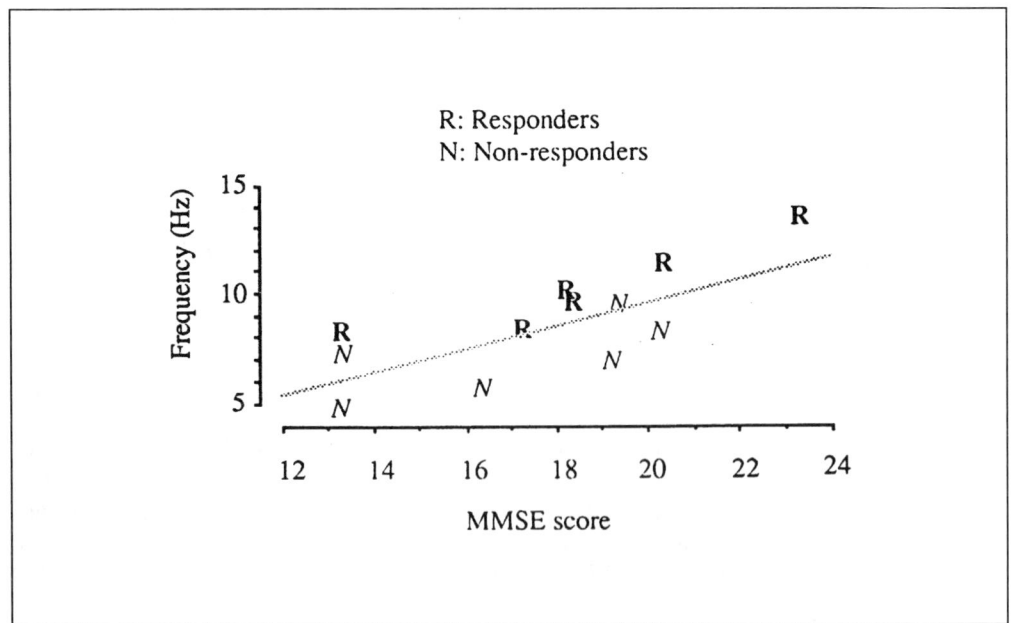

Figure 3. Correlation between MMSE score and mean dominant frequency in posterior areas for the whole population (grey line).

Table II. Sensitivity and specificity of cEEG parameters; number of correct classifications. MPF=mean frequency in O1 and O2 electrodes; L/R occipital alpha ratio=left/right occipital alpha power ratio.

	Cut-off value	Responders (n=5)	Non-responders (n=6)
MPF	< 7.8	0	5
	> 7.8	5	1
L/R occipital alpha ratio	< 1	3	1
	>1	2	5
Frontal α/θ ratio	<1	0	5
	> 1	5	1
C-EEGq index	< 0.7	5	0
	> 0.7	0	6

Event-related potentials (ERPs)

Introduction

As for cEEG, we tried to find the characteristic ERP profiles of depression and dementia in responders and non-responders. Such characteristic profiles have been described elsewhere for pure groups of major depressed and demented patients. More than 80% of demented patients had delayed P300 latencies. On the other hand, P300 latency in depressed patients fell within normal limits. Reports on P300 amplitude in depression are inconclusive; some authors have noted reduced amplitudes whereas others have found no difference between depressed patients and control subjects (review in Morault et al., 1993)

Methods

Four hundred binaural tone bursts (50 msec, 65dB SL, 5 msec rise-fall times) were presented through an earphone at a rate of 1/1.5 sec in each run. Eighty percent (320) of the bursts had a frequency of 1000 Hz and 20 percent (80) a frequency of 2 000 Hz. The stimulus sequence was random with the precondition that no two rare stimuli should appear in succession (usual «odd-ball paradigm»). Before the run, the patient was instructed to keep a mental record of the rare bursts and to report the number at the end of the run. A good ability to perform the task correctly was necessary. Additional electrodes were positioned superior and lateral to the right eye in order to monitor eye-related potentials. Amplification parameters were: band pass = 0.3-70 Hz, time of analysis = 750 msec. Averaged evoked potentials were computed separately for all rare and frequent stimuli in each condition. Four components were usually recorded: N100 (75-150 msec), P200 (120-250 msec), N250 (150-350 msec) and P300 (250-700 msec).

Results

No ERP modification was noted in future responders. Comparisons between the two groups exhibited significant delayed latencies of N100 (P< 0.01) and P200 (P< 0.05) components in future non-responders. No differences in P300 latencies were noted. These ERP components are not specific but are sensitive to cognitive processes and to vigilance, and may reflect information processing (Sutton, 1965). We hypothesize that increased N100 and P200 latencies in non-responders may reflect attentional impairment in such demented patients.

Discussion

Our study confirms than neither classical clinical examination, Wells' specific list of pseudodementia versus dementia features, nor paraclinical data (dexamethasone suppression test, CT scan, ERPs) have proved conclusive for diagnostic purposes. This is congruent with other studies (review in Azorin *et al.* 1990). Conventional EEG exhibits slightly better performances in the same task.

The major finding of this study is that cEEG may provide a safe, simple and effective probe for reversibility of cognitive disturbances in dementia-like patients, before any therapeutic trial. Significant group differences exist in cEEG between patients whose cognitive disturbances will improve after treatment for depression (depressive pseudodementia) compared to patients who will remain unimproved after treatment (dementia). In future responders, alpha power in posterior areas, and mean dominant posterior frequency is higher than in future non-responders. A 100% discriminant sensitivity and specificity is obtained by the combination of two cEEG parameters and one clinical parameter (symmetry of alpha power in posterior areas-alpha/theta power ratio in anterior areas-MMSE score). To avoid averaging of electrode values across scalp areas, we propose a more simple index which only requires measurement of electrode values as given by any cEEG equipment. This index is the ratio (O1/O2 alpha power) (F7 alpha/theta power). With a cut-off value of 0.7, it discriminates the two groups with the same sensitivity and specificity of 100%. Discriminant stepwise analysis does not take account of mean dominant frequency in posterior areas because of the strong correlation with the index of symmetry of alpha power in the posterior areas.

Finally, differences in cEEGs in our two groups of patients are similar to those classically found in pure demented and depressed groups. Similarly, Brenner *et al.* (1989) found the same similarities in waking EEGs. Reynolds *et al.* (1988) and Buysse *et al.* (1988), utilizing EEG sleep data, found that differences between the pure demented and depressed groups also reliably characterized mixed groups of patients (i.e., pseudodemented v.s. demented with secondary depression).

Further studies on a wider sample are necessary. Their aim would not be to provide arguments for a dichotomy between irreversibility and reversibility of cognitive disturbances in the elderly, but rather a rationale for more aggressive treatment of «excess disability».

References

1. Azorin JM, Donnet A., Habib M. Critères pour le diagnostic de pseudodémence dépressive. *L'Encéphale*, 1990; XVI:31-34.
2. Wells CE. Pseudo-dementia, *Am J Psychiatry*, 1979; 136:895-900.
3. Palem E. La Pseudo-démence dépressive. Revue de la littérature et étude personnelle. Thèse de Doctorat en Médecine, Université de Bordeaux II, 1991; N°3038.
4. Nott PN, Fleminger JJ. Presenile dementia: the difficulties of early diagnosis. *Acta Psychiat Scand*, 1975; 51:210-217.
5. Ron MA, Toone BK, Garralda ME, Lishman WA. Diagnostic accuracy in presenile dementia. *Brit J Psychiatry*, 1979; 134:161-168.
6. Brenner RP, Reynolds III Ch F, Ulrich RF. EEG findings in depressive pseudodementia and demantia with secondary depression. *EEG Clin Neurophysiol*, 1989; 72:298-304.
7. Folstein M, Folstein S, Mc Hugh P. «Minimental state»: a practical method for grading the cognitive state of patients for clinician. *J Psychiatry Res*, 1975; 12:189-198.
8. Blessed G, Tomlison BE, Roth M. The association between quantitatives measures of dementia and senile change in the cerebral grey matter of elderly subjects. *Br J Psychiatry*, 1968; 114:797-811.
9. Montgomery SA, Asberg M. A new depression scale designed to be sensitive to change. *Brit J Psychiatry*, 1976; 134:382-389.
10. Timsit-Berthier M. Approche neurophysiologique des états dépressifs. *Psychol Med*, 1990; 22(8):757-763.
11. Duffy FH, Albert MS, Mc Anulty G. Brain electrical activity in patients with senile and presenile dementia of the Alzheimer's type. *Ann Neurol*, 1984; 16:439-448.
12. Coben LA, Danziger WL, Storandt M. A longitudinal EEG study of mild senile dementia of the Alzheimer's type: changes at 1 year and at 2,5 years. *EEG Clin Neurophysiol*, 1985; 61:101-112.
13. Pentilla M, Partanen JV, Soininen H, Riekkinen PJ. Quantitative analysis of occipital EEG in different stages of Alzheimer's disease. *EEG Clin Neurophysiol*, 1985; 60:1-6.
14. Samson-Dollfuss D, Bertoldi I, Hannequin D, Senant J, Denis P, Samson M, Clerc I. Apport de l'EEG quantitatif au diagnostic de maladie d'Alzheimer. In: Leys D, Petit H (éds). *Congrès de Psychiatrie et de Neurologie de langue française: la maladie d'Alzheimer et ses limites*. Masson, Paris, 1989; 271-274.
15. Gueguen B. Aspects électrophysiologiques du vieillissement normal et pathologique. In: *Investigations cliniques et paracliniques dans le vieillissement cérébral*. Doin, Paris, 1987; 199-219.
16. Gueguen B, Derouesné C, Bourdel MC, Guillou S, Landre E, Gaches J, Hossard H, Ancri D, Mann M. Apport de l'EEG quantifié au diagnostic de démence de type Alzheimer. *Neurophysiol Clin*, 1991; a, 21:357-371.
17. Gueguen B, Derouesné C, Bourdel MC, Guillou S, Rahal A, Landre E, Gasnault J, Ancri D. Intérêt de l'EEG pour la prédiction de l'évolution des démences de type Alzheimer. *Neurophysiol Clin*, 1991; b, 21:389-400.
18. Hjorth B. EEG analysis based on time domain properties. *EEG Clin Neurophysiol*, 1975; 29:306-310.

19 Morault P, Bourgeois M, Paty J. *L'électrophysiologie cérébrale en psychiatrie.* Masson, Paris, 1993.
20 Sutton S, Braren M, Zubin J, John ER. Evoked potential correlates of stimulus uncertain. *Science,* 1965; 150: 1187-1188.
21 Reynolds III Ch F, Kupfer DJ, Houck CC, Stack JA, Berman SR, Zimmer B. Reliable discrimination of elderly depressed and demented patients by EEG sleep data. *Arch Gen Psychiatry,* 1988; 45:258-264.
22 Buysse DJ, Reynolds III Ch F, Kupfer DJ, Houck PR, Hoch CC, Stack JA, Berman SR. EEG sleep in depressive pseudodementia. *Arch Gen Psychiatry,* 1988.

16

Phenomenology of aging

O. DOERR-ZEGERS

Psiquiatria y Psicoterapia Luis Thayer, OJEDA n° 0115 of 502, CL, Santiago de Chile, Chili.

In Spanish as in other romance languages, like French, there are two expressions used for referring to the also called «third age», old age or senescence and senility. The first one points to the normal process of aging and the second one to its pathological forms. This distinction is, according to Pelicier, particularly important, since old age or senescence encloses possibilities of compensation, «while in senility, the organism abandons itself to the deficitary process». According to the same author, every approach to the problem of aging will have to take into account the fact that the biological model is not the only possible one and that the notion of old age is closely linked to the cultural and social context, since it is the rest of society who determines at what age and who will have to be considered «old», when somebody must retire from work, cease his/her teaching functions, stop driving a car, etc. In this sense, it is of great value for a modern and scientific approach to the problem of old age to become aware of and, if possible, to eliminate the long series of pre-judices with which our western society still overburden the aged. About this and other general aspects of the problem of old age I will remit particularly to the contributions of the already mentioned French author, as well as to the capital work of the German authors Ursula Lehr.

But today we will not refer to these general aspects of old age. Nor to the social and economic impact that the sustained increase of the population older than 65 years in the modern world means. Our interest is rather directed to certain fundamental aspects which are however somehow forgotten among writers of treatises about the theme, as is the case of certain anthropological radicals such as time and space, or, more precisely, temporality and spatiality of the normal senescent. To determine the essential features of these structural and structuring dimensions of the human world in old age seems to us of the greatest importance, both for a better knowledge of this stage of human life as well as for a better organisation of the corresponding rehabilitating measures, more and more necessary in modern society.

The study of temporality and spatiality in the world of each different mental disease begins around the thirties, together with the development of the phenomenologic-anthropological orientation in psychiatry, and it is linked in its beginnings to the names of Binswanger, V.E. von Gebsattel, E. Minkowski, Erwin Straus and J. Zutt. All of them are in turn tributaries of the analysis of spatiality and temporality of Dasein performed by Martin Heidegger in his capital work «Being and Time». Subsequently the studies about spatiality in melancholic of Tellenbach appeared, being these fundamental to determine the features of the «typus melancholicus» described by this same author and today almost universally accepted as a clinical reality. We have also made some contributions to the problem of spatiality in epilepsy (see Dörr-Zegers, 1981) and in schizophrenia. Likewise other authors have collaborated in establishing the way these existential dimensions are modified in the different mental diseases and their respective premorbid personalities. It is the case, for example, of A. Kraus, B. Kiura, and Y. Pelicier.

Finally, one may mention our attempts to determine both the spatiality and the temporality of certain universal human phenomena not related to pathology, as is the case of love, violence, work and the feminine. We do not know of a similar attempt in the field of normal and/or pathological aging, except what was developed by Buytendijk in relation to body movement in the aged in comparison with the adult and the child, characteristics which in some way come in contact with spatial aspects.

Spatiality of old age

Spatiality is not just one more characteristic of the human being, that he could have or not. As Heidegger says, the human existent or Dasein is spatial from his very structure as being-in-the-world. Human space has little or nothing to do with the space of dimensions, which is measured in centimetres, meters or kilometers. That friend living in Paris, thousand of kilometers away according to geographic space, is much closer than my neighbour, from whom, according to that same space, I am separated by only a few centimetres of wall. The picture hanging from the wall to so many meters of distance away is much closer than the glasses resting on my nose, at an almost care distance of my body. It is the concern or cure (die Sorge) which determines the nearness or distance to something or somebody, according to Heidegger *(op. cit.)*. Now, the human existent is spatial, as we said, but at the same time he/she is permanently granting, giving space (einräumen in German), letting things be in their spatiality. Only in that way is knowledge of things and consequently their management possible; and in the case of others, that giving space to the other, is the basis of respect, of friendship and of love. However, in daily life, men are permanently removing space from each other. This is the fight for vital space, the world of competition in general, so characteristic of commercial activity, but above all, origin of lawsuits (for the limits of a property, for the distribution of an inheritance, etc.) and of wars, where whole populations fight for a determined territory in dispute. Love would be the only exception to this fight for vital space, because in it there is a fusion of the respective spaces of the beings who love each other into one only space which is ours and in a certain way angelical; whose most typical concretion is the embrace, but which is also expressed through sharing the bread, the money and the bed. The aggressive and violent act, instead, would represent the extreme form of the fight for vital space which characterizes daily life of individuals and populations. In this, the other is not raised to a higher dimension, as in love, nor displaced, as in competition, but overwhelmed and destroyed.

Just as there is a space characteristic of commercial activity, another of love and another of violence, as we have recently outlined, there are many other spaces, such as the religious one, the artistic one or the mathematical one, about which we will not be able to extend ourselves; but there are also different spaces according to the stage of life, and so we could distinguish at least an infantile space, an adult one and another one characteristic of old age. And what would be that which more properly characterizes the space of old age ?

Distance

Unlike the child, who lives linked to what is immediate, and the adult, who lives thrown into determined short and long term projects, and that spatially are, let us say, at an intermediate distance between what is distant and what is near, the aged lives in a world of retreat, of keeping one's distance (die Distanzierung), as Buytendijk says. This keeping one's distance is not only referred to his abandonment of work and duties, but also to moving away from every activity and in a certain way from every active participation in life. Ambition, eagerness and desire are more or less quiet. Now, this does not mean laziness or death; it is rather a new way of being in the world, easily expecting what life can give, without having to obtain it by means of work and effort. Buytendijk says with respect to this: «... it is not sleeping, but watching in legitimate quietness...». The description of behavior of the aged seated in parks can help us determine the essential characteristics of their spatiality. Unlike children with their permanent restlessness and the youth who soon get tired of inactivity, the aged can stay seated for a long time. They enjoy being seated, because that way they reach the plenitude of life through the easy contemplation of what happens in their surroundings. We owe Hamburger the observation of how the aged who stay long hours seated in parks follow the movement of life around them (children playing, walkers passing by, noises and conversations) «only with slight changes in the position of the head, while the trunk remains in a sort of immobility. The eyes express opposed feelings of approval or rejection, joy or irritation, and that expression of the eyes is accompanied by movements of the head». This description of Hamburger allows us to recognize something that is typical of the aged in his way of being in the world, of his spatial being: the fact that the events around him are lived as if they occurred on a stage. Hence that apparent contradiction between the great interest that anything happening around him, however banal it may be, awakens (perceived in his curious look, permanently approving or disapproving) in contrast with his almost immobility. This image clearly reminds the spectator of a dramatic piece and has to do, for sure, with that feature of moving away, so characteristic of the spatiality of the aged.

This remoteness begins to gradually increase in normal old age till arriving, in the confines of death, to a sort of «transfiguration» of the body. How many times have we had a premonition of the death of some beloved or known person of advanced age only because the way of being distant had become more marked, because it seemed to us that his/her body somehow floated between heaven and earth. This phenomenon is also observed in adults close to death, be it known or not hat it is coming. Naturally, we can only check this retrospectively. We find out about the sudden death of So-and-so and if we are rigorous with our memories and experiences, we will have to recognize that the last time we saw him/her, a few days or perhaps the same day before his/her death, he/she was like distant, his/her greeting had something special, as if worldly things did not touch him/her anymore, as if he/she were already halfway between heaven and earth. Unfortunately we do not have the possibility of knowing how they, the dead before dying, lived those moments that for us were felt as, remoteness, as a sort of farewell.

Immobility

Together with the remoteness of daily eagerness, of fights, purposes and plans, there is a sort of poverty of movement in the elderly. Movements which naturally accompany a determined action and which are not completely necessary gradually disappear with age. Unlike a young man who at the same time can walk, greet and exchange a package from one hand to the other, the aged can only make these different movements one after the other. The same occurs to him with eating and talking at the same time, thing that in the youth, but also in the mature adult is still perfectly possible. The motor excess of the child or of the youth has completely disappeared in the aged. This motor activity, characteristic of aging, shows an unmistakable similarity with what occurs in Parkinson's disease. Rigidity, hypominima and absence of accessory and expressive movements, which characterize this disease, would be an extreme version of this motor and consequently spatial reduction that we observe in the elderly. And here we find another apparent paradox in the spatiality of old age: the coexistence of a reduction of space with a withdrawal from the world, that at the same time means an opening towards a wider space, a transcendent space: the body has been becoming immobilized, the space becoming reduced, in the sense that the things that attract and interest are less; simultaneously, however, that look which scarcely rests over the surrounding objects begins to open itself towards a wider horizon, towards a space in a certain way angelical, greater than all the known spaces, which is the sacred space. It is frequent to observe an increase of religiosity in the aged, which has not necessarily to do with fear of death. As we will see with respect to temporality of aging, death can be seen in the aged, as in the young subject, like something very distant, although it is chronologically near. The greater religiosity of the aged (how do the old ladies fill the churches in the morning ! How do we find a message of eternity in each piece of advise from grandparents to grandchildren !) is rather related to the different characteristics that we have described with respect to the spatiality of senescence : withdrawal from the eagerness of the world, diminution of mobility, that in a certain way prepares for retreat and opening of the glance towards the space of transcendence.

Coexistence of what is essential and what is accessory

The fact that the world of the aged is so full of trifles, of useless objects, of unnecessary arrangements, of all kinds of collections, is curious. This is very evident in senility and particularly in Alzheimer's dementia of tardive onset, but it is also observed in the normal senescent. Little things acquire disproportionate importance, and so they suffer with the loss of objects, which makes them emphasize the measures of order, which in turn produces new losses because of natural forgetfulness, and so on. It is not unfrequent to attribute such losses to mnestic failures, and that sticking to material and dispensable things to a loss of the abstract attitude in the sense of Goldstein. However, this is not necessarily so. In the first place, because it is a selective phenomenon. The elderly does not stick to any object or trifle as if it were the most important in the world but to all that which has had a particular significance in his life: photographs of his ancestors, maybe forgotten during the years of activity and production and that now reappear again, as to accompany his in his last stage; objects which belonged to his mother or to a prematurely dead son; but also determined objects of personal use, such as a fountain pen, radio or watch, that at his age are not so easily purchasable or changeable anymore as in the productive stage of life.

Second, and this seems the most important thing to us, because this apparent remaining imprisoned in the space of what is little and accessory is closely related with an exactly opposite phenomenon: a great capacity to grasp and communicate essential things, condition that since unmemorable times has made them deserve the attribution of «wise». Let us remember the assembly of Geronts in Greece, but also in Medieval stories the aged appear full of wisdom and powers (let us recall Merlin the Magician), while in the Catholic Church the Cardinalate is only reached at an advanced age. The same occurs with the members of the Academies of Arts or of Sciences or with those of the Supreme Courts of Justice, etc. When wisdom is required, more even, when one speaks of wisdom, when one wants to represent it, the figure of the older man appears in first place. In fact, with aging a process of «essentialization» (forgiving the neologism), a greater capacity to apprehend eternal values, as well as to transmit them, begins to take place. All that is superfluous begins to be left aside. According to the pet Antonio Machado, he would want, in the closing stages of life, that death find him «light of burdens». The fact that with the years most people begin to loose weight and that the obese aged are an exception, is curious. It is as if nature itself became part of this process of «lightening» of the body and of the space, necessary when nearing the boundaries of death.

In summary, spatiality in the person of advanced age is marked by three pairs of opposed elements: nearness and distance; reduction of space till the almost immobility of Parkinson's disease and opening up to the widest of spaces, the space of transcendence; fixation to what is little and accessory in objects of the environment and at the same time, capacity to grasp essential things and then transmit them.

Temporality in old age

With time it happens as with space. Chronological time is only a derivative, an abstraction of existential time. In contrast with the uniformity of chronological time, in human life there are many different times, according to the age and/or the circumstances. The time of joy is different to the time of pain, the one of waiting is endlessly large, while we always find the time of the happy encounter short. How fast does time pass in the days and how slow does it appear in depression. Now, it occurs that the human existent is temporal from his/her very structure as being-in-the-world, since the motor of this structure is the cure, worry or care (die Sorge) in which the instances of future, present and past are articulated. In each «addressing to something», in each interest in something that faces us in the world, we are already anticipating and interpreting the future, from a certain way of being in our body and in our past (al that has been lived and experienced before that moment and that is determining my way of interpreting that future that approaches me) and carrying out the act of meeting with something or with someone in the present. The basis of temporality is death. As Heidegger says, the human being (the Dasein) is a «being-relatively-to-death». Time is constituted from finitude (death) and its central character is transitoriness. In the way of assuming this condition of «being-relatively-to-death» the ultimate reasons of why there are achieved and miscarried lives are hidden. But in addition to the possibilities of deviation that the human being has according to his/her capacity of being faithful to this particular temporality, the different stages of life have each their own temporality. Nobody could discuss that the time of childhood is very different from the time of the adult or to the one of the elderly. We will try to outline the main characteristics of time in old age.

Slowing

Who could deny the fact from general experience that as a child one lives time as a slow passing, and that between the beginning of classes and the next holidays the space of time seemed infinite to us? And what occurs instead with the adult? Exactly the opposite: time is found faster and faster each year, up to the point that we confuse summers, the one when we went to the beach with the other spent in the mountains. The more projects we have, the more realisations and trips and engagements we write down on our agenda, the faster we lose our time, our days, weeks and years. In old age, work already abandoned, without having to make an effort to earn their sustenance, concerned with the grandchildren and with a few innocent amusements, time becomes slow again, and infinite distance interferes again between spring and the next fall, and consequently, death withdraws again, that limit situation that approached us so closely in the adult age, in the middle of responsibilities with children and work, when we got ill of anything and felt for the first time the limits set by the body and were taken by anguish. In old age, time flows slowly again and resembles, also because of this fact, to our childhood. Nothing urges us, nobody needs us anymore, as before in the office or in the hospital, but nobody forces of commands us either. We have all the time in the world at our disposition and although we do much less than when we were adults, we have again this childish feeling old omnipotence: any day we will do this or that.

Contemporaneity of essential and trivial moments

Another characteristic phenomenon occurs parallel to this slowing: each moment acquires a very big and almost equivalent importance. It is as if the elderly lost his capacity to distinguish between moments that are essential and the ones that are not, and thus, he gives the same important to the loss of any object than to the visit of a son or to the initial symptoms of an illness. At least the emotional engagement observed in him in each one of these circumstances of such different significative value is very similar. A version pertaining to a caricature of the mentioned phenomenon would be the known «catastrophic behavior» presented by the elderly with sign of deterioration or dementia faced with overloads or frustrations in daily life. Without distinguishing, in a certain way, the different value that an exam situation, not finding a lost object or not receiving something that you wanted to eat in a given moment may have, the deteriorated patient reacts with the same anguish and irritation. This lack of discrimination between different moments of daily life has, however, its positive side which is the level of devotion that can be reached by the elderly, specially in the relationship with his grandchildren and relatives or with animals. The adult, always taken by obligations and engagements, lacks the necessary time to devote completely to a moment of the present, as can be done by the elderly, while the child, with his high degree of distraction, jumps from one interest to another, from a moment to the following, without being able to pause in that sort of interested and loving state of rest that can be reached by the elderly. Whoever has had the luck of enjoying his/her grand-parents for a long time will be able to testify about what I am describing. How many time did they dedicate themselves to us in childhood, as if we were the most important being in the world for them. In literature there are innumerable descriptions about the richness that those moments near the elderly can reach. In this context I remember the case of that wonderful subject, quite eccentric and elderly, who was Godfry, uncle of the immortal character of Romain Rolland, John Christopher, and of how the long talks between both of them were determinant in the life and creations of his nephew. And let us not forget that this novel is inspired nothing less than in Beethoven's life.

Making present

The third element which characterises temporality of normal aging, which has a lot to do with the previous point, is something like «making» life «present». In certain way the future fades away by not having obligations to fulfil nor projects to realise; it is also a way of placing death at a distance when one has it so near from the point of view of chronological time. All that strength invested by the youth, but also by the adult, in a future that does not exist yet, that being thrown towards the future which characterizes the human being in his/her stage of work and creation, is concentrated in the present moment, making it richer, more intense and more prolonged, as we saw previously. The past, instead, so quickly forgotten by both youth and adults, is made clearly present in the aged through that extraordinary memory for remote events, which, more than a more mechanical capacity to revive images, is another way of being in the world and orienting oneself in it. All the pas experiences, all that which for the adult seems to have retired to a remote past, is made so alive and clear until its smallest details, that it acquires the strength of what is contemporary. This making present the past explains the capacity of the aged to devoting for hours to a present without activities nor achievements, apparently empty. Nothing is further from reality than this very common opinion. In those long contemplative presents the elderly lives those distant memories intensely, he reviews his childhood, youth and maturity moment to moment as well as the historic circumstances which respectively surrounded those stages, and he/she uses, fat the same time, all the vital strength otherwise spent in projects by the adult to live with redoubled intensity, and some times also deepness, the present that he/she has before him a landscape, a grandchild, a conversation.

Maybe it is this phenomenon of concentration of all the vital strength in a present penetrated by the past, removing every dream about unreachable futures, that gives the healthy elderly that consistency, that roundness that in some reaches the level of wisdom. The origin of the Spanish word for wisdom (sabiduria) is «sapere», which in classic Latin means to know in the sense of savouring, of tasting. Who knew how to distinguish savours, wines and foods was a wise in the classic world. To be taster or gourmet is a condition that one can not simply acquire by more personal decision, the same as being wise. It is as if nature also manifested itself through those beings who are able to distinguish the infinite nuances of the things offered by it. The community between the taster or the gourmet, on one side, and the wise, on the other, goes farther than the fact of being able to distinguish nuances. If there is something characteristic of the taster or of the gourmet it is his capacity to find the right measure, the exact median, the perfect measure, something he has in common with the an of good taste and that affiliates him with the man of common sense. The wise is all this in a superlative form, while the elderly arrives naturally to wisdom from this phenomenon of making present pointed out by s. Since, removing the future as empty expectatives, or what is the same, using all the strength that usually is spent in projects, in living the present, together with assuming the best from the past, allows the aged to completely devote himself to that concentrated and enriched present, and that way to savour it well, to discover its measure, its good taste and from there to be able to act in front of others with the most perfect common sense, that is to say, with wisdom.

17

An ammonia hypothesis of Alzheimer disease

N. SEILER

Marion-Merrell Dow Research Institute,
16, rue d'Ankara,
67009 Strasbourg Cedex, France.

There is little doubt that dementia of the Alzheimer type (DAT) is a multifactorial disease. The opinion about the existence of a major gene for DAT is equivocal (Tzourio *et al.*, 1992, Farer *et al.*, 1991), however, a genetic predisposition is considered to be likely from the high concordance rate for monozygotic and dizygotic twins (Jarvik *et al.*, 1980), and an increased frequency of the disease in relatives of affected patients (Heston *et al.*, 1980). The long arm of chromosome 21 is considered to be the locus of predisposition (St. George-Hyslop *et al.*, 1987), but the expression of a number of genes encoding for various neuronal and non-neuronal proteins is also changed in DAT brains (Boyes *et al.*, 1992) and may be of importance in the etiology of the disease.

In Table I suggestions regarding pathogenetic events and factors which may contribute to the etiology or progression of DAT have been summarised. The list is still growing, and it is becoming more and more difficult to decide which factors are potentially of importance. Among the numerous hypotheses, the formation of neurotoxic amyloid depositions due to abnormal processing of the precursor protein of ß-amyloid (ßAPP) has attracted by far the greatest interest, because plaques and fibrillary tangles are hallmarks of DAT. The fact that certain mutations in the ßAPP are known to lead to familial forms of DAT (Selkoe, 1991), is the most convincing argument in favor of the ß-amyloid hypothesis, although it has repeatedly been shown that plaque formation is not correlating well with the severity of cognitive impairment in aged people (Lassmann *et al.*, 1993, Delaere *et al.*, 1989, Terry *et al.*, 1991).

Table I. Potential pathogenetic events and factors, respectively, of Alzheimer disease.

Genetic predisposition:	Tanzi et al., 1991; Farrer, 1991; Jarvik et al., 1980; Heston and White, 1980; Jarrett and Lansbury, 1993; Yankner et al., 1990.
Formation of neurotoxic β-amyloid depositions:	Hardy and Alsop, 1991; Pike et al., 1993; Neurofibrillary degeneration abnormal phosphorylation of Tau protein: Crowther, 1993.
Impairment of neuronal functions:	Fowler et al., 1992; Christensen et al., 1992. Degeneration of selected neurons (cholinergic, serotoninergic, noradrenergic, somatostatinergic). Palmer and Dekosky, 1993; Davies and Maloney, 1976; Benton et al., 1982; McGeer et al., 1984.
Changes in receptor density or function:	(serotonin, dopamine, glutamate, etc.): De Keyser, 1992; Giacobini, 1991; Greenamyre and Marages, 1993; Blin et al., 1993; Joyce et al., 1993.
Impairment of glial functions :	Astroglia: Frederickson, 1992. Microglia: McGeer et al., 1993.
Lack of trophic factors :	Nerve growth factor : Hefti and Schneider, 1991.
Neurotoxins :	Cytokines : Vandenbeele and Fiers, 1991. Aluminium: Deloncle and Guillard, 1990; Markesbery et al., 1981; Thompson et al., 1988; Good et al., 1992. Radicals: Jeandel et al., 1989; Evans et al., 1989; Volicer and Crino, 1990. Glutamate: Lawlor and Davis, 1992; Maragos et al., 1987. Colchicine-like factor: Gorenstein, 1987. Ammonia: Seiler 1993.
Infections :	Treponema pallidum : Miklossy, 1993. Viral agents: Prusiner, 1984.

It has been hypothesised that risk factors in DAT increase with age (Henderson, 1988). If this is true, we have to consider consequences of general age-related changes in organ functions as potential contributing factors, among which the impairment of the blood brain barrier function (Alafuzoff et al., 1987) is of especial importance. Indeed pathogenetic effects of environmental factors, such as aluminium, and infection with spirochetes (Miklossy, 1993) have been considered a consequence of the dysfunction of the blood brain barrier.

Enhanced exposure of the organism to oxygen free radicals, e.g. due to the impairment of catalase and superoxide dismutase, may be another general noxious event, although direct evidence for the validity of this idea with respect to DAT is scarce. But oxygen free radicals have nevertheless been implicated as etiological agents in the process of aging, (Harman, 1984), and in several neurodegenerative disorders (Lohr, 1991) including DAT (Jeandel et al., 1989, Volicer and Crino, 1990).

Ammonia, a neurotoxic agent, is a normal metabolite in virtually all tissues, but it is also taken up by the body from the Gi tract. In Figure 1, ammonia movements in the vertebrate organism are shown. At pH 7.4, 1.7 % of ammonia is present in non-protonated form (NH$_3$), while 98.3 % are protonated (NH$_4^+$) (Benjamin, 1982). Most tissues take up ammonia from the arterial blood and release corresponding amounts of glutamine. Final detoxification occurs in liver by urea formation. Since NH$_3$ easily passes cell membranes the blood-brain barrier can also be passed by diffusion.

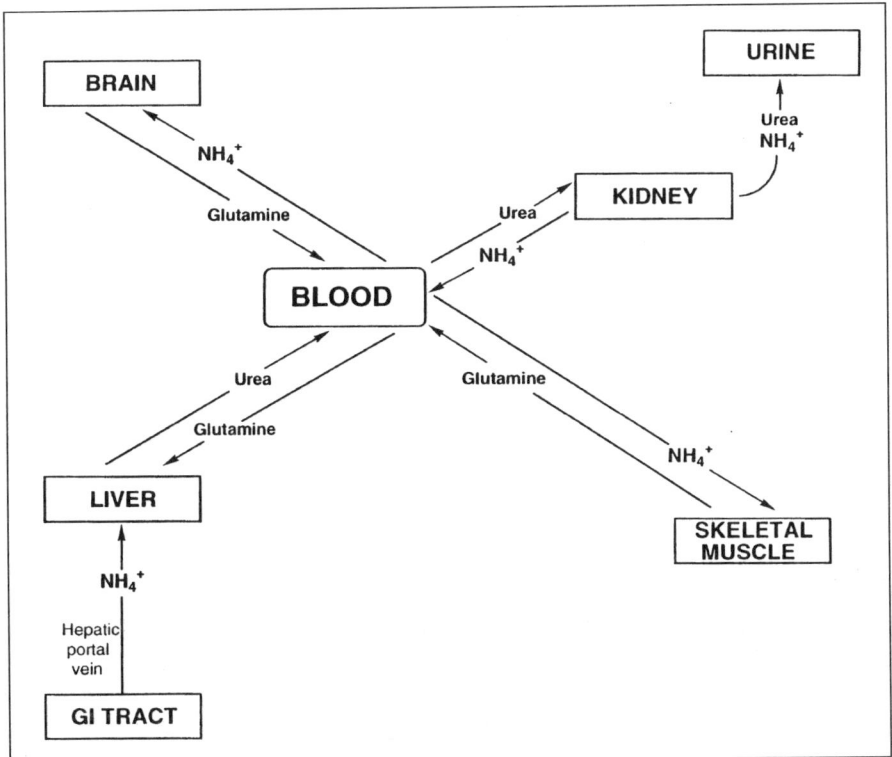

Figure 1. Ammonia movements in the vertebrate organism.

Our present knowledge of ammonia as neurotoxin in humans are mainly based on observations of patients with impaired liver function (fulminant hepatic failure, liver cirrhosis), and of children with hereditary deficiencies of urea cycle enzymes. It is evident from the course of these diseases, that DAT is not a direct consequence of hyperammonemia. However, as will be shown in the following, hepatic encephalopathy and DAT have common features. It seems conceivable that chronic elevation of brain ammonia, together with other factors, may determine severity and progression of DAT.

Evidence for elevated ammonia concentrations in blood and brain in DAT

Owing to technical difficulties, data on ammonia concentrations in blood and CSF show considerable variation (Table II). The brain values have been extrapolated from animal studies, since ammonia concentrations are rapidly increasing after death (Benjamin, 1982).

Table II. Ammonia in human brain and body fluids.

Brain	100-300 nmol/g
CSF	20-100 nmol/ml
Arterial blood/plasma	70-113 nmol/ml
Venous blood/plasma	20-100 nmol/ml

Data from Cooper and Plum (1987).

Observations which directly suggest a role of ammonia in DAT are scarce. Since, however, ammonia has not attracted attention in this regard, no systematic studies are available.

Fisman et al. (1985, 1989) demonstrated in two reports that post-prandial blood ammonia levels were significantly higher in DAT patients than in appropriately matched control subjects. Some DAT patients had triphasic waves on EEG, a waveform suggestive for metabolic encephalopathy (Conn and Kieberthal, 1979). The fasting blood ammonia levels in those patients were significantly higher than in the other DAT patients.

Branconnier et al. (1986) found in patients who met the diagnostic criteria of DAT, but had no liver disease, nor urinary tract infections, 122 ± 80 nmol ammonia per ml of plasma. The normal range in this study was found to be 12-55 nmol/ml; 83 % of the patients had blood ammonia concentrations above the normal limit.

Hoyer et al. (1990) determined arterio-venous differences of ammonia in patients suffering from advanced DAT, and in patients clinically diagnosed as having incipient dementia, in all probability DAT of early onset. Healthy volunteers showed an average ammonia uptake by the brain of 72 ± 7 $\mu g.kg^{-1}.min^{-1}$. in striking contrast, 27 ± 3 $\mu g.kg^{-1}.min^{-1}$ of ammonia was released from the brains of patients with advanced DAT. Patients with presumed early-onset DAT released even 256 ± 162 $\mu g.kg^{-1}.min^{-1}$ ammonia into the circulation. These findings suggest excessive ammonia production within the brain, with or without a deficient mechanism of ammonia detoxification.

From the above cited reports it seems evident that in addition to usual age-related impairments of liver function (i.e. reduction of the hepatic detoxification capacity), there are disease-related causes for hyperammonemia in DAT, which are not of hepatic origin.

Sources of brain ammonia, and ammonia detoxification mechanisms

Ammonia concentrations in vertebrate brains seem to be correlated with the functional state of the brain : reduction in functional activity is associated with a reduced concentration of ammonia, and functional activity, electrical stimulation and many convulsant agents produce elevated brain ammonia levels (Benjamin, 1982).

In Figure 2, the major sources of ammonia of the vertebrate brain have been summarised. A significant proportion of the ammonia of the vertebrate organism originates from the gastrointestinal tract. Deficient hepatic detoxification due to the impairment of liver function causes hyperammonemia, and since ammonia easily passes the blood brain barrier (Benjamin, 1982), elevated brain ammonia concentrations are a result. In hepatic encephalopathy resulting from acute or chronic liver disease, exogenous (gastrointestinal) ammonia is a key factor in the pathogenesis of the disease (Butterworth et al., 1987, Butterworth, 1992, Zieve, 1987). Bacterial infections of the urinary tract (e.g. the neurogenic bladder) is another potential cause for hyperammonemic encephalopathy (Drayna et al., 1981). Proteins, nucleic acids and hexosamines have long been suggested as sources of cerebral ammonia (Vrba and Folberg, 1959, Vrba et al., 1957, Weil-Malherbe and Drysdale, 1957). Hydrolysis of glutamine and asparagine, oxidative deaminations of primary amines (monoamines, diamines and polyamines), glycine catabolism via the glycine cleavage system, deaminations of purines and pyrimidines and glucosamine-6-phosphate, among others, are well known ammonia generating reactions, which may contribute to the steady-state level of brain ammonia (Kvamme, 1983).

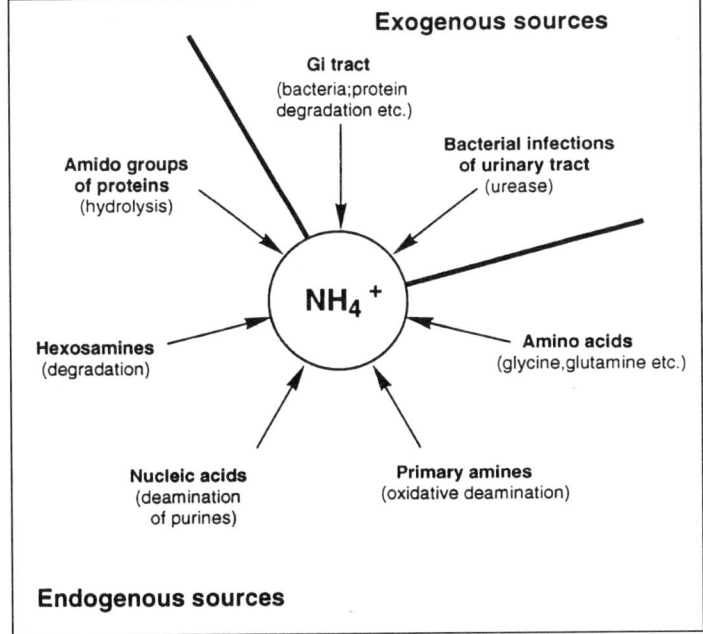

Figure 2. Ammonia sources of the vertebrate brain.
«Endogenous sources» denote ammonia forming reactions within the vertebrate organism. Most ammonia generating reactions are, however, also active within the CNS.

Glutamate dehydrogenase is a major mitochondrial enzyme, which links the tricarboxylic acid cycle with ammonia. The direction of the neural glutamate dehydrogenase-catalysed reaction appears to be regulated by the intracellular (NAD(P)+/NAD(P)H-ratio : when the ration is high, e.g. in the absence of glucose, when this ratio falls, and 2-oxoglutarate is not rate limiting, reductive amination of 2-oxoglutarate to glutamate seems favored (Benjamin, 1982). Paradoxically, in hyperammonemic states the synaptic (in contrast with non-synaptic) mitochondrial glutamate dehydrogenase is stimulated in the direction of glutamate oxidation (Faff-Michalak and Albrecht, 1993). One may assume that this reaction counteracts the hyperammonemia-induced decrease of cerebral α-ketoglutarate production in other metabolic pathways, i.e. it supports energy production via the tricarboxylic acid cyle.

Hepatic urea formation is the most important ammonia detoxifying reaction of the mammalian organism. In brain ornithine-carbamyl transferase is present only at low activity (Jones *et al.*, 1961), therefore, the urea cycle is not functional. The ATP-dependent formation of glutamine (Figure 3) in astrocytes, and its release into the

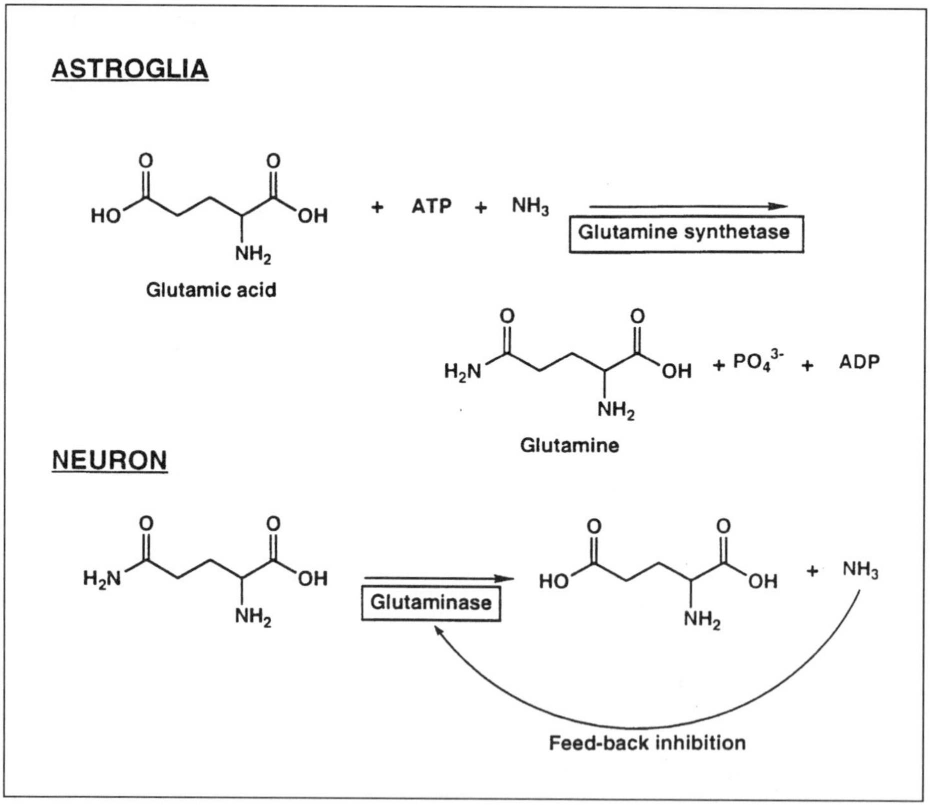

Figure 3. Glutamine formation and hydrolysis. The energy dependent formation of glutamine from glutamate is nearly the exclusive ammonia detoxification reaction of the vertebrate brain; it takes place within the astroglia.
Enzymatic hydrolysis of glutamine is the major ammonia generating reaction in neurons. Neuronal glutaminase is phosphate-activated, and controlled by ammonia via a feedback mechanism.

circulation is nearly exclusively responsible for the limitation of brain ammonia concentrations (Benjamin, 1982, Kvamme, 1983).

Brain ammonia metabolism in DAT

Elevation of brain ammonia with age in vertebrates is presumably a general phenomenon (Kirzinger and Fonda, 1978). The release of ammonia from the brain of DAT patients (Hoyer et al., 1990) suggest the pathologic enhancement of ammonia formation, or a deficient detoxification, or both.

Age-related gradual reduction of glutamine synthetase activity has been reported, with a significantly lower activity of this enzyme in the brains of DAT patients than in age-matched controls (Oliver et al., 1990, Smith et al., 1991).

In contrast, phosphate-activated glutaminase, the enzyme responsible for intraneuronal liberation of glutamate from glutamine, is not changed in DAT (Procter et al., 1988). It is known that ammonia is involved in the regulation of the (phosphate-activated) glutaminase (Figure 3). In the brains of young rats glutaminase activity is reduced in the presence of ammonia. In aged animals, however, glutamine hydrolysis was significantly less sensitive to inhibition by ammonia than in the brains of young rats, indicating the presence of an isoenzyme which is less responsive to feed-back regulation (Wallace and Dawson, 1992).

The reduction of glial glutamine formation, and the impaired regulation of ammonia release from glutamine are most probably the major aberrations of the key ammonia detoxification mechanism of the aged vertebrate brain. They are expected to be the most important cause for the observed elevation of brain ammonia and glutamic acid concentrations.

A major reason for the loss of glutamine synthetase during aging is presumably the sensitivity of this enzyme against damage by oxygen free radicals. This is suggested by the greatly reduced activity of glutamine synthetase in the brains of aged gerbils (Carney et al., 1991), the rapid loss of glutamine synthetase during ischemia/reperfusion - induced brain injury (Oliver et al., 1990) and during hyperoxia in neonatal rats (Schor et al., 1991). Deloncle and Guillard (1990) suggested a role for aluminium, which is passing the blood-brain barrier as complex with glutamate, in the impairment of ammonia detoxification.

Whether the imbalance between glutamine formation and its hydrolytic cleavage is a sufficient explanation for an ammonia excess in the brain of DAT patients, is not known. It is also unknown, whether any other ammonia generating reaction is active above physiological level. Although speculative, one type of potential ammonia generating reaction, namely oxidative deaminations of primary amines, is nevertheless briefly considered in the following, because the underlying hypothesis can be tested in humans.

Among the enzymes involved in oxidative deaminations of primary amines, monoamine oxidase (MAO) is most important. In brain, monoamine oxidase B (MAO-B) is mostly extraneuronally localised (Student and Edwards, 1977) and represents in the human CNS over 80 % of MAO (Garrick and Murphy, 1980). An age-related increase of this enzyme by about 50 % has been demonstrated (Robinson et al., 1971). This increase was more marked in the brains of DAT patients than in age - matched controls (Adolfsson *et al.*, 1980, Rainikainen *et al.*, 1988), and has been related to gliosis involving astrocytes (Nakamura *et al.*, 1990). The enhancement of MAO-B activity seems to be due to the presence of more MAO-B molecules, not due to a high-activity isoform of the enzyme (Jossan *et al.*, 1991).

MAO-B deaminates oxidatively numerous endogenous and exogenous primary amines (e.g. dopamine, tyramine, tryptamine, ß-phenyl-ethylamine, benzylamine) to form ammonia, hydroperoxide and the aldehyde corresponding to the amine substrate, as is depicted in Figure 4. Not only hydroperoxide, a source of oxygen free radicals, but all three reaction products of MAO (and of all oxidative deaminations in general) are noxious agents that need to be inactivated by the mammalian organism. All enzymes involved in oxidative deaminations, that use molecular oxygen, as well as their substrates and products of their reactions, deserve our special attention as potential pathogenetic factors.

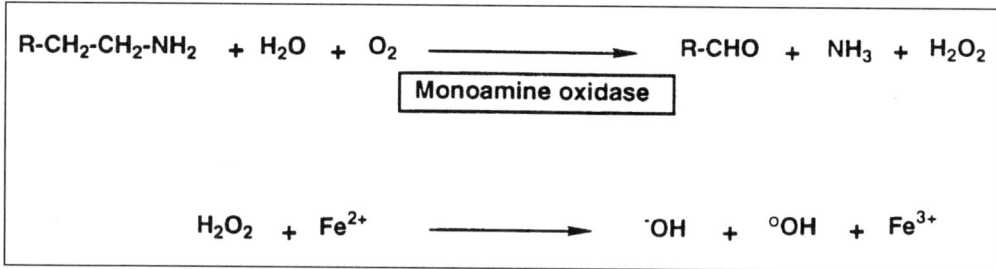

Figure 4. The oxidative deamination of primary amines is a source of hydroperoxide and of ammonia. Monoamine oxidases A and B are the most important enzymes in the brain, which catalyze oxidative deaminations.

The physiologic rate of MAO-B-catalysed reactions (and of related oxidative deaminations) in brain is not known. In DAT patients the impaired blood-brain barrier (Alafuzoff *et al.*, 1987) may allow the enhanced intrusion of substrates of MAO-B and related oxidase from the blood into the brain and consequently oxidative deaminations may occur at a very high rate. It seems not unlikely that the recent reports on the improvement of cognitive functions of DAT patients by treatment with an inactivator of MAO-B (Falsaperla *et al.*, 1990, Campi *et al.*, 1990, Mangoni *et al.*, 1991) are due to the reduction of ammonia formation (in addition to reduced ammonia formation there are of course several other potential explanations for the beneficial effects of MAO-B inhibition et DAT).

Toxic effects of ammonia and Alzheimer pathology

In experimental animals key toxic manifestations of enhanced brain ammonia concentrations are independent of the genesis of the state of hyperammonemia, i.e. the symptoms are much the same after impairment of liver function (e.g. by portacaval shunting), hyperammonemia produced by unease injections, or by inactivation of glutamine synthetase, using methionine sulfoximine (Raabe and Onstad, 1982, Yamamoto *et al.*, 1989, Jessy *et al.*, 1990), and resemble pathophysiological

observations in the brains of patients with hepatic encephalopathy and hereditary defects of urea cycle enzymes (Butterworth *et al.*, 1987, Butterworth, 1992). Based on these facts, it may not surprise that a number of features of hyperammonemic states are also observed in patients with DAT:
Impaired cognitive functions
Impaired blood-brain barrier
Astrocytosis
Impaired glucose utilisation
Impaired energy metabolism
Reduced glutamine synthetase activity
Enhanced extracellular glutamate
Loss of glutamate receptors (NMDA-type)
Enhanced MAO-B activity
Impaired lysosomal processing of proteins

Ammonia intoxication and synaptic transmission

Based on experimental results it was calculated that an increase of ammonia to about 0.5 $\mu mol.g^{-1}$ brain i.e. a 2 - 5-fold increase, is sufficient to disturb excitatory and inhibitory synaptic transmission and to initiate the encephalopathy related to acute ammonia intoxication (Raabe, 1987). Thus, it seems likely that slowly progressing pathogenetic mechanisms may be initiated even at brain ammonia concentrations only slightly above physiological levels.

Glutamate-mediated excitatory synaptic transmission is decreased by ammonia (Raabe, 1987). Inhibitory synaptic transmission is also decreased by ammonia due to hyperpolarization of Cl-dependent inhibitory (e.g. GABAergic and glycinergic) neurons. This effect is related to the inactivation of the extrusion of Cl- from neurons by ammonia. By the same action ammonia also decreases the hyperpolarizing action of Ca^{2+} and voltage dependent Cl^--currents (Raabe, 1987). Since a large proportion of the GABAergic and other inhibitory neurons control inhibitory inputs, ammonia produces and increase in neuronal excitability by «disinhibition» (Roberts, 1976).

The fact that ammonia is capable of interfering with the function of the major excitatory (glutamatergic), and the major inhibitory (GABAergic) neuronal systems of the vertebrate CNS should be sufficient reason to attract our especial interest.

Reduced glucose utilisation

The reduced utilisation of glucose is one of the most conspicuous findings in experimental (Jessy *et al.*, 1990) and disease-related hyperammonemic states, with concomitantly decreased rates of energy metabolism (Hawkins and Mans, 1990, Lockwood *et al.*, 1991). Analogous observations have been made in DAT: In PET studies (McGeer *et al.*, 1989, Foster *et al.*, 1984, Fukuyama *et al.*, 1991) cerebral glucose utilisation was found to be predominantly reduced in the parieto-temporal cortex. Overall cerebral glucose utilisation was diminished by about 50 %, with normal oxygen consumption in early-onset (Hoyer *et al.*, 1988, Hoyer and Nitsch, 1989, Hoyer, 1991), but reduced oxygen consumption in late onset DAT (Frackowiak *et al.*, 1981). The impairment of brain energy metabolism in DAT, and of enzymes involved in energy metabolism, has subsequently been reported by several investigators (e.g. *see ref.* Heiss *et al.*, 1991, Parker, 1991, Liguri *et al.*, 1990).

Impairment of astroglia function and excitotoxicity

Astrocytic alterations, characterised as «Alzheimer type II gliosis» are an invariable, most characteristic histopathological consequence of sustained hyperammonemia, both in experimental animals (Gibson *et al.*, 1974) and in patients with hepatic encephalopathy (Martin *et al.*, 1987, Lavoie *et al.*, 1987).

Frederickson (1992) summarised observations supporting the idea that reactive astrocytes may mediate neuropathologic events of DAT, including the facilitation of extracellular depositions of ß-AP.

Astrocytic damage by ammonia is followed by a decrease of glutamine synthetase activity, as was evidenced from the reduction of the activity of this enzyme by 15 % in rats with portacaval shunts (Butterworth *et al.*, 1988). However, this decrease in synthetase activity may cause further damage to astrocytes. It is well established that glutamine synthethase is critically involved in the regulation of intracellular ammonia and acid-base balance (Benjamin, 1982). Any derangement of the function of this enzyme will be followed by the amplification of ammonia toxicity. Therefore, it is not surprising that an increased intracellular pH, and swelling of astrocytes was observed in hyperammonemic rats (Swain *et al.* 1991).

Presumably the most conspicuous difference between the amino acid patterns of cirrhotic (Butterworth *et al.*, 1987) and DAT patients (Procter *et al.*, 1988) is the several-fold increase of glutamine in all brain regions of cirrhotics, but no change in the concentration of this amino acid in the brains of DAT patients. Likewise, no increase of glutamine was detected in the CSF of patients with DAT (Pomara *et al.*, 1992), whereas the levels of this amino acid were elevated in the CSF of experimental animals with portal-systemic encephalopathy (Therrien and Butterworth, 1991). These findings suggest the inability of the brains of DAT patients to enhance glutamine formation above a certain level, and may be taken as an indication for a considerable sensitivity of DAT brains even to small increases in the rate of ammonia formation.

Glutamate concentrations are lower in the brains of DAT patients than in age-matched controls, due to losses of glutamatergic neurons (Procter *et al.*, 1988), but CSF levels of glutamate are elevated, both in DAT (Pomara *et al.*, 1992) and in portal systemic encephalopathy (Therrien and Butterworth, 1991). The elevation of extracellular glutamate has been directly demonstrated in rats with porta-caval shunts (Moroni *et al.*, 1983, Tossman *et al.*, 1987). It is a major effect of ammonia-induced astrocytosis, and most probably due to the impaired glutamate uptake by the functionally compromised astrocytes. Neuronal degeneration is the logical consequence of enhanced glutamate. Based on different considerations several authors have suggested glutamate-induced excitotoxicity as potential pathogenetic mechanism in

Alzheimer disease (Lawlor and Davis, 1992, Maragos *et al.*, 1987, Frederickson, 1992). Excitotoxic mechanisms in the pathogenesis of DAT are especially attractive, since they are able to explain symptoms of cortical disconnection (e.g. aphasia), and memory dysfunction.

From the key observations reported in the preceding sections the scenario schematised in Figure 5 seems evident: Damage of glutamine synthetase (and of other proteins) e.g. by oxygen free radicals, or the impairment of astroglia function by toxins could provoke the reduction of the capacity of the brain to detoxify ammonia, which then initiates vicious circles. These result in the progressively increasing accumulation of ammonia with progressive astrocytosis, and direct disturbance of synaptic functions by ammonia as a consequence. Impairment of astrocyte function favors, as has been mentioned, the accumulation of extracellular glutamate, which may initiate neuronal damage mediated by glutamate receptors.

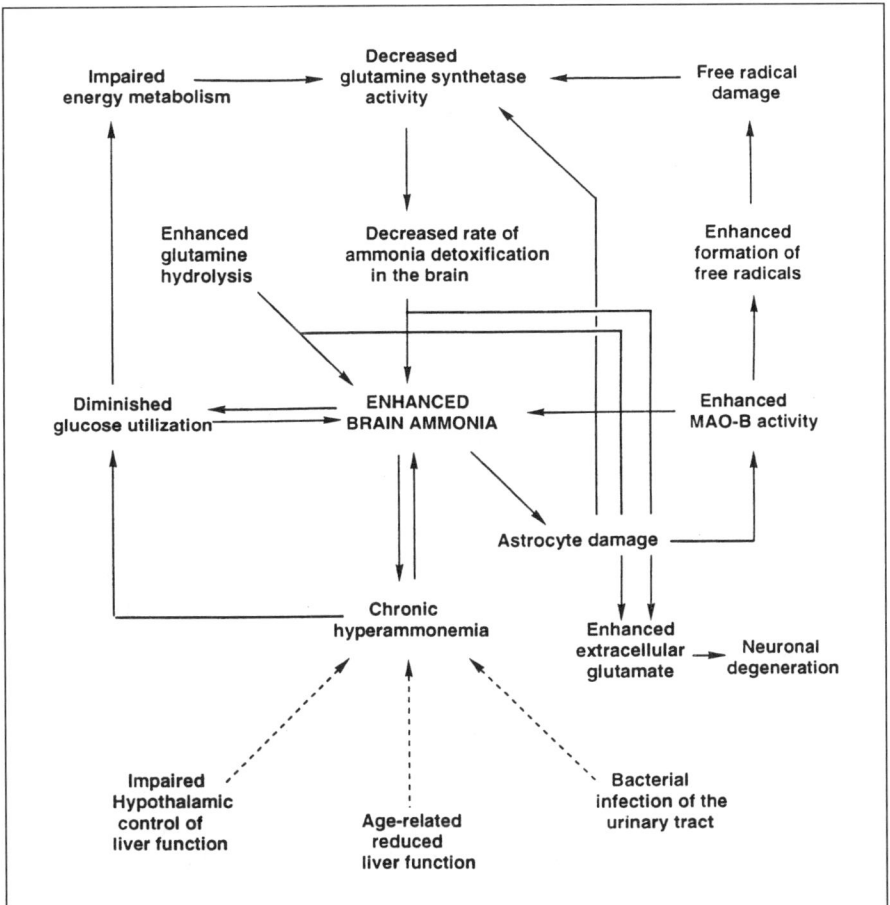

Figure 5. Some potential consequences of chronic hyperammonemia. Positive feedback regulatory cycles are induced in states of enhanced brain ammonia concentrations, which may lead to progressive functional impairment of astroglia cells and neuronal damage.

The impairment of glucose utilisation is a potential primary event (Hoyer *et al.*, 1988, Hoyer, 1991), expected to have similar consequences as the impairment of ammonia detoxification (Figure 5).

Lysosomes, ß-amyloid precursor protein and ammonia

The prevailing opinion concerning the role of lysosomes in the processing of ßAPP has repeatedly changed in the past; nevertheless, several lines of evidence are in favor of a role of the endosomal-lysosomal system in the pathogenesis of DAT:

a) Using an antibody, ß-APP was localised to lysosomes (Benowitz *and al.*, 1989, Cole *et al.*, 1989, Cataldo and Nixon, 1990, Kawai *et al.*, 1992).

b) Lysosomal proteinase antigens are prominently localised within senile plaques (Cataldo *et al.*, 1990).

c) The degradation but not the secretion of ß-APP by PC12 cells was impaired by inhibitors of lysosomal function (i.e. ammonium chloride, leupeptine and chloroquine), (Cole *et al.*, 1989, Caporaso *et al.*, 1992).

d) Golde *et al.* (1992) generated deletion mutants of CEP4ß cells that produced the normal set of carboxyl-terminal derivatives of ß-APP, and shortened secreted derivatives were analysed. It was shown that secretase cleaved ß-APP at a single site within the ß-amyloid region, and generated one secreted derivative and one non-amyloidogenic carboxyl-terminal fragment. In contrast, a complex set of carboxyl-terminal derivatives was produced by the endosomal-lysosomal system that included potentially amyloidogenic forms. Exposure of the cells to 50 mM ammonium chloride reduced the entire set of 8-12 kD carboxyl-terminal derivatives and almost abolished the two largest forms; at the same time it augmented the cell content of the full length ß-APP. Treatment with ammonium chloride had, however, no effect on secretase cleavage. Thus, it appears that ß-APP may be internalised from the cell surface and targeted to lysosomes, where an array of potentially amyloidogenic carboxyl-terminal fragments are generated.

A number of studies suggested that the transport of ammonia follows the pH gradient, due to the higher permeability of membranes for NH_3 than for NH_{4+} (Benjamin, 1992). Owing to their low pH, lysosomes are the organelles in which ammonia will preferentially accumulate, even at moderately elevated intracellular ammonia concentrations. It has been mentioned that in the brains of hyperammonemic rats the intracellular pH is increased (Swain *et al.*, 1991).

Ammonia (and other weak bases) interfere with lysosomal proteolysis most probably due to elevation of the intralysosomal pH (Segelen, 1983). It has been shown, for example that human glial cells in culture, if exposed to glycosaminoglycans and ammonium acetate, assume the appearance of cells of patients with mucopolysaccharidosis (Glimelius *et al.*, 1977). In hyperammonemic rats hepatic lysosomal proteolysis is diminished (Felipo *et al.*, 1988).

From the above mentioned observations the impairment of lysosomal proteolysis instates of hyperammonemia is to be expected, with gradual accumulation of certain proteins, including ß-APP. This does, however, not imply that hydrolytic cleavage of all proteins will be equally affected. On the contrary, it is more likely that some of the lysosomal hydrolases are more sensitive than others to the ammonia induced changes of their environment, and the impairment of the cleavage of selected proteins may be more important than that of others.

Ammonia is known to release lysosomal enzymes from cells (Tsuboi et al., 1993, Leoni and Dan, 1983), and different classes of lysosomal enzymes have been localised in extra-lysosomal compartments of Alzheimer brains (e.g. in perikarya and proximal dendrites of many cortical neurons and in senile plaques (Cataldo et al., 1991, Nakamura et al., 1991).

It is tempting to speculate that the fragile lysosomal membrane is affected in its function due to ammonia accumulation, and the metabolic derangements following abnormal ammonia accumulation, so that lysosomal hydrolases are able to pass the membranes and exert detrimental effects in various parts of the cells (and the brain, respectively) to which they normally do not have access. This idea is supported by the observation that ß-glucuronidase (a lysosomal enzyme) measured post-mortem in DAT brains, and the metabolic rates for glucose, determined pre-mortem by PET in the same patients, were inversely correlated (McGeer et al., 1989), and the fact that proteolysis of MAP-2 (a protein controlling together with Tau protein the polymerisation of microtubules) in rats with severe hyperammonemia is enhanced (Felipo et al., 1993). The invasion of microglia into cortical and other brain areas with prevailing neuronal degeneration is a potential source of lysosomal components of senile plaques (Dickson et al., 1988).

Potential consequences of enhanced brain tryptophan metabolism

The enhanced uptake and turnover of tryptophan in hepatic failure (Curzon et al., 1973) was considered a pathogenetic factor in hepatic encephalopathy (Record, 1991). But hyperammonemia in the absence of any derangement of liver function also causes the enhancement of tryptophan uptake by the brain (Bachmann and Colombo, 1983). The reports concerning the rate of tryptophan and serotonin metabolism in DAT are controversial (Martignoni et al., 1991). The following considerations may nevertheless be valid in view of the data which support a role of hyperammonemia in the pathogenesis of DAT.

Kynurenine is a toxic (Lapin, 1989) metabolite of tryptophan. It is formed by oxidative cleavage of the pyrrole ring to N-fromyl kynurenine and enzymatic removal of the formyl residue (Bender, 1989). Quinolinic acid is formed from kynurenine (Figure 6). It is excitotoxic, similar to glutamate and kainic acid (Foster and Schwarcz, 1989). Enhanced kynurenine concentrations in plasma, CSF, and brains of hyperammonemic patients (with liver cirrhosis) have been recognized as a consequence of enhanced tryptophan levels (Körnhüber et al., 1989). Increased quinolinic acid formation in brain seems not to be a direct consequence of enhanced kynurenine formation. However, quinolinic acid concentrations were found to be elevated in the brains of aged rats (Moroni et al., 1989). Therefore, they may be a consequence of enhanced quinolic acid formation in liver, and enhanced uptake due to the age-related impairment of the blood-brain barrier (Alafuzoff *et al.*, 1987).

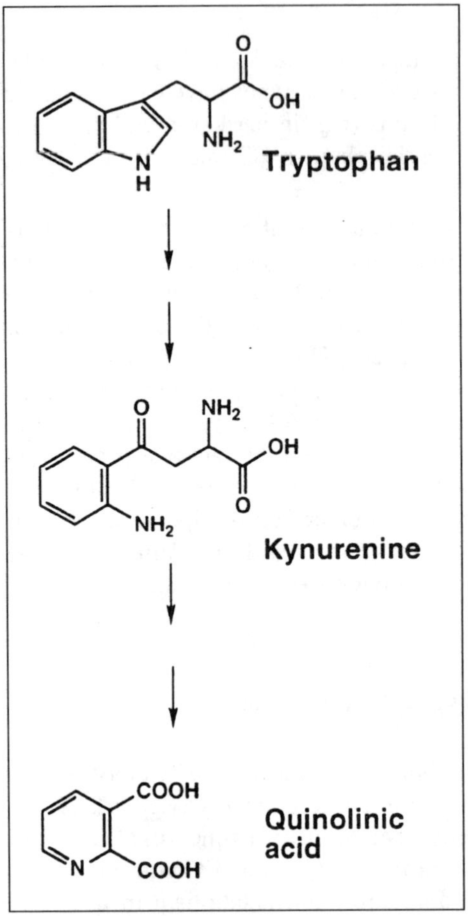

Figure 6. Structural formulae of tryptophan, kynurenine and quinolinic acid.

Based on this information it is not difficult to imagine a scenario for aged with chronic hyperammonemia, as is depicted in Figure 7. In addition to excitotoxic damage generated by quinolinic acid and kynurenine, the impairment of lysosomal proteolysis by both, tryptophan and kynurenine (Grinde, 1989) is a likely consequence of chronically elevated brain ammonia concentrations.

Conclusions

It is not generally recognized that there is considerable evidence in favor of the idea that hyperammonemias differ considerably from DAT with respect to disease progression and symptoms. However, the derangement of astrocyte metabolism and

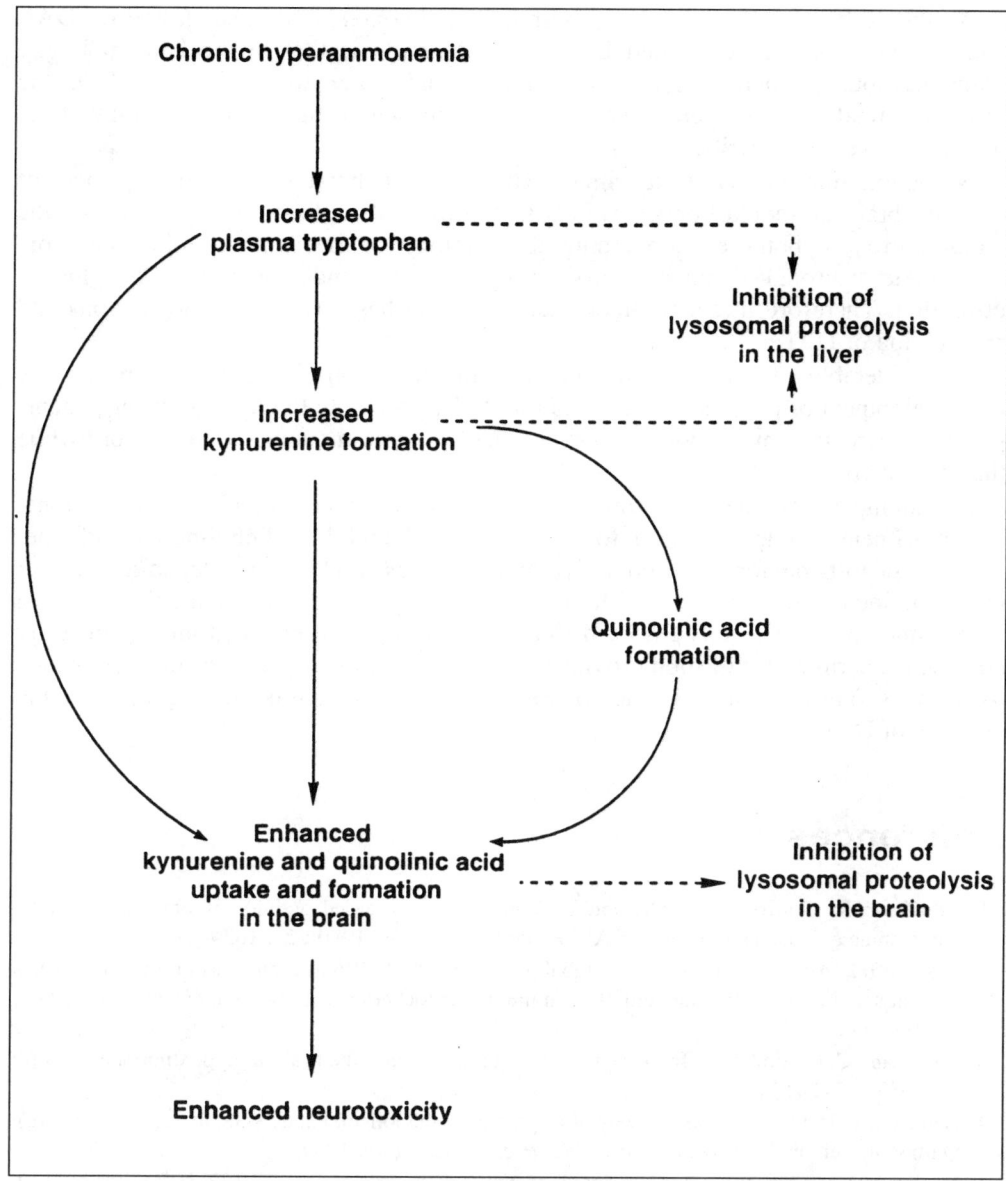

Figure 7. Potential pathologic consequences of enhanced tryptophan metabolism along the kynurenine-quinolinic acid pathway.

astrocytosis, the decrease in glucose utilisation rate and energy metabolism, the enhanced formation and release of excitotoxic amino acids, and the presumptive derangement of neurotransmission in GABAergic, glycinergic and glutamatergic neurons are common to both diseases, and may hint at a common source, ammonia.

A major difference between brain-born hyperammonemia, as is suggested for DAT, and hyperammonemia generated by liver dysfunction is that in the latter not only ammonia, but aliphatic amines, mercaptans and other toxins generated in the gastrointestinal tract, may enter the brain and contribute to the pathophysiology of the disease (Zieve, 1987, Uribe, 1989).

No doubt, ammonia is not a primary cause of DAT, however, the consequences of elevated brain ammonia concentrations have obvious implications in several of the major current hypotheses concerning the etiology of DAT: ß-amyloid formation, excitotoxic neuronal damage, astrocyte dysfunction, and impairment of glucose utilisation. Therefore, it seems likely that ammonia has a role in manifestations and progression of DAT.

A considerable effort is presently put on the identification of targets which may allow the development of preventive therapies for DAT patients. In the light of the arguments presented here, the amelioration or prevention of hyperammonemia seems a worthwhile therapeutic effort.

No attempts were made in this review to connect hyperammonemia to regional aspects of neuronal degeneration, to the selective vulnerability of cholinergic and other neurons, or to behavioral and cognitive abnormalities in DAT, in order to avoid over interpretation of the scarce data. But, once a role of ammonia in the pathophysiological manifestations of DAT has attracted more general attention, refined and specifically designed experiments will soon provide answers to those open questions that are needed to allow us to draw a more detailed picture of the role that ammonia might play in the etiology of DAT.

References

1. Adolfsson R, Gottfries CG, Oreland L, Winblad B. Increased activity of brain and platelet monoamine oxidase in dementia of Alzheimer type. *Life Sci* 1980 ; 27: 1029-1034.
2. Alafuzoff I, Adolfsson R, Grundke-Iqbal I, Windblad B. Blood-brain barrier in Alzheimer's dementia and in non-demented elderly. An immunocytochemical study. *Acta Neuropathol* 1987 ; 73: 160-160.
3. Bachmann C, Colombo JP. Increased tryptophan uptake into the brain in hyperammonemia. *Life Sci* 1983 ; 33: 2417-2424.
4. Bender DA. The kynurenine pathway of tryptophan metabolism. Pages 3-38, in Stone, T.W. (ed.). Quinolinic acid and the kynurenines. *CRC Press, Boca Raton* 1989.
5. Benjamin A.M. Ammonia. In: Handbook of Neurochemistry, pages 117-137, in Lajtha, A. (ed.). vol.1. Plenum Press, *New York* 1982.
6. Benowitz L-I, Rodriguez W, Paskevich P, Mufson EJ, Schenk D, Neve R.L. The amyloid precursor protein is concentrated in neuronal lysosomes in normal and Alzheimer disease subjects. *Exp. Neurol* 1989 ; 106: 237-250.
7. Benton JS, Bowen DM, Allen SJ, Haan EA, Davison AN, Neary D, Murphy RP, Snowden JS. Alzheimer's disease as a disorder of isodendritic care. *Lancet ii* 1982 ; 456.
8. Blin J, Baron JC, Dubois B, Crouzel C, Fiorelli M, Attar-Levy D, Pillon B, Fournier D, Vidailhet M, Agid Y. Loss of brain 5-HT2 receptors in Alzheimer's disease. *Brain* 1993 ; 116: 497-510.

9. Boyes BE, Walker DG, McGeer PL, McGeer EG. Identification and characterisation of a large human brain gene whose expression is increased in Alzheimer disease. *Mol. Brain Re* 1992 ; 12: 47-57.
10. Branconnier RJ, Dessain EC, McNiff ME,Cole JO. Blood ammonia and Alzheimer's disease. *Am. J. Psychiatry* 1986 ; 143: 1313.
11. Butterworth RF. Pathogenesis and treatment of portal-systemic encephalopathy: an update. *Dig. Dis. Sci.* 1992 ; 37: 321-327.
12. Butterworth RF, Giguere JF, Michaud J, Lavoie J, Pomier-Layrargues G. Ammonia: Key factor in the pathogenesis of hepatic encephalopathy. Neurochem. *Pathol* 1987 ; 6: 1-12.
13. Butterworth RF, Girard G, Giguère JF. Regional differences in the capacity for ammonia removal by brain following portacaval anastomosis. *J. Neurochem* 1988 ; 51: 486-490.
14. Campi N, Todeschini GP, Scarzella L. Selegiline versus L-acetylcarnitine in the treatment of Alzheimer-type dementia. *Clin. Ther* 1990 ; 12: 306-314.
15. Caporaso GL, Gandy SE, Buxbaum JD, Greengard P. Chloroquine inhibits intracellular degradation but not secretion of Alzheimer ß-A4 amyloid precursor protein. *Proc. Natl. Acad. Sci., USA* 1992 ; 89: 2252-2256.
16. Carney JM, Starke-Reed PE, Oliver CN, Landeem R, W Cheng MS, Wu JF Floyd RA. Reversal of age-related increase in brain protein oxidation, decrease in enzyme activity, and loss in temporal and spatial memory by chronic administration of the spin-trapping compound N-tert.butyl-α-phenylnitrone. *Proc. Natl. Acad. Sci. USA* 1991 ; 88: 3633-3636.
17. Cataldo AM, Nixon RA. Enzymatically active lysosomal proteases are associated with amyloid deposits in Alzheimer brain. *Proc. Natl. Acad. Sci. USA* 1990 ; 87: 3861-3865.
18. Cataldo AM, Thayer CY, Bird ED, Wheelock TR, Nixon RA. Lysosomal proteinase antigens are prominently localised within senile plaques of Alzheimer's disease: evidence for a neuronal origin. *Brain Res* 1990 ; 513: 181-192.
19. Cataldo AM, Paskevich PE, Kominami E, Nixon RA. Lysosomal hydrolases of different classes are abnormally distributed in brains of patients with Alzheimer disease. *Proc. Natl. Acad. Sci. USA* 1991 ; 88: 10998-11002.
20. Christensen H, Maltby N, Jorm AF, Creasey H, Broe GA. Cholinergic «blockade» as a model of the cognitive deficits in Alzheimer's disease. *Brain* 1992 ; 115: 1681-1699.
21. Cole GM, Huynh TV, Saitoh T. Evidence for lysosomal processing of amyloid beta-protein precursor in cultured cells. *Neurochem. Res* 1989 ; 14: 933-939.
22. Conn HO, Kieberthal MM. The hepatic coma syndromes and lactulose. Pages 22-27. Williams & Wilkins, *Baltimore* 1979.
23. Cooper AJL, Plum F. Biochemistry and physiology of brain ammonia. *Physiol. Rev* 1987 ; 67: 440-519.
24. Crowther RA. Tau protein and paired helical filaments of Alzheimer's disease. *Current Opinion Struct. Biol* 1993 ; 3: 202-206.
25. Curzon G, Kantamaneni BD, Winch J, Rochas-Bueno A, Murray-Lyon IM, Williams R. Plasma and brain tryptophan changes in experimental acute hepatic failure. *J. Neurochem* 1973 ; 21: 137-145.
26. Davies P, Maloney AJR. Selective loss of central cholinergic neurons in Alzheimer's disease. *Lancet ii* 1976 ; 1403.
27. De Keyser J. Loss of high-affinity agonist receptor binding in Alzheimer's disease. *Ann. Neurol* 1992 ; 31: 231-231.
28. Deleare P, Duyckaerts C, Brion JT, Poulain V, Hauw JJ. Tau, paired helical filaments and amyloid in the neocortex: a morphometric study of 15 cases with graded intellectual status in ageing and senile dementia of Alzheimer type. *Acta Neuropathol* 1989 ; 77: 645-653.
29. Deloncle R, Guillard O. Mechanism of Alzheimer's disease: Arguments for a neurotransmitter-aluminium complex implication. *Neurochem. Res* 1990 ; 15: 1239-1245.

30. Dickson DW, Farlo J, Davies P, Crystal H, Fuld P, Yen SH. Alzheimer's disease: a double-labeling immunohistochemical study of senile plaques. *Am. J. Pathol* 1988 ; 132: 86-101.
31. Drayna CJ, Titcomb CP, Varma RR, Soergel KH. Hyperammonemic encephalopathy caused by infection in a neurogenic bladder. N. Engl. J. *Med* 1981 ; 304: 766-768.
32. Evans PH, Klinowski J, Yano E, Urano N. Alzheimer's disease: a pathogenetic role for aluminosilicate-induced phagocytic free radicals. *Free Radic. Res. Commun* 6: 1989 ; 317-321.
33. Faff-Michalak L, Albrecht J. Hyperammonemia and hepatic encephalopathy stimulate rat cerebral synaptic mitochondrial glutamate dehydrogenase activity specifically in the direction of glutamate oxidation. *Brain Res* 1993 ; 618: 299-302.
34. Falsaperla A, Monici Preti PA, Oliani C. Selegiline versus oxiracetam in patients with Alzheimer-type dementia. *Clin. Ther* 1990 ; 12: 376-384.
35. Farrer LA, Myers RH, Connor L, Cupples LA, Growdon JH. Segregation analysis reveals evidence of a major gene for Alzheimer disease. Am. J. Hum. *Genet* 1991 ; 48: 1026-1033.
36. Felipo V, Minana MD, Wallacer R, Grisolia S. Long-term ingestion of ammonium inhibits lysosomal proteolysis in rat liver. *FEBS Lett* 1988 ; 234: 213-214.
37. Felipo V, Grau E, Minama MD, Grisolia S. Ammonium injection induces an N-methyl-D-aspartate receptor-mediated proteolysis of the microtubule-associated protein MAP-2.J. *Neurochem* 1993 ; 60: 1626-1630.
38. Fisman M, Ball M, Blume W. Hyperammonemia and Alzheimer's disease. *J. Am. Ger. Soc* 1989 ; 37: 1102.
39. Fisman, M., Gordon, B., Felcki, V., Helmes, E., Appell, J., and Rabhern, K. 1985. Hyperammonemia in Alzheimer's disease. Am. J. Psychiatry 142: 71-73.
40. Foster AC, Schwarcz R. Neurotoxic effects of quinolinic acid in the mammalian central nervous system. Pages 173-192, in Stone, T.W. (ed). Quinolinic acid and the kynurenines. CRC Press, *Boca Raton* 1989.
41. Fowler CJ, Cowburn RF, O'Neill C. Brain signal transduction disturbances in neurodegenerative disorders. *Cell. Signal* 1992 ; 4: 1-9.
42. Frackowiak RS, Possili C, Legg NJ, Du Boulay GH, Marshall J, Lenzi GL, Jones T. Regional cerebral oxygen supply and utilisation in dementia. A clinical and physiological study with oxygen-15 and positron tomography. *Brain* 1981 ; 104: 753-778.
43. Frederickson RCA. Astroglia in Alzheimer's disease. *Neurobiol. Aging* 1992 ; 13: 239-253.
44. Fukuyama H, Harada K, Yamauchi H, Miyoshi T, Yamagushi S, Kimura J, Kameyama M, Senda M, Yonekura Y, Konishi J. Coronal reconstruction images of glucose metabolism in Alzheimer's disease. *J. Neurol. Sci* 1991 ; 106: 128-134.
45. Garrick N, Murphy DL. Species differences in the deamination of dopamine and other substrates for monoamine oxidase in brain. *Psychopharmacology* 1980 ; 72: 27-33.
46. Giacobini E. Nicotinic cholinergic receptors in human brain: effects of aging and Alzheimer. Adv. Exp. *Med. Biol* 1991 ; 296: 303-315.
47. Gibson GE, Zimber A, Krook L, Richardson EP, Visek WJ. Brain histology and behavior of mice injected with urease. *J. Neuropathol. Exp. Neurol* 1974 ; 33: 201-211.
48. Glimelius B, Westermark B, Wasteson A. Ammonium ion interferes with the lysosomal degradation of glycosaminoglycans in cultures of human glial cells. Exp. *Cell Res* 1977 ; 107: 207-217.
49. Golde TE, Estus S, Younkin LH, Selkoe DJ, Younkin SG. Processing of the amyloid protein precursor to potentially amyloidogenic derivatives. *Science* 1992 ; 255: 728-730.
50. Good PF, Perl DP, Bierer LM, Schmeidler J. Selective accumulation of aluminium and iron in the neurofibrillary tangles of Alzheimer's disease: a laser microprobe (LAMMA) study. *Ann. Neurol* 1992 ; 31: 286-292.

51. Gorenstein C. A hypothesis concerning the role of endogenous colchicine-like factors in the etiology of Alzheimer's disease. Med. *Hypotheses* 1987 ; 23: 371-374.
52. Greenamyre JT, Maragos WG. Neurotransmitter receptors in Alzheimer disease. Cerebrovasc. *Brain Metab. Rev* 1993 ; 5: 61-94.
53. Grinde B. Kynurenine and lysosomal proteolysis. Pages 91-97, in Stone, T.W. (ed.). Quinolinic acid and the kynurenines. CRC Press, *Boca Raton* 1989.
54. Hardy J, Allsop D. Amyloid deposition as the central event in the aetiology of Alzheimer's disease. *TIPS* 1991 ; 12: 383-388.
55. Harman D. Free radical theory of aging: The «free radical» diseases. *Age* 1984 ; 7: 111-131.
56. Hawkins RA, Mans M. Cirrhosis, hepatic encephalopathy and ammonium toxicity. *Adv. Exp. Med. Biol* 1990 ; 272: 1-22.
57. Hefti F, Schneider LS. Nerve growth factor and Alzheimer's disease. Clin. Neuropharmacol. 14, *Suppl* 1991 ; 1, S62-S76.
58. Heiss WD, Szelies B, Kessler J,Herholz K. Abnormalities of energy metabolism in Alzheimer's disease studied with PET. Ann. N.Y. *Acad. Sci* 1991 ; 640: 65-71.
59. Henderson AS. The risk factors of Alzheimer's disease: a review and an hypothesis. *Acta Psychiatr. Scand* 1988 ; 78: 257-275.
60. Heston LL, White J. A family study of Alzheimer disease and senile dementia an interim report. Pages.63-72, in Cole, J.O., and Barrett, J.E. (ed.). American Psychopathological Association series: Psychopathology in the aged. Raven Press, *New York* 1980.
61. Hoyer S. Abnormalities of glucose metabolism in Alzheimer's disease. Ann. N.Y. *Acad. Sci* 1991 ; 640: 53-58.
62. Hoyer S, Nitsch R. Cerebral excess release of neurotransmitter amino acids subsequent to reduced cerebral glucose metabolism in early-onset dementia of Alzheimer type. *J. Neural. Transm* 1989 ; 75: 227-232.
63. Hoyer S, Oesterreich K, Wagner O. Glucose metabolism as the site of the primary abnormality in early-onset dementia of Alzheimer type ? *J. Neurol* 1988 ; 235: 143-148.
64. Hoyer S, Nitsch R, Oesterreich K. Ammonia is endogenously generated in the brain in the presence of presumed and verified dementia of Alzheimer type. *Neurosci. Lett* 1990 ; 117: 358-368.
65. Jarrett JT, Lansbury Jr PT. Seeding «one-dimensional crystallisation» of amyloid: a pathogenic mechanism in Alzheimer's disease and Scrapie. *Cell* 1993 ; 73: 1055-1058.
66. Jarvik LF, Ruth V, Matsuyama, SS. Organic brain syndrome and aging. A 6 year follow-up of surviving twins. *Arch. Gen. Psychiatry* 1980 ; 37: 280-286.
67. Jeandel C, Nicolas MB, Dubois F, Nabet-Belleville F, Penin F, Cuny G. Lipid peroxidation and free-radical scavengers in Alzheimer's disease. *Gerontology* 1989 ; 35: 275-282.
68. Jessy J, Mans AM, De Joseph RM, Hawkins A. Hyperammonemia causes many of the changes found after portacaval shunting. *Biochem. J* 1990 ; 272: 311-317.
69. Jones ME, Anderson D, Anderson C, Hodes S. Citruline synthesis in rat tissues. *Arch. Biochem. Biophys* 1961 ; 95: 499-507.
70. Jossan SS, Gillberg PG, Gottfries CG, Karlsson I, Oreland L. Monoamine oxidase B in brains from patients with Alzheimer's disease: a biochemical and autoradiographical study. *Neurosci* 1991 ; 45: 1-12.
71. Joyce JN, Kaeger C, Ryoo H, Goldsmith S. Dopamine D2 receptors in the hippocampus and amygdala in Alzheimer's disease. Neurosci. *Lett* 1993 ; 154: 171-174.
72. Kawai M, Cras P, Richey P, Tabaton M, Lowery DE, Gonzalez-de-Whitt PA, Greenberg BD, Gambetty P, Perry G. Subcellular localisation of amyloid precursor protein in senile plaques of Alzheimer's disease. Am. J. *Pathol* 1992 ; 140: 947-958.

73. Kirzinger SS, Fonda ML. Glutamine and ammonia metabolism in the brains of senescent mice. *Exp. Geront* 1978 ; 13: 255-261.
74. Körnhüber J, Wichart I, Riederer P, Kleinberger G, Jellinger K. Kynurenine in hepatic encephalopathy. Pages 275-281, in Stone, T.W. (ed.). Quinolinic acid and the kynurenines. CRC Press, *Boca Raton* 1989.
75. Kvamme E. Ammonia Metabolism in the CNS. Progr. Neurobiol. 20 Lohr, J.B. 1991. Oxygen radicals and neuropsychiatric illness. Some speculations. Arch. Gen. *Psychiatry* 1983 ; 48: 1097-1106.
76. Lapin IP. Behavioral and convulsant effects of kynurenines. Pages 193-211, in Stone, T.W. (ed.). Quinolinic acid and the kynurenines. CRC Press, *Boca Raton* 1989.
77. Lassman H, Fischer P, Jellinger K. Synaptic pathology of Alzheimer's disease in: Alzheimer's Disease. Amyloid Precursor Proteins, Signal Transduction and Neural Transplantation. Proc. 7th Meeting of the Intern. *Study Group on the Pharmacology of Memory Disorders Associated with Aging* 1993 ; pp. 41-47.
78. Lavoie J, Giguère JF, Pomier Layrargues G, Butterworth RF. Amino acid changes in autopsies brain tissue from cirrhotic patients with hepatic encephalopathy. J. *Neurochem* 1987 ; 49: 692-697.
79. Lawlor BA, Davis KL. Does modulation of glutamatergic function represent a viable therapeutic strategy in Alzheimer's disease. Biol. *Psychiatry* 1992 ; 31: 337-340.
80. Leoni P, Dean RT. Mechanisms of lysosomal enzyme secretion by human monocytes. Biochim. Biophys. *Acta* 1983 ; 762: 378-389.
81. Liguri G, Taddei N, Nassi P, Latorraca S, Nediani C, Sorbi S. Changes in Na^+, K^+-ATPase, Ca^{2-} ATPase and some soluble enzymes related to energy metabolism in brains of patients with Alzheimer's disease. Neurosci. *Lett* 1990 ; 112: 338-342.
82. Lockwood AH, Yap EWG, Wong WH. Cerebral ammonia metabolism in patients with severe liver disease and minimal hepatic encephalopathy. J. *Cerebral Blood Flow Metab* 1991 ; 11: 337-341.
83. Lohr JB. Oxygen radicals and neuropsychiatric illness. Some speculations. Arch. Gen. *Psychiatry* 1991 ; 48: 1097-1106.
84. Mangoni A, Grassi MP, Frattola L, Piolti R, Bassi S, Motta A, Marcone A, Smirne C. Effect of an MAO-B inhibitor in the treatment of Alzheimer disease. Eur. *Neurol* 1991 ; 31: 100-107.
85. Maragos WF, Greenamyre T, Penney Jr. JB, Young AB. Glutamate dysfunction in Alzheimer's disease: an hypothesis. *TINS* 1987 ; 10: 65-68.
86. Markesbery WR, Ehmann WD, Hossain TIM, Alauddin M, Goodin DT. Instrumental neutron activation analysis of brain aluminium in Alzheimer disease and aging. Ann. *Neurol* 1981 ; 10: 511-516.
87. Martignoni E, Bono G, Blandini F, Sinforiani E, Merlo, P, Nappi G. Monoamines and related metabolite levels in the cerebrospinal fluid of patients with dementia of Alzheimer type. Influence of treatment with L-deprenyl. J. *Neural Transm* 1991 ; 3: 15-25.
88. Martin H, Voss K, Hufnagl P, Wack R, Wassilew G. Morphometric and densitometric investigations of protoplasmic astrocytes and neurons in hepatic encephalopathy. Exp. *Pathol* 1987 ; 32: 198-237.
89. McGeer PL, McGeer EG, Suzudi J, Dolman CE, Nagai T. Aging, Alzheimer disease and the cholinergic system of the basal forebrain. *Neurology* 1984 ; 34: 741-745.
90. McGeer EG, McGeer PL, Akiyama H, Harrop R. Cortical glutaminase and glucose utilisation in Alzheimer's disease. J. Canad. Sci. *Neurol* 1989 ; 16: 511-515.
91. McGeer PL, Kawamata T, Walker DG, Akiyama H, Tooyama I, McGeer E. Microglia in degenerative neurological disease. *Glia* 1993 ; 7: 84-92.
92. Miklossy J. Alzheimer's disease, a spirochetosis ? *Neuro Report* 1993 ; 4, 841-848.

93. Moroni F, Lombardi G, Moneti G, Cortesini C. The release and neosynthesis of glutamic acid are increased in experimental models of hepatic encephalopathy. J. *Neurochem* 1983 ; 40: 850-854.
94. Moroni F, Lombardi and Carlà V. The measurement of quinolinic acid in the mammalian brain: neuropharmacological and physiopathological studies. Pages 53-62, in Stone, T.W. (ed.). Quinolinic acid and the kynurenines. CRC Press, *Boca Raton* 1989.
95. Nakamura S, Kawamata T, Akiguchi I, Kamayama M, Nakamura N, Kimura H. Expression of monoamine oxidase B activity in astrocytes of senile plaques. *Acta Neuropathol* 1990 ; 80: 419-425.
96. Nakamura Y, Takeda M, Suzudi H, Hattori H, Tada K, Hariguchi S, Hashimoto S, Nishimura T. Abnormal distribution of cathepsins in the brain of patients with Alzheimer's disease. *Neurosci. Lett* 1991 ; 130. 195-198.
97. Oliver CN, Starke-Reed PE, Stadtman ER, Liu GJ, Carney JM, Floyd RA. Oxidative damage to brain proteins, loss of glutamine synthetase activity and production of free radicals during ischemia/perfusion-induced injury to gerbil brain. *Proc. Natl. Acad. Sci. USA* 1990 ; 87: 5144-5147.
98. Palmer AM, Dekosky ST. Monoamine neurons in aging and Alzheimer disease. J. *Neural. Transm* 1993 ; 91: 135-139.
99. Parker Jr. WD. Cytochrome oxidase deficiency in Alzheimer's disease. *Ann. N.Y. Acad. Sci* 1991 ; 640: 59-64.
100. Pike CJ, Burdick D, Walencewicz AJ, Glabe CG, Cotman CW. Neurodegeneration induced by beta-amyloid peptides in vitro: The role of peptide assembly state. J. *Neurosci* 1993 ; 13: 1676-1687.
101. Pomara N, Singh R, Deptula D, Chou JCY, Banay Schwartz M, Le Witt PA. Glutamate and other CSF amino acids in Alzheimer's disease. *Am. J. Psychiatry* 1992 ; 149: 251-254.
102. Procter AW, Palmer AM, Francis DT, Low SL, Neary D, Murphey E, Doshi R, Bowen DM. Evidence of glutamatergic denervation and possible abnormal metabolism in Alzheimer's disease. J. *Neurochem* 1988 ; 50: 790-802.
103. Prusiner SD. Some speculations about prions, amyloid, and Alzheimer's disease. *N. Engl. J. Med* 1984 ; 310: 661-663.
104. Raabe W. Synaptic transmission in ammonia intoxication. *Neurochem. Pathol.* 6: 145-166.
105. Raabe, W.A., and Onstad, G.A. 1982. Ammonia and methionine sulfoximine intoxication. *Brain Res* 1987 ; 242: 291-298.
106. Rainikainen KJ, Paljärvi L, Halonen T, Malminen O, Kosma VM, Laakso M, Riekkinen PJ. Dopaminergic system and monoamine oxidase-B activity in Alzheimer's disease. *Neurobiol. Aging* 1988 ; 9: 245-252.
107. Record CO. Neurochemistry of hepatic encephalopathy. *Gut* 1991 ; 32: 1261-1263.
108. Roberts E. Disinhibition as an organising principle in the nervous system. The role of the GABA system. Application to neurologic and psychiatric disorders. Pages 515-539, in Roberts, E., Chase, T.N., and Tower, D.B. (eds.). GAB in Nervous System Function. Raven Press, *New York* 1976.
109. Robinson DS, Davis JM, Nies A, Ravaris CL, Sylwester D. Relation of sex and aging to monoamine oxidase activity in human brain, plasma and platelets. *Arch. Gen. Psychiatry* 1971 ; 24: 536-539.
110. Schor NF, Ahdab-Barmada M, Nemoto E. Brain glutamine synthetase activity and hyperoxia in neonatal rats. *Brain Res* 1991 ; 566: 342-343.
111. Segelen PO. Inhibitors of lysosomal function. *Meth. Enzymol* 1983 ; 96: 737-765.
112. Seiler N. Is ammonia a pathogenetic factor in Alzheimer's disease ? *Neurochem. Res* 1993 ; 18: 235-245.
113. Selkoe DJ. The molecular pathology of Alzheimer's disease. *Neuron* 1991 ; 6: 487-498.

114. Smith CD, Carney JM, Starke-Reed PE, Oliver CN, Stadtman ER, Floyd RA, Markesbery WR. Excess brain protein oxidations and enzyme dysfunction in normal aging and in Alzheimer disease. *Proc. Natl. Acad. Sci. USA* 1991 . 88: 10540-10543.
115. St. George-Hyslop PH, Tanzi RE, Polinsky RJ, Haines JL, Nee L, Watkins PC, Myers RH, Feldman RG, Pollen D, Drachman D, Groxdon J, Bruni A, Foncin JF, Salmon D, Frommet P, Amaducci L, Sorbi S, Piacentini S, Stewart GD, Hobbs WJ, Conneally PM, Gusella JF. The genetic defect causing familial Alzheimer's disease maps on chromosome 21. *Science* 1987 ; 235: 885-890.
116. Student AK, Edwards DJ. Subcellular localisation of types A and B monoamine oxidase in rat brain. Biochem. Pharmacol. 1977 ; 26: 2337-2342.
117. Swain MS, Blei AT, Butterworth RF, Kraig RP. Intracellular pH rises and astrocytes swell after portacaval anastomosis in rats. Am. J. *Physiol* 1991 ; 261: 51494-51496.
118. Tanzi RE, St. George-Hyslop P, Gusella JF. Molecular genetics of Alzheimer disease amyloid. J. *Biol. Chem* 1991 ; 266: 20579-20582.
119. Terry RD, Masliah E, Salmon DP, Butters N, De Theresa R, Hill R, Hausen LA, Katzman R. Physical basis of cognitive alterations in Alzheimer's disease: synaptic loss is the major correlate of cognitive impairment. *Ann. Neurol* 1991 ; 30: 572-580.
120. Therrien G, Butterworth RF. Cerebrospinal amino acids in relation to neurological status in experimental portal-systemic encephalopathy. *Metabolic Brain Dis* 1991 ; 6: 65-74.
121. Thompson CM, Markesbery WR, Ehmann WD, Mao YX, Vance DE. Regional brain trace element studies in Alzheimer's disease. *Neurotoxicology* 1988 ; 9: 1-8.
122. Tossman U, Delin A, Eriksson LS, Ungerstedt U. Brain cortical amino acids measured by intracerebral dialysis in portacaval shunted rats. *Neurochem. Res* 1987 ; 12: 265-269.
123. Tsuboi M, Harasawa K, Izawa T, komabayashi T, Fujinami H, Suda K. Intralysosomal pH and release of lysosomal enzymes in the rat liver after exhaustive exercise. J. Appl. *Physiol* 1993 ; 74: 1628-1634.
124. Tzourio C, Bonaiti C, Clerget-Darpoux F, Alperovitch A. Segregation analysis in Alzheimer disease: No evidence for a major gene. Am. J. *Hum. Gen* 1992 ; 50: 645-646.
125. Uribe. Nutrition, diet and hepatic encephalopathy. ages 529-547, in Butterworth R.F., and Pomier Layrarges G. (eds.). Hepatic encephalopathy: Pathophysiology and treatment. Humana Press, *Clifton* 1989.
126. Vandenbeele P, Fiers W. Is amyloidogenesis during Alzheimer's disease due to IL-1-/IL-6 mediated acute phase response in the brain ? Immunol. *Today* 1991 ; 12: 217-219.
127. Volicer L, Crino PB. Involvement of free radicals in dementia of the Alzheimer type: a hypothesis. Neurobiol. *Aging* 1990 ; 11: 567-571.
128. Vrba R, Folberg J. Endogenous metabolism in brain in vitro and in vivo. J. *Neurochem* 1959 ; 4: 338-349.
129. Vrba R, Folberg J, Kanturek V. Ammonia formation in brain cortex slices. *Nature* 1957 ; 179: 470-471.
130. Wallace DR, Dawson Jr. R. Ammonia regulation of phosphate-activated glutaminase displays regional variation and impairment in the brain of aged rats. *Neurochem. Res* 1992 ; 17: 1113-1122.
131. Weil-Malherbe H, Drysdale AC. Ammonia formation in brain. III. Role of the protein amide groups and of hexosamines. J. *Neurochem* 1957 ; 1: 250-257.
132. Yamamoto T, Iwasaki Y, Sato Y, Yamamoto H, Konno H. Astrocytic pathology of methionine sulfoximine-induced encephalopathy. *Acta Neuropathol* 1989 ; 77: 357-368.
133. Yankner BA, Duffy LK, Kirschner DA. Neurotrophic and neurotoxic effects of amyloid beta protein: reversal by tachykinin neuropeptides. *Science* 1990 ; 250: 279-282.
134. Zieve L. Pathogenesis of hepatic encephalopathy; *Metabolic Brain Dis* 1987 ; 2: 147-165.

18

Pattern recognition techniques in MRI Brain disease diagnosis : a quantified approach

A. ALAUX

Université de Montpellier I, Faculté de Médecine
Département de biophysique
Institut de biologie, Boulevard Henri IV, 34080 Montpellier Cedex, France.

Today magnetic resonance imaging techniques yield tomograms of impressive visual quality.

However, with the movement toward a rich radiological technique, MRI has suffered the loss of its development as quantitative diagnostic test. The majority of the MRI research to date has been geared toward producing aesthetically pleasing images with higher signal to noise ratio, finer resolution and faster scan times. While these are laudable goals in the context of imaging it is not clear how to transform improvements in these attributes into improvements in diagnostic performance.

If we want to improve the MRI diagnostic performance we have to introduce the concept of limit and apply it to MRI and the MRI user.

MRI possesses :
• several physical parameters,
difficulties in computing and exploiting these parameters,
the possibility to derive a multivariate test.
MRI clinicians :
• know very well : anatomy, physiology and pathology,
• they are unable to differentiate 4095 grey levels in an MR Image,
• they are unable to make correlations if the number of images per anatomical slice exceeds 3,

• the main concern of a clinician is to improve the sensitivity and the specificity of a diagnostic test.

Next point is that accurate tissue discrimination may require increased dependence on computer based image analysis techniques to extract tissue specific information. Finally I would say that it may be advantageous to develop new image products and image presentation to facilitate interpretation.

Our approach to these problems has been through pattern recognition techniques.

Pattern recognition

What is pattern recognition ?

Pattern recognition is a general term assigned to a large group of techniques pertaining to decision making.

In the case of MR image data sets, pattern recognition refers to finding rules that allow a mapping of pixel intensity values onto different tissue type.

When MR image intensities for a particular anatomical location are considered, then these values may allow us to decide that a pixel contains a particular tissue type.

Since the theories and techniques of pattern recognition are largely mathematical in nature I would say that the mathematical level of this presentation will be very low.

I am today far more interested with providing insight and understanding than with establishing rigorous mathematical foundation.

The use of many illustrative examples and plausibility arguments reflect our concern.

As a general comment we have to say that considering MR Image intensities, high sensitivity is required, so avoidable variations due to both data acquisition and data analysis must be minimised. Variations due to the imager, must be small with respect to the intrinsic variability of the tissue and data analysis must introduce no extra source of variability. Quality assurance methods suited to quantification have been developed. Three aspects of the MR imager are monitored : stability, precision and accuracy.

Let us turn our attention to the pattern recognition techniques of MR images.

Materials and methods

Our study includes twenty four normal volunteers and eighteen patients with various axial and extra axial brain lesions.

MR images of the brain were acquired on MR imaging systems at 0.5 and 1.5 T (Gyroscan 55 and S15; Philips Medical) using a spin echo multislice 2DFT technique (5mm thickness, 256 x 256 matrix, 2,5 mm interslice) namely a T1, T2 and spin echo weighted image and a Fast Field echo technique.

Our procedure can be divided into three main steps :
• the pre-processing step,
• the processing step,
• the post-processing step.

Pre-processing step

The pre-processing step includes the calibration of the signal intensity, the correction of intensity non uniformities and the registration.

For pattern recognition techniques it is essential to correct image intensity non uniformities and there are several possible sources of non uniformity in clinical images :
1. the transmitted B1 field which determines flip angle.
2. the received B1 field which determines sensitivity.
3. the receiver filter : an analogue filter in the receiver chain used to limit bandwidth encode direction.
4. uncompensated gradient eddy currents.

Among these sources, the coils can give rise to marked image intensity non uniformities. This is most apparent in image of uniform phantoms, where the signal intensity varies across the field of view and from slice to slice with high regions close to the coil winding.

Several approaches can be used for correction of the RF coil non uniformities. Our correction is based on the response of a system to a uniform phantom. That approach determines the actual non uniformities shown in an image of a uniform phantom and use this image to produce a correction matrix which can be divided from a patient or object to correct for its non uniformities.

The next pre-processing step occurs when there has been displacement of the head during scan time of the image components. The term image component denotes a single image from a given slice acquired by a fixed setting of the extrinsic parameters. So using different settings of the pulse timing parameters but keeping the other parameters constant will thus results in a set of image components.

All the image components must overlap as perfectly as possible, the quality of image registration having a significant effect on quantitative image analysis and pattern recognition techniques.

The transformation is done to align T1 weighted and fast field echo images with proton density weighted image. In all cases, two majors steps are required to do the transformation.

- First the warping or deformation to apply is specified. This is done by specifying a mathematical deformation model defining the relation between the line and sample co-ordinates in the corrected image and the line and sample co-ordinate in the input image.
- Secondly using the model the corrected image is generated from the input image. The most common method of doing this second step is to resample the input image.

The deformation model is computed by using control points. The control points are anatomical features located both in the input and the reference images. Once computed the deformation model, we can map pixel locations from the corrected image to the input image and we are ready to consider the «picking up» of a pixel value. This is the resampling.

Three resampling algorithms are available :
- nearest neighbour
- bilinear interpolation
- cubic convolution

Once this preparation work is done we can turn our attention to the processing step of the MR corrected data.

Processing step

MR imaging systems measure spatial distribution of several distinct physical parameters. The relative pixel intensities in the MR data set for each tissue class result in the formation of related tissue clusters in feature space. If image intensity based methods are used and a large number of image components are generated for each anatomical slice using different radio frequency pulse sequences, a higher order feature space is obtained that further improves segmentation, not possible by visual evaluation of the individual image component.

Pattern recognition techniques can be used to locate tissue clusters in feature space and hence can inherently provide a greater confidence level of image interpretation than simplistic grey scale approaches used for X-ray CT or single MR images.

Many pattern recognition methods used for image segmentation require training data sets to identify each tissue type and are referred to as supervised segmentation techniques.

Methods of unsupervised classification attempt to find clusters in the feature space. The tissues and lesions are determined within the algorithm by locating clusters in feature space and assuming that each cluster corresponds to a tissue or lesion.

Supervised classification

Among the families of supervised pattern recognition techniques the maximum likelihood method is a representative for the parametric method.

We consider several MR image intensities for a particular anatomical location then these values may allow us to decide that a pixel contains a particular tissue type. The decision is based on the prior knowledge of the above intensity values determined by the selected training ROIs and how close the training data sets are compared to the measured pixel intensity values.

The method can be stated as a sequence of conceptual steps necessary to classify an image.

– First we select training areas for each candidate tissue. These are areas known to contain pixels representative of a tissue type. Training ROIs are defined over various components of the image : white matter, grey matter, fat, CSF muscle and diploe. We have to know that training ROIs may be selected within the same image slice, adjacent slice or slice from a different imaging session or patient.

– A high order dimensional histogram is computed for the training data for each tissue. The normalised histograms are considered as estimates of the conditional probability density functions.

– The conditional probability density functions are scaled by the a priori probabilities assumed to be equal in order to derive a set of decision functions : called likelihood functions.
– Finally a decision is made for the classification of each pixel : each pixel being assigned to the tissue for which the likelihood function is maximum. This gives the method its name: maximum likelihood classification.

The result of the classification is theme maps in which each colour represent a particular tissue. Once derived, the set of decision functions may be applied for the classification of the adjacent slice or a slice from a different imaging session or patient.

Unsupervised classification

Until now we have assumed that the training samples used to design the bayesian classifier were labelled to show their category membership.

Now we shall investigate unsupervised procedures that use unlabelled samples. That is we shall see what can be done when all one has is a collection of samples without being told their classification. One might wonder why anyone is interested in such an unpromising problem and whether or not it is even possible to learn anything of value from unlabelled samples.

There are two basic reasons for interest in unsupervised techniques.
– First the collection and labelling of a large set of sample patterns can be costly and time consuming.
– Second the MR physical parameters of the tissues can change with time.

So, methods of unsupervised classification attempt to find clusters in the distribution of the pixels in feature space. Although clusters are often fairly easy for a human to identify in one and two dimensional plots, their centres and boundaries are difficult to identify mathematically, and cluster analysis is a field of study all its own.

In feature space points or vectors coming from fat will form a cluster that will be different from that one of muscle, or grey mater and so on... The clustering problem is that of finding natural groupings in a set of MR intensity values. We are obliged to define what we mean by a «natural grouping». In what sense are we to say that the points in one cluster are more like one another than like points in other clusters.

This question actually involves two separate issues :
• how should one measure the similarity between samples,
• and how should one evaluate a partitioning of a set of samples into clusters.

Viewed geometrically these pixels form cloud of points. The most obvious measure of the similarity between two pixels is the distance between them. One way to begin a clustering investigation is to define a suitable distance function and compute the matrix of distances between all pair of pixels.

Our iterative clustering method is called the K-means algorithm. Expressed in terms of the MR image data it has the following steps.

Initially the user supplies a set of means, or clusters centres... and thus implicitly the number of tissues. Then :
– For each pixel in the image, assign the pixel to the tissue to whose mean it is closest.
– Recompute the mean of each class as the average of the pixels assigned to it.

– If any of the tissue means has changed significantly go to the second step, otherwise stop.

In fact we use the Isodata algorithm which is a modified version of the k-means algorithm that allows classes to be split and merged. Even with this version, best results are usually obtained when running this unsupervised classifier in a «supervised» mode. In this case, after each iteration, the user views the results, adjusts parameters to control the splitting and merging and stops the iterations when satisfactory classes have been obtained.

For the normal head we generally stop the process when we have got 8 or 9 clusters.

Clinical evaluation and inter observer inter patient analysis

Evaluated were twenty four studies of normal and eighteen patient studies. Three parameters were assessed on each image : conspiscuity of the lesion, extension of the lesion and edge detection and the number of differentiable components within the lesion.

Correctness of segmentation was evaluated by two teams of two experienced MR radiologists by comparison of the segmentation with the MR films. One team was blinded to the patient history. Although disagreement between the radiologist existed on points, there was a consensus on the overall ranking of the segmentation methods.

Statistical validity cannot be assured from such a small sample. However we can give partial answers to the three following questions :

1. Does our pattern recognition technique perform comparably with the radiologist as far as the lesion detectability is concerned ?

Segmentation techniques can detect lesions as well as the radiologist in 87 % of all cases. As for as the size of the lesion is concerned these techniques are able to detect a lesion whose size is larger than 0.5 cm^2. Results are variable for smaller lesions but can be improved.

2. Do segmentation techniques perform comparably with the radiologist as far as the extension of the lesion and edge detection are concerned ?

Regarding extension and delineation the supervised technique rated better than the radiologist in 44 % of all cases, identically in 50 % and worse in 6 %.

The clustering technique rated better than the radiologist in 56 % of all cases and identically in 44 %.

3. Do segmentation techniques perform comparably with the radiologist as far as the number of differentiable components are concerned ?

The number of identifiable structures was identical on supervised theme maps and acquired images. The number of differentiable components was greater on 8 non supervised theme maps than on acquired images. In all other the identifiable components were identical on unsupervised theme maps and acquired images.

Conclusion

We have shown that computer analysis can provide improved lesion detection, improved boundary definition between tissues and some confidence level in the detection of the differential components.

This presentation focuses on several steps of the procedure for pattern recognition techniques of MR images that affect the correctness of the segmentation results. Other factors affects it too, such as imaging protocols and patient related factors and have to be explored.

We have shown that intensity distortions can be corrected using derived correction matrices. Registration correction is necessary too.

However, advances in MR technology may probably, reduce many of the instrument related factors that can affect the stability of segmentation such as rapid 2D or 3DFT imaging methods.

Alternative supervised-segmentation methods as k-nearest neighbours and artificial neural net work techniques with fixed or dynamic architecture has to be explored.

Similarly, alternative unsupervised segmentation methods are possible such as fuzzy clustering techniques.

Pattern recognition methods should therefore play an increasingly important role for image fusion of multispectral 3D data sets and provide an improved confidence level for image interpretation using a 3D workstation for MRI data analysis.

References

1. Alaux A. *Multispectral analysis of MR. Images, internal paper : MR.* Centre 1988, Trondhein - Norway.
2. Alaux A.M. Dalati. Multispectral analysis of MR. Images. Berlin 1988 Second European Congress of NMR in Medicine and Biology.
3. Alaux A. et Al. *Pattern classification techniques in cardiac magnetic resonance imaging. First results.* ICR, 1989, Paris.
4. Alaux A., Rinck P. Principal component analysis and MR image synthesis. A clinical evaluation SMRM Congress, 1989; Amsterdam.
5. Alaux A., Dalati M., Rinck P. Supervised and unsupervised classification techniques in MRI. New developments I.C.R., 1989; Paris.
6. Alaux A., Rinck P. Supervised and unsupervised classification in MRI. A clinical evaluation. In *Tissue characterisation in MR imaging* (H.P. Higer and G. Bielke, Eds). Springer, Berlin, Heidelberg, New York, 1990.
7. Alaux A., Myrheim J., Rue H. Coil sensitivity correction in MRI. European Congress of NMR in Medicine and Biology, 1990; Strasbourg.
8. Alaux A., Kvaerness J., Rinck P. Pattern recognition techniques in cardiac magnetic resonance imaging. European Congress of NMR in Medicine and Biology, 1990; Strasbourg.
9. Alaux A., Myrheim J., Rinck P. Improvement of the MRI diagnostic performance by using pattern recognition techniques. European Congress of NMR in Medicine and Biology, 1990; Strasbourg.
10. Alaux A. *L'image par Resonance Magnétique.* Sauramps Medical, Montpellier 1994.

11. Alaux A. Transformations géométriques, chapitre 20, pp 471-484, l'*Image par Résonance Magnétique*. Sauramps Médical, Montpellier, 1994.
12. Alaux A. Segmentation, description, Chapitre 21, pp 485-520, l'*Image par Résonance Magnétique*. Sauramps Médical, Montpellier, 1994.
13. Alaux A. La Reconnaissance des formes en IRM, Chapitre 22, pp 521-554, l'*Image par Résonance Magnétique*. Sauramps Medical, Montpellier, 1994.
14. Alaux A. Le diagnostic assisté par ordinateur en Imagerie Médicale, chapitre 22, pp 555-608, l'*Image par Résonance Magnétique*, Sauramps Medical Montpellier, 1994.
15. Alpert N.M., Bradshaw J.F., Kennedy D., Correia J.A. The principal axes transformations - a method for image registration. *J. Nucl. Med.* 31 : 1717-1722, 1990.
16. Bensaid A.M., Hall L.O., Clarke L.P., Velthuizn R.P. MRI Segmentation using supervised and unsupervised methods. Proceedings of the 13th Annual IEEE Eng. Med et Biol. Orlando, FL, Oct 31-Nov. 3: 1991.
17. Bezdek J.C. A convergence theorem for the fuzzy ISODATA clustering algorithms. IEEE Trans on Pattern Analysis and machine Intelligence PAMI-2(1): 1-8, 1980.
18. Choi H.S., Haynor D.R., Kim Y. Multivariate tissue classification of MRI images for 3-D volume reconstruction a statistical approach, SPIE 1092, 183-193 (1989).
19. Fahlman S., Hinton G. Connectionist architectures for artificial intelligence. IEEE Computer 20(1): 100-109, 1987.
20. Glennon D.T. Correction of magnetic resonance image non-uniformity. University of south Florida, December 1991, Masters Thesis.
21. Hu X., Johnson V., Wong W.H., Chen C.T. Bayesian image processing in magnetic resonance imaging. *Magn. Reson. Imaging* 9: 611-620 (1991).
22. Hyman T.J., Kurland R.J., Levy G.C., Shoop J.D. Characterisation of normal brain tissue using seven calculated MRI parameters and a statistical analysis system. *Magn. Reson. Med.* 11:22-34, 1989.
23. Jungke M., Von Seelen W., Bielke G., Meindi S., Krone G., Gricat M., Higer P., Pfannenstiel P. Information processing in nuclear magnetic resonance imaging. *Magn. Reson. Imaging* 6: 683-693, 1988.
24. Menhart W., Schmidt K.H. Computer vision on magnetic resonance images. *Pattern Recogn. Lettr.* 8: 73-85, 1988.
25. Merickel M.B., Carman C.S., Brookeman J.R., Ayers C.R. Image analysis and quantification of atherosclerosis using MRI. Comput. *Med. Imaging. graph.* 15(4): 207-216, 1991.
26. O'Donnell, MM Gore J.C., Dams W.J. Toward an automated analysis system for nuclear magnetic resonance imaging. II. Initial segmentation algorithm. *Med. Phys.* 13(3): 293-297, 1986.
27. Sclove S.L. Application of the conditional population-mixture model to image segmentation. IEEE Trans. Pattern Anal. Machine Intell. PAMI-5(4): 428-433 (1983).
28. Windham J.P., Soltanian-Zadeh H., Peck D.J. Delineation of internal structure in cerebral tumors using MRI. *Med. Phys.* (19(3), 844 (1992).

19

Relevance of psychiatric rating scales : what do they measure ?

P.E. BAILEY

FORENAP, Secteur VIII, Centre Hospitalier, 68250 Rouffach, France.

The search for neuroanatomical and neurophysiological correlates of psychiatric symptoms and syndromes demands more than sophisticated methods of mapping brain structure and function. It also requires reliable, valid methods for ascertaining the presence or absence and, where possible, the intensity of psychiatric phenomena. Psychiatric rating scales are generally used for this purpose.

A complete review of the topic is beyond the scope of a short paper. I should therefore like to offer a few remarks on some problems and limitations of psychiatric rating scales. As an example I shall take the rating of the negative symptoms of schizophrenia, since this has been one focus of interest in brain-imaging studies (*see* e.g. Lewis, 1990).

Rating scales in psychiatry are traditionally divided into those filled out by the patient himself (self-rating scales) and those filled out by a doctor, nurse or other professional (observer-rating scales). For reasons of space I shall not discuss self-rating scales, nor scales assessing cognitive function.

Rating scales and their uses

Diagnosis

Much progress has been made in recent years in the search for biological markers of psychiatric disorder. Nonetheless there is still no psychiatric disorder for which the anatomical and physiological basis has been precisely defined. Thus psychiatric diagnosis consists in the identification of psychiatric symptoms (some of which are just the extremes of normal experience, e.g. sadness, whilst others are clearly abnormal, e.g. hallucinations) and their assembly into one (or several) more or less generally recognized syndromes.

One way of increasing agreement about diagnosis is to use diagnostic criteria, such as the Diagnostic and Statistical Manual (DSM) of the American Psychiatric Association. These criteria can be regarded as logically-linked multiple rating scales. For example, consider Criterion A for Schizophrenia in the DSM-IV (American Psychiatric Association 1994):

Two (or more) of the following, each present for a significant portion of time during a one-month period (or less if successfully treated):
  1. delusions,
  2. hallucinations,
  3. disorganized speech (e.g. frequent derailment or incoherence),
  4. grossly disorganized or catatonic behaviour,
  5. negative symptoms, ie affective flattening, alogia or avolition.

This can be regarded as a rating scale. Score 0 if the symptom is absent, score 1 if present; add the scores; if total is two or more go to criterion B, otherwise go to next diagnosis. (DSM experts will realise that, to clarify the argument, I have oversimplified: under some circumstances a total of one is sufficient.)

The more conventional use of rating scales in diagnosis is simply to define a threshold total score and regard the diagnosis as established if the patient scores higher than the threshold. The popularity of this procedure has often been allowed to obscure its methodological drawbacks. For example, patients with multiple somatic complaints and high anxiety levels will have high scores on the Hamilton Depression Rating Scale but they may not be depressed. This is probably one reason why Hamilton himself (1960) explicitly stated that his scale was not to be used for diagnostic purposes - an observation which has often passed unnoticed.

Severity

Quantification of severity is the more frequent use for psychiatric rating scales. In everyday clinical practice we may wish to follow change in a patient's clinical state over time by rating him regularly, say once a week. Thus the apparent effectiveness of clinical interventions (psychotherapy, medication, etc.) can be assessed. In a research setting we may wish to compare the efficacy of two or more treatments, correlate a symptom or syndrome with a biological measure, and so on.

To use a rating scale in such circumstances rather than relying on clinical acumen implies that the scale offers some advantages. These are usually described in terms of reliability and validity.

Reliability and validity

Stated informally:
Reliability is the extent to which two (or more) raters agree.
Validity is the extent to which the rating measures what it claims to measure.

Reliability is interesting in its own right, but the most important aspect of reliability in the practical application of rating scales is this: stated once again informally, validity is always lower than reliability. Reliability is the "noise" in measurement introduced by inter-rater variability. For example, if the true difference between patient A and patient B on some scale is three points, and if rater X and rater Y disagree randomly on their ratings by up to five points, then, if X and Y both rate A and B, the true difference is likely to be obscured by the random variation. If X rates only A and Y rates only B then the situation is even worse.

It is a common misconception that *the* "reliability" of a scale can be measured. Reliability is context-dependent. If X and Y are together when they rate A, their ratings will agree more than if they rate A on separate occasions (even assuming that A himself does not change). If X and Y work in the same unit, their ratings will agree more than if they work in different centres. But "the most important point, least welcome to medical researchers, is the suggestion that one needs a matrix... to describe the reliability of a categorical measure. A single summary index will not do." (Kraemer 1992; see also the article by Agresti in the same volume for a discussion of reliability of non-categorical measures.)

If estimating *the* reliability of a scale is problematic, estimating the validity is even more so. Different types of validity have been identified, but for the purposes of this discussion they can be reduced to three forms: criterion validity, face validity and construct validity.

Criterion validity involves direct comparison with an external measurement standard. Thus I might validate a one-meter ruler by taking the ruler to Paris and comparing it directly with the international Standard Meter. The equivalent in psychiatry would presumably be to compare the rating with some direct measure of the underlying biological pathology. This is clearly impossible at present but, even worse, I shall suggest in a moment that it is conceptually impossible too. *Faute de mieux*, criterion validity of psychiatric rating scales is often presented in terms of the correlation between the sum score of the new scale and that of a "standard" scale. Since the criterion validity of the "standard" scale can by definition never be established in this way, such a procedure seems hard to justify. Predictive validity, in which the scale score is shown to correlate with some measure of outcome, is simply a form of criterion validity, since it depends on the existence of previous studies showing a correlation between outcome and a standard scale.

Face validity describes the extent to which accepted features of the entity to be measured are reflected in the scale. Thus a depression rating scale without an item assessing depressed mood would have low face validity. However establishing face validity for syndromes whose content is controversial (e.g. negative schizophrenia) is problematic.

So more or less by a process of elimination it is construct validity which generally plays an important role in the validation of psychiatric scales. Construct validity is the use of mathematical measures internal to the scale itself to justify the construction of the scale, usually by demonstrating that it is in some sense unidimensional. There are many such measures available, such as split-half coefficients, Cronbach's alpha, Rasch analysis, and factor analysis. Some of these measures are interrelated: for example, Cronbach's alpha is an average of all possible split-half coefficients. The precise application of these measures to a given problem raises mathematical as well as clinical questions: see for instance McDonald (1981) for a discussion of such measures and their relationship to the problem of unidimensionality. But the general approach is to appeal to a mathematical entity (a factor, a high correlation ...) as a kind of proxy for the unobservable psychiatric pathology.

I would suggest that this approach is open to the same conceptual difficulties as criterion validity. The difficulties arise from trying to form a notion of a "depression score" or a "schizophrenia score". Consider these three statements:

1. A is less depressed than one week ago.
2. A is less depressed than B.
3. A is exactly as depressed as B.

(1) is straightforward. This is the kind of assessment that we make all the time in our clinical practice, the assessment that guides our treatment plan. The fact that it may be difficult from time to time to judge if it is true or not does not mean that the statement is meaningles, (2) is seductive because it looks similar to (1), but at the very least it seems difficult to decide how the truth of such a statement could be verified, (3) is even more problematic. Substitute «schizophrenic» for «depressed» in (2), and then in (3), and the problem becomes clearer: A, an acutely-ill, excited, hallucinating patient may have the same score on a rating scale as B, a passive, withdrawn, apathetic chronic patient. I suggest that it makes no sense at all to state that one is "exactly as ill" as the other. If A and B are both assigned the same number by a rating scale, it is not clear to me how this number can be a proxy for their clinical state. Clinical states are not unidimensional; schizophrenia almost certainly is not and depression probably is not either.

To ask why rating scales have achieved such widespread popularity in the face of such methodological adversity is to venture into psychological and philosophical questions far beyond the remit of this paper. One possible answer has been outlined by Walker (1994): "Standard clinical practice leans heavily toward the realist view of diagnostic criteria having a contingent relationship to a presumed underlying process, whereas DSM [...] remains stuck within a now outmoded empiricist philosophy of science."

An example: negative symptoms of schizophrenia

One of the oldest and most widely-used rating scales is the Brief Psychiatric Rating Scale (BPRS) of Overall and Gorham. It illustrates another problem of rating scales not yet alluded to: that of multiple versions. In its original form (Overall and Gorham, 1962) the BPRS had 16 items, but the authors later added another two ("Excitement" and "Disorientation"). The 18-item version (Overall and Gorham 1976) is now standard, but studies using the longer version often incorrectly cite the reference to the 16-item scale.

The authors of the BPRS performed a factor analysis on ratings from 3 596 patients and described an "Anergia" (negative symptom) factor consisting of the items "Emotional Withdrawal", "Motor Retardation", "Blunted Affect" and "Disorientation". Most subsequent factor analyses of the BPRS have also found this factor, which thus has a certain construct validity. However some clinical studies of negative symptoms have omitted the "Disorientation" item or added the item "Depression", apparently on the basis of face validity (Möller et al., 1994). The BPRS full scale total score is often taken as a measure of criterion validity for new scales.

The best-known scale devoted entirely to negative symptoms is the Scale for the Assessment of Negative Symptoms (SANS; Andreasen, 1981). The items of this scale were originally selected on the basis of face validity; some items were then eliminated on the grounds of poor reliability and/or poor correlation with other items (construct validity). Nonetheless a recent multicentre study (Mueser Sayers Schooler et al., 1994) reported considerably lower item reliability (using a single-index measure) than that obtained by Andreasen's group. Furthermore, the construct validity of the scale has been questioned on two grounds. First, the original version of the scale included five items tapping the patient's subjective awareness of negative symptoms; these correlated poorly with other items and were later dropped. Second, the scale includes at least two items ("Inappropriate Affect" and "Poverty of Content of Speech") which appear not to form part of a "core" negative syndrome. These two items form a separate factor in a three-factor model of the SANS which has been found to be superior to the subscale structure proposed by Andreasen (Keefe Harvey Lenzenweger et al., 1992).

The Positive and Negative Syndrome Scale (Kay Fiszbein and Opler, 1987) is a development and extension of the BPRS: to the 18 BPRS items the authors added a further 12 which they considered important in the assessment of the schizophrenic patient (face validity) and then gave definitions for the rating of each item, in order to improve inter-rater reliability. Studies by the authors and by independent groups (e.g. Bell Milstein Beam-Goulet et al., 1992) suggest that single-index measures of reliability do indeed favour the PANSS over the BPRS. Negative symptoms are assessed by means of the 7-item Negative Scale, of which five items load heavily on a single factor (construct validity). The authors found a correlation of 0.77 between the Negative Scale and the SANS total score (alleged criterion validity).

The item content of the SANS and of the Negative Scale of the PANSS have been compared with six other negative symptom scales by Fenton and McGlashan (1992). Substantial differences were found, the SANS being the most inclusive. This suggests that assessment of face validity of these scales is subject to great variation. Of course face validity is also context-dependent. If the intention of a rating is to capture the broadest possible range of negative symptomatology, at the risk of including some symptoms peripheral to the true negative syndrome (ignoring questions as to how its "truth" might be established...), then the SANS is clearly the instrument of choice;

however it would be viewed better as a symptom checklist than as a scale. If the intention is to maximize rater reliability and sum the item scores to arrive at a "negative score" then it would be preferable to choose a scale which is more limited in scope and which is in some sense unidimensional.

Conclusion

The use of psychiatric rating scales is not as straightforward as it may appear at first sight. However, in the absence of identified causative pathology in psychiatric disorders, such scales provide our only approach to the quantification and objectification of symptoms which, by their very nature, are subjective. That indeed is the curse and the fascination of clinical psychiatry.

References

Andreasen N (1982). Scale for the Assessment of Negative Symptoms (SANS). University of Iowa, Iowa City.
American Psychiatric Association (1994). Diagnostic and statistical manual of mental disorders. Fourth edition. *American Psychiatric Association*, Washington, DC.
Bell M, Milstein R, Beam-Goulet J *et al.* (1992). The Positive and Negative Syndrome Scale and the Brief Psychiatric Rating Scale. *Journal of Nervous and Mental Disease* 180: 723-728.
Fenton WS, McGlashan TH (1992). Testing systems for assessment of negative symptoms in schizophrenia. *Archives of General Psychiatry* 49: 179-184.
Hamilton M (1960). A rating scale for depression. *Journal of Neurology Neurosurgery and Psychiatry* 23: 56-62.
Kay SR, Fiszbein A, Opler LA (1987). The Positive and Negative Syndrome Scale (PANSS) for schizophrenia. *Schizophrenia Bulletin* 13: 261-276.
Keefe RSE, Harvey PD, Lenzenweger MF *et al.* (1992). Empirical assessment of the factorial structure of clinical symptoms in schizophrenia: negative symptoms. *Psychiatry Research* 44: 153-165.
Kraemer HC (1992). Measurement of reliability for categorical data in medical research. *Statistical Methods in Medical Research* 1: 183-199.
Lewis SW (1990). Computerised tomography in schizophrenia. 15 years on. *British Journal of Psychiatry* 157 (suppl. 9): 16-24.
McDonald RP (1981). The dimensionality of tests and items. *British Journal of Mathematical and Statistical Psychology* 34: 100-117.
Möller H-J, van Praag HM, Aufdembrinke B *et al.* (1994). Negative symptoms in schizophrenia: considerations for clinical trials. *Psychopharmacology* 115: 221-228.
Mueser KT, Sayers SL, Schooler NR *et al.* (1994). A multi-site investigation of the reliability of the Scale for the Assessment of Negative Symptoms. *American Journal of Psychiatry* 151: 1453-1462.
Overall JE, Gorham DR (1962). Brief Psychiatric Rating Scale. *Psychological Reports* 10: 799-812.
Overall JE, Gorham DR (1976). Brief Psychiatric Rating Scale. In: Guy W (ed), *ECDEU assessment manual for psychopharmacology*. Revised edition. Rockville, Maryland, pp 157-169.
Walker C (1994). From empiricism to neural networks: a philosophical analysis of the basis of psychiatric practice. *Current Opinion in Psychiatry* 7: 411-413.

20

Comparing cerebral blood flow response (FMRI) and neuronal response (MEG) to motor activation

R. BEISTEINER[1], G. GOMISCEK[2,3], M. ERDLER[1], C. TEICHTMEISTER[2], E. MOSER[2,3], L. DEECKE[1]

[1] Neurological University Clinic
[2] NMR Group, Institute for Medical Physics
[3] Magnetic Resonance Institute
University of Vienna, Vienna, Austria.

Functional Magnetic Resonance Imaging (FMRI) has proven to be a valuable tool for monitoring brain activity during various tasks (Belliveau et al. 1991; Kwong et al. 1992; Bandettini et al. 1992; McCarthy et al. 1993). The underlying principle for the signal increase measured by gradient-echo FMRI is twofold. Firstly, the mere increase of inflow of blood into an activated region produces a signal increase when using conventional (flow compensated) gradient-echo measurement sequences (Gomiscek et al. 1993; Frahm et al. 1994). Secondly, the decrease of the local deoxyhemoglobin concentration due to increased inflow of oxyhemoglobin leads to a reduction of local magnetic field inhomogeneities and thus an increase in signal intensity (Ogawa et al. 1990). Using the high spatial resolution, the non invasiveness and the potential to monitor brain responses in 3D, FMRI studies tried to show the locations of taskspecific brain activation. However, a most important question concerning the reliability of such localizations has not yet been addressed; how is the cerebral blood flow response spatially related to the centers of neuronal activity?

Methods

Paradigm

Eight healthy righthanded subjects (mean age 25, range 22 to 29, 4 female, 4 male) had to perform voluntary tapping of the right index finger for approximately 3 seconds, then relax for about 3 seconds before starting the next self-paced finger movements.

MEG Experiment

Using BTI Model 607 (7 channels), finger movement-related magnetic fields were recorded from 28 positions over the left central hemisphere (high pass filter 0.1 Hz, low pass filter 50 Hz, 150 samples/sec). In total 300 epochs of 1.5 sec before and 1.5 sec after electromyogram onset were recorded at every of the 28 positions.

FMRI Experiment

3 min complete rest alternated with 3 min of motor activity (3 resting and 2 activation periods, start by light signal). Motor activity was defined as 3 sec rest followed by 3 sec finger tapping. During each 3 min period 5 FMRI images were taken. Three parallel transversal slices tilted laterally were investigated over the left central hemisphere. Measurements were performed on a commercially available MR-system (MAGNETOM SP 1.5 T, SIEMENS AG Erlangen, Germany) with the standard CP head coil using a first order flow compensated gradient echo sequence with TE = 60 ms, TR = 91 ms, Flip Angle = 40°, Matrix = 256*256 pixel, FOV = 230 mm and 3 mm slice thickness.

Data analysis MEG

Artefact free epochs were averaged and then further processed. We took the magnetic field distribution somewhere between -200 ms before EMG onset to +100 ms after EMG onset for analysis. This time period was chosen because the synchronisation of brain activity within the various epochs averaged is best at the beginning of the movement sequence. Within the time window chosen, neuronal activity should comprise pre- and postcentral activity. The dipole locations found accounted for 80-90% of the data variance and two left central dipoles represented the centers of contralateral primary motor and primary sensory cortex activation. Since we didn't divide the blood flow data into precentral/postcentral activation, we also took the middle between both dipoles to compare with the blood flow center.

Data analysis FMRI

Pixel accepted as responding to the motor stimulation had to fulfill two criteria. Firstly, the signal increase during motor activation had to be in a range of 0%-10%. This was chosen to exclude artefacts and signals resulting from within a large vessel (>10%). As is theoretically expected and as it was confirmed by a separate analysis using various amplitude thresholds, the larger vessels yield the larger signal amplitudes. Large supplying and draining vessels are most probably not very closely related to the primary center of brain activation and its corresponding microvasculature (Lai et al. 1993, Segebarth et al. 1994). Our approach excludes all those large vessels which pass the measured slice more or less perpendicularly.

The second criterion accepts only pixel showing a correlation with the stimulation course of at least 60% of the maximum correlation occurring within all pixel of an image. This was done to select only specific signal changes and to rule out random fluctuations. The center of gravity of all pixel fulfilling both criteria was marked and overlayed on an anatomical image of the measured slice (Figure 1). We did not try to separate precentral and postcentral vascular activity since the individual vascular networks and blood flow patterns were not known. The positions of the flow response center and the neuronal center was calculated relative to the head references.

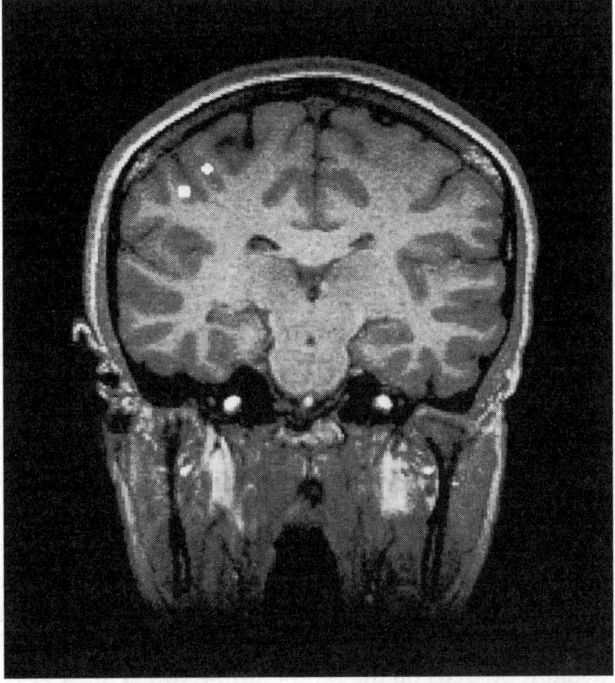

Figure 1. Coronal section of one subject. Up is up, left is left. The common center of neuronal activation is shown by the white square. The center of the blood flow response is shown by the white cross.

Results

The distance between the MEG center and the FMRI center was calculated independently for every FMRI slice. Concerning FMRI results, we found between 5 and 50 pixel showing up in the 8 best MEG correlated slices of the 8 subjects. Their mean distance from the MEG center is shown in Table I.

Table I.

Subject #, age, gender	Absolute distance between the centers of neuronal and blood flow response in mm	Maximum distance in x, y or z direction in mm
1. 22, f	27,8	19,7
2. 26, m	18,3	12,9
3. 27, m	12,8	10,9
4. 29, m	11,9	8,4
5. 24, f	13,5	9,7
6. 26, f	8,5	6,0
7. 23, f	25,4	17,9
8. 24, m	15,1	10,7
Arithmetic mean	16,66	12,03

Discussion

This study provides a first multi subject estimation to what extent functional cerebral blood flow changes are spatially related to their cause, namely neuronal activation. By using fixed analysis parameters for every FMRI image we tried to avoid any operator related bias concerning the analysis process. Our results indicate, that the mean distance between centers of blood flow and neuronal response may be between 1-2 cm in the given task. Although dipole models as used in the MEG data analysis bear some uncertainties due to the inverse problem, the longstanding experiences and the known spatial resolution in the millimeter range legitimate MEG to be regarded as a valid reference. So, what about the localization qualities of conventional FMRI? The answer must be twofold. Concerning definition of spatially well separated brain areas, e.g. distinction of hand and foot areas on the motor strip (Kim et al., 1994) this task may be solved reliably. Since cortical activation of a specialized area usually comprises several square cm, an uncertainty of 1-2 cm concerning it's center should still depict activated regions reasonably well. However, separation of more closely related areas like neighbouring sensory areas of the hand (Yang et al., 1993) or even simultaneously active pre- and postcentral gyri may show considerable blood supply overlap. Defining separate and specific blood flow centers here may be limited, even more so given the neuronal/vascular mismatch found.

References

1. Bandettini P.A., Wong W.C., Hinks R.S., Kikofsky R.S., Hyde J.S. Time course EPI of human brain function during task activation. Magn. Reson. Med. 25: 390-398, 1992.
2. Belliveau J.W., Kennedy D.N., McKinstry R.C., Buchbinder B.R., Weisskoff R.M., Cohen M.S., Vevea J.M., Brady T.J., Rosen B.R. Functional mapping of the human visual cortex by magnetic resonance imaging. Science 254: 716-719, 1991.
3. Frahm J., Merboldt K.D., Hänicke W., Kleinschmidt A., Boecker H. Brain or vein - oxygenation or flow? On signal physiology in functional MRI of human brain activation. NMR in Biomedicine 6, 1994.
4. Gomiscek G., Beisteiner R., Hittmair K., Mueller E., Moser E. A possible role of inflow effects in functional MR-imaging. MAGMA 1: 109-113, 1993.
5. Kim S.G., Hendrich K., Hu X., Merkle H., Ugurbil K. Potential pitfalls of functional MRI using conventional gradient-recalled echo techniques. NMR in Biomedicine 7: 69-74, 1994.
6. Kwong K.K., Belliveau J.W., Chesler D.A., Goldberg I.E., Weisskoff R.M., Poncelet B.P., Kennedy D.N., Hoppel B.E., Cohen M.S., Turner R., Cheng H.M., Brady T.J., Rosen B.R. Dynamic magnetic resonance imaging of human brain activity during primary sensory stimulation. Proc. Natl. Scad. Sci. U.S.A. 98: 5675-5679, 1992.
7. Lai S., Hopkins A.L., Haacke E.M. *et al.* Identification of vascular structures as a major source of signal contrast in high resolution 2d and 3d functional activation imaging of the motor cortex at 1.5T: preliminary results. Magn. Res. Med. 30: 387-392, 1993..
   McCarthy G., Blamire A.M., Rothman D.L., Gruetter R., Shulman R.G. Echo-planar magnetic resonance imaging studies of frontal cortex activation during word generation in humans. Proc. Natl. Acad. Sci. USA 90: 4952-4956, 1993.
8. Ogawa S., Lee T.M., Nayak A.S., Glynn P. Oxygenation sensitive contrast in magnetic resonance images of rodent brain at high magnetic fields. Magn. Res. Med. 14: 68-78, 1990.
9. Segebarth C., Belle V., Delon C., Massarelli R., Decety J., Le Bas J.F., Décorps M., Benabid A.L. Functional MRI of the human brain: predominance of signals from extracerebral veins. NeuroReport 5: 813-816, 1994.
10. Yang T.T., Gallen C.C., Schwartz B.J., Bloom F.E. Noninvasive somatosensory homunculus mapping in humans by using a large-array biomagnetometer. Proc. Nat. Acad. Sci. U.S.A. 90(7): 3098-3102, 1993.

ved # 21

Functional MRI studies of spatial working memory and language

A. M. BLAMIRE

Department of Neurosurgery, Yale University, New Haven CT, USA.

Functional magnetic resonance imaging was performed in 14 normal right-handed subjects performing tasks known to involve the frontal and temporal lobes. Images were acquired using the Echo-Planar imaging technique with a gradient echo time of 50 ms to provide blood oxygen level dependent (BOLD) contrast. A limited number of imaging slices were chosen based on information from prior studies by other modalities. Subjects performed either of the following tasks: a spatial working memory task (remembering the location of visually presented objects); overt repetition of visually presented nouns, overt and covert generation of a verb to match a visually presented nouns. Consistent activation was observed in all subjects in the frontal and temporal lobe slices selected. Restudy of a subset of the subjects showed the activations to be reproducible.

Functional MRI (fMRI) is a relatively new concept in *in vivo* MR. Changes in the apparent transverse relaxation time (T_2^*) of the water signal have been linked to blood oxygenation levels via the paramagnetic/diamagnetic properties of the haemoglobin molecule in the respective deoxygenated and oxygenated forms [1]. The relative concentration of each form is linked to local cerebral blood flow and metabolism. Thus changes in CBF and metabolism are reflected in altered image intensity in gradient echo images. The precise mechanisms relating these parameters are still under investigation, however the methodology is undergoing rapid development with final goals being both non-invasive clinical assessment of patients and neuro-psychological research. Extensive studies have been performed in the visual cortex [2-5], in part because of the accessibility of the occipital lobe to the MR experiment but also because of the wealth of understanding already available for comparison with new MR results. We describe here initial studies of more complex cognitive processes which have been performed with the aims of increasing the spatial selectivity of previous measurements by Positron Emission Tomography (PET, 6) and examination of possible limitations of the fMRI technique. The paradigms used were as follows. Spatial working memory (SWM): being the capacity to maintain a mental ongoing record of the location of visually presented information, Generation of verbs to match presented nouns.

Methods

All imaging experiments were performed using a Bruker Biospec Spectrometer operating at 2.1 Tesla. A plexiglass cylinder lined with high-density foam shaped to receive a head was used to minimize subject movements. MR signals were transmitted and received using a linear birdcage resonator. Subject positioning within the magnet and anatomy of the selected slices was determined using a T_1 weighted, multislice inversion recovery sequence (TIR = 760 ms, TE = 17 ms, TR = 2.1 s). Slices for functional imaging were positioned relative to the anterior commissure defined in the sagittal plane. Selected slices were shimmed to reduce macroscopic B_o field inhomogeneities and maximize functional signal changes [4]. Two dimensional time-of-flight angiograms (TE = 17 ms, TR = 70 ms, flip angle = 45°) were obtained to show the location of major vessels which are known to give large BOLD effects [7]. Functional images were then acquired using the Echo-Planar Imaging sequence (EPI, 8) as previously described [9]. A spin-echo version of the sequence was modified to include a gradient-echo delay (asymmetric spin-echo) and hence introduce BOLD contrast into the images. Spin-echo time was 26 ms and subsequent gradient-echo (TE) was 50 ms. Image repetition time varied with each study and was between 3 and 6 seconds. All subjects studied were normal right-handed volunteers from within the University community and gave informed consent for all imaging procedures which were approved by the Human Investigation Committee of Yale School of Medicine.

Tasks

Spatial working memory

Irregular shapes from a pool of 20 were presented visually at a rate of 1 shape every 1.5 s. Shapes appeared in any of 20 locations distributed randomly throughout the field of view. Subjects were required to respond when any shape appeared at a location which had previously been occupied in that trial. The subjects therefore had an increasing number of locations to memorize as each trial progressed. Control tasks were a «dot detection» task in which the subject responded whenever a small dot appeared within any of the shapes, and a «colour detection» task in which the subject responded if any object was red in colour. Eight subjects (5 restudies) were studied using a single coronal slice placed 40 mm anterior to the anterior commissure. Each task was repeated 3 - 6 times. A full description of the study is given in [10].

Language production

Stimuli were common English nouns presented visually at a rate of one word every 3 s. In separate trials subjects were to either overtly repeat the noun, overtly generate a matching verb or covertly generate a matching verb. «Probe» words which consisted of verbs or nouns surrounded by «? ?», were added randomly to each task to allow monitoring of subject response in the covert verb generation condition. Subjects compared the probe words with the last word they had repeated or generated and gave a yes/no finger response indicating the match. Eight subjects were studied using 4 coronal slices spanning the anterior commissure to 10 mm anterior to the corpus callosum in the midline. Each trial was repeated 4 times.

Data processing

Contamination of functional images by subject movement was assessed by examining the data in cine mode and the centre-of-mass of each image as a function of time. Trials in which subject movement was suspected were discarded prior to data analysis. Each trial was analyzed by t-tests as previously described [10)]. Resulting activation images were averaged across task replications to increase signal to noise ratio.

Results

The foci of the largest activations for each task are shown in Figure 1. Data are from single typical subjects in each study. SWM activity is marked with triangles and overt verb generation is marked by squares. For clarity control task activations are not included in the Figure 1.

Spatial working memory

Focal activation was observed in middle frontal gyrus (Brodmanns area 46) in both the SWM and control tasks. The magnitude of the functional signal change was however larger in the SWM task than the dot and colour detection tasks. Activation of the right hemisphere was greater and more consistent than in the left hemisphere.

Language

Activity was observed in regions of frontal cortex. Bilateral activation was observed in area 47 but this was generally greater in the left than right hemisphere. This confirms our earlier fMRI observations [11]. Consistent activation was also observed in left area 44 and the anterior cingulate in good agreement with previous PET data [6].

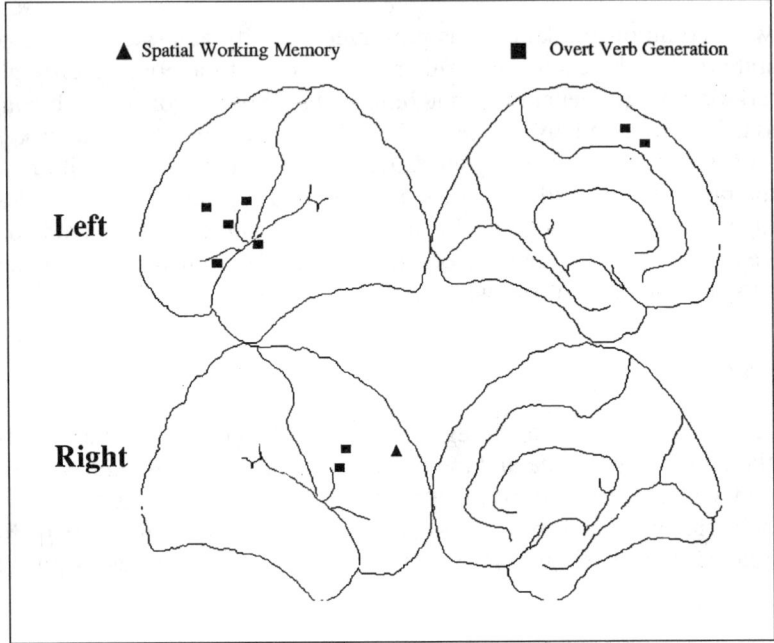

Figure 1. Presentation of the major activations observed for two individual subjects performing the spatial working memory (SWM) and overt verb generation tasks. Activation in the SWM is marked by triangles and for verb generation by squares. Symbols mark the centre of each individual activated areas. Activation was determined relative to non-stimulated resting conditions.

Discussion

The language experiments have closely followed studies by PET which used inter-subject averaging of data [6]. In general our results in individual subjects are in good agreement with the previous PET data. Similarly, the results in spatial wording memory agree well with a PET study of a different working memory task [12] which also found right hemisphere activation of area 46. The non-invasive nature of the fMRI method has allowed the restudy of subjects with both sets of tasks and the results are qualitatively reproducible. Quantitative assessment of intra-subject variability remain to be made. While there is inter-subject variability in anatomy, the locations of activated areas are consistent across subjects. Some differences have been noted between the fMRI and PET data. These may be due to the differences in signal to noise ratio and spatial resolution between the methods.

Functional MRI is sensitive enough to detect BOLD changes in normal subjects associated with the cognitive processes studied here and signal changes of 5 - 10 % have been observed at 2.1T. Functional image quality is highly dependent on subject compliance and data must be rigorously assessed for movement and artefacts from large vessels in order to obtain reliable results. Such studies of normal subjects lead the way for studies of patient groups.

Acknowledgements

The author acknowledges his collaboration with Drs Robert G. Shulman, Gregory McCarthy and Bruce Wewler at Yale University in performing this work.

References

1. Ogawa S., Lee T.-S., Nayak A.S., Glynn P., Magn. Reson. Med. 1990; 14: 68-78.
2. Kwong K.K., Belliveau J.W., Chesler D.A., Goldberg I.E., Weisskoff R.M., Poncelet B.P., Kennedy D.N., Hoppel B.E., Cohen M.S., Turner R., Cheng H.-M., Brady T.J., Rosen B.R., Proc. Natl. Acad. Sci. USA, 1992; 89: 5675-5679.
3. Ogawa S., Tank D.W., Menon R., Ellermann J., Kim S.-G., Merkle H., Ugurbil K., Proc. Natl. Acad. Sci. USA. 1992; 89: 5951-5955.
4. Blamire A.M., Ogawa S., Ugurbil K., Rothman D., McCarthy G., Ellermann J.M., Hyder F., Rattner Z., Shulman R.G., Proc. Natl. Acad. Sci. USA. 1992; 89: 11069-11073.
5. Schnieder W., Noll D.C., Cohen J.D., Nature, 1993; 365: 150-153.
6. Petersen S.E., Fox P.T., Posner M.I., Mintun M., Raichle M.E., Nature, 1988; 331: 585-588.
7. Menon R.S., Ogawa S., Tank D.W., Ugurbil K., Magn. Reson. Med., 1993; 30: 380-386.
8. Mansfield, p., J. Phys C, 1977; 10: L55-L58.
9. Blamire A.M., Shulman R.G. Magn. Reson. Imag., 1994; 12: 669-673.
10. McCarthy G., Blamire A.M., Puce A., Nobre A.C., Bloch G., Hyder F., Goldman-Rakic P., Shulman R.G., Proc. Natl. Acad. Sci. USA, 1994; 91: 8690-8694.
11. McCarthy G., Blamire A.M., Rothman D.L., Gruetter R., Shulman R.G. Proc. Natl. Acad. Sci. USA, 1993; 90: 4952-4956.
12. Petrides M., Alivasatos B., Meyer E., Evans A.C.Proc. Natl. Acad. Sci. USA, 1993; 90: 878-882.

22

Parametric imaging : application to Parkinsonism

J.M. BONNY, J.Y. BOIRE, F. DURIF[1], D. SINARDET[1], A. VEYRE, M. ZANCA

ERIM-INSERM U71, [1] Service de Neurologie, Clermont-Ferrand, France.

Previous works have shown that multispectral analysis - i.e. multiparametric - in MRI should distinguish normal from pathological tissues [6,13,15]. Most obvious classification parameters are *T1, T2* relaxation times and proton density, even if other criteria have shown to be discriminant (textural analysis) [8,11]. Parkinson's disease is a degenerative affection with dopaminergic neuronal loss in the *substantia nigra (pars compacta)*.with, as consequence, a dopamine amount decrease in the *striatum (putamen and caudate nucleus)*. Our aim is to look for any MRI parameter change in *basal ganglia* of Parkinsonian patients. Finally, we want to evaluate if a *T1, T2, M0* multispectral analysis could differentiate patients with Parkinson's disease from control subjects. The object of this paper is to describe the methodological aspects we used in our work ; details on clinical results are expanded elsewhere (Durif, 1994).

Methods

Protocol

On clinical MR imagers, *in vivo* accurate measurements of *M0, T1* and *T2* parameters in a reasonably short acquisition time is a tough problem. Our protocol has been determined in order to acquire the minimum set of data capable of generating accurate *T1, T2* and *M0* parametric images in approximately 30 minutes. For *T1*, the most efficient sequences in terms of propagated noise per unit imaging time are theoretically inversion recovery (IR) and TOMROP (T One by Multiple Read Out Pulses) (Crawley, 1988). The conventional IR sequence requires prohibitive imaging time for our 256x256 matrix sampling needed for basal ganglia examination ; for example, *T1* calculated from 5 points using a repetition time of 2500 ms lasts as long as 53 minutes. Using TOMROP, this imaging time could be notably reduced ; anyway, *T2* measurement needs another protocol based on Carr-Purcell-Meiboom-Gill (CPMG) multi-echo sequence with a large repetition time. Thus, we did prefer the use of the high signal to noise ratio (SNR) CPMG sequence both for *T2* and *T1* estimation. Our approach consists in four Spin-Echo acquisitions with different repetition times (t_R=4000, 1000, 600, 200 ms). The first one with t_R=4000 is a multi-echo CPMG (t_E=22,60,120 ms) whereas the three others are a single-echo SE (t_E=22 ms). Finally, the proton density can ever be estimated from *T1* and *T2* weighted densities (Rajanayagam, 1991).

The slice orientation has been chosen parallel to the bicommisural line. After visual inspection of all images, three planes were selected for parametric reconstruction, through the *substantia nigra,* the *striatum* (i.e. *putamen* and *caudate nucleus*), the *pallidum* and the *thalamus*. These parametric images are simultaneously reconstructed on a workstation before measuring each parameter in several manually placed regions of interest (ROI). With a field of view of 250x250 mm^2, the nominal size of voxel is 1x1x5 mm^3.

This protocol, applied on 30 healthy subjects and 41 Parkinsonian patients, takes about 40 minutes for one patient on a MAGNETOM (Siemens, Erlangen) 1T superconducting whole body imager. The head coil used is both emitter and receiver.

Parametric imaging

Principle of parametric imaging

For two-dimensional spin-warp imaging, the magnitude image signal in a given voxel can be written as :

$$I_i = GM_{SEQ}(\mathbf{xi},\mathbf{a}) + b_i \qquad (1)$$

The used *SEQ* sequence is represented by a *MSEQ* model and a vector **xi** of experimental parameters (*tE, tR*, flip angle, ...). *G* and **a** correspond respectively to the receiver head coil response and the unknown parameters *[M0,T1,T2]T*. If mean SNR is larger than 5, the centered additive noise *b* (*bi* being a sample of *b*) can be regarded as Gaussian. An estimation of **a** is obtained by acquiring *N* images with different parameters **xi** (with different *T1* and *T2* weightings), thus a vector **I** of measurements. An estimation â is given by :

$$\arg\max_{\hat{a}} L(\mathbf{I}/\mathbf{a}) \qquad (2)$$

This approach is the well known maximum likelihood (ML) method where L is a likelihood function which proceeds from noise statistics. L yields the probability that the data set **I** occurs given **a** parameters. When b is Gaussian and independent, ML is equivalent to a least squares fitting of vector **I** to *GMSEQ* model.

Advantages of parametric imaging

To evaluate **a** from a MRI set of acquisition, one classical way is to extract the signal mean in a manually placed ROI from each image, and then fit the chosen parametric model on the obtained values. The interest of such spatially averaged signal is to limit noise effects, nevertheless the obtained mean depends in this case slightly on G heterogeneity. Moreover, it is impossible to accurately know how large the deviations of parameter estimation are in the studied region. On the contrary, results obtained inside ROI directly placed on parametric images are mean values and standard deviations of the parameter (*T1* or *T2* or *M0*). Moreover, these measurements are independent on G modulations.

T2 estimation

Estimator expression

A monoexponential behavior is assumed for the decay curves of the three CPMG echoes in basal ganglia ; then, for the ith echo :

$$I_i = GM_{SE}(\mathbf{x_1},\mathbf{a}) + b_i = a_1 \exp c(-\frac{x_{i1}}{T2}) + b_i \qquad (3)$$

Following measurements vector **I** and parameter matrix **x** (limited to the variable parameters *(tE,tR)*) can mathematically describe our protocol :

$$\mathbf{I}\begin{bmatrix} I_1 \\ I_2 \\ I_3 \end{bmatrix} \mathbf{x} \begin{bmatrix} 22 & 4000 \\ 60 & 4000 \\ 120 & 4000 \end{bmatrix} (N=3) \qquad (4)$$

The pseudo-density *a1* is defined as the signal mean at an echo time of zero ; thus it corresponds to the product of *T1* weighting by proton density, modulated by G. Our *T2* estimator consists in performing a weighted linear least squares regression on the signal logarithms [9]. Without any minimization procedure, *T2* estimation is given by :

$$\widehat{T2} = \widehat{R2}^{-1} = \left[-\frac{\sum_{i=1}^{N} I_i^2 \sum_{i=1}^{N} I_i^2 x_{i1} \ln I_i - \sum_{i=1}^{N} I_i^2 x_{i1} \sum_{i=1}^{N} I_i^2 \ln I_i}{\sum_{i=1}^{N} I_i^2 \sum_{i=1}^{N} I_i^2 x_{i1}^2 - \left(\sum_{i=1}^{N} I_i^2 x_{i1} \right)^2} \right]^{-1} \quad (5)$$

T1 and GM0 estimation

Estimator

[T1,GM0]T vector is estimated from SE sequences with different repetition times. The signal is described by :

$$I_i = GM0[1 - \exp(-\frac{x_{i2}}{T1})]a_2 + b_i \quad (6)$$

a2 is the T2 weighting at the echo time of 22 ms for whole repetition times. Rewrite measurements vector **I** and parameter matrix **x** as :

$$\mathbf{I}\begin{bmatrix} I_1 \\ I_2 \\ I_3 \\ I_4 \end{bmatrix} \mathbf{x} \begin{bmatrix} 22 & 4000 \\ 22 & 1000 \\ 22 & 600 \\ 22 & 200 \end{bmatrix} (N=4) \quad (7)$$

In this case, ML estimation is strictly equivalent to minimizing the classical chi-square criteria given by :

$$\chi^2 = \sum_{i=1}^{N} \left\{ I_i - GM0[1 - \exp(-\frac{\chi_{i2}}{T1})]\widehat{a2} \right\}^2 \quad (8)$$

An approximation of a2 is obtained from previous T2 estimation. In each image, standard deviation of noise is constant ; then, a weighted criteria is unnecessary. From stationary conditions, we obtain likelihood equations which must hold at the chi-square minimum :

$$\left.\frac{\partial \chi^2}{\partial T1}\right|_{\widehat{a1}} = 0 \quad \left.\frac{\partial \chi^2}{\partial GM0}\right|_{\widehat{GM0}} = 0 \quad (9)$$

Roots finding of a non-linear function in each voxel is a time consuming procedure, especially when generic algorithms are used (Müller, Brent or Newton-Raphson methods). For that reason, we have developed a modified version of the Newton-Raphson algorithm [2] which converges slightly quicker than the dichotomic reference method [4].

Principle of bias and confidence level analysis

When the number of samples is reduced ($N=3$ for $T2$ and $N=4$ for $GM0$ and $T1$), the best way to evaluate bias and confidence level of a parameter estimation is to simulate a large number Q of data sets (Monte-Carlo methods). Thus, the corresponding Q estimations allows to determine uncertainties and the difference between mean and true values of the different parameters. In order to fit to experimental conditions, noise standard deviation is estimated from image background mean values [5]. The simulation is done by choosing the larger one, i.e.=30. Moreover, each sample is the result of a magnitude reconstruction of two independent channels corrupted by independent Gaussian noises.

Effects of RF receiver coil response variations

Whatever the sequence used, $M0$ and G will always be two indistinguishable unknown constants. Then, proton density is always modulated by G which never is perfectly homogeneous. $M0$ can be estimated only by *a priori* knowledge of G receiver head coil response. For that purpose, one among the possible efficient ways is to acquire uniform phantom images [12]. In order to evaluate coil uniformity, our protocol has been applied on an uniform phantom ($NiSO4$ solution).

Results

Bias and confidence level for T2 estimation

Bias

Two bias have to be considered :
When taking the logarithm of the signal, the noise is no more additive and its statistic is no more Gaussian but becomes asymmetric ; thus, $T2$ estimate cannot strictly come from ML approach. The asymmetric noise distribution should be expressed by a non-zero error mean, i.e. the bias. From both numerical simulation and theoretical approximation, we have shown that this quantity can be considered as negligible (less than 0,5%), essentially because of large SNR of the three echoes. Although, large bias can be notice for $T2$ values between 20 and 30 ms. In this case, the late echo signal rapidly decreases to low SNR (less than 5) from which noise distribution becomes

asymmetric [10] ; then, monoexponential fitting to a non zero asymptotic mean value gives the observed overestimation of $T2$.

Moreover, a systematic underestimation of about 20% in our $T2$ values, due to the refocusing pulses imperfections [3], is observed when comparing our protocol to a multi-echo CPMG limited to even echoes.

Confidence levels

Noise effect seems to explain a large part of $T2$ deviations measured inside a ROI. In our experimental conditions, simulated standard deviations are currently less than 10%. Only $T2$ values between 20 and 30 ms have shown a large noise sensitivity.

Bias and confidence level of *T1* and *GM0* estimation

Bias

By considering that expression [6] is an accurate model of signal, our ML application yields an unbiased estimation of $T1$. Moreover, we can see in chi-square expression [8] that $T2$ and $GM0$ are dependent ; then, underestimation of $T2$ induces an overestimation of $GM0$. By considering that the product of $GM0$ by $T2$ weighted density is a constant, the resulting bias is about 5%.

Confidence levels

For $T1$, simulations are performed for a realistic range of $GM0$ by $T2$ weighting product (signal mean at a repetition time of zero). Parameter standard deviation is always below 10%.

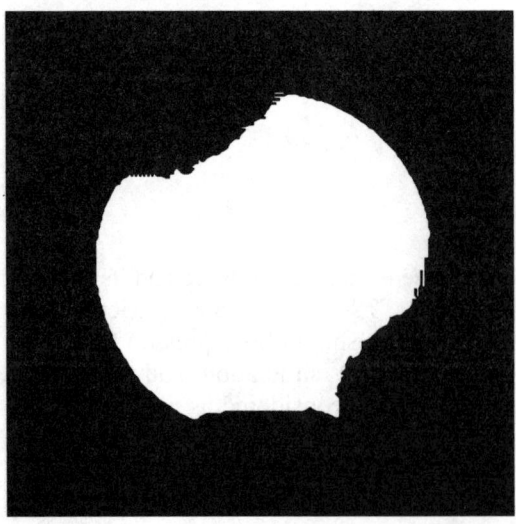

Figure 1. Proton density weighted image (SE4000/22) of a uniform phantom in our RF head coil.

RF receiver coil response analysis

Figure 1 shows that G modulation is smooth compared to voxel size, even for the areas used in our ROI. Moreover, G can be considered as homogeneous near its center. Both in the bicommisural plane and in the direction of selection, signal deviates by a maximum of 10% from areas close to coil wires toward center. Thus, it seems difficult to concede a large signification to $GM0$ when measured in a ROI far from coil center ; indeed, positioning is not perfectly reproducible between the different patients.

$M0$, $T1$ and $T2$ differences between Parkinsonian's patients (PP) and control subjects (CS)

For PP, statistical analysis shows a significant decrease of $M0$ in the two parts of the *substantia nigra (pars compacta* and *pars reticulata*) and a significant increase of $T1$ in the *putamen* (Durif, 1994).

Discussion

Even if systematic errors could not be avoided in our protocol, especially for $T2$, our interest was first of all in a comparative analysis of parameters between PP and CS. Regarding bias, we just checked that no observable $T2$ values lower than 30 ms existed, and took care for GM0 measurement to keep ROI only located near the coil center. We then controlled for each parameter that experimental deviations inside the chosen ROI was of the same order as the one simulated. It was thus reasonable to consider that partial volume effect in our ROI is negligible.

For example, in the left superior *putamen* (LSP), right posterior *putamen* (RPP) and left white matter (LWM), $T1$ criterion estimated by mean-fitting approach (see 2.2.2) gives no difference between PP and CS. While, our parametric way gives around a half the interindividual standard deviation of $T1$ (difference is not significant) ; furthermore, $T1$ in LSP and RPP now enables to significantly differentiate PP from CS (*see* Table I). Moreover, interindividual standard deviation for $T1$ is significantly larger for PP than for CS. This suggests a $T1$ scattering in the PP sample and thus a more heterogeneous population. It could be interesting to correlate $T1$ increases observed in PP with a more selective sorting from clinical and pharmacological criteria. The future trends of this work is to improve the parameters measurement technique by mono-parametric imaging. This could be of interest, especially for $T1$ by using TOMROP, to confirm or infirm a possible sensitive gradation of Parkinson's disease from $T1$ criterion.

Table I. T1 variations between control subjects (n=21) and Parkinsonian's patients (n=25) in LSP, RPP and GM (significant changes are mentioned in parenthesis by giving p and deviation in percent).

ROI	T1 mean (CS)	SD (CS)	T1 mean (PP)	SD (PP)
LSP	1046	63	1096 (p=0.02, +5%)	76
RPP	1024	62	1079 (p=0.03, +5%)	98 (p=0.04, +58%)
GM	831	71	866	92

Contrary to the *T2* shortening reported in the literature [1], our protocol has not pointed out any significant change in *T2*. Indeed, simultaneous estimation of *M0*, *T1* and *T2* parameters prevents any refined or multiexponential analysis of *T2*. Moreover, it is not clearly demonstrated that the known different iron content in basal ganglia involves a measurable monoexponential *T2* shortening [14, 16].

Finally, we obtain 77% of true classification by a progressive discriminant analysis using significant variables.

References

1. Antonini A., Leenders K.L., Meier D., Oertel W.H., Boesiger P., Anlikze M., «T2 relaxation time in patients with Parkinson's disease», Neurology, 1993; 43: pp 697-700.
2. Erbland E., Bonny J.M., Boire J.Y., Veyre A., Zanca M., «An efficient Newton-Raphson algorithm for T1 parametric image estimation with MR Spin-Echo acquisitions», 13th Annual International Conference of the IEEE EMBS, Baltimore, 1994
3. Fransson A., Ericsson A., Jung B., Sperber G.O., «Properties of the phase-alternating phase shift (phaps) multiple spin-echo protocol in MRI : a study of the effects of imperfect RF pulses», Magnetic Resonance Imaging, 1993; 11: pp 771-784.
4. Gong J., Hornak J.P., «A fast T1 algorithm», Magnetic Resonance Imaging, 1992; 10: pp 623-626.
5. Henkelman R.M., «Measurement of signal intensities in the presence of noise in MR images», Medical Physics, 1985; 12: pp 232-233.
6. Jungke M., Von Seelen W., Bielke G., Meindl S., Krone G., Grigat M., Higer P., Pfannenstiel P., «Information processing in nuclear magnetic resonance imaging», Magnetic Resonance Imaging, 1988; 6: pp 683-693.
7. Kapouleas I., «Automatic detection of white matter lesions in magnetic resonance brain images», Computer Methods and Programs in Biomedecine, 1900; 32: pp 17-35.
8. Lerski R.A., Straughan K., Shad L.R., Boyce D., Blüml S., Zuna I., «MR image texture analysis - an approach to tissue characterization», 1993; 11: pp 873-887.
9. Liu J., Nieminen A.O.K., Koenig J.L., «Calculation of T1, T2, and proton spin density images in nuclear magnetic resonance imaging», Journal of Magnetic Resonance, 1989; 85: pp 95-110.
10. Miller A.J., Joseph P.M., «The use of power images to perform quantitative analysis on low SNR MR images», Magnetic Resonance Imaging, 1993; 11: pp 1051-1056.
11. Schad L.R., Blüml S., Zuna I., «MR tissue characterization of intracranial tumors by means of texture analysis», Magnetic Resonance Imaging, 1993; 11: pp 889-896.

12. Simmons A., Tofts P.S., Barker G.J., Arridge S.R., «Source of intensity nonuniformity in spin echo images at 1.5T», Magnetic Resonance in Medicine, 1994; 32: pp 121-128.
13. Taxt T., Lundervold A., Fuglaas B., Lien H., Abeler V., «Multispectral analysis of uterine corpus tumors in magnetic resonance imaging», Magnetic Resonance in Medicine, 1992; 23: pp 55-76.
14. Tosk J.M., Holshouser B.A., Aloia R.C., «Effects of interaction between ferric iron and L-dopa melanin on T1 and T2 relaxation times determined by magnetic resonance imaging», Magnetic Resonance in Medicine, 1992; 26: pp 40-45.
15. Vannier M.W., Pilgram T.K., Speidel C.M., Neumann L.R., Rickman D.L., Schertz L.D., «Validation of magnetic resonance imaging (MRI) multispectral tissue classification», Computerized Medical Imaging and Graphics, 1991; 15: pp 217-223.
16. Vymazal J., Books R.A., Zak O., «T1 and T2 of ferritin at different field strengths. Effect on MRI», Magnetic Resonance in Medicine, 1992; 27: pp 368-374.

23

How to take advantages of gradients ? Fundamentals and some applications

A. BRIGUET, M. BOURGEOIS, O. BEUF

*Laboratoire de Résonance Magnétique Nucléaire
Chimie Physique Electronique, Université Claude-Bernard Lyon-I,
43, boulevard du 11-Novembre-1918, 69622 Villeurbanne Cedex, France.*

It is well known that the discovery of magnetic resonance imaging was based on the generation of the spatial linear variation of the main static field along a particular direction of the sample [1]. Simultaneously the NMR signal was acquired, so space to frequency encoding could be achieved. This prolific idea was in fact very simple. Nevertheless the applications of gradients during a sequence as well as the building of a gradient unit may still pose problems because now fast imaging, ultra-fast imaging and spectroscopy require high performance gradient systems. Moreover the concept of gradient is no longer limited to the spatial control of the static field value. Local gradient effects caused by magnetic susceptibility variations within the sample, may be also turned to profit to get informations by the NMR way. The following note starts with a presentation of the magnetic gradient techniques : the concept of gradients, mathematical support of gradient coil design, operating gradients requirements. Classically such gradients are used for imaging. Moreover it will be shown that natural magnetic gradients occurring within the sample, lead to extract supplementary informations : susceptibility measurements, contents of contrast agents which may be correlated to functional image analysis.

What are gradients ?

For imaging and for volume selection gradients used are particular magnetic fields having a linear dependence with respect to the X, Y, Z coordinates of the laboratory frame. A very strong distinction exists between the three first order gradients and higher order gradients, the last ones are unable to produce image easily. The necessity to employ first, order gradients is illustrated by the basic formula of NMR : $\omega=\gamma B$ (where w is the Larmore angular frequency, γ is the gyromagnetic ratio of the resonant nuclei and B the magnetic field). This formula clearly shows that frequency is linearly dependent on the position of the object in the presence of a perfectly linear gradient. Consequently it is possible to determine this position by simple spectral analysis. For this reason it is said that gradients define the reciprocal space (or k-space) of the object. The generation of linear gradient stands on fundamental properties of static magnetic fields summarized as it follows [2] :

and
$$\text{div}(\mathbf{B}) = 0 \quad (1)$$
$$\text{curl}(\mathbf{B}) = 0 \quad (2)$$

for a current-free space.

The first equation states that a magnetic unique pole cannot exist. The second one gives very particular relationships between the magnetic field components :

$$\delta B_z/\delta x = \delta B_x/\delta z \; ; \; \delta B_z/\delta y = \delta B_y/\delta z \; ; \; \delta B_x/\delta y = \delta B_y/\delta x$$

Eq. (3) may be advantageously used to design transverse gradients coils since a gradient of the X component along the Z direction is also a gradient of the Z component along the X direction (resp. Y, Z). From Eq.(3) it must be pointed out that gradient generation creates a new component of the magnetic field. Fortunately this inhomogeneity may be usually neglected. Finally by combining Eq. (1) and (2), the Laplace's equation is obtained :

$$\Delta \mathbf{B} = 0 \quad (4)$$

The universality of this equation is useful to derive analytical expressions for magnetic fields and gradients, then it may serve as a guide for gradient coils design.

Gradients generation

Spherical harmonics or Legendre's polynomials represent the most suited basis set to express efficiently a magnetic field. Inside a current coil system, the general expansion of the created magnetic field which defines the Z direction, may be written as :

$$B_z = \Sigma_l \Sigma_m B_{lm} r^l P_{lm}(\theta, \phi) \cos(m\phi - \phi_{lm}) \quad (5)$$

where $\mathbf{B}_{lm}$ are numerical coefficients, $\mathbf{P}_{lm}$ is the Legendre's polynomial of order l and degree m, (r,θ,ϕ) are the spherical coordinates and f_{lm} a constant value depending of l (l is varying from zero to infinity) and ϕ_{lm} (from zero to l).

The number of degrees increases rapidly when the order increases (at a given degree may correspond several orders). The higher the order and the degree are, the smaller the expansion coefficients $\mathbf{B}_{lm}$ are. The zero order term represents the homogeneous component of the field and inhomogeneities are depicted by other terms. So gradients are the first order terms of the inhomogeneity and these terms must be specifically created when energizing a gradient coil. Moreover the generation of a gradient and the gradient coil design may be based on symmetry consideration [3]. Symmetry must be taken with respect to the XY plane while the main static field is along Z. Symmetrical sets of currents generate even terms; it is the basis of magnet design. On the opposite anti-symmetrical sets of currents generate odd terms. Keeping a first order term ($l = 1$). with a degree $m = 0$ leads to a Z-gradient, and $m = 1$ terms give X- or Y- gradients according to the value of f_{lm} (zero or ninety degree). In practice playing with geometry is a way to reduce high order terms, especially orders three and five. Wirings and currents values have to be arranged to reinforce the first order terms with respect to the other terms.

The generation of a gradient oriented along the main field direction can be treated by this method. Since this gradient corresponds to m equal to zero, a cylindrical symmetry around the Z axis is required and circular loops may be employed efficiently. Drawings in Figure 1 illustrate this principle. One may focus attention on the half-opening angle denoted as θ_0. Choosing $\theta_0 = 49°$ leads to an approximately linear variation of the Z-component along Z since third order terms are cancelled out. Moreover it is possible to suppress the fifth order contribution if $\theta_0 = 32°$ or $62°$. Then the gradient systems sketched in Figure 1 are obtained by the combination of two pairs of coils having such opening angles and by proper adjustment of the currents ratio in order to eliminate the third order terms. The gradient coils in Figure 1 (left) are designed for cylindrical magnets having axial access, and the second system shown in Figure 1 (right) works for magnet with transverse access.

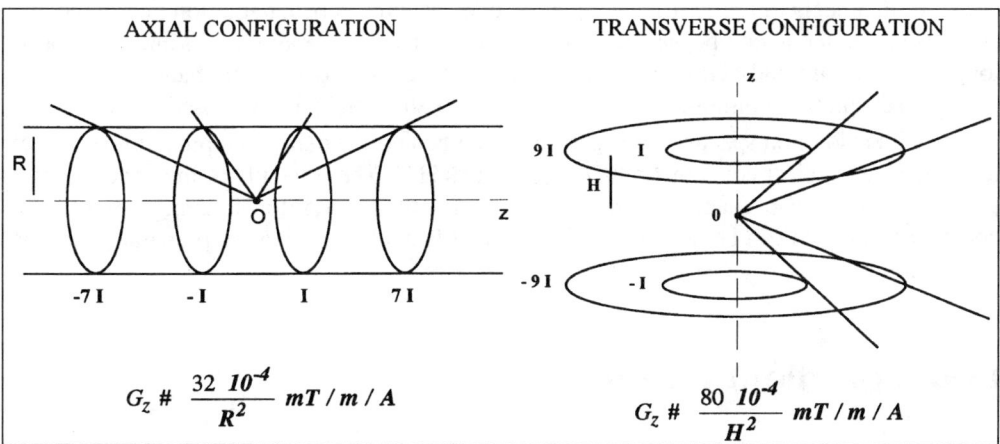

Figure 1. Two designs of z gradient with third and fifth order correction.

The problem is fundamentally different for gradients oriented orthogonally with respect to static field direction. The first and clearly expressed solution to this problem has been indicated many years ago [4]. Most of the transverse gradients employed are inspired from the Golay's proposals [5]. A reliable transverse gradient may be also produced by a quadrupolar set up [6]. In this case, a gradient requires a four rectangular coil design, each coil being tilted by 90° with respect to its neighbours. Improvements of the gradient uniformity depend on the length to width ratio of the gradient value within a given sphere surrounded by the gradient coil.

The use of gradients for imaging and spectroscopy

The ancient imaging experiments based on projection-reconstruction technique could employ static gradient generation during each step of the imaging sequence. Fourier transform techniques and volume selection - i.e. slice selection for imaging and sensitive volume selection for localized spectroscopy had led to impose several changes of the gradient sense and magnitude after the radiofrequency pulse. Finally the advent of fast and ultra-fast imaging techniques had considerably increased the ratio between the number of gradients switches and the number of radiofrequency excitations. Consequently the switch time of a gradient appears to be a determining feature. It may be defined by the time necessary to reach ninety per cent of the desired gradient variation. The amount of energy required enlights the actuality of the problem. The classical expression of the magnetostatic density of energy shows that the results is proportional to the square of the gradient amplitude and to the power five of the gradient coil size. For a common gradient value (10 mT/m), a switch time equal to 1 ms and for a 1m size, the required power is about 40 kW. Then very powerful electrical supplies are required. A pre-emphasis command of the gradient is generally performed to anticipate the opposing effect of eddy currents due to electrical coupling between the gradient wirings and surrounding materials. A single conductive shield having an appropriate thickness may be inserted between the gradient coils and the magnet in order to decouple the two systems. A better solution is provided by currents monitored to compensate magnetic effects outside the gradient coils and to suppress long time constant eddy currents in materials. Several techniques (self-shielded gradients, multiple screening, minimum energy coils, resonant structures) are proposed [7-10].

For high resolution spectroscopy, gradients can be applied during the preparation step of the sequence to select coherence transfer pathways [11]. The principle of the experiment is similar to transverse magnetization spoiling as encountered for imaging : particular coherence transfers can be destructed if a gradient is applied during the preparation period of the sequence.

Local gradient effects

Besides gradients generated by well controlled currents, natural magnetic gradients due to physical non uniformities within the sample may be considered. Susceptibility differences create magnetic field variations which may be approximated by linear gradients at the submillimetric scale. Passing through the interface between two tissues or through the interface between a living tissue and a biomaterial represents well the situation because the magnetic field lines are refracted according to the susceptibilities ratio. This explains well image artefacts observed in the vicinity of dental implants or near interventional materials. Shifts of the resonance frequency due to susceptibility effects in liquids or tissues [12] and image intensity distortions caused by materials [13] are now well documented. Nevertheless it must be pointed out that a very straightforward application consists to measure the susceptibilities values [14]. Using cylindrical samples, the principle of the experiment is illustrated in Figure 2. It may be observed that the experiment is able to provide also the sign of the difference between the susceptibility of the sample (let be χ) and the susceptibility of its surrounding medium χ_e :

$$\chi = \chi_e \pm 2\left[H - \left(1 + \sqrt{2}/2\right)a\right] G/B \qquad (6)$$

where a is the radius of the cylinder, G is the read gradient amplitude, B is the static field and H is the distance between the high intensity spots. This distance is measured along the read gradient direction (vertical direction in Figure 2). The plus sign is for the picture on the left and minus sign for the picture on the right.

Figure 2. Image distortion of paramagnetic sample (left) and diamagnetic sample (right).

Combination of susceptibility and diffusion effects may play an important role in functional imaging [15]. Moreover local susceptibility effects associated to blood oxygenation are time dependent and they create relatively small intensity fluctuations within tissues [16]. Consequently it can be looked for a method that emphasizes such local variations. Figure 3 illustrates the principle of the detection of a susceptibility phantom (capillar tubes in water). The NMR sequence was designed in order to enhance distortion created by the object and to eliminate automatically signal due to the rest of the sample.

Figure 3. Enhancement of susceptibility effects (left) and corresponding magnetic field plot (right).

Conclusion

Gradients are the key for NMR imaging but they are also the source of several difficulties when using imaging sequences. Some fundamentals of gradients have been recalled; showing that mathematical basis is necessary to take advantages of gradients. At sample or at patient scale, gradient systems building and improvement are well documented. Moreover it has been shown that internal gradients may act at the millimetric or submillimetric scale so they represent a new way to detect abnormalities in samples. The enhancement of intensity variations observed in images has been indicated to detect local gradients.

References

1. Lauterbur PC, *Nature* 1973 ; **242** : 190.
2. Jackson JD, Classical Electrodynamics, John Wiley and Sons 1975.
3. Roméo F, Hoult DI, *Magn Reson Med* 1984 ; **1** : 44.
4. Anderson WA, *Rev Sci Instrum* 1961 ; **32** : 241.
5. Golay MJ, *Rev Sci Instrum* 1958 ; **29** : 313.
6. Briguet A, Chakji J, *Rev Sci Instrum* 1985 ; **56** : 1626.
7. Turner R, Bowley RM, *J Phys E* (Sci. Instrum.) 1986 ; **19** : 876.
8. Mansfield P, Chapman B, *J Magn Reson* 1986 ; **66** : 573.
9. Mansfield P, Harvey PR, Coxon RJ, *Meas Sci Techn* 1991 ; **2** : 1051.
10. Pissanetzky S, *Meas Sci Techn* 1992 ; **3** : 667.
11. Bax A, De Jong PG, Mehlkopf AF, Smidt J, *Chem Phys Letters* 1980 ; **69** : 567.
12. Chu SCK, Xu Y, Balschi JA, Springer CS, *Magn Reson Med* 1990 ; **13** : 239.
13. Henkelmann RM, Bronskill MJ, *Rev Magn Reson Med* 1987 ; **2** : 1.
14. Weisskopf RM, Kiihine S, *Magn Reson Med* 1992 ; **24** : 375.
15. Callaghan PT, Forde LC, Rofe JR, *J Magn Reson* 1994 ; **B104** : 34.
16. Kennan RP, Zhong J, Gore JC, *Magn Reson Med* 1994 ; **31** : 9.

24

Neuronal integrity in the frontal cortex of schizophrenics evaluated by ^{1}H magnetic resonance spectroscopy

G.CALABRESE, A. FALINI[1], S. LIPARI[1], D. ORIGGI[1], C. COLOMBO,
A. BONFANTI, G. SCOTTI[1], S. SCARONE

*Department of Neurosciences and [1]Department of Neuroradiology,
San Raffaele Hospital, University of Milan, Italy.*

Psychiatrists have been always searched for a structural and/or functional brain abnormality underlying mental disorders. Like other technical development in the area of brain imaging, Magnetic Resonance Spectroscopy (MRS) has been looked at with great interest and expectation for its possibility to evaluate brain metabolites *in vivo* and non invasively, adding functional data to the morphological ones of the MR imaging.

The first application of MRS to psychiatry was presented at the meeting on Schizophrenia Research in 1989 from Keshavan (1989) who studied the frontal cortex, and O'Callagan (1989) who evaluated the temporal lobes of schizophrenic patients using phosphorous MRS (^{31}P-MRS).

As far as the frontal lobe studies are concerned, Keshavan observed a phosphomonoesters (PME) reduction and a phosphodiesters (PDE) increase in the dorsolateral prefrontal cortex of first episode never treated schizophrenic patients. Subsequent studies confirmed the initial results of membrane phospholipid levels alteration in the frontal cortex (Pettegrew 1991, Williamson 1991 and Stanley 1992). Stanley reported not only decreased PME levels but a shift of this resonance as well, further suggesting a decrease of phosphorilethanolamine. Both in the longitudinal study by Pettegrew and in the transversal studies by Williamson and Stanley the PDE increase observed at the onset was not present in chronic patients, treated with neuroleptic therapy. PME and PDE peaks have been shown, by experimental evidences to be involved in the synthesis and catabolism of cell membrane, so that their levels are considered an index of membrane turnover rate (Bottomley 1985). The results of these works were interpreted as an other support to the hypothesis of schizophrenia as a neurodevelopmental disorder, involving abnormal neuronal development in the frontal cortex (Pettegrew 1993).

Proton MRS (1H-MRS) not only gives information on cell membrane turnover, like ^{31}P-MRS, but provides data on neuronal density and status as well. In fact in a proton spectra besides the choline (Cho) resonance, containing signal from several membrane phospholipid constituent, there is the peak from N-acetylaspartate (NAA), considered to be a neuronal marker and shown to be decreased in neurodegenerative diseases. Moreover a proton spectrum acquired using short echo times contains more peaks such as myoinositol (Ins), which function as a second messenger, glutamate and glutamine and other neuroexcitatories aminoacids.

We used proton MRS to test the specific hypothesis of a neuronal alteration in the frontal cortex of schizophrenics.

Subjects and method

We evaluated 12 chronic schizophrenic patients (8 males and 4 females, mean age 25 years) and 8 normal subjects (5 males and 3 females, mean age 28 years) as control group. All patients were on neuroleptic treatment.

MR T1 sagital and coronal and T2 axial images were acquired prior to spectroscopy for localization purposes. A modified STEAM sequence (TR=1600 msec, TE=20 msec, 256 acq.) was used to study a volume of 8 cc positioned in the interemispheric frontal cortex just above the orbital gyrus (Figure 1). Spectra were processed on the software provided by Siemens applying a Gauss filter of 256 Hz at half bandwidth. From the FFT spectra peak areas were calculated for the metabolic ratios.

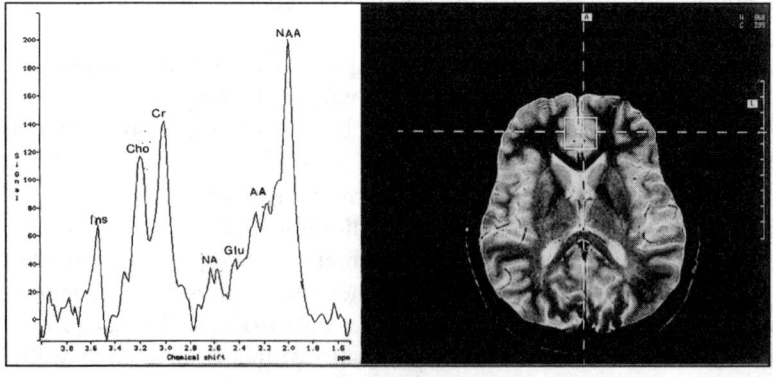

Figure 1: b) MRI section, through the basal ganglia levels, with the volume of interest localized in the frontal cortex. a) short echo time (TE = 20 msec.) proton spectra acquired from the VOI; from left to right the following peaks may be identified: Inositol (Ins), Choline containing compounds (Cho), Creatine-Phosphocreatine (Cr), N-acetylaspartate at 2.7 and 2 ppm (NA and NAA respectively), glutamate-glutamine (Glu) and various amminoacid (AA).

Results

Table I shows the metabolic ratios for the two groups.

The only difference between the two groups was increased choline containing compounds levels in the schizophrenic group compared to controls, eventhough this did not reach statistical significance. No other differences were observed for the other metabolites, in particular no variation in the NAA levels was noted in our sample of schizophrenic patients.

Table 1. Metabolite ratios (mean values ± SD) in the schizophrenic and the contol group.

Metabolite ratios	Controls	Schizophrenics
INS/CR	0.30 ± 0.13	0.36 ± 0.16
CHO/CR *	0.63 ± 0.06	0.71 ± 0.07
NAA/CR	1.79 ± 0.39	1.78 ± 0.50
NAA/CHO	2.89 ± 0.69	2.52 ± 0.61
NA/CR	0.41 ± 0.20	0.39 ± 0.18
GLU/CR	0.41 ± 0.39	0.16 ± 0.09
AA/CR	1.36 ± 0.59	1.18 ± 0.47

* Mann-Whitney U test: Z = -0.15, p = 0.08

Discussion

There are several compounds contributing to the choline resonance at 3.2 ppm. Experimental studies demonstrated that the constituents of cell membrane containing a choline group, mainly phosphatidil-choline and sphingomyeline, are the principal metabolites resonating at this frequency *in vivo* (Miller 1991). Increased Cho levels have been shown to occur in reactive gliosys and in condition of rapid cell proliferation like in neoplastic lesions. This increment is generally considered as an expression of increased cell membrane turnover. The increased cell turnover rate we observed in the frontal cortex of schizophrenic patients is in agreement with the ^{31}P-MRS study. As no differences were observed for the NAA, considered a marker of neuronal viability, our study do not support the hypothesys of pathological processes causing a reduction of neurons.

In conclusion, these results suggest that in schizophrenia there might be a pathological process involving neuronal cells in the frontal cortex, with a modification of cell membrane structure and neuronal pattern alteration, without loss of neurons itself.

While it is aknowledged the value of MRS to invastigate, *in vivo* and non invasively, brain metabolism at various levels (i.e. cell membrane turnover, energy production, neuronal density) its application in psychiatry is still limited to the research field and more studies need to be done in association with other imaging techniques to confirm pathogenetic hypothesis of major psychiatric deseases.

References

1. Bottomley PA. Human *in-vivo* NMR spectroscopy in diagnostic medicine:clinical tool or research probe? *Radiology* 1989 ; 170 : 1-15.
2. Keshavan MS *et al. In vivo* ^{31}P nuclear magnetic resonance (NMR) spectroscopy of the frontal lobe metabolism in neuroleptic naive first episode psychoses: preliminary studies. *Schizophrenia Research* 1989 ; 2 : 122.
3. Miller BL. A review of chemical issues in H1 NMR spectroscopy: N-Acetyl-L-Aspartate, creatine and choline. *NMR Biomed* 1991 ; 4;47-52.
4. O'Callagan E *et al.* ^{31}P magnetic resonance spectroscopy of the left temporal lobe in schizophrenia: procedures and preliminary results. *Schizophrenia Research* 1989 ; 2 :125.
5. Pettegrew JW *et al.* Alterations in brain high-energy phosphate and membrane phospholipid metabolism in first-episode, drug naive schizophrenics. *Arch Gen Psy* 1991 ; 48 : 563-8.
6. Pettegrew JW *et al.* ^{31}P Nuclear Magnetic Resonance Spectrosocpy: Neurodevelopment and Schizophrenia. *Schizophrenia Bullettin* 1993 ; 19(1) : 35-53.
7. Stanley J.A. *et al.* In vivo ^{31}P NMR spectroscopy study of schizophrenics at different stages of illness. *Abstract at the Eleventh Annual meeting of Society Magnetic Resonance in Medicine* 1992 ; 756.
8. Williamson P *et al.* Localized phosphorus 31 magnetic resonance spectroscopy in chronic schizophrenic patients and normal controls. *Arch Gen Psy* 1991 ; 48;578.

25

Evaluation of multiple sclerosis with magnetization transfer

A. CAMPI

Department of Neuroradiology, Scientific Institute Ospedale S Raffaele, University of Milan, Italy.

Magnetization Transfer (MT) is a technique of recent application which evaluates the in vivo *water content of tissues and its relationship to macromolecules or membranes. This technique provides the possibility of having some tissue specificity particularly in demyelinating diseases. MT could provide indirect evaluation of the characteristics of multiple sclerosis (MS) lesions. MT is induced by applying a radiofrequency pulse to saturate the energy level of bound protons, this irradiation causes exchange of magnetization and a decrease in the net magnetization of free protons. The extent of magnetization transfer effects was quantified by the magnetization transfer ratio (MTR). MTR was calculated by the equation of Dousset et al. To calculate Mo and Ms, regions of interest were chosen within the lesions and in the white matter by using cursors of 0.04-0.02 cm^2. The aims of the study were: 1) to characterize brain MS lesions and to compare MTR values for enhancing lesions with different patterns of enhancement, 2) to define the role of subtle changes in the normal appearing white matter (NAWM) in the development of disability in MS. Twenty-nine clinically definite MS patients, with either relapsing-remitting or chronic-progressive courses, and 10 sex- and age-matched controls entered the study. In MS patients we evaluated the MTR for 65 Gadolinium-enhancing and 292 non-enhancing lesions. For each patient and control, two NAWM areas in the frontal lobe were also studied with MT. For patients, MTR values were also calculated for three contiguous areas of NAWM progressively further from «isolated» lesions visible on conventional magnetic resonance imaging (MRI) scans. Lesions had significantly lower MTR than the NAWN of the patients or the normal white matter of healthy controls. There was no difference in MTR of enhancing and non-enhancing lesions. Enhancement was homogeneous in 45 and ring-*

like in 20 lesions. MTR values were lower for ring-like than homogeneous lesions. These differences are due to the variability of the pathological features of both enhancing (different amounts of proteins and inflammatory cells, edema and demyelination) and non-enhancing (gliosis, demyelination and axonal loss) lesions. Frontal NAWM had lower mean MTR than the frontal white matter of the controls (p=0.02). MTR in the NAWM adjacent to «isolated» lesions increased with distance from them towards the cortical grey matter (p=0.04). This pattern was typical for patients with chronic-progressive MS, whose MTR in the first two regions of NAWM adjacent to lesions were lower than those of the same regions of patients with relapsing-remitting MS. This study confirms the supposed reactivated chronic nature of ring-like lesions and the presence of subtle changes in the NAWM of MS patients indicating that such changes could play a role in the development of disability in MS, the MT technique, by providing MTR values within standardized narrow ranges (related to the different pathological characteristics of the lesions), could help us to differentiate edematous from demyelinated or gliotic lesions. In combination with a standardized clinical evaluation, it should help us to select appropriate groups of patients to enter therapeutic trials and to monitor the effects of treatment.

Conventional MR is very sensitive for providing the anatomical details and pathological changes of the majority of neurological diseases. MR is the main diagnostic support for the diagnosis of multiple sclerosis (MS). In conventional MR imaging, the image contrast depends on spin-lattice (T1) and spin-spin relaxation times (T2) of protons in tissue molecules, and on the proton density [1]. The signal mostly comes from hydrogen nuclei in water. Therefore, an increased water load in lesions is easily detected by current MR imaging. However, its capacity for characterizing the pathological nature of the tissues is poor. Use of alternative techniques such as magnetization transfer, T2 relaxation decay curves and spectroscopy has recently been proposed to achieve tissue specificity [2-5]. MT is based on interactions between protons which are immobile or closely bound to macromolecules and the free protons of tissues [6]. MT is induced by applying an off-resonance radiofrequency pulse strong enough to saturate the energy level of bound water population protons. This pulse is applied at the frequency far from resonance peak of free water protons and when magnetization transfer effects occur, partial saturation and reduction of signal are observed in the non-irradiated pool of free water spins. Magnetization transfer effects can be quantified by the MTR, calculated by comparing the signal intensities of saturated and unsaturated images [6-7].

In a previous report [6], patients with MS had a significant decrease in the MTR of lesions, which was more evident in patients with chronic-progressive MS. A smaller but still significant reduction of mean MTR values was also found for the normal-appearing white matter (NAWM) of such patients. There is Gadolinium enhancement in MS lesions with abnormal blood-brain barrier (BBB) permeability. Two typical patterns of enhancement in MS brain lesions have been described: homogeneous and ring-like [8]. The first pattern of enhancement seems to be related to fresh new active lesions, the second to reactivation on the periphery of chronic lesions.

There are some discrepancies between the extent of lesions seen on conventional MR imaging (MRI) scans and the clinical status of the patients [9]. Several biological explanations and methodological limitations may account for this lack of correlation [8-9]. One of these possible explanations is that the NAWM might be more diffusely and severely affected in more disabled patients, contributing along with other factors to determining the disability in MS. Previous MR studies evaluating this issue have given conflicting results. On the one hand, several authors found no difference in the relaxation times of NAWM of MS patients with different disease courses [10] and disabilities [11]. On the other hand, Thompson et al. [12] demonstrated higher T1 values for the NAWM of patients with secondary progressive MS than those of patients with primary progressive MS and Dousset et al. [6] found lower MT ratios for the NAWM of patients with chronic-progressive MS than those with relapsing-remitting MS. Finally, a recent pixel-by-pixel relaxation time (RT) study [13] found a significant proportion of the NAWM in MS to be discretely involved by multiple small areas, often of one or two pixels, suggesting once again a possible role of the «invisible» lesion load in the evolution of MS.

The aims of this study were the following:

a) To characterize brain MS lesions by calculating MTR values

b) To compare the MTR values of enhancing lesions with the two different patterns of enhancement

c) To define the role of subtle changes of the NAWM in the development of disability in MS.

Patients and methods

Twenty-nine (10 male, 19 female) patients with clinically definite multiple sclerosis [14] entered the study. Twentyone had relapsing-remitting (RR) MS and 8 secondary-progressive (SP) MS. The mean age was 39 (30 for RR and 48 for SP), the mean duration of the disease was 4.7 years (SD + 1.3). The median disability score measured with the Expanded disability status scale (EDSS) [10] was 3.0 (range=1.5-7.5) All patients had MR images obtained at 1.5T. Axial 5-mm section (0.1 gap) spin-echo (SE) T2-weighted images were obtained using parameters of 2500/40/80 (TR/TE) at 192x256 acquisition matrix. Axial 5-mm section SE T1-weighted images (0.1 gap) 500/17 were obtained after Gadolinium-DTPA infusion. Two concurrently obtained 2D gradient-echo images, (600/12/20°) (0.4 gap) with and without saturation pulse were obtained before the T1WI. An 1.5-KHz off-resonance RF pulse frequency of 16.384 ms was used. The bandwidth of the pulse was 250 Hz.

The extent of magnetization transfer effects was quantified by the magnetization transfer ratio (MTR). MTR was calculated by the equation of Dousset et al. [6] : MTR = Mo-Ms/Mo, in which Mo represents the signal amplitude without saturation and Ms represents the signal amplitude with application of the saturation impulse. To calculate Mo and Ms, regions of interest were chosen within the lesions and in the white matter by using cursors of 0.04-0.02 cm^2. In the patients, we evaluated 65 Gadolinium-enhancing and 292 non- enhancing lesions. Enhancement was homogeneous in 45 and ring-like in 20 lesions. The MTR of 41 «isolated» unenhancing lesions and of the adjacent NAWM were also measured. «Isolated» lesions were those which were surrounded on the same slice and in at least the two adjacent ones by macroscopically normal white matter in order to avoid partial volume effects from other lesions. Two-mm round regions of interest (ROI) were placed in the center of the lesion, and 3 others in contiguous NAWM areas, starting from the external edge of the lesions and progressing towards the cortical grey matter (first, second and third NAWM ROIs). In addition, for each patient MTR was calculated for 2 regions of NAWM in the frontal lobes. In the same areas, MTR were also calculated in 10 age- and sex-matched healthy volunteers.

The data were analyzed statistically by the Student t Test or one-way ANOVA. When the data sets were not distributed normally, the Mann-Whitney Test was used.

Results

The average percentage values for MTR are reported in Table I. Mean MTR values for the MS lesions were significantly lower than those for the NAWM ($p<0.0001$) and for normal white matter of healthy subjects ($p<0.0001$). There was no significant difference between MTR values of Gadolinium-enhancing and non-enhancing lesions. The 65 Gd-enhancing lesions were divided according to the pattern of enhancement into two subgroups: A) 45 with homogeneous enhancement, B) 20 with ring-like enhancement. MTR values were significantly lower ($p= .0167$) in subgroup B: 34.3 + 7.2(SD)%, than in subgroup A: 38.2+ 5.4 % (Table II).

Table I. Mean MTR (± standard deviation) for enhancing and non-enhancing lesions in MS patients.

Patients number	MTR of enhancing lesions	MTR of non-enhancing lesions
All = 29	37±6.2	41±6.7
Relapsing-remitting = 21	36.9+6.7	41.2+6.1
Chronic-progressive = 8	37.4+5.5	40.5+7.7

Frontal NAWM had lower mean MTR than the frontal white matter of the controls (mean MTR+SD=49.8+1.6% vs 50.8+1.7%, p=0.02).

For the group as a whole, the MTR in the NAWN adjacent to isolated lesions increased progressively from the NAWM contiguous to the lesions towards the cortical grey matter (p=0.04). At post-hoc analysis, the MTR obtained for the first NAWM ROI were significantly lower than those of the third NAWM ROI (p=0.02) (Table III). This pattern of increased MTR in NAWM moving away from the lesions was found to apply to patients with chronic-progressive MS (mean+SD = 46.2+3.8% in the first NAWM

ROI and 47.5+2.8% in the third NAWM ROI; p=0.05), but not to patients with relapsing-remitting MS.

Table II. Mean MTR values of lesions with homogeneous and ring-like enhancement.

Enhancement	Homogeneous	Ring-like	p
MTR (standard deviation)	38.2 (5.4)	34.3 (7.2)	< 0.02

Table III. MTR of «isolated» lesions and different NAWM regions.

	«Isolated» lesions	1° NAWM ROI	2° NAWM ROI	3° NAWM ROI	p*
Mean MTR (SD)	40.7 (4.1) %	48.1 (3.0) %	48.8 (2.3) %	49.5 (2.1) %	0.0001

*Statistical analysis: one-way ANOVA. At post-hoc analysis (Student t Test): first NAWM ROI MTR vs third NAWM ROI MTR p=0.02.

Discussion

The significantly low in MTR values in all patients confirm previously published data [6,16]. Previous studies have already demonstrated that MTI is useful for evaluation of the pathological features of both chronic [6, 16 and new active [17] MS lesions and that the average MTR of all the brain lesions is correlated with the degree of disability in patients with MS [16].

MTR of enhancing lesions

The lack of significant difference in MTR values between enhancing and non-enhancing lesions is not surprising. In fact, Gadolinium DTPA can only differentiate lesions in which there is breakdown of the blood-brain barrier (BBB) (enhancing) from lesions with intact BBB (non-enhancing). Abnormality of the BBB is usually found in active lesions both new and peripheral zones of old reactivated lesions [18]. Enhancement is not related to the amount of cells in MS plaques [19]. Enhancing lesions probably include plaques with different degrees of demyelination, with various inflammatory components and different durations [20]. This is the reason for the variability of MTR values.

The pathological correlate of Gd-DTPA enhancement in MS is largely unknown. One group did autopsy studies of the brain of a patient after his last fatal exacerbation of an MS in which MR had shown Gd-DTPA enhancing lesions. Neuropathological examination of the enhancing areas displayed acute demyelination with a striking perivascular inflammatory response consisting of lymphocytes, monocytes and plasmacells. The borders of the lesions consisted of a dense mononuclear wall, the center showed a nearly complete loss of myelin. In another enhancing lesion, the central area contained a multitude of foamy macrophages or ameboid microglia, oligodendrocytes, demyelinated axons, and axonal spheroids, with active demyelination evident at the margins [19]. In a large study correlating MR and computed tomography (CT) with MS lesions, all histologically «active lesions», despite the variety of their radiological appearances, showed some type of contrast enhancement [21]. More specifically, all ring lesions with peripheral enhancement showed inflammatory activity and relatively prominent macrophage infiltration.

Histological characteristics of homogeneous and ring-like lesions probably differ in the entity of tissue loss and inflammatory cell presence, therefore they have different MTR values. The lower MTR values of ring-like lesions seem to confirm their supposed reactivated chronic nature, since they are characterized by greater expansion of the extracellular spaces. There is probably a correlation between the rims of monocytes at the margin of the lesion and the appearance of the ring enhancement in MR [19]. At the early phase of the disease, enhancing lesions may have a separate mechanism for alteration of the brain barrier or perhaps a few invading lymphocytes might be responsible for the change in the BBB. They could be the histological correlate of homogeneous enhancing lesions. Correlation of Gd-DTPA enhancement with histology in the experimental allergic encephalytis (EAE) model support the association of inflammation with enhancement in new lesions and suggests a primary role for inflammatory cells [22].

MTR of the frontal NAWM

The results obtained for the NAWM are still conflicting [6, 16]. Dousset *et al.* [6] reported that the MTR of the NAWM was significantly lower, particularly in patients with chronic-progressive MS, than that of the white matter of controls, while this difference was not found by Gass *et al.* [16]. There are several possible explanations for this discrepancy, such as the MR methodology, the extent of white matter disease and the clinical characteristics of the patients. However, it is possible that another factor might be responsible for these conflicting results. It has been suggested recently by a pixel-by-pixel RT study [13] that microscopic changes in the NAWM of MS do not occur randomly and diffusely but seem to be related to the presence of small, discrete abnormalities, often only one to two pixels in size. If this is the case, when NAWM is studied the MTR might vary significantly in relation to the number of pixels which are involved by the pathological process within the region of interest.

The analysis of the NAWM far away from visible lesions was restricted to the frontal lobe, since MT is known to change in different brain regions [16], depending on the extent of myelination and/or the varying amounts of bound water in myelin and/or the density of nerve fibers.

The pathological nature of the decrease in MT is still unknown. It might derive in part from small lesions that are beyond the resolution of the system [13] and in part to the widespread abnormalities described by pathological studies [23]. These abnormalities, which include diffuse astrocytic hyperplasia, patchy edema and perivascular cellular infiltration [23, 24], can modify the relative proportions of mobile and immobile protons, thus inducing changes in MT. In this respect, it is of particular interest that a post-mortem study demonstrated water content in the brain NAWM of MS patients to be 4% greater than that of normal controls [25].

NAWM adjacent to the lesions

MTR of the NAWM were found to be the lowest around the lesions visible on conventional MR scans and to increase progressively moving away from the lesions to values similar to those found in the NAWM of the frontal lobes.

Since we have considered in this evaluation only NAWM around lesions which were not surrounded on the same slice and in at least the two adjacent ones by other visible lesions, partial volume effects from other lesions can be reasonably excluded. This is even more evident when the small size of the ROIs (0.2 mm^2) is compared to the larger thickness of the slices (5 mm) and of the interslice gap (2 mm).

Therefore, two other explanations seems to be more likely. First, there might be a partial volume effect from the same lesion surrounded by the NAWM studied. Even if no abnormalities at all were visible on conventional MR scans around these lesions, it is known that microscopically the shapes of such lesions are not so well-defined [26]. Second, the presence of small lesions or widespread abnormalities might be more frequent and severe in NAWM closer to lesions, thus causing a «penumbra» around the visible lesions. Our results seem to confirm that there is an «invisible» lesion load in patients with MS that might at least partially account for some of the discrepancies beween the clinical and MR findings in MS reported by several studies using conventional MR scans [8, 9].

Our study also indicates that the abnormalities of the NAWM adjacent to the lesions are more striking in patients with chronic-progressive MS than in those with relapsing-remitting MS. A recent longitudinal MRI study demonstrated that new lesion formation is correlated with changes in disability in relapsing-remitting MS, while such parameters do not correlate at all in patients with chronic-progressive MS, raising the possibility that other mechanisms might be related to the development of the disability in such patients [27]. One of these possible factors might be the presence of repeated or continuous activity in chronic lesions which, on the one hand, might lead to greater degrees of axonal loss and/or demyelination in the chronic lesions and, on the other, might be responsible for a diffusion of the pathological process into the macroscopically NAWM.

On the basis of the different MTR values, we could consider highly demyelinated plaques those with markedly decreased MTR to be chronic, while slightly higher, but still low MTR are observed in acute inflammatory-edematous lesions, such as EAE and the acute phase of MS plaques [6]. During remyelination, we could theoretically expect increases in MTR values, from low to normal. MT has the potential to detect subtle changes of the NAWM in MS. These NAWM abnormalities seem to be greater in more disabled patients and therefore seem to be meaningful in influencing the natural history of the disease.

The usefulness of the MT technique is supported by a recent study [16] which has shown that clinical disability is correlated more strongly with the average lesion MT ratio than with total lesion volume. The MT technique, by providing MTR values within standardized narrow ranges (related to the different pathological characteristics of the lesions), could help us to differentiate edematous from demyelinated or gliotic lesions. It could also provide prognostic information about the possibility of complete or partial regression of symptoms. In combination with a standardized clinical evaluation, it should help us to select appropriate groups of patients to enter therapeutic trials and to monitor the effects of treatment.

References

1. Lundbom N. Determination of Magnetization Transfer Contrast in tissue : An MR imaging study of brain tumors. *AJR* 1992; 159: 1279-1285.
2. Wolff SD, Balaban RS. Magnetization Transfer Contrast (MTC) and tissue water proton relaxation in vivo. *Magn Reson Med* 1989; 10: 135-144.
3. Balaban RS, Ceckler TL. Magnetization Transfer Contrast in magnetic resonance imaging. *Magn Res Quat* 1992; 2: 116-137.
4. Larsson HBW, Frederiksen J et al. Assessment of demyelination, edema, and gliosis by in vivo determenation of T1 and T2 in the brain of patients with acute attack of multiple sclerosis. *Magn Reson in Med* 1989; 11: 337-348 .
5. Fullerton DG, Potter JL, Dornbluth NC. NMR relaxation of protons in tissues and macromolecular water solutions. *Magn Reson Imag* 1982; 1209-1226.
6. Dousset V, Grossman RI et al. Experimental allergic encephalomyelitis and Multiple Sclerosis: Lesion characterization with Magnetization Transfer imaging. *Radiology* 1992; 182: 483-491.
7. Mittl RLJr, Gomori JM, Schnall MD, Holland GA, Grossman RI, Atlas SW. Magnetization Transfer Effects in MR Imaging of in vivo intracranial hemorrhage. *AJNR* 1993; 14: 881-891.
8. Mc Donald WI, Miller DH, Barnes D. The pathological evolution of multiple sclerosis. *Neuropathology Applied Neurobiology* 1992; 18: 319-334.
9. Kermode AG, Thompson AJ, Tofts P, *et al.* Brekdown of blood-brain barrier precedes symptoms and other MRI signs of new lesions in multiple sclerosis: pathogenetic and clinical implications. *Brain* 1990; 113: 1477-1489.
10. Ormerod IEC, Johnson G, MacManus D, du Boulay EPGH, McDonald WI. Relaxation times of apparently normal cerebral white matter in multiple sclerosis. Acta Radiol 1986; 369: 382-384.
11. Haughton VM, Zerrin Yetkin F, Rao SM, *et al.* Quantitative MR in the diagnosis of multiple sclerosis. *Magn Reson Med* 1992; 26: 71-78.
12. Thompson AJ, Kermode AG, Wicks D, *et al.* Major differences in the dynamics of primary and secondary progressive multiple sclerosis. *Ann Neurol* 1991; 29: 53-62.
13. Barbosa S, Blumhardt LD, Roberts N, Lock T, Edwards RHT. Magnetic resonance relaxation time mapping in multiple sclerosis: normal appearing white matter and the «invisible» lesion load. *Magn Reson Imaging* 1994; 12: 33-42.
14. Poser CM, Paty DW, Scheinberg L *et al.* New diagnostic criteria for multiple sclerosis: guidelines for research protocols. *Ann Neurol* 1983; 13: 227-231.

15. Kurtzke JF. Disability rating scales in multiple sclerosis. In *Annals NY Academy of Sciences* 1983.
16. Gass A, Barker, Kidd D *et al*. Correlation of magnetization transfer ratio with clinical disability in multiple sclerosis. *Ann Neurol* 1994; 36: 62-67.
17. Hiehle JF, Grossman RI, Ramer KN, Gonzales-Scarano F, Cohen JA. Comparison of gadolinium enhanced spin-echo imaging versus magnetization transfer imaging in the evaluation of magnetic resonance detected lesions in multiple sclerosis. *AJNR* 1994 (in press).
18. Paty DW. Magnetic resonance imaging in demyelination. In: Kim SU, (ed) *Myelination and demyelination, implications for multiple sclerosis*. New York, Plenum 1987 ; pp 259-272 .
19. Katz D, Taubenberger JK, Cannella B *et al*. Correlation between magnetic resonance imaging findings and lesion development in chronic active multiple sclerosis. *Ann Neurol* 1993; 34: 661-669.
20. Bruck W, Schmied M, Suchanek G *et al*. Oligodendrocytes in the early course of multiple sclerosis. *Ann Neurol* 1994; 35: 65-73.
21. Nesbit GM, Forbes GS, Scheithauer BW *et al*. Multiple sclerosis: histopathology and MR and/ or CT correlation in 37 cases at biopsy and three cases at autopsy. *Radiology* 1991; 180: 467-474.
22. Hawkins CP, Munro PMG, MacKenzie F *et al*. Duration and selectivity of blood-brain barrier breakdown in chronic relapsing experimental allergic encephalomyelitis studied by Gadolinium-DTPA and protein markers. *Brain* 1990; 113: 365-378.
23. Allen IV, McKeown SR. A histological, histochemical and biochemical study of the macroscopically normal white matter in multiple sclerosis. *J Neurol Sci* 1979; 41: 81-91.
24. Adams CWM. Pathology of multiple sclerosis: progression of the lesion. *Br Med Bull* 1977; 33: 15-20.
25. Bruhn H, Frahm J, Merboldt KD, *et al*. Cerebral metabolic alterations monitored by localised proton magnetic resonance spectroscopy in vivo. *Ann Neurol* 1992; 32: 140-150.
26. Allen IV. Pathology of multiple sclerosis. In: Matthews WB, ed. McAlpine's Multiple Sclerosis. 2nd ed.Edinburgh: Churchill Livingstone, 1991: 341-378.
27. Filippi M, Miller DH, Paty DW, *et al*. Correlations between changes in disability and MRI activity in multiple sclerosis: a two year follow up study [abstract]. *Neurology* 1994; 44 (suppl 2): 339.

26

Blood oxygenation and NMR signal changes

J. CHAMBRON

Institut de Physique Biologique, Strasbourg, France.

The use of an intravascular MR contrast agent has allowed the functional mapping of cerebral areas in which, for instance, flow changes are induced by visual stimulation [1].

PET studies have shown that physiological neuronal activity increases glucose uptake and blood flow (by 51% and 50%, respectively) much more than oxygen consumption (5%), leaving oxygen in excess in the venous blood - compared to the basal state [2]. This focal transient decrease in paramagnetic hemoglobin explains the increase in NMR signal intensity, known as Blood Oxygen Level Dependent (BOLD) contrast. The magnetic susceptibility of hemoglobin, depending on its oxygenation state makes a endogeneous contrast agent of it suitable for the purpose of blood flow monitoring [3].

Magnetic susceptibility of the hemoglobin in various states of oxygenation

The correlation between the oxygenation state of the hemoglobin and its magnetic susceptibility was established over five decades ago by Pauling and Coryell [4]. From their measurements they were able to derive a value for the magnetic moment of deoxyhemoglobin of 5.46 $\mu\beta$, the above value would indicate a complex with four unpaired electrons, and a slight orbital contribution to the total magnetic moment.

The value of $-0.5 \cdot 10^{-6}$ reported by Fabry and San George [5] for the volume magnetic susceptibility of a 5mM solution of deoxyhemoglobin, corresponding to the concentration of hemoglobin in the red blood cell (RBC). This value of 0.219 is less than the susceptibility of pure water, which is in agreement with the value of 0.2×10^{-6} for the susceptibility difference between the plasma and packed deoxygenated RBC reported by Thulborn et al. [6].

Effects of the compartmentation of the hemoglobin by the erythrocyte on the relaxation rate in blood

The early studies on suspensions of RBC containing the paramagnetic form of the heme have established that the observed increase in transverse relaxation rate or linewidth of water protons, in such samples, compared to oxygenated saturated samples, is dependent on the presence of intact cells, corresponding to a compartmented paramagnetic substance.

The paramagnetic agent alters the magnetic susceptibility of the solution, and thus changes the inducible bulk magnetization of the compartment containing it. Indeed, this magnetization does not only contribute to the total magnetic field strength experienced by a nucleus within the compartment, but also influences the magnetic field beyond the boundaries of the compartment giving rise to local magnetic field gradients.

Basically, the compartmentation of paramagnetic substances can affect the chemical shift or relaxation rates of a nucleus in two ways : [7]

1. through a direct dipolar or/and scalar coupling interaction between the water proton and the unpaired electron, where the signal change is quantified by a natural relaxation rate R_2;

2. by altering the bulk magnetic susceptibility homogeneity, where the signal change is quantified by the increased water (proton) linewidth or its equivalent R_2 relaxation rate,

3. by a combination of both processes with a signal change quantified by

$$R_2^* = R_2 + R_2'$$

While direct paramagnetic relaxation is considered as negligible, because the unpaired electrons are sequestered within a hydrophobic region of deoxyhemoglobin molecules, the second mechanism, which does not require a direct interaction mechanism has been considered as predominant.

On the basis of volume susceptibility measurements and of the dependence of R_2 on the pulse rate in Carr-Purcell-Meiboom-Gill (CPMG) sequences, Thulborn et al. [7] in their pioneering work have explained why R_2 enhancement with decreasing blood deoxygenation arises from the diffusion of water through those local field gradients. These effects were first mentioned in the radiological literature, by Gomori et al [8] who emphasized the importance of high field, and by R.R. Edelmann et al [9] by showing that when using a gradient echo sequence which is more sensitive to field heterogeneity than a spin echo sequence, the signal loss is even stronger and can occur at low field.

heterogeneity than a spin echo sequence, the signal loss is even stronger and can occur at low field.

Since then, functional MRI studies by Gradient Echo (GE), Echo Planar Imaging (EPI) or Spin Echo (SE) EPI have largely demonstrated that the intrinsic BOLD contrast is lesser in SE sequences than in GE sequences.

Effects of the compartmentation of blood in the vasculature on the relaxation rates of tissues (flow effects excluded)

The changes in oxygen level-dependent signal amplitude are rather complex in tissues due to susceptibility effects induced by the compartmentation of blood in the vasculature. According to the works of Ogawa *et al* [10], the degree of oxygen saturation of blood in a vessel is suggested to make the tissues surrounding it more or less magnetically homogeneous, introducing geometrical factors to explain tissue relaxivity as a function of the size of the vessel, its orientation relative to the main field, and the vessel density in voxels.

The extra phase f of a spin randomly walking by path steps of length $\delta\rho$ and duration $\delta\tau$ according to the Einstein relation $\delta_r = \sqrt{6D\delta_t}$ (D = diffusion constant), in a field heterogeneity characterized by its z microscopic component variation ΔB_z or this equivalent Larmor frequency $\delta\omega = \gamma\Delta B_z$, is given by $\phi = \Sigma\gamma\Delta B_z\delta t$ with $\Delta B_z = \alpha M$, where a is the geometrical factor and M the corresponding magnetic moment, $M = \Delta_x B_0$, where Δ_x is the microscopic susceptibility heterogeneity and B_0 the polarizing main field.

The diffusion process, characterized by its constant D, introduces for the loss of coherence in the framework of the geometrical system, three regimes characterized most easily by the product $\tau_D\delta\omega$, where τ_D is the correlation time given by

$$\tau_D = R_2 / D$$

where R is the dimension of the diffusion space.

These regimes, which we shall term motionnally averaged, intermediate, and static, are most easily defined in terms of the diffusion correlation τ_D of water molecules in the presence of a magnetic inhomogeneity and dw the characteristic variation in the Larmor Frequency due to the field perturbation.

The dependence on the vasculature size of the magnetic susceptibility effects created by deoxyhemoglobin are schematically very well summarized by Hoppel *et al* [12].

• In the intravascular environment, representing blood, the field inhomogeneities are averaged by the diffusional motion of the protons through the dense packing of the erythrocytes. The system is said to be in a motionally narrowed regime. The diffusion rate $1/\tau_D$ is much greater than $\delta\omega$; diffusion is fast, with respect to the spatial variations of the field perturbations $\delta\omega\tau_D \ll 1$. The notion of water protons produces a loss of phase between spins with little net phase shift within the vessel, so $\Delta R_2 / \Delta R'_2 \gg 1$.

• In tissues surrounding the capillaries, the diffusion distance is comparable to the extent of the field gradient; the diffusion rate is comparable to the frequency shift created by deoxygenated blood, therefore, an intermediate regime $\tau\Delta\delta\omega$ ª 1 is expected. The loss of coherence in tissue water due to the diffusional motion ΔR_2 is of the same order than the net phase shift accumulation ΔR_2, so $\Delta R_2 / \Delta R_2 \approx 1$.

• Finally, in tissues surrounding a veinule or a vein, the gradient extent produced by the blood is very large as compared with the diffusion distance of the protons, producing a large shift in frequency ΔR_2 with a small loss in phase coherence ΔR_2, so $\Delta R_2 / \Delta R_2 << 1$. Diffusion is slow enough, so that the spin echo effectively refocuses the magnetization. The regime is slow or static : $\tau\Delta\delta\omega >> 1$.

Quantitative approach of the relaxivity of tissues by computer imulation and relaxivity theories

The different models, characterised in terms of diffusion coefficient, voxel size, magnetization, and blood volume, have been validated recently by Hennan et al. [11] by applying the Anderson-Weiss mean theory and compared, to obtain a better quantitative understanding, to a computer simulation of the phase loss of a spin randomly walking in field heterogeneity, based on the classical theory of macroscopic magnetism.

In short, the susceptibility effect governed by diffusion will produce both spin echo and gradient echo attenuations in different fashions, depending on the regime of the spin motion. Within the range of physiological diffusion coefficient in tissues (10^{-5} cm² sec.), and for a reasonable echo time of 20 to 50 msec, a spin echo measurement will be more sensitive to small vessel environments such as capillaries, while a gradient echo sequence is sensitive to both capillaries and any larger vessel environments in which loss of phase in static or slow regime would be refocused, in spin echo measurements.

Finally, if the signal changes came purely from the intravascular water signal, a high $\Delta R_2 / \Delta R_2'$ ratio would be expected, as observed with blood phantoms by Hoppel et al. (12), due to the large number of red blood cells averaged by a diffusing spin, hence a very little phase shift with loss of spin echo signal intensity within the vessel, as measured in whole blood experiments.

These results have been recently confirmed by *in vivo* studies performed in order to assess the respective ability and advantages of SE and GE sequences to discriminate activated brain areas relying on BOLD contrast.

R.A. Bandettini et al., have shown that while greater BOLD contrast is observed in Gradient Echo sequences, Spin Echo sequences are preferentially more sensitive to smaller vessels. Moreover changes in R_2 in large vessels may be greater because of the fast diffusion of water in gradients induced by dense packing of erythrocytes. This implies that if draining veins are large enough to fill a voxel, the intrinsic R_2 changes in the blood cause significant signal changes.

Is the oxygen-dependent relaxivity enhancement of blood samples only a susceptibility effect, governed by the molecular diffusion of water ?

Finally, current thinking is focusing on the magnetic susceptibility mechanism of the relaxivity enhancement induced by deoxygenation of the blood at once in the blood itself and in the surrounding vessel.

But natural water relaxation processes governed by diffusion and exchange, in the blood compartment and their propagation in tissues, implying membrane and endothelial vascular permeability cannot be excluded.

In their pioneering work, Thulborn et al., on the basis of volume susceptibility measurements and of the dependence of R_2 on pulse rate in CPMG sequences, have shown that the increase in R_2 with increasing blood oxygenation in unstirred blood samples arises from the diffusion of water through field gradients. These authors have found a correlation time τ_D of 0.6 msec. and a quadratic dependence of R_2 on the hematocrit. Since these studies, many research works have been published, but the results are not in full agreement as to the nature of the diffusion process, i.e. whether it is an intra- or extracellular process, or a combination of both. Gillis and Koenig, Gomori, re-interpreting the data of Thulborn et al., had attributed this 0.6 msec. correlation time to an intravascular diffusion process; but recently, Gillis (personal communication) [13] on the basis of further research performed with computer simulations as described by Kennan et al., came to the conclusion that both intra and extracellular diffusion contribute to the relaxivity enhancement.

Discrepancies have also been found concerning the relationship between R_2 and the hematocrit, which should be quadratic, according to Thulborn et al., but linear according to Bryant et al.

Bearing in mind that Herbst and Goldstein [15] observed wide discrepancies between NMR data obtained on circulating and unstirred blood mainly because of the aggregation of red blood cells which takes place during sedimentation, and also bearing in mind the fact that, in circulating blood, the motion of red blood cells can modulate the local field gradients as well as the molecular diffusion [7,19], our group, Meyer et al [20], studied the relaxivity of moving blood samples (2-20 ml/m) on an NMR probe, as a function of the oxygenation degree of a sample previously equilibrated in an extracorporeal oxygenator. Our results showed a linear regression of R_2 versus the fraction Ds of deoxyhemoglobin, even though T_1 is insensitive to the oxygenation degree. The hypothesis of a molecular diffusion process through an inhomogeneous local magnetic field has been tested with Hahn echoes.

The data was correctly adjusted with a single exponential, but further fitting using a second order diffusion-dependent coefficient in the exponential yield a large error, compatible with a negligible diffusion effect.

T_2 decays were obtained by varying the pulse rate from 1 to 14 msec in GMPG sequences. The T_2 values plotted versus the echo time τ was adjusted by Luz and Meiboom's relation [21]. An exchange time of 1.2 msec was found for a PO_2 ranging from 3 to 290 mmHg.

Discrepancies arise in the literature, concerning the significance of this correlation time, as determined in the chemical exchange model worked out by Luz and Meiboom [21]. General expressions have been developed to account for the dephasing effect of field gradients, monitored by diffusion or exchange, but a mathematical model incorporating both effects has not yet been established. The various diffusion regimes are approximately described by the Anderson-Weiss mean field theory [22] and the exact formulation of the dependence of R_2 on diffusion in a complex and restricted water compartment, like erythrocytes or blood vessels, is not really known. In this very complicated theoretical situation, investigators, as Brooks *et al.* have explained, [23] have borrowed theories developed for chemical exchange to analyse their experimental data. They have made a translational diffusion process to be similar to a chemical exchange process, except however Bryant *et al.* [15], who effectively underline the physical differences between them.

Being unable to clearly demonstrate by Hahn echo experiments the existence of a net diffusion effect, and displaying a 1.2 msec. chemical exchange time in the true sense of the Luz-Meiboom theory, [21] close to that found for amino-acid solutions [24] suggested to us a complementary way of explaining the oxygen-dependent relaxivity of blood.

Previous studies by Eisenstadt and Fabry [24] on blood relaxivity have established the evidence of cross-relaxation between heme protein and water, effective enough to cause a solute solvent to relax as one whole, implying the T_2 of water to be less than its T_1. Such a mechanism can be involved in the case of the globin molecule, which contains exchangeable protons, particularly of the histidine residue situated on the opposite side to the oxygen binding site, close to the iron atom. The histidine proton could be considered as a relaxation sink for bulk water protons, in which they are transferred by cross relaxation and spin diffusion. The relaxivity of the histidine proton would be enhanced by the interaction with a thermal average electron spin, or Curie spin [25].

In conclusion, further experiments could be performed to refine our understanding of blood oxygen level dependent relaxivity processes. These should allow to explain the results obtained in clinical applications and improve the best experimental conditions as well.

References

1. Belliveau JW, Kennedy DN, McKinstry RC, Buchbinder BR, Weisshoff RM, Cohe MS, Vevea JM, Brady TJ, Rosen B.R. Functional mapping of the hyman visual cortex by magnetic resonance imaging. *Science* 1991 ; 254, 716-718.
2. Fox PT, Raichle ME, Mintun MA, Dence C. Nonoxidative glucose consumption during focal physiologic neural activity *Science* 1988 ; 241, 462-463.
3. Ogawa S, Tank DW, Menon R, Ellermann JM, Kim SG, Merkle H, Ugurbil K. Intrinsic signal changes accompanying sensory stimulation: Functional brain mapping with magnetic resonance imaging. *Proc. Natl. Acad. Sci* 1992 ; 89, 5951-5955.
4. Pauling L, Coryell CD. The magnetic properties and structure of hemoglobin, oxyhemoglobin and carbon monocyhemoglobin. *Proc. Natl. Acad. Sci., USA* 1936 ; 22, 210-216.

5. Fabry M, San George RC. Effect of magnetic susceptibility on nuclear magnetic resonance signals arising from Red Cells: A waring. *Biochemistry* 1983 ; 22. 4119-4125.
6. Thulborn KR, Wterton JC, Matthews PM, Radda GK. Oxygenation dependence of the transverse relaxation time of water protons in whole blood at high field. Biochim. Biophys. *Acta* 1982 ; 714, 265-270.
7. Gasparovic C, Matwiyoff MA. The magnetic properties and water dynamics of red blood cell: A study by proton-NMR. Lineshape analysis. Magn. Reson. *MEd.* 1992 ; 26, 274-299.
8. Gomori JM, Grossman RI, Goldberg HI, Zimmerman RA, Bilaniuk LT. Intracranial hematomas: imaging by high field MR. *Radiology* 1985 ; 157, 87-93.
9. Edelman RR, Johnson K, Buxton R, Shoakimas C, Rosen BR, Davis KR, Brady TJ. MR of hemorrhage: a nex approach. Amer. J. *Neuroradiol* 1986 ; 7, 751-756.
10. Ogawa S, Lee TM, Nayak AS, Glynn P. Oxygenation-sensitive contrast in magnetic resonance image of rodent brain at high magnetic fields. Magn. Reson. *Med.* 1990 ; 14, 68-78.
11. Kennan RP, Zhong J, Gore JC. Intravascular susceptibility contrast mechanisms in tissues. Magn. Reson. *Med.* 1994 ; 31, 9.
12. Hoppel BE, Weisshoff RM, Thulborn KR, Moore JB, Kwong KK, Rosen BR. Measurement of Regional Blood oxygenation and cerebral hemodynamics. Magn. Reson. *Med.* 1993 ; 30, 715-723.
13. Gillis P, Pétö S, Moiny F, Mispelter J, Cuenod C.A. Proton transverse nuclear magnetic relaxation in oxidized Blood: a numerical approach (in press - Magn. Reson. Med.).
14. Bandettini PA, Wong EC, Jesmanowick A, Hinks RS, Hyde JS. Spin Echo and Gradient Echo EPI of human brain activation using BOLD contrast: a comparative study at 1.5T. *NMR in Biomed* 1994 ; 7, 12-20.
15. Bryant RG, Marril K, Blackmore C, Francis C. Magnetic relaxation in blood and blood clots. Magn. Reson. *Med.* 1990 ; 13, 133-144.
16. Gomori JM, Grossman RI, Yu Ip C, Asakura T. NMR Relaxation times of blood: Dependence on field strength, oxidation state, and cell integrity. J. *Comp. Assist. Tom.* 1987 ; 14, 684.
17. Gillis P, Koenig SH. Transverse relaxation of solvent protons induced by magnetized spheres: application to ferritin, erythrocytes, and magnetite. Magn. Reson. *Med.* 1987 ; 5, 323-345.
18. Herbst MD, Goldstein JH. A review of water diffusion measurement by NMR in human red blood cells. Am. J. *Physiol* 1989 ; 256, C1097-C1104.
19. Turner R, Serrard P, Hertz Pannier L, Le Bihan D, Feinberg D. Functional Neuroimaging with EPI: Sequence issues. Abstract book pp 163-169. Functional MRI of the Brain - Workshop of SMRM SMRI, *Arlington USA* 1993.
20. Meyer ME, Yu O, Eclancher B, Grucker D, Chambron J. NMR relaxation rates and blood oxygenation level. Submitted to Magn. Reson. Med.
21. Luz Z, Meiboom S. Nuclear Magnetic Resonance study of the protolysis of trimethylammonium ion in aqueous solution - order of the reaction with respect for solvent. J. *Chem. Phys* 1963 ; 39, 366-370.
22. Anderson PW, Weiss PR. Exchange narrowing in paramagnetic resonance. *Rev. Mod. Phys* 1953 ; 25, 269-276.
23. Brooks RA, Di Chiro G. Magnetic Resonance imaging of stationary blood: a review. *Med. Phys* 1987 ; 14, 903-913.
24. Eisenstadt M, Fabry ME. NMR Relaxation of the Hemoglobin-water proton spin system in red blood cells. J. *Magn. Res* 1978 ; 29, 591-297.
25. Grucker D, Steibel J, Dumitresco B, Armspach JP, Chambron J. Proton nuclear magnetic resonance relaxation rates in aqueous solutions of amino-acids. *Molec. Phys* 1990 ; 70, 903-919.
26. Gueron M. Nuclear relaxation in macromolecules by paramagnetic ions: a novel mechanism. J. *Magn. Reson* 1975 ; 19, 58-66.

27

Visualisation of vein effect in functional imaging using phase gradient methods

G. CROS, F. HENNEL, N. BOLO, F. GIRARD, C. LABADIE,
J. F. NEDELEC, J. P. MACHER, M. DÉCORPS*

FORENAP, Unité de Résonance Magnétique, Centre Hospitalier, 68250 Rouffach, France
* INSERM U318, GARN, CHU Nord, BP 217X 38043 Grenoble Cedex, France.

The performance of a given cognitive task produces local brain activation : there are local increases in the cerebral metabolism, blood flow, blood volume and blood oxygenation level. Since the transverse relaxation time T2* depends on this oxygenation level, methods which provide images with T2* based contrast, demonstrate local blood oxygenation level changes, therefore cerebral activity.

T2* depends on the blood oxygenation level, because of the magnetic properties of blood : oxyhemoglobin is diamagnetic like plasma and cerebral tissue whereas deoxyhemoglobin is paramagnetic. Therefore when blood is deoxygenated there is a difference of magnetic susceptibility between blood and tissue. This difference generates static magnetic field variations at the vessel-tissue interfaces. The magnitude of these variations depend on the vessel's size, the angle between the static magnetic field Bo and the vessel's axis, the value of the difference of magnetic susceptibility, the strength of Bo and the coordinates of the observed point.

In the presence of this field gradient the signal decreases by loss of phase coherence on T2* weighted images. So in standard functional studies based on T2* contrast the signal increases with the stimulus because of the increase of the blood oxygenation level.

But functional MRI methods based on T2* contrast are sensitive to blood oxygenation changes in both capillaries, where plasma-tissu exchange occurs, and larger veins which drain the tissue where exchanges have occured. Since only the capillary effect is directly related to cortex activity, it is important to distinguish it from the vein response in functional studies. Recently, the venous contribution to activation maps has been demonstrated [1] by comparison of functional imaging with MR angiography. In the present work, the distinction between vein and capillary responses is studied using MR venography based on phase gradient.

Methods

Excitation pulse

MR venography can be realized by using a pulse which has a bilinear phase distribution around the slice center along the slice selection direction. This method has been described by Z. H. Cho and his collaborators [2]. With this kind of excitation pulse one obtains images weighted by the field variation at the vein-tissue interfaces. The signal from spins which do not experience the field gradient is cancelled by the phase distribution. However the signal from spins which experience the field gradient due to the paramagnetic properties of deoxyhemoglobin, is refocused by this phase distribution. So when this type of venographic image is used in a functional study, the vein response in the image is opposite that observed with standard gradient echo imaging. In other words the signal drops when the blood oxygenation level increases during stimulus.

For low flip angles, the theory of linear response applies, and thus we determined an analytic expression of the pulse generating the bilinear phase distribution by executing the inverse Fourier transform of the desired magnetization amplitude and phase distribution. The result is an amplitude and phase modulated pulse (assuming a low flip angle) which we call BILI in the following.

But, a similar effect can be obtained by a pulse modulated only in amplitude without refocusing the slice gradient [3]. Indeed if the slice gradient refocusing is cancelled, there is a linear phase distribution along the slice selection direction which cancels the signal in an homogeneous static magnetic field. According to the same principle described above, venography can be realized by using this method.

VISUALISATION OF VEIN EFFECT IN FUNCTIONAL IMAGING

Examples of phase venography applied on a phantom (an air filled tube in water)

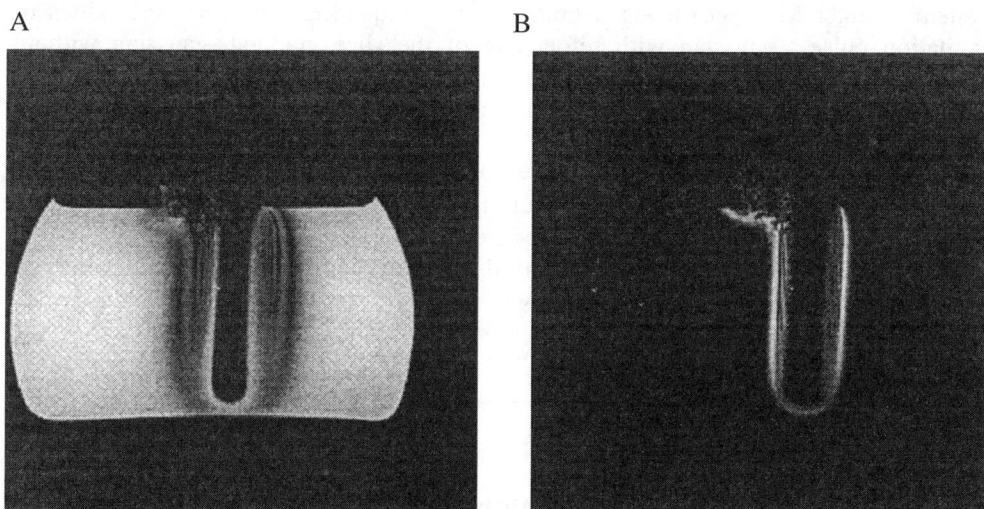

Figure 1. Sagittal slice of an air filled tube in water obtained using a gradient-echo sequence with an amplitude-only modulated pulse (a gaussian). (A) with refocusing the slice gradient, (B) without refocusing the slice gradient.

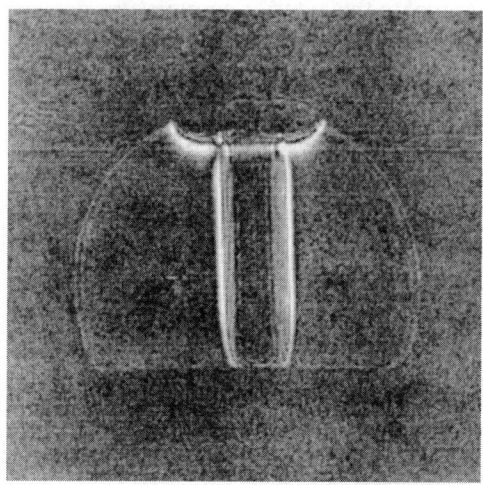

Figure 2. Sagittal slice of an air filled tube in water obtained using a gradient-echo sequence with an amplitude and phase modulated pulse (BILI).

Functional imaging

Functional imaging experiments were carried out on a 3T whole body imaging system (Bruker Medspec) using a gradient echo sequence. We used three kinds of excitation pulse : gaussian with refocusing of the slice gradient, gaussian without refocusing of the slice gradient and the amplitude and phase modulated pulse. The activation task was finger tapping with right or left hand executed by a right-handed volunteer.

The acquisition parameters were : TE = 40 ms, TR = 100 ms, voxel size = 1.4*1.4*3 mm^3, spectral bandwidth = 31.25 Hz/pixel, image size = 128*128 and flip angle = 35° (angle for which the theory of linear response can still be applied).

The activation paradigm was two periods of rest conditions interleaved with one period of finger tapping ; as shown below :

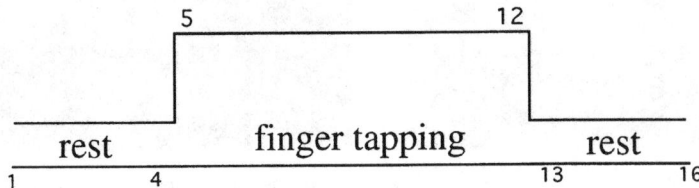

Results

Figure 3 shows the location of the studied slice which is a transverse oblique one whose orientation is parallel to the anterior commissure-posterior commissure axis. The functional results are presented on functional images (Figure 4 to Figure 6) which are calculated as the sum of activated states minus the sum of rest states.

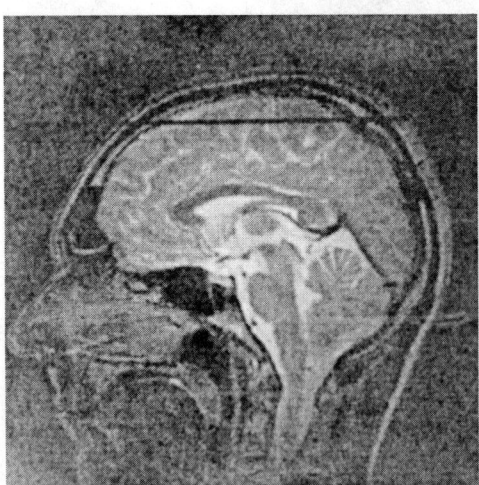

Figure 3. Location of the studied slice for functional imaging.

VISUALISATION OF VEIN EFFECT IN FUNCTIONAL IMAGING 255

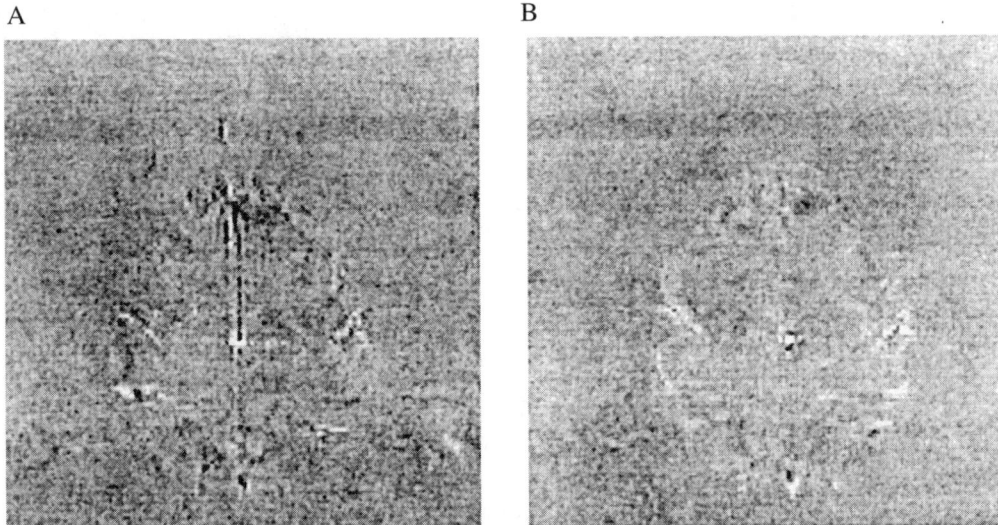

Figure 4. Functional images obtained with a gradient-echo sequence with a gaussian excitation pulse with refocusing of the slice gradient, on these two images activated regions are visible, for the two cases we observe an ipsilateral and contralataral responses. (A) left hand task, (B) right hand task.

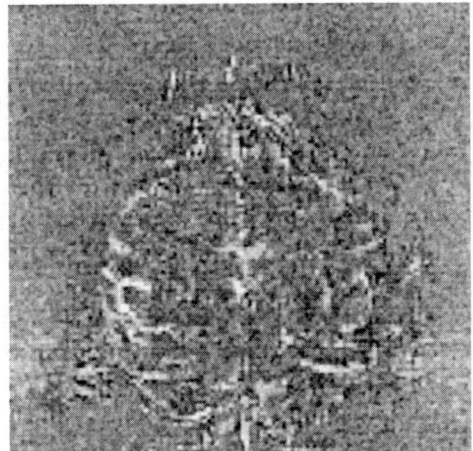

Figure 5. Maximun Intensity Projection of the functional images from 4 contiguous slices with a left hand task, obtained with a gradient-echo sequence with a gaussian excitation pulse with refocusing of the slice gradient. Active regions from the different slices are contiguous, suggesting the visualisation of veins.

A 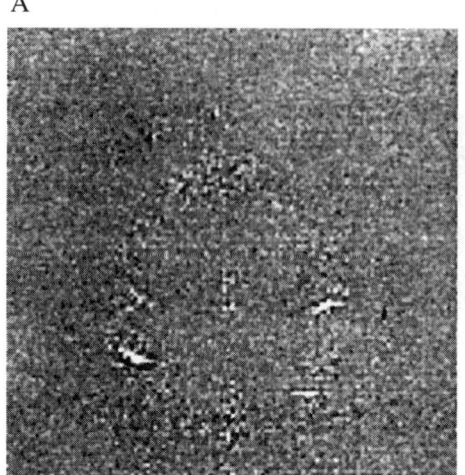 B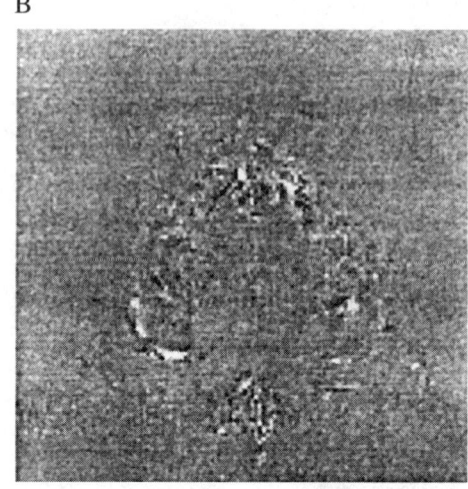

Figure 6. MR venography functional studies obtained with a gradient-echo sequence, left hand task. (A) gaussian excitation pulse without refocusing the slice gradient, (B) BILI excitation pulse with refocusing the slice gradient.

Discussion

• With venographic functional images we detect dark regions probably corresponding to the blood-tissue interface. Indeed with activation the blood oxygenation level increases therefore the field gradient decreases and the signal drops.

• Bright regions contiguous to dark ones are visible as well. This result is probably due to the increased blood flow during activation which generate gradients inside veins. These gradients increase the signal in the case of the venographic technique.

• A response was observed with the three methods. Each activated region of the motor cortex in standard imaging was also visible in functional venography.

• Use of the amplitude and phase modulated pulse, makes another region of activation appear. Indeed with this pulse B_0 gradients are compensated independently of their direction because of the bilinear phase distribution. This region could therefore correspond to a vein whose gradient direction is opposite to that of veins visible when using the gaussian without refocusing slice gradient method.

• These results suggest that all active regions observed in our functional studies with gradient echo methods contain macroscopic veins. Their location may therefore not directly correspond to the cortical tissue where activity is present, but to venous areas that drain the active cortex regions.

References

1. Segebarth C, Belle V, Delon C, Massarelli R, Decety J, Le Bas JF, Décorps M, Benabid AL. *NeuroReport* 1994 ; 5, 813.
2. Cho ZH, Ro YM, Lim TH. *Magn. Reson. Med.* 1992 ; 28, 25.
3. Frahm J, Merboldt KD, Hönicke W. *Magn. Reson. Med.* 1988; 6, 474.

28

Methodological difficulties in localized spectroscopy

M. DÉCORPS, A. ZIEGLER, C. RÉMY

*Groupe d'Application de la RMN à la Neurobiologie,
Unité INSERM U. 318,
Université Joseph-Fourier,
Hôpital Albert-Michallon, Pavillon B, BP 217 X,
38043 Grenoble, France.*

Spatial localization of the signal is a crucial point in *in vivo* Magnetic Resonance Spectroscopy (MRS) of a specific organ or of a lesion in human beings or animals. It is necessary to differentiate signals arising from the different organs or from lesioned and normal tissues. The simplest spatial localization technique uses a surface coil placed over the region to be explored. The signal comes roughly from a half sphere under the surface coil whose diameter is equal to the coil diameter. The spatial localization is thus coarse and partial volume effects generally occur. Only superficial organs and tissues can be studied with this technique. Thus surface coil studies are mainly focused on brain studies with animal models and muscle studies in human. When more precise spatial localization is needed, techniques deriving from Magnetic Resonance Imaging (MRI) are used. These methods are based on the use of gradients in the static magnetic field B_0.

Techniques based on the use of B_0 gradients

Excellent techniques now exist which can be divided into two groups (for references see [1]). In the *first group*, spatial encoding is achieved by gradients applied in the presence of frequency selective rf pulses, resulting in spatially selective excitation. Spectroscopic information from one voxel in human subjects or animals is generally obtained after the normal one-dimensional Fourier transform and without further signal processing. The size of the region of interest can be modified by varying the pulsed gradient strength, and its position moved within the object by changing on the frequency of the selective pulses. An important advantage of these methods is that a localized spectrum may be obtained in a single scan. In the *second group*, gradients are generally applied during a free precession delay [2], resulting in a spatially dependent modulation of the Free Induction Decay (FID). Successive acquisitions are made using different amplitudes of the phase encoding gradient. After processing of the data array resulting from N spatially encoded experiments, spectroscopic information can be obtained from N voxels simultaneously. The spatial localization properties of Fourier methods are best described by the use of the spatial response function which gives the contribution of a point sample at $z = z_0$ to the spectrum from a voxel at z_m. The shape of the spatial response can be modified by using k-space filters which act both on the shape of the spatial function and on signal to noise ratio. Spectroscopic Imaging (SI) is increasingly used in clinical research as well as for animal model studies.

Spectroscopic images have one additional dimension compared to a classical MR image : the frequency dimension. This property leads to some difficulties for the image presentation. Two types of spectroscopic image presentation can be used. The *first one* consists in displaying each spectrum arising from each voxel. The large quantity of informations contained in such a presentation make it difficult to analyze, especially to follow the variation of a resonance line intensity as function of the voxel position. The *second one* is the image presentation where the intensity, or area, of each peak is determined and associated to a grey or colored level in an image matrix. SI seems to be an advantageous localization technique since spectra are simultaneously obtained from a number of volume elements, the position of which can be shifted after acquisition. The spatial distribution of each metabolite can be obtained and analyzed at various locations in an heterogeneous organ, tissue or lesion.

The main problems of phase encoding techniques are the minimum duration of the experiment which can be large, the B_0 homogeneity over the region of interest and the shape of the sensitivity profile. Moreover the spatial localization achieved with a spectroscopic imaging technique is based on an add process of FIDs. Motion and instrumental instabilities can produce localization errors. Single voxel experiments offer the advantage to work with one single scan, allowing shimming in the Volume Of Interest (VOI). Motion or instrumental instabilities may produce some signal loss but the signal from the VOI remains relatively free from contamination. In principle, techniques based on selective excitation in the presence of gradients have the advantage of complete phase coherence and provides well-delimited volumes.

^{1}H spectroscopy

Since the early experiment in Yale, *in vivo* proton spectroscopy has developed rapidly. Proton spectroscopy has numerous advantages : the NMR-active $_1$H is the natural isotope (98.98% natural abundance) has a high sensitivity and is present in most molecules of biological interest. However *in vivo* proton MRS has to face two difficulties.

The *first one* is due to the intense water signal. The concentration of the water protons in tissues (between 60 and 100 M) is around 10^4 times higher than those of the mobile low molecular weight metabolites which are MRS-detectable (between several 100 µM to 10 mM). The observation of these metabolites thus requires the selective suppression of the water signal to avoid problems of dynamic range. A number of water suppression techniques now exist which work reasonably well (for references *see* [3]). The water line saturation technique can be used, which resembles spatial localization techniques employing a saturation of the outer volume. One can also use a selective excitation of the resonances of interest which leaves the water magnetization unchanged ; this method resembles spatial localization methods using direct excitation of the spins from inside the VOI. Note that the acquisition of a spectrum from a 1 ml VOI in the human brain requires a suppression of the signal from the outer volume by a factor much greater than 10^3. This is quite similar to the requirements for water suppression in ^{1}H spectroscopy.

The *second difficulty* is due to the intense lipid signal which may arise from fat located inside the region of interest or adjacent to it. Most organs or tissues contain a high amount of NMR visible lipids. Whatever the spatial localization technique used, the lipid resonances can overlap the metabolite resonances. This is the reason why most proton MRS studies are performed on brain which does not contain high concentration of NMR visible lipids. However due to imperfect localization, lipid signals from surrounding regions can contaminate spectra of voxels which are deeply seated. This occurs with bone marrow and subcutaneous fat surrounding the brain. Several techniques have been developed for avoiding such contaminations. The usual solution consist in selecting a volume of interest well inside the brain, inside which a spectroscopic image is acquired. This approach leaves a substantial proportion of the brain unsampled. A more satisfactory approach could be using spatially tailored outer volume signal presaturation [4] which was shown to be efficient for both, minimizing lipid contamination and permitting the use of short echo times.

^{31}P spectroscopy

From some points of view, ^{31}P MRS is easier to perform : no need of solvent suppression techniques and no contamination by subcutaneous signals. Cardiac and skeletal muscles, and subcutaneously implanted tumors were largely studied *in vivo*. However, compared to ^{1}H, ^{31}P suffers from the low sensitivity of this nucleus and thus ^{31}P MRS from a lower spatial resolution. Nevertheless, the informations gained by ^{31}P MRS may be valuable. Recently pH images were obtained at 2 T from *in vivo* three dimensional ^{31}P chemical shift images in an ischemia-reperfusion model of diabetic rat calf muscles [5]. Chemical shift images were acquired during the reperfusion period and lasted 43 min. The pH map (nominal voxel size : 3x3x5 mm^3) showed that the pH of the anterior tibial muscle was more acidic than that of the gastrocnemius muscle. In clinical studies, SI tends now to supersede single voxel techniques. Brain but also muscles and heart diseases are studied in order to evaluate the interest of ^{31}P MRS for diagnosis and therapy control. In the case of heart, the acquisition of the SI need to be gated with the cardiac rythm to avoid movement artefacts.

^{13}C MRS

This nucleus has still a lower sensitivity than ^{31}P. In addition, ^{13}C represents only 1.1% of the carbon nuclei present in the tissues. Its main interest is the use of ^{13}C labelled molecules allowing to study the metabolism in which they are involved. The advantage of this labelling compared to the radioactive one, is that the metabolites containing the nuclei and even their position in the molecules can be determined *in vivo*. Techniques based on polarization transfer from ^{1}H to ^{13}C or from ^{13}C to ^{1}H can be used in order to increase the sensitivity of the method.

Spatial resolution

Magnetic Resonance Imaging gives mainly anatomical information (organization of normal tissue, localization and extension of a lesion) and MRS information about the energetic and lipid metabolisms. The concentrations of the nuclei observed by MRS are about 10^4 times lower than those of the water protons which are imaged by MRI. The MRS signal is thus reduced in the same proportion. In order to obtained the same signal-to-noise ratio, the acquisition time and/or the size of the observed voxels has to be increased. Thus the spatial resolution of MRS is much lower than that of MRI, which is of the order of 1 mm^3 in humans. Nuclei such as ^{31}P which have a lower sensitivity than that of the proton require larger voxels to be analyzed. The spatial resolutions obtained in human studies using ^{1}H and ^{31}P MRS are respectively around 1 and 3 cm^3. Due to the reduced size of the NMR probe, the resolution achieved on experimental models can be much better (around 5 µl in the rat brain using ^{1}H MRS). Recently spectroscopic images of 1-^{13}C glucose and 3- and 4-^{13}C glutamate/glutamine have been obtained *in vivo* at 4.7 T in the cat brain with a spatial resolution of 200 mm^3 and a time resolution of 34 min [6].

Methodological progress and prospects

A number of high quality ^{1}H or ^{31}P spectra have now been obtained on humans and animals. However, experimenters have still to deal with a number of difficulties, which require further methodological advances : B_0 inhomogeneities over the volume of interest which can impair spectral quality ; suppression of signals from lipid-rich regions located along the periphery of the brain (^{1}H SI) ; sensitivity to motion which motivates research for rapid spectroscopic imaging and phase tracking techniques ; short echo times which are still difficult to use routinely, etc.

The difficulties related to the low signal to noise ratio suggest to develop techniques based on a best exploitation of the experiment time. For example a technique was demonstrated [7] for dual chemical shift imaging acquisitions, where advantage is taken of the protons smaller T_1 values to interleave an ^{1}H acquisition in the ^{31}P recycle time. Furthermore proton-decoupling increases the signal to noise ratio of ^{31}P spectra. The advantage of this approach is significant time saving, but its clinical potential has still to be evaluated.

A significant reduction of the measurement time may be obtained by acquiring multiple spin echoes within a single repetition time [8]. The increased efficiency may be applied to increase the signal to noise ratio in a given measurement time. Spectroscopic imaging techniques based on the use of phase encoding the chemical may also allow for a dramatic reduction of the measurement time [9].

The long imaging times mean that patient motion (respiration, cardiac motion, blood flow, peristaltic motion, or restlessness of the patient) causes blurring and ghosting artefacts. In imaging much effort is being focused on the development of fast techniques which solve motion problems by permitting scan times that are short compared with physiological motion. The concept of navigator echoes [10] which was initially introduced in the context of MRI can be efficiently used for correcting motion artefacts in spectroscopic imaging.

Finally the spectral resolution of *in vivo* spectra is generally low. Two-dimensional spectroscopy [11] and spectral editing imaging techniques [12] may become increasingly important in studies where peak overlap and broadening are significant.

In conclusion, *in vivo* localized spectroscopy is still evolving. A number of new developments have been proposed for circumventing some of the difficulties. Clinical usefulness however remains to be established.

References

1. Décorps M, Bourgeois D. *Localized Spectroscopy Using Static Magnetic Field Gradients : comparison of techniques.* NMR Basic Principles and Progress 1992 ; 27, 119-149.
2. Brown TR, Kincaid BM, Ugürbil K. *NMR chemical shift imaging in three dimensions.* Proc. Natl. Acad. Sci. USA 1982 ; 79, 3523-3526.
3. Guéron M, Plateau P, Décorps M. *Solvent Signal Suppression in NMR.* Prog. NMR Spectr. 1991 ; 23, 135-203.
4. Shungun DC, Glikson JD. *Sensitivity and localization enhancement in multinuclear in vivo NMR spectroscopy by outer volume presaturation.* Magn. Reson. Med. 1994 ; 30, 661-671.

5. Morikawa S, Inubish T, Kito K, Kido C. *pH mapping in living tissues : an application of in vivo 31P NMR chemical shift imaging. Magn Reson Med.* 1993 ; 29, 249-251.
6. Zijl PCM van, Chesnick AS, DesPres D, Moonen CTW, Ruiz-Cabello J, Gelderen. P. van. *In vivo proton spectroscopy and spectroscopic imaging of {1-13C}-glucose and its metabolic products. Magn Reson Med* 1993 ; 30, 544-551.
7. Gonen O, Hu J, Murphy-Boesch J, Stoyanova R, Brown TR. *Dual interleaved 1H and proton-decoupled-31P in vivo chemical shift imaging of human brain. Magn. Reson. Med* 1994 ; 32, 104-109.
8. Duyn JH, Moonen CTW. *Fast proton spectroscopic imaging of human brain using multiple spin-echoes. Magn. Reson. Med* 1994 ; 30, 409-414.
9. Jakob PM, Ziegler A, Doran SJ, Décorps M. *Echo-timed-encoded burst imaging (EBI) : a novel technique for spectroscopic imaging. Magn Reson Med,*1995, in press.
10. Anderson AW, Gore JC. *Analysis and correction of motion artifacts in diffusion weighted imaging. Magn. Reson. Med* 1994 ; 32, 379-387.
11. Brereton IM, Galloway GJ, Rose SE, Dodrell DM. *Localized two-dimensional shift correlated spectroscopy in humans at 2 Tesla. Magn. Reson. Med* 1994 ; 32, 251-257.
12. Böhlen JM, Izquierdo M, Décorps M. *Simultaneous observation of Single and Multiple-Quantum coherence Images by gradient Proportional Phase Incrementation (GPPI). J. Magn. Reson.* A110 1994 ; 106-108.

29

Functional MRI in Parkinson's disease

F. DURIF, D. SINARDET, J.M. BONNY, J.Y. BOIRE, A. VEYRE, M. ZANCA

Department of Neurology, INSERM U 71, Biostatistic department.
CHRU Clermont-Ferrand, France.

Parkinson's disease (PD) is characterized pathologically by Lewi body degeneration of the dopaminergic neurons of the substantia nigra compacta, with as consequence a decrease of the amount of dopamine in the striatum (putamen + caudate nucleus), and clinically by akinesia, rigidity and rest tremor which are markedly improved by levodopa therapy. MRI studies (A. Antonini *et al.*) have reported several patterns of decrease of the T_2 parameter in the striatum and in the substantia nigra (SN) of patients with PD, possibly explained by an increase in iron concentration and in other metals in these structures. The aim of this study was to estimate the T_1 and T_2 relaxation parameter times and the proton density in parkinsonian patients and in control subjects 1) to explore the consequences of the dopaminergic denervation in the striatum on these biophysical parameters and 2) to try to differentiate patients with PD from control subjects.

Methods

41 patients with PD (17 male and 24 female) and 30 healthy volunteers (15 male and 15 female) were included in this study. The age of parkinsonian patients was 65 ± 8 years (mean ± SD) and the duration of disease was 11 ± 6 years. The healthy volunteers were relatives of the parkinsonian patients, and had a mean age of 63 ± 10 years.

Motor parkinsonian disability was assessed by the motor part of the Unified Parkinson's disease rating scale (UPDRS) (maximal score 108) which was performed both at the time of maximal effect of levodopa treatment (treated score) and a least 12 hours after withdrawal of antiparkinsonian treatment (basal score). Percentage improvement induced by antiparkinsonian treatment was calculated for the UPDRS using formula : (baseline score - treated score) / baseline score x 100.

CHARACTERISTICS OF PARKINSONIAN PATIENTS

AGE (years)	65 ± 8
SEX (M/F)	17/24
DURATION OF DISEASE (years)	11 ± 6
Levodopa dose (+ IDC)mg	757 ± 365
MOTOR SCORE (basal)	41 ± 17
MOTOR SCORE (treated)	17 ± 8
% improvement induced by levodopa	58 ± 14

4 spin-echo sequences were performed using a Siemens Magnetom operating at 1 T to obtain simultaneously the estimation of Mo, T_1 and T_2. Contiguous axial sections, 5 mm thick, were parallel to the bicommissural plane. All images were acquired using 256 x 256 matrix, and transferred on a DEC workstation. Then, parameter images (Mo, T_1, T_2) were reconstructed from the original images (J.M. Bonny et al.). The measurement of Mo, T_1 and T_2 parameters was performed from the corresponding parametric images by placing on each hemisphere the following circular regions of interest : SN (compacta and reticulata), thalamus, pallidum, putamen (anterior, posterior, upper), caudate nucleus and white matter. In each subject, Mo, T_1 and T_2 values obtained from the right and left brain hemispheres were pooled.

Results were expressed as the mean +/- SD. The comparison of the relaxation time parameters and the proton density between the 2 groups of patients was performed using ANOVA, Student t test and Chi-2 test, depending on the data. A progressive discriminant ANOVA, Student t test and Chi-2 test, depending on the data. A progressive discriminant analysis using the significant variables as explicative variables was performed to classify patients in their respective diagnosis group. Principal component factor analysis with varimax rotation was performed to evaluate the relationships between the biophysical parameters and clinical data in parkinsonian patients. Interfactor association was determined by Spearman rank-order correlation of the mean of those variables that attained factor loadings greater than 0.60 within a given factor. Regression analysis was also performed. Significance was at $p<0.05$.

Results

Age and sex were not statistically different between the parkinsonian patients and the healthy volunteers. Mo was significantly shorter in the substantia nigra pars compacta (- 3.3 %, $p < 0.05$) and in the pars reticulata (- 4.3 %, $p < 0.02$) in patients with PD than in healthy volunteers.

Mo PARAMETER

	Volunteers	Parkinsonian patients	Difference (%)	P
Substantia nigra (pc)	1 740 ± 88	1 683 ± 128	- 3.29	0.039
Substantia nigra (pr)	1 509 ± 106	1 444 ± 115	- 4.29	0.013
Putamen (anterior)	1 898 ± 103	1 863 ± 133	- 1.86	0.21
Putamen (posterior)	1 862 ± 92	1 828 ± 121	- 1.79	0.19
Putamen (upper)	1 829 ± 218	1 837 ± 158	0.43	0.86
Pallidum	1 753 ± 90	1 714 ± 119	- 2.20	0.13
Caudate nucleus	1 337 ± 228	1 843 ± 162	0.35	0.89
Thalamus	1 679 ± 101	1 652 ± 151	- 1.64	0.39
White matter	1 570 ± 97	1 526 ± 131	- 2.83	0.11

T_1 was significantly longer in the upper putamen (4.7 %, $p < 0.05$) and was longer in the anterior part of the putamen and in the caudate nucleus with a difference close to the significance in parkinsonian patients than in healthy volunteers.

T_1 PARAMETER

	Volunteers	Parkinsonian patients	Difference (%)	P
Substantia nigra (pc)	945 ± 45	945 ± 38	0.04	0.97
Substantia nigra (pr)	868 ± 63	885 ± 47	1.97	0.22
Putamen (anterior)	1 133 ± 78	1 169 ± 86	3.22	0.07
Putamen (posterior)	1 038 ± 88	1 069 ± 73	2.95	0.12
Putamen (upper)	1 030 ± 125	1 078 ± 69	4.70	0.04
Pallidum	936 ± 64	964 ± 84	2.98	0.12
Caudate nucleus	1 156 ± 150	1 205 ± 76	4.24	0.07
Thalamus	1 021 ± 58	1 023 ± 62	0.21	0.88
White matter	845 ± 73	838 ± 74	- 0.87	0.68

No significant difference between the 2 groups of subjects was observed for the T_2 parameter.

T₂ PARAMETER

	Volunteers	Parkinsonian patients	Difference (%)	P
Substantia nigra (pc)	65 ± 4	64 ± 4	- 1.00	0.49
Substantia nigra (pr)	73 ± 5	75 ± 5	3.10	0.08
Putamen (anterior)	64 ± 3	64 ± 3	- 0.58	0.62
Putamen (posterior)	61 ± 4	61 ± 4	- 0.03	0.98
Putamen (upper)	61 ± 7	62 ± 4	1.97	0.35
Pallidum	60 ± 5	60 ± 5	0.38	0.85
Caudate nucleus	66 ± 7	67 ± 4	1.65	0.40
Thalamus	68 ± 5	68 ± 3	- 1.14	0.37
White matter	6 ± 4	65 ± 3	- 1.39	0.30

A progressive discriminant analysis using significant variables as explicative variables correctly classified 77 % of subjects in their respective own group with a significant difference ($p < 0.01$).

CLINICAL GROUP	PREDICTED NUMBER	
	PARKINSON'S DISEASE	VOLUNTEERS
Parkinson's disease	29	10
Volunteers	6	24

Oververall correct classification : 77 %, p = 0.006
Statistical significant variables are used as dependant variables

A significant relationship was observed between the treated motor score evaluated by the UPDRS and the T_2 relaxation parameter time from the posterior part of the putamen ($p < 0.01$).

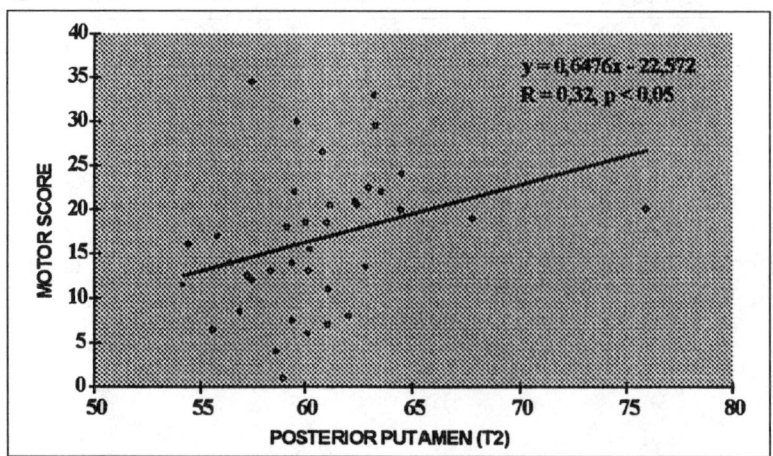

Discussion

These results indicate that Mo and T_1 parameters were significantly modified in the basal ganglia of parkinsonian patients, and could reflect the dysfunction of these structures. The decrease of Mo could reflect the gliosis of the substantia nigra, observed in deceased patients who had Parkinson's disease. The increase of T_1 parameter in the putamen could be in relation with the change of the striatal neuronal activity secondary to the decrease of the dopamine amount in the striatum. Moreover, the estimation of these parameters could be useful to help the clinician to differentiate patients with Parkinson's disease from healthy subjects.

References

1. Antonini A. *et al.* : T_2 relaxation time in patients with Parkinson's disease. *Neurology* 1993 ; 43: 697-700.
2. Bonny J.M. *et al.* : Parametric imaging : application to Parkinsonism. Rouffach, 1994.

30

Functional imaging and functional spectroscopy during motor activation

E. FEIFEL[1], N. BOLO[3], J. HENNIG[2], TH. ERNST[2], J. F. NEDELEC[3], F.HENNEL[3], G. DEUSCHL[1], J-P. MACHER[3]

[1]Neurologische Klinik und [2]Radiologische Klinik der Universität Freiburg, Germany.
[3]FORENAP, Centre Hospitalier Rouffach, France.

Recently numerous attempts to investigate cerebral activity during motor activation have been performed using Functional MR at different field strengths. In our experiments we examined cerebral activity during simple and complex finger movements at 2 and 3 Tesla with Functional Imaging and Functional Spectroscopy.

Methods

Experiments were performed using a 2 Tesla (T) whole body scanner (Bruker S 200 F) with shielded gradients and the standard head coil. Experiments could also be performed in identical volunteers on a 3 T whole body scanner (Bruker S 300). 18 volunteers were examined at 2 T, 5 at 3 T. 17 Imaging series were obtained from 8 volunteers at 2 T, 22 from 5 volunteers at 3 T. 72 spectroscopy examinations were performed in 18 volunteers at 2 T.

Functional Imaging was performed using a gradient echo experiment with 40 ms echo time. Transverse sections through the sensorimotor cortex and the supplementary motor cortex (SMA) as well as coronal slices along the central sulcus were acquired. Simple repetitive Finger-Opposition-Movements and complex sequential Finger Movements were performed. The activation task protocol was made up of 4 rest periods interleaved with 4 activation periods, 2 images being acquired per 20 second period. Images of cerebral activity were obtained by 2 methods:

a. subtraction of the sum of rest-period images from the sum of active period images.
b. Correlation of pixel intensity to a square activation function by a modified method based on reference (Bandettini).

Functional Spectroscopy was performed using a PRESS experiment without water suppression. The water signal was recorded with a TE between 20 and 270 ms. TR was normally set to 3-5 s to exclude saturation effects. Alternating repetitive stimulation was applied during 64 spectra. (Figure 1).

Data points during rest and activation were calculated into mean values resulting in an 8 point-curve indicating the difference between rest and activation during the time course.

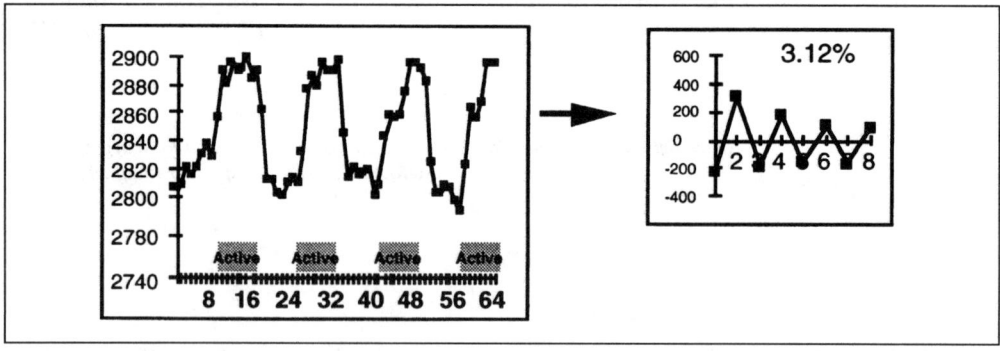

Figure 1. Repetitive finger movement.

Results

Activation in the Sensorimotor cortex could be shown with Functional Imaging during simple and complex finger movements. Imaging proved to be far more conclusive at 3 T with a signal increase of 2-6 % in the regions of interest during stimulation. While of 18 examinations at 2 T only 3 showed an effect, at 3 T activation was seen in 3 out of 5 examinations. At 3 T differentiation between simple and complex finger movements was possible. Statistical evaluation by a correlation function was possible at 3 T and resulted in localised activation areas (*see* Figure 3 c-f). Over all, great interindividual differences were noted.

Functional Spectroscopy showed a considerably better signal-to-noise ratio compared to imaging methods. During simple and complex finger movements at 2 T activation with signal changes of 1-6 % could be observed in the Sensorimotor cortex (Figure 2 a).

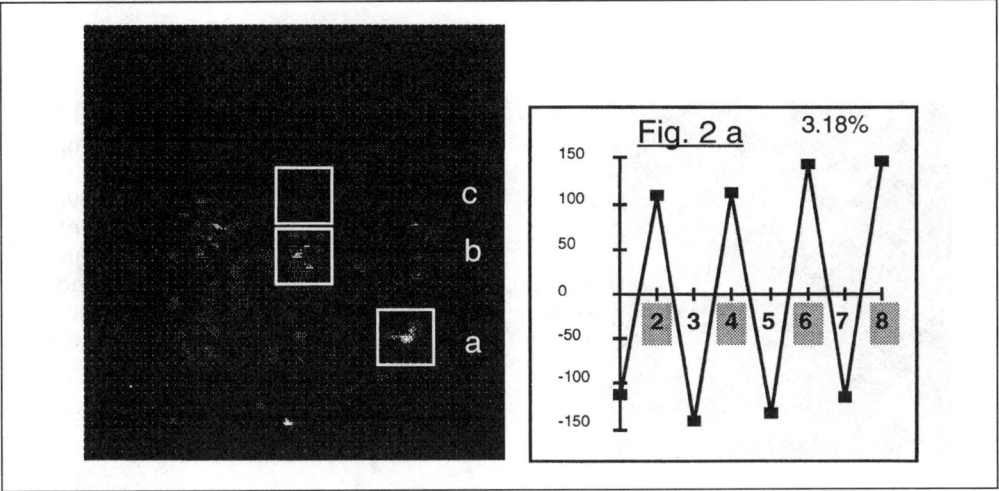

Figure 2. Functional imaging and functional spectroscopy at 2 Tesla.

Exemplary spectroscopy results (Figures 2 a-c) were acquired in regions a-c (volunteers not identical).

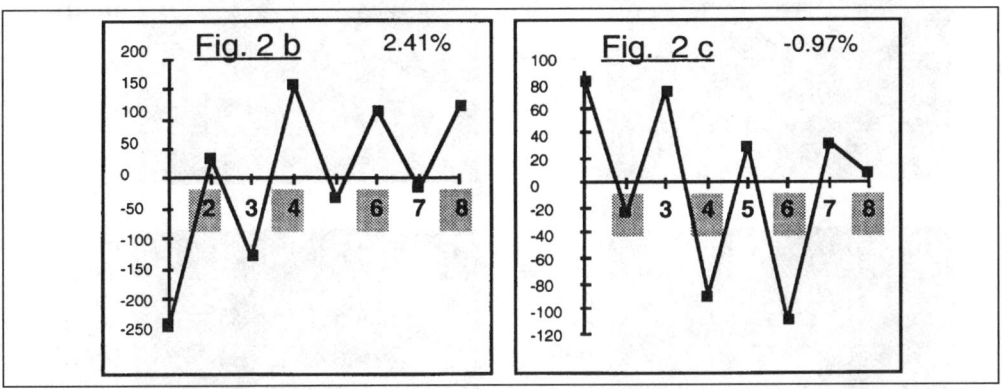

Degree of activation indicated in %.
x-Axis: Number of trials 1-8, 8 Spectra per Trial. Activated trials (2, 4, 6, 8) indicated gray.
Figure 2a: complex finger movement, voxel located in sensorimotor cortex.
Figure 2b: complex finger movement, voxel located in SMA.
Figure 2c: complex finger movement, voxel located in area rostrally of SMA.

In the SMA (located 1.5-2.5 cms rostrally of the central sulcus close to the midline) activation with signal increases of 1 - 3.5 % was seen (Figure 2 b). In an area 1 cm rostrally to the SMA in 9 of 11 volunteers a reproducible negative activation during simple finger movements could be demonstrated (Figure 2 c). At 3T, the localisation of the voxel for spectroscopy could be based on activity observed in the functional difference image.

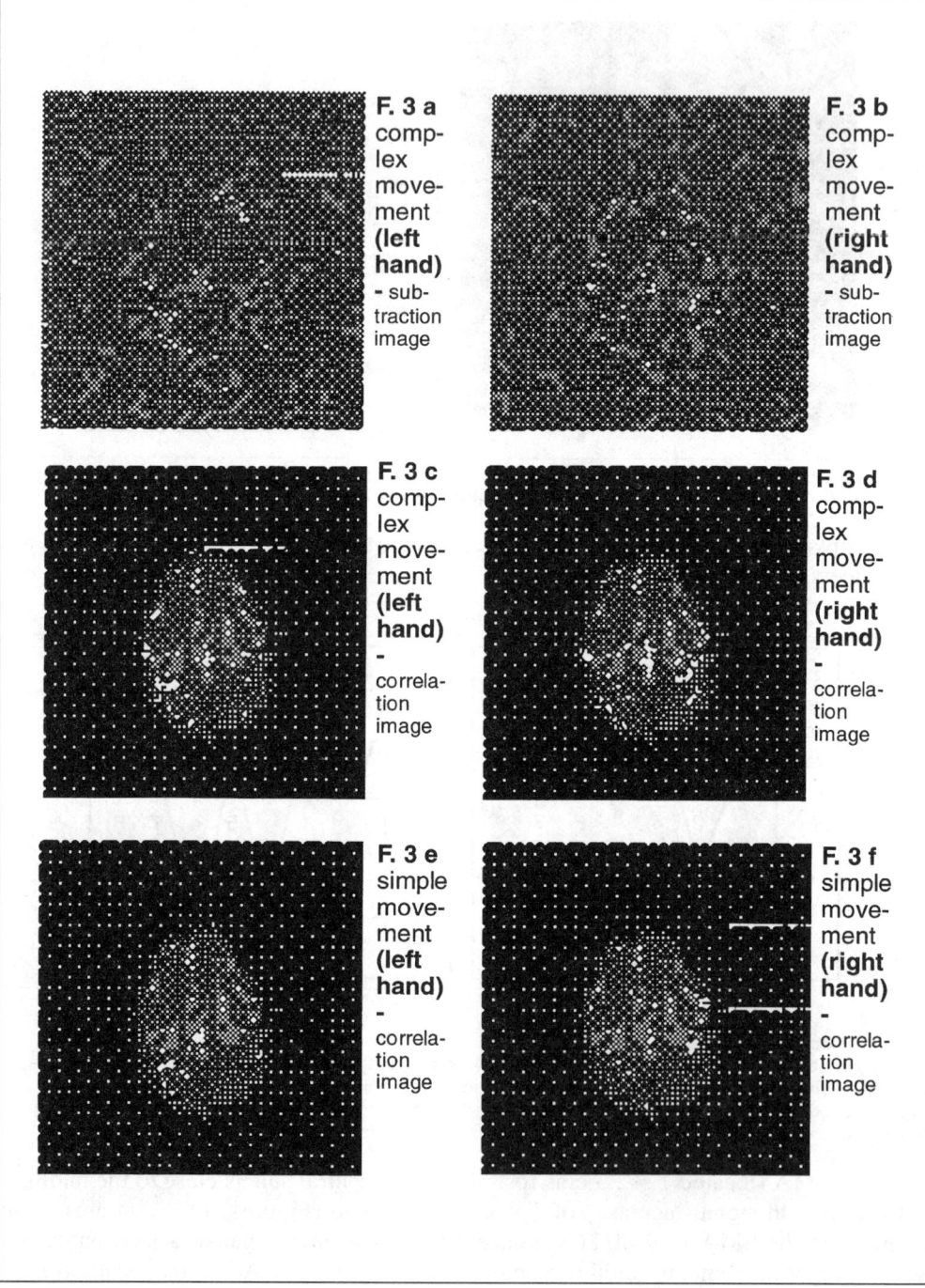

Figure 3. Functional Imaging at 3 Tesla.

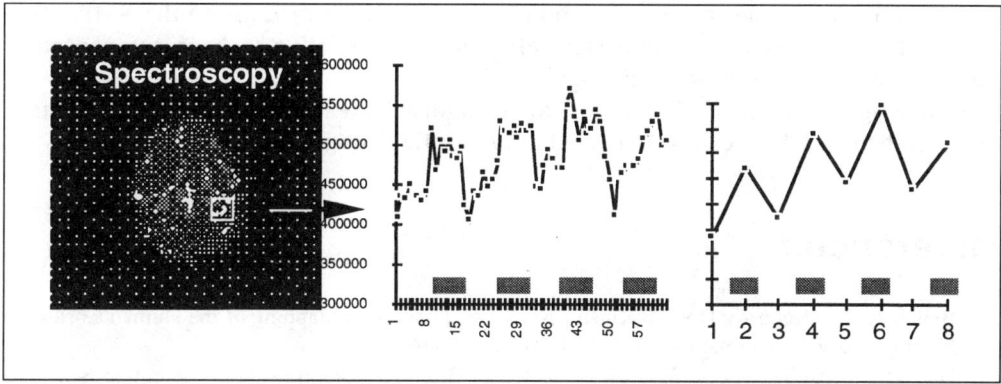

Figure 4. Functional spectroscopy at 3 T (on line-spectroscopy).

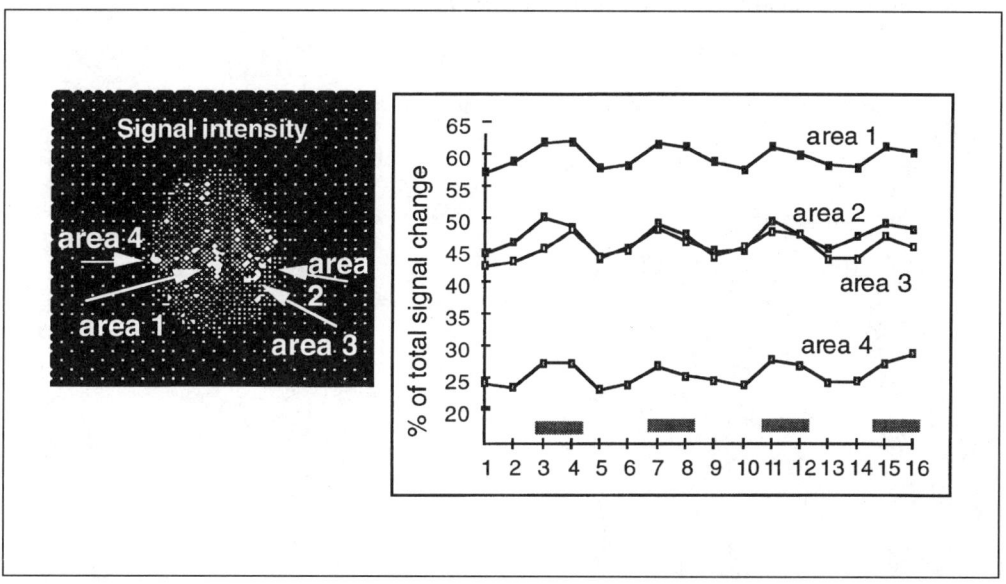

Figure 5. Signal intensity changes at 3 T.

Conclusions

• Functional Spectroscopy using motor activation has been compared to Functional Imaging. Functional Spectroscopy has been shown to be a sensitive and reliable tool to examine cortical activation in different areas.

• Activation in SMA and sensorimotor cortex during simple and complex finger movements could be shown with Functional Spectroscopy and Imaging at 2 and 3 Tesla.

• Negative activation has been demonstrated in an area rostrally to the SMA. This might be caused by a perfusion steal effect or by a relative lack of compensatory perfusion during activation in this region.

• Imaging performed at 3 T was able to distinguish better between different activation patterns than at 2 T, as can be expected at higher field strengths.

References

1. Belliveau JW, Kennedy DN, McKinstry RC, *et al.* Functional Mapping of the Human Cortex by Magnetic Resonance Imaging, *Science* 1991 ; 254 : 716.
2. Hennig J, Ernst Th, Speck O, *et al.* Detection of Brain Activation using Oxygenqtion Sensitive Functional Spectroscopy. *MRIM* 1994 ; 31 : 85-90
3. Bandettini PA, Jesmanowicz A,Wong EC, Hyde JS. Processing Strategies for Time-course Data-Sets in Functional MRI of the Human Brain. *MRIM* 1993 ; 30 : 161-173.

31

Quantitative assessment of MRI lesion load in multiple sclerosis

M. FILIPPI

*Department of Neurology, Scientific Institute, Ospedale San Raffaele, University of Milan,
Via Olgettina 60, 20132 Milan, Italy.*

Brain magnetic resonance (MRI) has proven to be very sensitive in diagnosing multiple sclerosis (MS) [1-2] and, more recently, in providing important insight into the natural history of the disease [3-4]. This is why brain MRI is increasingly being used in studying MS, expecially for monitoring the treatment [5-7]. However, several cross-sectional [8-10] studies found little or even no correlation between brain MRI findings and clinical features and the majority of the longitudinal studies [11-19] failed to demonstrate a relationship between the development of disability and the increase of MRI lesion load.

There are several explanations for these clinical/MRI discrepancies.

First, the way in which disability is assessed, usually by the Kurtzke's Expanded Disability Status Scale (EDSS) [20]. This scale is a mixture of impairment and disability, is mainly weighted towards locomotor disability (which might be mainly related to spinal cord damage) and is characterized by high intra- and inter-rater variability [21].

Second, previous studies have some methodological limitations [22]. Usually, patients with widely differing disease duration have been studied [9-19]. It is indeed possible that the time taken to develop a given lesion load, with possibly different effects on reparative mechanisms, known to occur from the first stages of lesion formation [22], might be more relevant than the actual lesion load in determining disability. In addition, these studies [11-19] considered small numbers of patients (tipically 10-20), followed up for short periods of time (usually 6 months or less). Given the highly variable course of MS, which occurs over years rather than months, it is not surprising that no correlation was seen.

Third, all these studies [8-19] used conventional brain MRI sequences which give no information about two of the potentially more disabling aspects of the disease. It is conceivable that much of the disability might be due to spinal cord involvement and/or to the amount of demyelination and axonal loss in chronic lesions. The first aspect (i.e., spinal cord damage) has not been systematically studied until recently [24], due to major technical limitations [25]. The second aspect (i.e., pathological characteristics of the lesions) is not investigated by conventional unenhanced MRI. Lesions are seen by this technique because of an increased water content and this is a consequence of any of the major pathological features of MS (i.e., edema, inflammation, gliosis, demyelination and axonal loss), which can cause highly different clinical outcomes.

Finally, inaccurancies in measuring lesion load on T_2-weighted images must also be considered. Many studies [9, 10, 16-18] measured brain lesion load in a crude semiquantitative fashion, by an arbitrary scoring system weighted for the number and the largest diameter of lesions [26]. This system is clearly inaccurate (e.g., 1 point is given to a lesion of 3X3X3 mm which, therefore, is considered smaller than a lesion of 6X1X1 mm which is scored 2 points; lesions greater than 10 mm and confluent lesions are scored 3 and 4 points, regardless their actual size) and has proven to have poor reproducibility [27]. Lesion load can be measured more objectively and reliably by calculating lesion area on a computerized image, outlining manually the lesions or using more automated techniques, such as thresholding, edge detection, and other segmentation strategies [28-31].

This review will consider the main contributions given by quantitative techniques for assessing lesion load to the understanding of the evolution of MS and the possible role of such techniques in monitoring treatment trials. The answers to four crucial questions will be the content of the review:

1. Are these techniques more reliable and reproducible than other system currently used?

2. Do these techniques increase the strenght of clinical/MRI correlation?

3. Is what we measure with these techniques (i.e., the extent of lesions) related to other aspects of the complex pathological process of MS?

4. Which is the role of quantitative assessment of MRI lesion load in the evaluation of treatment efficacy?

First question. Are these techniques more reliable and reproducible than other systems currently used?

Quantification of lesion load was first obtained by manual outlining. An operator draws the border of the lesions using a mouse-controlled cursor on a computer display. Once the border of each lesion is defined, each outline is stored on computer disk before automatic computation of total lesion area in square millimiters. This technique has been extensively used by the MS/MRI Study Group of the University of British Columbia in Vancouver, who have shown an intra-rater reproducibility of 6% in experienced hands [6], and a highly reproducible measure of lesion load increase (about 10% per annum) in the placebo groups of three different clinical trails [32-37]. In our MS Centre, the intra and inter-rater variability of this technique was measured and compared to those of a widely used arbitrary scoring system. We found the manual tracing technique to have a inter-rater variability of 14.14% and an inter-rater variability of 6.54%. This latter variability was significantly lower of that obtained using the arbitrary scoring system [27].

However, this technique still requires major human interaction. This has two main consequences. First, it is time-consuming. Second, its reproducibility is suboptimal. This is clearly demonstrated in the recent beta-interferon study [37], where there was a 10% reduction in lesion loads measured after 3 years in all patients (treated and untreated) compared to the 2-year lesion load. This has been attributed to a systematic change in the manual technique applied by the single observer who performed the measurements. At present, more fully automated techniques have been developed [28-31], which should overcome these limitations, by reducing the human interaction.

The semi-automated technique operating at our center was developed by the NMR Research Group in London [31] and is based on simple intensity threshold segmentation. The image processing software works in two stages and is fully described by Wicks et al. [31}. The first uses a combination of thresholding and knowledge of the 3D structure of the brain to remove subcutaneous fat and much of the other soft tissue. The remaining brain structure is eroded from the edge to remove some of the brighter grey matter. Next, a simple intensity threshold is applied to identify the hyperintense white matter lesions. The threshold for the identification of lesions is chosen interactively by the observer on a patient-by-patient basis. After automatic lesion detection, a manual review is always performed to remove spurious lesions, to add low-intensity lesions which were undetected, or to modify the boundary of poorly-defined or confluent lesions.The lesion volume is calculated simply as the lesion area multiplied by the slice thickness. The assumption here is that the lesion is of constant thickness and has sharply-defined edges.

We calculated the intra- and inter-rater variability of such technique by measuring the lesion load in 20 patients with either relapsing-remitting or secondary progressive MS and EDSS scores between 3.0 and 5.5 (these patients are those that for their clinical characteristics are tipically eligible for clinical trials). Three observers were used who previously reached a consensus about the choice of threshold for segmentation and the independently rewieved the computed lesion load. The intra- and inter-rater variability of the technique were 1.64% and 5.40%. These variabilities were significantly lower compared to those obtained using both the arbitrary scoring system and the manual tracing technique [27]. These results agree with those by Wicks et al. [31] who found this semi-automated technique to achieve a precision of 6% compared to a range of 12-33% for the manual tracing method.

It would appear that this quantitative technique allows the evaluation of the actual lesion load in MS more objectively and precisely than in the past. However, for three reasons it is also obvious that the lesion loads measured with this technique are not the true volumes of MS lesions present. First, cortical lesions, which are commonly found at post-mortem [38, 39], are rarely seen on T_2-weighted MRI, perhaps because many cortical lesions and normal cortex have similar proton density and relaxation times. Secondly, the assumption that lesions have a constant cross-section through the slice is made, without allowance for partial volume effects. Finally, the "invisible" lesion load (40), which comprises microscopic lesions below the resolution of the scanner, cannot be distinguished and quantified using the simple lesion volume approach. These limitations will be partly overcome by using thinner slices - with the new 3D fast spin echo sequence, it will be possible to obtain 1 mm thick slices. The FLAIR sequence is another approach which needs evaluation, as it has been reported to improve the detection of some MS lesions [41]. In addition, the implementation of more sophisticated techniques for lesion segmentation may be helpful [28, 29]. However, the fundamental requirement for a technique for assessing lesion load in MS is that it should be reliable and reproducible over time, allowing accurate quantification of changes in lesion load and the comparison of lesion load between patients with different courses of the disease.

Second question. Do these techniques increase the strenght of clinical/MRI correlation?

Given the clinical evolution of MS, the problem raised by this question must be divided into two other groups of questions:

a) Does quantitative assessment of brain MRI lesion load increase the predictive value of brain MRI abnormalities at presentation with a clinically isolated syndrome (CIS) suggestive of MS? Is it useful to predict the development of disability and of new lesions in such cases?

b) Does quantitative assessment of brain MRI lesion load allow to explain better the clinical manifestation of clinically definite MS? Can it be useful to predict the development of disability in such patients?

The clinical relevance of these questions is readily apparent, considering that the extra-time and the extra-costs needed to perform this measures, must be counterbalanced by additional information regarding the natural history of MS these techniques might provide. In addition, instrumental measures to evaluate the activity and the evolution of a disease and the effects induced by treatment can be realistically used only when they are related to the clinical outcome measures.

Question 2a

Does quantitative assessment of brain MRI lesion load increase the predictive value of brain MRI abnormalities at presentation with a clinically isolated syndrome (CIS) suggestive of MS? Is it useful to predict the development of disability and of new lesions in such cases?

These questions have been recently addressed in a paper by Filippi et al. [42]. In this study, using the thresholding technique described previously, the authors performed quantitative assessment of brain MRI abnormalities seen at presentation and at 5 year follow up in 84 patients presenting with an acute CIS of the optic nerves, brainstem, or spinal cord suggestive of MS. Patients who developed MS during follow up had a higher lesion load at presentation than those who did not. In addition, the MRI lesion load at presentation was strongly correlated with both the increase in lesion load over the next 5 years and disability at follow up, and was inversely correlated with the time to development of MS clinically. In detail, patients with a lesion load greater than 1.23 cm^3 had a 90% chance of developing MS, 86% chance of increasing their lesion load of at least 1 cm^3 during the follow up and 52% chance of accumulating moderate to severe disability over the next 5 years. These chances dropped to 55%, 35% and 23% in patients with abnormalities smaller than 1.23 cm3 at initial MRI and to 6%, 6% and 0% in those with normal MRI at presentation.

Several previous studies had already demonstrated that patients who presented with such syndromes and who had abnormalities on brain MRI are more likely to develop MS than those with normal MRI [43-51]. In all these studies, MRI abnormalities were not measured quantitatively and, therefore, it was not possible to identify patients with higher probability to developing more aggressive forms of the disease both clinically and pathologically. On the contrary, the results of the study by Filippi et al. [42] establish that MRI at presentation with CIS is useful in predicting the subsequent clinical course and the development of new MRI lesions. This suggests that quantitative brain MRI will be helpful in selecting patients with early clinical MS for clinical trials and for subsequent monitoring of their response to treatment. This aspect is crucial given that an effective treatment would potentially be most beneficial at the very onset of the disease and in those patients who are likely to develop severe disability within a short period of time.

Question 2b

Does quantitative assessment of brain MRI lesion load allow to explain better the clinical manifestation of clinically definite MS? Can it be useful to predict the development of disability in such patients?

The results are less clear when the development of disability in patients with MS is considered. As already pointed out, previous cross-sectional and longitudinal studies found uncertain relationships of brain MRI and clinical feature [8-19], probably because of methodological limitations [22]. However, there are some recent studies in which at least some of these limitations are not present and correlation between the degree of disability and the extent of abnormalities on T_2-weighted MRI scans are emerging.

Rao et al. [52] and Swirski-Sacchetti et al. [53] overcome some of these limitations by correlating MRI lesion areas (obtained by manual outlining) with neuropsychological testing. In the study by Rao et al. [52], total lesion load predicted better than ventricular/brain ratio and size of the corpus callosum the presence of cognitive dysfunction, particularly for measures of recent memory, abstract/conceptual reasoning, language, and visuo-spatial problem solving. In detail, 10 of 12 (83%) patients with total lesion area greater than 30 cm^2 were cognitively impaired and, conversely, 32 of 41 (78%) patients with total lesion area less than 30 cm^2 were cognitively intact. Swirski-Sacchetti et al. [53] quantifiyed the topographic distribution of lesions and consequent effects on upon cognitive function. Once again, total lesion area was the best predictor of neuropsychological deficits (mean total lesion area for the cognitively impaired patients was 28.30 cm^2 versus 7.41 cm^2 for the cognitively intact group; $p<0.0001$). In addition, multiple regression analysis revealed that left frontal lobe involvement best predicted impaired abstract problem solving, memory, and word fluency, while left-parieto-occipital region involvement best predicted deficits in verbal learning and complex visual-integrative skills. That analysis of regional cerebral lesion load may assist in understanding the particular pattern and course of cognitive disability in MS is also demonstrated by data collected in our center (unpublished data). We performed a large battery of neuropsychological tests exploring "frontal" functions in patients with clinically definite MS and correlated the results with the lesion volumes measured in the frontal lobe and in the whole brain. Frontal and brain lesion loads were 8 770 mm^3 and 34 650 mm^3 in patients with severe frontal deficits, 3 700 mm^3 and 25 310 mm^3 in patients with mild frontal deficits and 1 160 mm^3 and 8 080 mm^3 in patients without such deficits. The percentage of total brain lesion volumes due to frontal lesion volume was 25% in the former group and decreased to 15% and 14% in the other two groups.

Relationships between quantitative measures of brain MRI lesion load and physical disability are also emerging. Koopmans et al. [8] and Filippi et al. [54] demonstrated higher brain lesion load, particularly in the infratentorial regions, in patients with chronic-progressive MS or secondary progressive compared to patients with benign MS. A significant correlation between disability and lesion area were found by Gass et al. ($r=0.33$) [55] in a sample of 43 MS patients with different disease courses and durations. Filippi et al. [42] demonstrated a higher correlation between these parameters in a more homogeneous group of 38 MS patients ($r= 0.57$).

Recent longitudinal studies are also demostrating significant correlations between changes in disability and quantitative MRI parameters.

At NIH [56] nine patients have been followed up over a mean period of 30 months to assess the relationship between the area of enhancing lesions and development of short-term disability. A significant relationship was observed between periods of clinical worsening and the total area of enhancement. In addition, logistic regression analysis showed a significant effect of the number and area of enhancing MRI lesions on both the onset and continuation of clinical worsening.

Finally, in studies with longer follow ups correlation between increase in disability and changes in lesion load on T_2-weighted images have been described. Filippi et al. [42] found a significant correlation ($r=0.62$) between the development of disability and lesion volume increase over 5 years in 84 patients with CIS suggestive of MS. Van

Walderveen et al. [57] found a similar correlation (r=0.53) in 49 patients with clinically definite MS followed up for 2 years.

These results, although encouraging, indicate that the correlation between clinical events and pathological changes as seen on MRI has to be further improved. However, the importance of assessing quantitatively brain MRI abnormalities to monitoring the natural history of MS is also evident and such results are crucial for using quantitative MRI as a marker of disease activity in clinical trials.

Question 3. Is what we measure with these techniques (i.e., the extent of lesions) related to other aspects of the complex pathological process of MS?

The extent of lesions as seen on brain T_2-weighted MRI scans is not the unique factor related to the development of disability in MS [3-4]. To this respect, other factors are also relevant and probably even more important. They may be the location of the lesions, the time taken to develop a given lesion load, the amount of spinal cord damage, the degree of axonal loss and demyelination in chronic lesions, the severity and extent of microscopic changes in normal-appearing white matter, the capacity for remyelination and the degree of conduction recovery in persistently demyelinated axons.

Several recent studies have demonstrated correlation of clinical disability with non-standard MR parameters thought to reflect MS destructive pathology in the brain [54, 55, 57-59] and spinal cord [24]. This is the reason why new non-conventional MR end points have been added in more recent clinical trials. However, definitive phase 3 trials in MS usually need multicenter cooperation in which context it would be very difficult to perform very complex and sophisticated MRI protocols. For the present, it is easier to measure brain lesion load on standard T_2-weighted images. Therefore, the demonstration that a relationship of extent of abnormalities on T_2-weighted images and other MR parameters evaluating disease activity and progression are extremely useful.

An inverse correlation (r=-0.32) between total lesion area and average magnetization transfer ratio (reduction of magnetization transfer ratio is related to tissue disruption, to which both demyelination and axonal loss may contribute) has been described [55]. Similarly, but using proton MR spectroscopy, Arnold et al. [60] found a correlation (r= -0.49) between changes in NAA/Cr ratio (an index of neuron dysfunction) and in total hemispheric lesion volume in 7 patients followed up for 18 months. It is of particular interest that this correlation was even stronger (r= -0.74) when the subgroup of patients with relapsing remitting MS was considered alone.

Some suggestions for a possible relationship between the extent of lesions and the presence of a more destructive pathological process come also from studies which did not attempt to correlate directly conventional and non-conventional MR findings. There is indeed evidence that patients with secondary progressive MS, compared to patients with benign MS, have higher brain lesion loads and proportions of lesions with a biexponential T_2 decay (which provides evidence for axonal loss; 61) [54] and that changes in disability are correlated with increase in both T_2 and in hypointense T_1 lesion load [58], which probably represents the chronic MS lesions where severe tissue damage might have been occured [62].

The relationship between the extent of the lesions and the severity of the pathological process in terms of amount of axonal loss and demyelination and in terms of lesion location (i.e., involvement of infratentorial regions and spinal cord) might simply be due to stochastic reasons. By chance, patients with more lesions might have higher probability that strategic locations producing clinical deficits will be affected and/or might tend to have a more aggressive disease, leading to tissue distruction and, consequently, to severe and permanent neurologic deficits.

Question 4. Which is the role of quantitative assessment of MRI lesion load in the evaluation of treatment efficacy ?

Brain MRI has been used in clinical trials to evaluate whether new putative therapies might favorably modify the evolution of the disease or as a secondary marker of disease activity in definitive phase III studies, in which clinical measures are the primary outcomes.

Usually, the monitoring of new treatment efficacy is made by counting the numbers of active brain lesions. The number of patients required is smaller and the length of follow up shorter than those necessary to evaluate the effects on clinical features [63], given the ability of enhanced MRI in detecting new pathological activity 5 to 10 times more frequently than clinical measures in patients with early relapsing remitting or secondary progressive MS [64}. Therefore, it is possible that in the near future quantification of the extent of enhancing lesion area might be prove to be helpful in increasing the value of MRI in such studies [56].

Changes in lesion load as seen on T_2-weighted images is the measure used for large scale phase III trials. In such trials, a quantitative assessment of brain MRI abnormalities is the preferred approach, for the reasons discussed in the previous paragraphs. Several studies have already been published, which used this measure as a secondary end-point to evaluate the efficacy of azathioprine [65], cyclosporin [35, 65], interferon-alpha [32], total lymphoid irradiation [66], and interferon-beta [37]. The latter study demonstrated a significantly smaller rate of increase in lesion load in patients with relapsing remitting MS treated with high-dose interferon-beta. This observation was useful to strengthen clinical results indicating a beneficial effect of interferon-beta on the frequency of relapses, but not on disability [36]. Since the nature of the disease, it is not surprising that a parameter as disability, which evolves over several years, was found not to be affected in a clinical trial that lasted 3 years. Therefore, the demonstration by quantitative MRI of a significant effect on a pathological feature of the disease (i.e., lesion formation), which several studies suggest to be related to the development of disability, is extremely interesting and encouraging confirming the utility of such an approach in clinical trials.

The possibility to quantify the abnormalities seen on T_2-weighted images adds another important role to MRI in clinical trials. The recent demonstration that having a lesion load greater than 1.23 cm^3 at presentation with a CIS suggestive of MS markedly increases the risk of a subsequent development of a clinically definite form of the disease associate with more severe clinical and pathological outcomes [42] indicates that, especially in the early phases of MS (when the modification of the clinical course of the disease might prove to be the most beneficial approach), quantification of brain MRI abnormalities might be useful in selecting patients at higher risk of worse evolution.

Conclusion

Quantitative assessment of brain MRI abnormalities is a reliable and reproducible technique to evaluate the natural history of MS and to monitor the efficacy of treatments. However, some problems still remain unsolved and future research is needed to define exactly the roles of quantitative MRI in studying MS.

The primary goal remain to improve the correlation between the extent of MRI abnormalities, the clinical evolution of the disease and other non-conventional MR markers of disease activity and progression. This may be achievable through improvements in the clinical scales to rate disability and in MR techniques that identify specific pathological features. However, major efforts are also required to improve quantification of lesion load. Human interaction should be reduced, the computed lesion load should be made as close as possible to the «true» lesion load and techniques to quantify cord lesion load should be developed. This means that data acquisition must be optimized, the automated parts of the programs increased and more sophisticated segmentation techniques developed.

References

1. Lukes SA, Crooks LE, Aminoff MJ, et al. Nuclear magnetic resonance imaging in multiple sclerosis. *Ann Neurol* 1983; 13: 592-601.
2. Gebarski SS, Gabrielsen TO, Gilman S, et al. The initial diagnosis of multiple sclerosis: clinical impact of magnetic resonance imaging. *Ann Neurol* 1985; 17: 469-474.
3. McDonald WI, Miller DH, Barnes D. The pathological evolution of multiple sclerosis. *Neuropathol Appl Neurobiol* 1992 ; 18: 319-334.
4. McDonald WI. The dynamics of multiple sclerosis. J Neurol 1993 ; 240: 28-36.
5. Miller DH. Magnetic resonance in monitoring the treatment of multiple sclerosis. *Ann Neurol* 1994 ; 36: S91-S94.

6. Paty DW, Li DKB, Oger JJF, et al. Magnetic resonance imaging in the evaluation of clinical trials in multiple sclerosis. *Ann Neurol* 1994 ; 36: S95-S96.
7. McDonald WI, Miller DH, Thompson AJ. Are magnetic resonance findings predictive of clinical outcome in therapeutic trials in multiple sclerosis? The dilemma of interferon-beta. *Ann Neurol* 199 4; 36: 14-18.
8. Koopmans RA, Li DBK, Grochowski E, et al. Benign versus chronic progressive multiple sclerosis: magnetic resonance imaging features. *Ann Neurol* 1989 ; 25: 74-81.
9. Baumhefner RW, Tourtellotte WW, Syndulko K, *et al.* Quantitative multiple sclerosis plaque assessment with magnetic resonance imaging. Its correlation with clinical parameters, evoked potentials and intrablood-brain-barrier IgG synthesis. *Arch Neurol* 1990 ; 47: 19-26.
10. Thompson AJ, Kermode AG, MacManus DG, *et al.* Patterns of disease activity in multiple sclerosis: clinical and magnetic resonance study. Br *Med* J 1990 ; 300: 631-634.
11. Isaac C, Li DBK, Genton M, et al. Multiple sclerosis: a serial study using MRI in relapsing patients. *Neurology* 1988 ; 38: 1511-1515.
12. Miller DH, Rudge P, Johnson G, *et al.* Serial gadolinium enhanced magnetic resonance imaging in multiple sclerosis. *Brain* 1988 ; 111: 927-939.
13. Willoughby EW, Grochowski E, Li DKB, *et al.* Serial magnetic resonance scanning in multiple sclerosis: a second prospective study in relapsing patients. *Ann Neurol* 1989 ; 25: 43-49.
14. Kermode AG, Tofts PS, Thompson AJ, *et al.* Heterogeneity of blood-brain barrier changes in multiple sclerosis: an MRI study with gadolinium-DTPA enhancement. *Neurology* 1990 ; 40: 229-235.
15. Harris JO, Frank JA, Patronas N, *et al.* Serial gadolinium-enhanced magnetic resonance imaging scans in patients with early, relapsing-remitting multiple sclerosis: implications for clinical trials and natural history. *Ann Neurol* 1991 ; 29: 548-555.
16. Thompson AJ, Kermode AG, Wicks D, *et al.* Major differences in the dynamics of primary and secondary progressive multiple sclerosis. *Ann Neurol* 1991 ; 29: 53-62.
17. Thompson AJ, Miller DH, Youl B, *et al.* Serial gadolinium-enhanced MRI in relapsing/remitting multiple sclerosis of varying disease duration. *Neurology* 1992 ; 42: 60-63.
18. Wiebe S, Lee DH, Karlik SJ, *et al.* Serial cranial and spinal cord magnetic resonance imaging in multiple sclerosis. *Ann Neurol* 1992 ; 32: 643-650.
19. Capra R, Marcianò N, Vignolo LA, *et al.* Gadolinium-pentetic acid magnetic resonance imaging in patients with relapsing remitting multiple sclerosis. Arch Neurol 1992; 49: 687-689.
20. Kurtzke JF. Rating neurological impairment in multiple sclerosis: an expanded disability status scale (EDSS). *Neurology* 1983 ; 33: 1444-1452.
21. Noseworthy JH, Vandervoort MK, Wong CJ, *et al.* Interrater variability with the expanded disability status scale (EDSS) and functional systems (FS) in a multiple sclerosis clinical trial. *Neurology* 1990 ; 40: 971-975.
22. Filippi M, Paty DW, Kappos L, *et al.* Correlations between changes in disability and T_2-weighted brain MRI activity in multiple sclerosis: a follow up study. *Neurology* 1994 (in press).
23. Prineas JW, Barnard RO, Kwon EE, *et al.* Multiple sclerosis: remyelination of nascent lesions. *Ann Neurol* 1993 ; 33:137-151.
24. Kidd D, Thorpe JW, Thompson AJ, *et al.* Spinal cord MRI using multi-array coils and fast spin echo. II. Findings in multiple sclerosis. *Neurology* 1993 ; 43: 2632-2637, 1993.
25. Thorpe JW, Kidd D, Kendall BE, *et al.* Spinal cord MRI using multi-array coils and fast spin echo. I. Technical aspects and findings in healthy adults. *Neurology* 1993 ; 43: 2625-2631.
26. Ormerod IEC, Miller DH, McDonald WI, *et al.* The role of NMR imaging in the assessment of multiple sclerosis and isolated neurological lesions. A quiantitative study. *Brain* 1987 ; 110: 1579-1616.

27. Filippi M, Horsfield MA, Bressi S, et al. Intra- and inter-observer variability of brain MRI lesion volume measurements in multiple sclerosis: a comparison of techniques. Neurology (submitted).
28. Cline HE, Lorensen WE, Kikinis R, et al. Three dimensional segmentation of MR images of the head using probability and connectivity. J Comput Assist Tomogr 1990 ; 14: 1037-1045.
29. Kapouleas I, Grossman RI, Kessler D et al. Techniques for quantitation and comparison of multiple sclerosis lesions in serial MRI studies [abstract]. Neurology 1993; 43 (suppl): 246.
30. Pannizzo F, Stallmeyer MJB, Friedman J, et al. Quantitative MRI studies for assessment of MS. Magn Reson Med 1992 ; 24: 90-99.
31. Wicks DAG, Tofts PS, Miller DH, et al. Volume measurements of multiple sclerosis lesions with magnetic resonance images: a preliminary study. Neuroradiology 1992; 34: 475-479.
32. Kastrukoff LF, Oger JJF, Hashimoto SA, et al. Systemic lymphoblastoid interferon therapy in chronic progressive multiple sclerosis. I. Clinical and MRI evaluation. Neurology 1990 ; 40: 479-486.
33. Koopmans RA, Li DBK, Redekop WK, et al. The use of magnetic resonance imaging in monitoring interferon therapy of multiple sclerosis. J Neuroimaging 1993 ; 3: 163-168.
34. The Multiple Sclerosis Study Group. Efficacy and toxicity of cyclosporine in chronic progressive multiple sclerosis: a randomized, double-blinded, placebo-controlled clinical trial. Ann Neurol 1990 ; 27: 591-605.
35. Koopmans RA, Li DBK, Zhao GJ et al. MRI assessment of cyclosporine therapy of MS in a multicenter trial [abstract]. Neurology 1992 ; 42 (suppl 3): 210.
36. The IFNB Multiple Sclerosis Study Group. Interferon-beta-1b is effective in relapsing-remitting MS.I. Clinical results of a multicenter, randomized, double-blind, placebo-controlled trial. Neurology 1993 ; 43: 655-661.
37. Paty DW, Li DBK, UBC MS/MRI Study Group, IFNB Multiple Sclerosis Study Group. Interferon beta-1b is effective in relapsing-remitting multiple sclerosis. II. MRI analysis results of a multicenter, randomized, double-blind, placebo-controlled trial. Neurology 1993 ; 43: 662-667.
38. Brownell B, Hughes JT. The distribution of plaques in the cerebrum in multiple sclerosis with special reference to cerebral plaques. Acta Neurol Scand 1962 ; 41: 1-161.
39. Lumdsen CE. The neuropathology of multiple sclerosis. In: Vinken PJ, Bruyn GW, eds. Handbook of clinical neurology, Vol 9. Amsterdam: North Holland, 1970 ; 296-298.
40. Barbosa S, Blumhardt LD, Roberts N, Lock T, Edwards RHT. Magnetic resonance relaxation time mapping in multiple sclerosis: normal appearing white matter and the "invisible" lesion load. Magn Reson Imaging 1994 ; 12: 33-42.
41. Thomas DJ, Pennock JM, Hajnal JV, Young IR, Bydder GM, Steiner RE. Magnetic resonance imaging of the spinal cord in multiple sclerosis by fluid-attenuated inversion recovery. Lancet 1993 ; i: 593-594.
42. Filippi M, Horsfield MA, Morrissey SP, et al. Quantitative brain MRI lesion load predicts the course of clinically isolated syndromes suggestive of multiple sclerosis. Neurology 1994 ; 44:635-641.
43. Miller DH, Ormerod IEC, McDonald WI, et al. The early risk of multiple sclerosis after optic neuritis. J Neurol Neurosurg Psychiatry 1988 ; 51: 1569-1571.
44. Miller DH, Ormerod IEC, Rudge P, Kendall BE, Moseley IF, McDonald WI. The early risk of multiple sclerosis following isolated acute syndromes of the brainstem and spinal cord. Ann Neurol 1989 ; 26: 635-639.
45. Frederiksen JL, Larsson HBW, Olesen J, Stigsby B. MRI, VEP, SEP, and biothesiometry suggest monosymptomatic acute optic neuritis to be the first manifestation of multiple sclerosis. Acta Neurol Scand 1991 ; 83: 343-350.
46. Martinelli V, Comi G, Filippi M, et al. Paraclinical tests in acute-onset optic neuritis: basal data and results of a short follow up. Acta Neurol Scand 1991 ; 84: 231-236.

47. Lee KH, Hashimoto SA, Hooge JP, *et al.* Magnetic resonance imaging of the head in the diagnosis of multiple sclerosis: a prospective 2-year follow-up with comparison of clinical evaluation, evoked potantials, oligoclonal banding, and CT. *Neurology* 1991 ; 41: 657-660.
48. Jacobs L, Munschauer FE, Kaba SE. Clinical and magnetic resonance imaging in optic neuritis. *Neurology* 1991 ; 41: 15-19.
49. Ford B, Tampieri D, Francis G. Long-term follo-up of acute partial transverse myelopathy. *Neurology* 1992 ; 42: 250-252.
50. Morrissey SP, Miller DH, Kendall BE, *et al.* Prognostic significance of brain MRI at presentation with a clinically isolated syndrome suggestive of MS - A five year follow up study. *Brain* 1993 ; 116: 135-146.
51. Filippini G, Comi GC, Cosi V, *et al.* Sensitivities and predictive value of paraclinical tests for diagnosing multiple sclerosis. *J Neurol* 1994 ; 241: 132-137.
52. Rao SM, Leo GJ, Haughton VM, StAubin-Faubert P, Bernardin L. Correlation of magnetic resonance imaging with neuropsychological testing in multiple sclerosis. *Neurology* 1898 ; 39: 161-166.
53. Swirski-Sacchetti T, Mitchell DR, Seward J, *et al.* Neuropsychological and structural brain lesions in multiple sclerosis: a regional analysis. *Neurology* 1992 ; 42: 1291-1295.
54. Filippi M, Barker GJ, Horsfield MA, *et al.* A quantitative brain MRI study in benign and secondary progressive multiple sclerosis. *J Neurol* 1994 ; 241: 246-251.
55. Gass A, Barker GJ, Kidd D, *et al.* Magnetization transfer rate correlates with clinical disability in multiple sclerosis. *Ann Neurol* 1994 ; 36: 62-67.
56. Smith ME, Stone LA, Albert PS, *et al.* Clinical worsening in multiple sclerosis is associated with increased frequency and area of gadopentetate dimeglumine-enhancing magnetic resonance imaging. *Ann Neurol* 1993 ; 33: 480-489.
57. Arnold DL, Matthews PM, Francis G, Antel J. Proton magnetic resonance spectroscopy of human brain in vivo in the evaluation of multiple sclerosis: assessment of the load of the disease. Magn Reson *Med* 1990 ; 14: 154-159.
58. van Walderveen MAA, Barkhof F, Hommes OR, Polman CH, Frequin STFM, Valk J. T1 SE more specific than T2 SE in identifying disabling lesions in multiple sclerosis. A quantitative follow up study. Proceedings of the Second Meeting of the Society of Magnetic *Resonance* 1994 ; 1: 536.
59. Dousset V, Grossman RI, Ramer KN, *et al.* Experimental allergic encephalomyelitis and multiple sclerosis: lesion characterization with magnetic transfer imaging. *Radiology* 1992 ; 182: 483-491.
60. Arnold DL, Riess GT, Matthews PM, *et al.* Use of proton magnetic resonance spectroscopy for monitoring disease progression in multiple sclerosis. *Ann Neurol* 1994 ; 36: 76-82.
61. Barnes D, Munro PGM, Youl BD, *et al.* The longstanding lesion in multiple sclerosis: a quantitative MRI and electron microscopic study. *Brain* 1991 ; 114: 1271-1280.
62. Uhlenbrock D, Sehlen S. The value of T1-weighted images in the differentiation between MS, white matter lesions, and subcortical arterosclerotic encephalopathy. *Neuroradiology* 1989 ; 31: 203-212.
63. Nauta JJP, Thompson AJ, Barkhof F, Miller DH. MR imaging in monitoring the treatment of MS patients: statistical power of parallel-groups and cross-over designs. *J Neurol Sci* 1994 ; 122: 6-14.
64. Miller DH, Barkhof F, Berry I, Kappos L, Scotti G, Thompson AJ. Magnetic resonance imaging in monitoring the treatment of multiple sclerosis: Concerted Action Guidelines. J Neurol Neurosurg *Psychiatry* 1991 ; 54: 683-688.
65. Kappos L, Stadt D, Ratzka M, et al. Magnetic resonance imaging in the evaluation of treatment in multiple sclerosis. *Neuroradiology* 1988 ; 30: 299-302.
66. Wiles CM, Omar L, Swan AV, et al. Total lymphoid irradiation in multiple sclerosis. J Neurol Neurosurg *Psychiatry* 1994 ; 57: 154-163.

32

2D localised spectroscopy on human brain

B. GILLET [1], B-T. DOAN [1], D. WECKER [2], J-F. NEDELEC [3], J-P. MACHER [3], J-C. BELOEIL [1]

[1]*Laboratoire de RMN biologique ICSN-CNRS, 91198 Gif-sur-Yvette Cedex, France.*
[2]*Bruker Medizintechnik, 76275 Ettlingen, Germany.*
[3]*FORENAP, 68250 Rouffach, France.*

Nuclear Magnetic Resonance (NMR) is a powerful non-invasive technique for studying living material. While the ^{1}H nucleus is present in a larger number of metabolites than is ^{31}P, it has been used very little because of two major drawbacks. First, the presence of water in all living material causes dynamic range problems and masks the presence of other metabolites. Second, one-dimensional spectra are complex and composed of overlapping signals from many metabolites, because of the limited chemical shift range. Developments in ^{1}H NMR spectroscopy, such as editing methods, selective solvent suppression sequences, and the use of two-dimensional NMR have overcome these drawbacks and revealed the advantages of ^{1}H for NMR studies on living material. Nevertheless, few 2D studies have been made on intact living animals [1-4] using a surface coil. We have previously demonstrated that 2D ^{1}H NMR is well suited to detecting and assigning small cerebral metabolites and that it is a powerful means of directly investigating the metabolism of the rat brain *in vivo* [5]. The COSY sequence can also be used to assign larger molecules such as fatty acids, and this technique has been used to compare, *in vivo*, the skeletal muscles of dystrophic (mdx) and normal (C57BL 10), mice, to determine the nature of the fatty acid in each muscle [6]. But before this type of study can be extended to human beings the measurements must be localized. One localized 2D sequence [7] has been performed on rat adipose tissues. This report describes the implementation of another 2D volume-selected sequence (VOSY-COSY) for human muscle and brain.

Material and methods

The sequence was implemented on a 2T and a 3T Bruker whole body system. The volume of interest was 32 cm³ for the muscle and 150 cm³ for the brain. Shimming was performed on this VOI with a standard VOSY sequence. The water signal was suppressed with three gaussian pulses prior to the 2D sequence. The «grasp-gradient» strength was 8mT/m over a period of 8ms. One 1K FID was acquired in the time domain t2 for each of the 128 increments in the time domain t1 for the muscle, and 32 1K FID were acquired in the time domain t2 for each of the 64 increments in the time domain t1 for the brain. The total measurement time was 4 min. for the muscle and 50 min. for the brain. The data were multiplied by an unshifted sine-bell function in the two dimensions and zero-filled to obtain a 1024 x 512 data point matrix before carrying out a 2D Fourier transform. The experiments were processed in absolute mode.

Results

The 2D localised sequence is shown in Figure 1. In this sequence, the water signal is suppressed using a CHESS sequence prior to the VOSY-COSY sequence. In the VOSY-COSY sequence, the VOSY provides «the first pulse» of the 2D sequence. It is followed by the second part of the GRASP-COSY sequence [8].

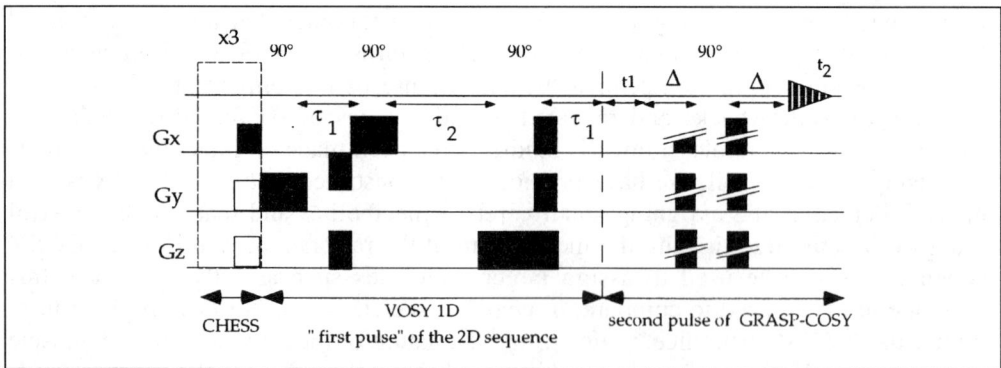

Figure 1. VOSY-COSY sequence.

The VOSY-COSY spectrum of a human calf muscle at 3T is shown in Figure 2. It was assigned by superimposing the 2D spectra of isolated fatty acids dissolved in CDC13. For example, the spectrum of linolenic acid is represented in Figure 3.

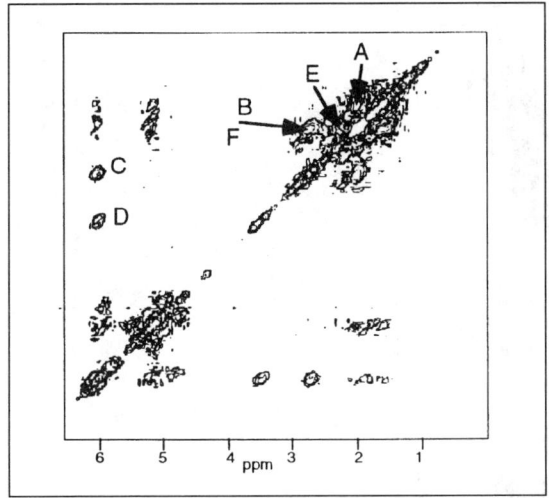

Figure 2. VOSY-COSY spectrum of a human calf muscle at 3T.

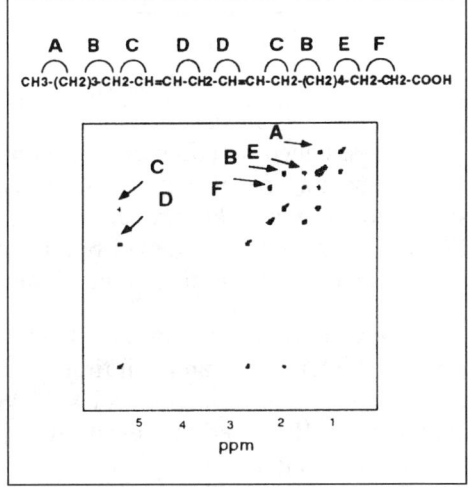

Figure 3. COSY of linolenic acid representative of lipid correlations.

Most types of correlation are present in this spectrum. E and F type correlations were found in the spectra of all fatty acids. There was also an A correlation in the spectra of fatty acids, except in those of unsaturated fatty acid, like linolenic acid. B, C and D are characteristic of unsaturated acyl chains.

All the correlations of the saturated and unsaturated fatty acyl chain are distinct in the VOSY-COSY spectrum of a human calf muscle at 3T (Figure 2), which could be useful for studies on muscles as has been shown for *mdx* mice [6]. With measurement times of less than 30 min. and low power deposit (less than 2 Watt/kg), this sequence could also be employed with patients. Figure 4 shows the VOSY-COSY spectrum of the brain of a volunteer.

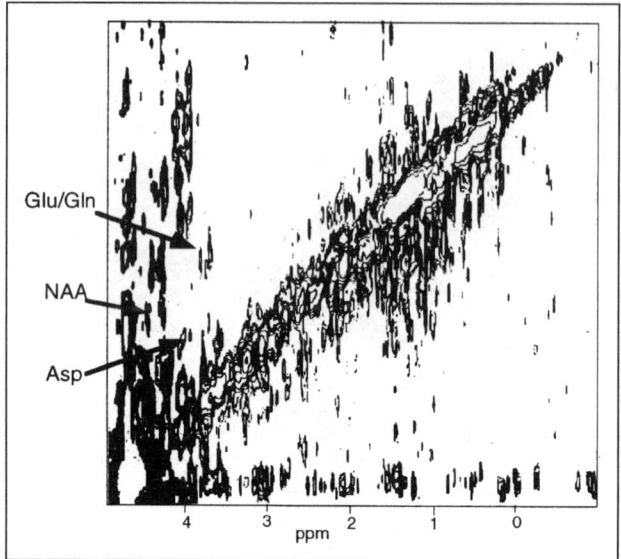

Figure 4. VOSY-COSY spectrum of a human brain at 2T.

It was assigned by comparing it with 2D spectra of rat brain and by superimposing the 2D spectra of isolated low molecular weight metabolites dissolved in a medium similar to the intracellular medium [4,5]. Some amino-acids correlations in the VOSY-COSY spectrum of this human brain can be detected. They have been assigned to N-acetyl-aspartate, aspartate and the glutamate/glutamine pool.

The low power deposit of the VOSY-COSY sequence allows it to be used on human beings. The total measurement time is less than 30 min., hence this sequence could be used for studies on human muscles. VOSY-COSY is clearly suitable for studies on the human brain. However, the sensitivity of the system must be improved, before it could be used with patients.

References

1. Berkowitz BA *et al.*, *Magn J. Reson.* 1988 ; 79, 547-553.
2. Berkowitz BA, Balaban RS, *Methods Enzymol* 1989 ; 176, 330-341.
3. Barrere B *et al.*, FEBS *Lett* 1990 ; 264, 198-202 .
4. Behar KL, Ogino T, Magn. Reson. *MEd* 1991 ; 17, 285-303.
5. Peres M *et al.*, Magn. Reson. *Med.* 1992 ; 27, 356-361.
6. Gillet B *et al.*, Neuromusc. *Disord.* 56, 1993 ; 433-438.
7. Desmoulin R *et al.*, Magn. Reson. *Med* 1990 ; 14, 160-168.
8. Brereton LM *et al.*, *Magn J. Reson* 1991 ; 93, 54-62.

33

^{13}C and ^{1}H NMR studies of glucose transport in the human brain

R. GRUETTER

Department of Molecular Biology and Biochemistry, Yale University, New Haven, CT and MR Center, Inselheimmatte, CH-3010 Bern, Switzerland.

Blood glucose is the major carbon source of energy in the normal human brain. Cerebral cell metabolism depends on an adequate transport of glucose across the blood-brain-barrier (BBB). The transport process has been shown to be by facilitated diffusion across the brain endothelial cell membranes [8]. Glucose transport across the BBB hence is a vital process which may become rate-limiting to metabolism in a variety of diseases such as seizures, hypoglycemia and Alzheimer's Disease. Glucose transport is difficult to measure in humans with radioactive tracers because of the need to know the cerebral glucose concentration for calculating the lumped constant or because the signal of labeled glucose cannot be distinguished from that of its metabolic products [19].

NMR spectroscopy has been shown to be a powerful non-invasive technique that can be used to quantify many metabolite concentrations *in vivo* (*for review see*, e.g. 1). In particular, due to the natural abundance of ^{13}C, administration of ^{13}C label can be used to measure specific metabolic rates non-invasively, such as the TCA cycle rate in heart and brain and glycogen synthesis rates (*for review see*, e.g. 3).

Most of the turnover studies in brain have concentrated on observing the proton coupled to the ^{13}C label [10, 27, 29]. Reports on direct ^{13}C NMR studies of the human brain have been scarce. Early ^{13}C NMR studies have shown that ^{13}C labeled substances can be observed in intact mammalian brain after [1-^{13}C] glucose infusion [4, 2, 22]. Recent advancements in shimming [17] together with decoupling gave improvements in sensitivity and spectral resolution which has extended theses studies considerably. This paper reviews the measurements of human brain glucose transport and metabolism we have made using direct ^{13}C NMR quantification and ^{1}H NMR of changes in cerebral glucose.

Methods

Subjects

Subjects were placed supine in a 2.1 Tesla whole-body magnet with the NMR transceiver beneath the occipito-parietal region of the brain. One arm as cannulated for the administration of glucose and insulin and the other was used to sample blood for the determination of plasma glucose and, if necessary, isotopic enrichment. Sensory stimulation was minimized by having the subjects wear ear plugs and eye-patches.

Infusion protocol

Plasma glucose levels were raised rapidly 5 or 10 mM above euglycemia using a primed variable-rate glucose infusion similar to the glucose-insulin clamp technique. In the studies involving ^{13}C labeled glucose, this initial infusion period was performed with 99%-enriched glucose in order to achieve rapidly a high isotopic fraction in plasma glucose. Hepatic output of unlabeled glucose during the study was minimized by infusing either insulin or by maintaining moderate hyperglycemia.

Localized 13C NMR measurement of metabolite concentrations

NMR signals were obtained from a 144 ml volume with a double-concentric $^{13}C(7\ cm)/^1H(14\ cm)$ surface coil using methods described previously [13, 14]. Localization in the occipital lobe excluded major blood vessels and the ventricles as judged from inversion recovery MRI. Quantification was achieved by comparing the *in vivo* measurement to that of the corresponding metabolite in an aqueous solution place in a 2l bottle. The solution measurements were obtained immediately after each *in vivo* measurement.

The quantification with external standards resulted in a volumetric measurement which is equivalent to the per wet weight measurement assuming a specific density of 1g/ml, and by taking the isotope enrichment of the metabolites into account.

Localized 1H NMR studies

The localization method for ^1H NMR was based on ISIS with outer volume suppression, as described by Gruetter *et al.* [15]. A volume of 36 ml in the occipito-parietal cortex was selected based on inversion recovery MRI. An elliptic 6 x 7 cm single frequency surface doil was used. Specta were collected with a 3-4 min time resolution. Difference spectra were obtained after zero-filling and digital frequency alignment.

Kinetic analyses

The steady-state relationship between brain and blood glucose concentrations can be analyzed with the symmetric Michaelis-Menten model of transport as in previous studies of animal brain [12, 22]. This model assumes glucose influx and efflux to be characterized by the same Michaelis-Menten kinetic parameters and that glucose is uniformly distributed in the aqueous phase of the brain, whose distribution volume is Vd =0.77 ml/g [11]. The time course of brain glucose is then given by the standard differential equation [21].

$$\frac{dG_{brain}(t)}{dt} = T_{max}\frac{G_{plasma}(t)}{K_t + G_{plasma}(t)} - \frac{G_{brain}(t)}{V_d K_t + G_{brain}(t)} - CMR_{glc} \quad (1)$$

Eq. [1] can be rewritten at steady-state to express the brain glucose concentration G_{brain} (µmol/g) as a function of the half saturation concentration K_t, the ratio of maximal transport rate to cerebral metabolic rate of glucose, T_{max}/CMR_{glc}, and the glucose concentration in plasma G_{plasma}, as

$$G_{brain} = V_d K_t \frac{\left(\frac{T_{max}}{CMR_{glc}} - 1\right) \times \frac{G_{plasma}}{K_t} - 1}{\frac{T_{max}}{CMR_{glc}} + \frac{G_{plasma}}{K_t} + 1} \quad (2)$$

Eq. [2] was fitted to the steady-state glucose measurements using non-linear, iterative numeric methods (Levenberg-Marquardt algorithm). T_{max} was calculated T_{max}/CMR_{glc} assuming $CMR_{glc} - 0.3 \mu mol\ g^{-1} min^{-1}$ reported for the human brain under sensory deprivation (28).

Results

Sensitivity considerations

Using localized natural abundance ^{13}C NMR, we have shown that signals from myo-inositol and other metabolites can be observed in the human brain (Figure 1). Quantification of these signals gave 7.2±0.5 µmol/g which is in good agreement with biopsy and autopsy data and subsequent ^1H NMR estimations and suggest a detection limit of 100µM ^{13}C for ^{13}C NMR *in vivo* [14]. The use of a three-dimensional localization scheme resulted in complete elimination of the scalp lipid signals over a 10-20 ppm wide chemical shift range, as indicated in Figure 1 by the elimination of glycerol signal intensity at 69.5 ppm. Our experience has shown that the absence of lipid signals is a very sensitive marker that the signals are localized to the brain tissue. Chemical shift displacement error was minimized by setting the spectrometer frequency within the chemical shift range studied.

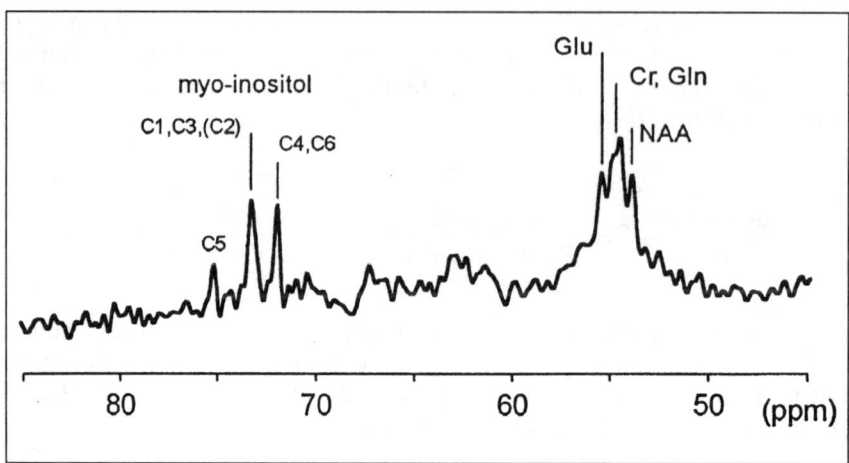

Figure 1. *In vivo natural abundance* spectra of *myo-inositol* from a 144 mol volume in the occipito-parietal region of the human brain. Shown is the sum of five measurements. Reproduced from. (14).

Measurement of glucose transport

The quantification of cerebral glucose by ^{13}C NMR resulted in a euglycemic plasma glucose concentration of 1.0±0.1 µmol/g (13). The quantification of brain glucose at different plasma glucose levels was used to determine transport kinetics by fitting Eq. [2]. The best fit to twelve measurements in six subjects is shown in Figure 2. The kinetic constants are consistent with transport not being rate-limiting for metabolism at plasma glucose levels above 2,3mM. A subsequent study showed that the relationship between plasma and brain glucose is not altered by chronic hyperglycemia over this range of plasma glucose values (26).

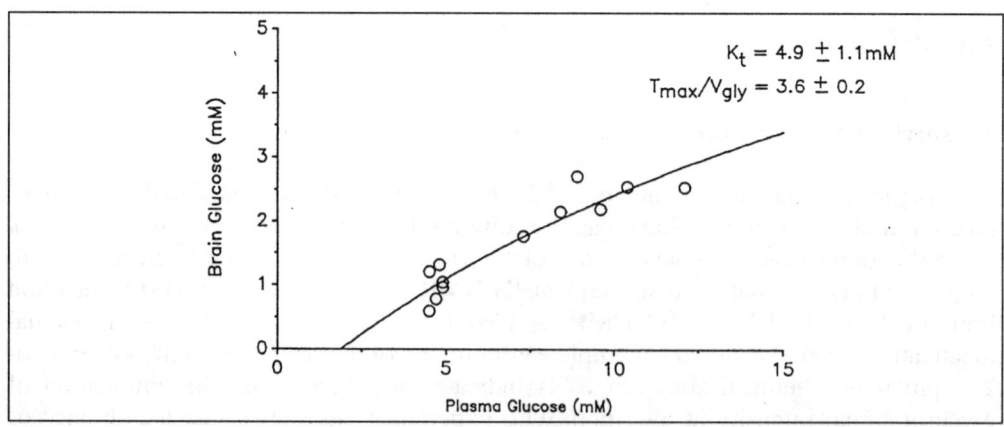

Figure 2. Determination of glucose transport kinetics from the steady-state quantification of cerebral glucose. Shown are the measurements from six subjects with the best fit of Eq. [2] indicated V_{gly} is equivalent to CMR_{glc}. Reproduced from (13).

^{1}H NMR has been used to observe changes in cerebral glucose during acute hyperglycemia and activation (15, 24, 20, 7). We have shown that the ^{1}H difference spectrum between eu- and hyperglycemia contains mainly peaks attributed to glucose (Figure 3). The time course of the change in cerebral glucose was consistent with the model described by Eq. [1] (25), assuming CMR_{glc}=0.3 µmol/g min in unstimulated human brain (28). To evaluate increases in glucose consumption during functional stimulation, the slight decrease in cerebral glucose observed can be modelled using Eq. [1] with a time-dependent CMR_{glc} (7).

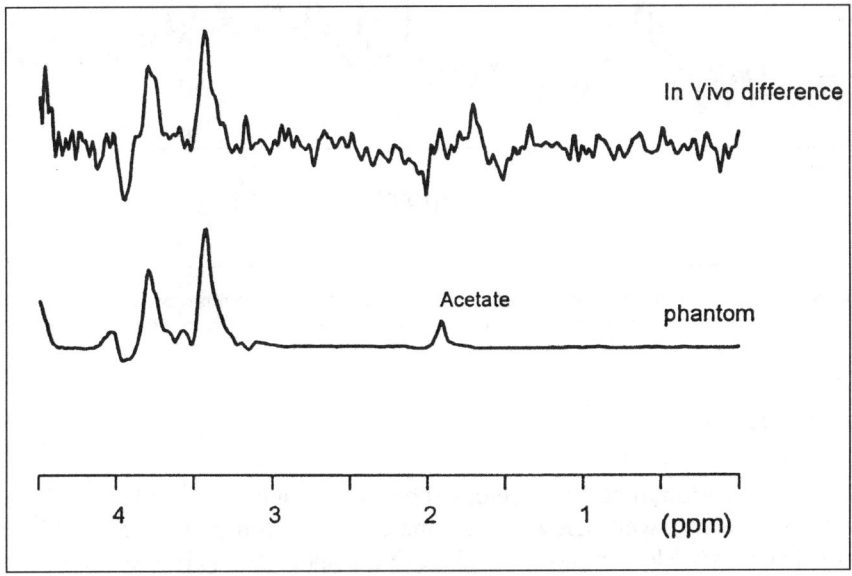

Figure 3. Assignment of ^{1}H NMR *in vivo* difference spectra of glucose from a 36 ml volume in the occipitoparietal region of the human brain. Shown is the difference spectrum between those acquired at hyperglycemia and euglycemia (top). The changes at 3.81 and 3.44 ppm are entirely attributed to glucose as shown by the identity of chemical shift and relative amplitudes with the solution spectrum (bottom). Modified from (15).

Observation of glucose metabolism by localized 13C NMR

Figure 4 shows a localized spectrum obtained after several hours of glucose infusion [16]. Linewidths were 2Hz for the glutamate resonances; which is sufficient to resolve glutamine from glutamate at this field strength. The resolved observation of carbon label at the C3 and C4 position of glutamate and glutamine, in conjunction with the above described quantification methods has permitted the assessment of cerebral amino acid pools and *in vivo* isotopic enrichment [18], TCA cycle rate, α-ketoglutarate, glutamate exchange and glutamine synthesis [23]. Glutamine synthesis was shown to lag slightly behind glutamate, which is consistent with rapid glutamine synthesis in human brain.

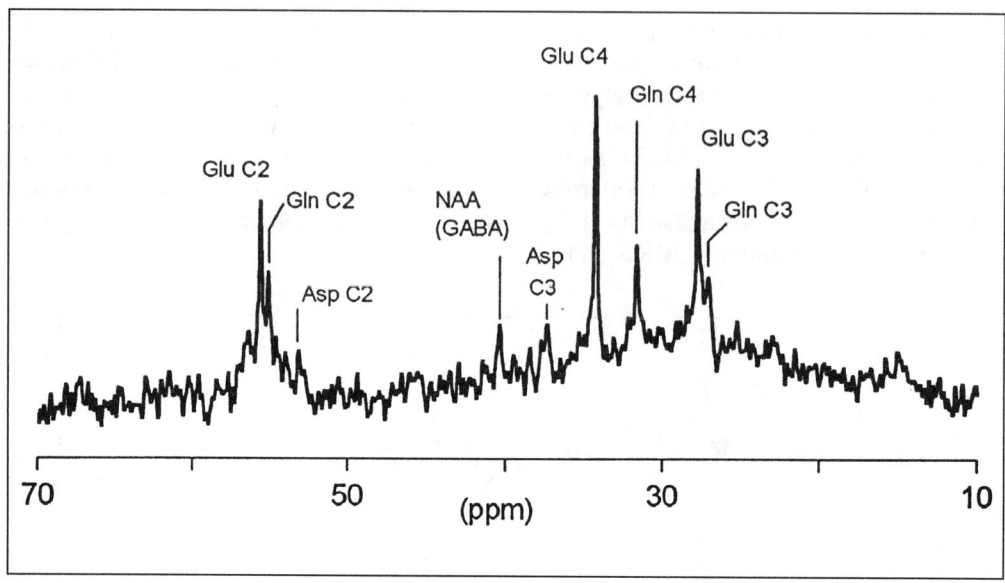

Figure 4. Observation of label incorporation in amino acids in the human brain. Shown is a spectrum obtained from a ml volume several hours after the start of the ^{13}C infusion. Reprinted from (16).

Discussion

The quantification of cerebral glucose concentration has shown levels of 1 µmol/g at euglycemia which is well below the plasma concentration of 4.8 mM and is consistent with the Michaelis-Menten model of glucose transport (Eq. [1]). Extension of ^{1}H NMR should permit a higher spatial and temporal resolution to study cerebral glucose transport and consumption, which should be useful to study cerebral glucose homeostasis.

The Michaelis-Menten constant of 4.9±1.1 mM (Figure 2) is in agreement with reports by positron emission tomography (5, 6, 9). The T_{max} and CMR_{glc} values reported by PET imply euglycemic cerebral glucose concentrations of 0.2 µmol/g [5] and 2.0 µmol/g [9], which are significantly different from the NMR measurements.

^{1}H NMR spectroscopy can alternatively be used to measure transient changes in cerebral glucose at a much higher spatial and temporal resolution (Figure 2) which offers the prospect of spatial and temporal mapping without using labeled substrate.

In addition to the study of glucose transport and metabolism, the observation of labeled products or intermediates of glucose metabolism in the human brain (Figure 4) in conjunction with improvements in sensitivity should permit the determination of several chemical reactions in the human brain, such as glutamine synthesis, TCA cycle rate and e.g. GABA synthesis. The differential localization of corresponding enzymes and the high synthesis rate of glutamine imply rapid neuronal-glial exchange in the intact, unstimulated human brain.

NMR studies such as those reviewed herein and extensions there of might provide a direct, non-invasive way to study the regulation of brain glucose homeostasis during e.g. drug intervention and functional stimulation, as well as cerebral glutamine synthesis in humans. The NMR measurements can be performed completely non-invasively and do not use ionizing radiation, which is particularly desirable for pediatric and longitudinal studies.

References

1. Bachelard HS, Badar-Goffer RS NMR spectroscopy in neurochemistry. J *Neurochem* 1993 ; 61:412.
2. Beckmann N, Turkalj I, Seelig J, Keller U 13C NMR for the assessment of human brain glucose metabolism *in vivo*. *Biochemistry* 1991 ; 30:6362.
3. Beckmann N In vivo 13C spectroscopy in humans. NMR *Basic Principles and Progress* 1992 ; 28:74.
4. Behar KL, Petroff OAC, Prichard JW, Alger JR, Shulman RG Detection of metabolites in rabbit brain by 13C NMR spectroscopy following administration of [1-13C] glucose. Magn. Reson. *Med* 1986 ; 3:911.
5. Blomqvist G, Gjedde A, Gutniak M, Grill V, Widén L, Stone-Elander S, Hellstrand E Facilitated transport of glucose from blood to brain in man and the effect of moderate hypoglycemia on cerebral glucose utilization. Eur. J. Nucl. *Med* (1991 ; 18:834.
6. Brooks KJ, Gibbs JSR, Sharp P, Herold S, Turton DR, Luthra SK, Kohner EM, Bloom SR, Jones T Regional cerebral glucose transport in insulin-dependent diabetic patients studied using [11C]3-O-methyl-D-glucose and positron emission tomography. J. Cereb. *Blood Flow Metabol* 1986 ; 6:240.
7. Chen W, Novotny EJN, Zhu XH, Rothman DL, Shulman RG. Localized 1H NMR measurement of glucose consumption in the human brain during visual stimulation. *Proc. Natl. Acad. Sci. USA* 1993 ; 90:9896.
8. Crone C. Facilitated transfer of glucose from blood into brain tissue. J. *Physiol* (London) 1965 ; 181:103.
9. Feinendegen LE, Herzog H, Wieler H, Patton DD, Schmid A. Glucose transport and utilization in the human brain: Model using carbon-11 methylglucose and positron emission tomography J. Nucl. *Med* 1986 ; 27:1867.
10. Fitzpatrick SM, Hetherington HP, Behar KL, Shuman RG. The fluc from glucose to glutamate in the rat brain in vivo as determined by 1H observed/13C edited NMR spectroscopy. J. Cereb. *Blood Flow Metab* 1990 ; 10:170.
11. Gjedde A, Diemer NH. Autoradiographic determination of regional brain glucose content J. Cereb. *Blood Flow Metabol* 1984 ; 3:303.
12. Gjedde A, Christensen O. Estimates of Michaelis-Menten constants for the two membranes of the brain endothelium J. Cereb. *Blood Flow Metabol* 1984 ; 4:241.
13. Gruetter R, Novotny EJ, Boulware SD, Rothman DL, Shulman GI, Mason GF, Shulman RG, Tamborlane WV. Direct measurement of brain glucose concentrations in humans by 13C NMR spectroscopy. Proc. Natl. Acad. Sci. USA 89:1109. *Erratum appears in vol* 1992 ; 89:12208.
14. Gruetter R, Rothman DKL, Novotny EJ, Shulman RG. Localized 13C NMR spectroscopy of myo-inositol in the human brain in vivo Magn. Reson. *med* 1992 ; 25:304.

15. Gruetter R, Rothman DL, Novotny EJ, Shulman GI, Prichard JW, Shulman RG. Detection and assignment of the glucose signal in 1H NMR difference spectra of the human brain Magn. Reson. *Med* 1992 ; 27:183.
16. Gruetter R, Novotny EJ, Boulware SD, Rothman DL, Tamborlane WV, Shulman RG. 11th Annual Meeting Soc. Magn. Reson. Med, Berlin, *August* 1992 ; 8-14, 1992, p. 1921.
17. Gruetter R. Automatic, localized in vivo adjustment of all first- and second- order shim coils. Magn. Reson. *Med* 1993 ; 29:804.
18. Gruetter R, Novotny EJ, Boulware SD, Mason GF, Rothman DL, Prichard JW, Shulman RG. Localized 13C NMR spectroscopy of amino acid labeling from [1-13C] D-glucose in the human brain. J. *Neurochem.* (in press) 1994.
19. Holden JE, Mori K, Diesel GA, Cruz NF, Nelson T, Sokoloff L. Modeling the dependence of hexose distribution volumes in brain on plasma glucose concentration: Implications for estimation of the local 2-deoxyglucose lumped constant. J. Cereb. *Blood Flow Metabol* 1991 ; 11:171.
20. Kreis R, Ross BD. Cerebral Metabolic Disturbances in Patients with Subacute and Chronic Diabetes Mellitus: Detection with Proton MR Spectroscopy, *Radiology* 1992 ; 184:123.
21. Lund-Andersen H. Transport of glucose from blood to brain *Physiol. Rev* 1979 ; 59:305.
22. Mason GF, Behar KL, Rothman DL, Shulman RG (1992) NMR determination of intracerebral glucose concentration and transport kinetics in rat brain. J. Cereb. Blood Flow Metabol. 12:448.
23. Mason GF, Gruetter R, Rothman DL, Behar KL, Shulman RG, Novotny EJ. Simultaneous determination of the rates of the TCA cycle, glucose utilization, ketoglutarate/glutamate exchange and glutamine synthesis in human brain by 13C NMR J. Cereb. *Blood Flow Metab* (in press) 1994.
24. Merboldt KD, Bruhn H, Hänicke W, Michaelis T, Frahm J. Decrease of Glucose in the Human Visual Cortex during Photic Stimulation. Magn. Reson. *Med* 1992 ; 25:187.
25. Novotny EJ, Gruetter R, Rothman DL, Boulware SD, Tamborlane WV, Shulman RG. 11th Annual Meeting, Soc. Magn. Reson. Med, Berlin, August 8-14, 1992, *Works-in-Progress* 1992 p. 1961.
26. Novotny EJ, Gruetter R, Rothman DL, Boulware SD, Tamborlane WV, Shulman RG. 12 th Annual Meeting Soc. Magn. Reson. Med. New York, *August* 1993 ; 14-20: p.324.
27. Rothman DL, Novotny EJ, Shulman GI, Howseman AM, Petroff OAC, Mason GF, Nixon T, Hanstock CC, Prichard JW, Shulman RG. 1H-[13C] NMR measurements of [4-13C] glutamate turnover in human brain. *Proc. Natl. Acad. Sci. USA* 1992 ; 82:1633.
28. Tyler JL, Strother SC, Zatorre RJ, Alivisatos B, Worsley KJ, Diksic M, Yamamoto YL Stability of regional cerebral glucose metabolism in the normal brain measured by positron emission tomography. *J. Nucl. Med* 1988 ; 29:631.
29. vanZijl PCM, Chesnick AS, Des Pres D, Moonen CTW, Ruiz-Cabello J, van Gelderen P. *In vivo* proton spectroscopy and spectroscopic imaging of [1-13C]- glucose and its metabolic products. *Magn. Reson. Med* 1993 ; 30:544.

34

Neurofunctional imaging and language

M. HABIB[1], M. DIDIC[1], O. LEVRIER[2], J.-F. DEMONET[3], P. SABBAH[2], G. SALAMON[2]

[1]Service de Neurologie, [2]Laboratoire de Neuroradiologie, CHU Timone, Marseille
[3]INSERM U 230 Toulouse, France.

The purpose of this paper is twofold : (1) to summarize some recent work devoted to *in vivo* imaging of language functions and (2) to delineate the most promising directions for future research in this domain, especially using functional Magnetic Resonance Imaging (fMRI). Instead of an exhaustive account, we will focus on some research published during the past few years which, to our opinion, illustrate well both the difficulties and promises of a new approach of brain/language relationships, which could lead to a new «cognitive anatomy» of language. Technical and methodological problems, in particular those encountered by positron emission tomography (PET) will not be considered here, the reader being refered to recent reviews on this subject (Démonet *et al.*, 1993; Frackowiak, 1994; Sergent, 1994).

The classical « anatomo-clinical » background

Most of our knowledge concerning brain-language relationships stems from studies of language breakdown (aphasia) in subjects suffering from left-hemisphere damage, which resulted in an anatomo-functional model of the role of a restricted region of the cortical mantle (the so-called «language area»). According to the aphasia model (*see for instance* Damasio, 1992), Broca's area, a small cortical zone occupying the ventro-caudal part of the frontal lobe (area 44), is specialized in expressive and articulatory aspects of speech and language, whereas Wernicke's area, a larger postero-dorsal region of the temporal lobe (area 22), is specifically involved in the receptive features of language and auditory comprehension. Extensions to this model have resulted in the widely admitted contention that there is in the left hemisphere, encompassing areas 22 and 44, a language-specific, perisylvian, continuous zone, also including : the opercular sensory-motor and insular regions, connecting the frontal and temporal zones, as well as the inferior parietal lobule (especially its most posterior part, the angular gyrus, whose role in written language was demonstrated by Dejerine more than a century ago). This continuous cortical zone is known as «the language area». More recent series of brain-damaged patients, explored by *in vivo* morphological imaging of the brain, have kept practically unaltered this general model, except perhaps for two points : the unexpected frequency of «exceptions to the rule» (*see for instance* Basso *et al.*, 1985), pointing to individual variations in anatomo-functional relationships, and the hitherto largely unravelled role of the right hemisphere in language (*see for instance* Joanette *et al.*, 1990). Finally, the role of mesial regions of the frontal lobes (supplementary motor area of SMA) in language has also been demonstrated from observations of patients with damage to this region.

The seminal work of the saint-Louis group (Petersen *et al.*, 1988, 1989, 1990)

The Saint-Louis group has been the first to apply the most recent technical advance in PET methodology (the use of ^{15}O to label intravenously injected H_2O) to the neurobiology of language. Although the method they used has been since then considerably improved, their work still stands as a reference in this domain. Petersen *et al.* (1988) conducted a parallel study of brain processing of single words in two modalities (visual and auditory). The experiment included several steps along a hierarchical design, each of them being compared to the previous one by subtracting functional maps obtained at each step.

Among various results obtained with this method, we will focus on the two most often referred to in subsequent papers. Probably the most widely used paradigm is that of verb generation. Subjects are presented with series of nouns and are requested to provide a semantically associated verb on each noun presented to them (e.g. apple : eat). These authors found a specific activation of an area (Figure 1) situated in the left infero-lateral frontal region (Brodmann's area 47). This location was somewhat unexpected in regard to classical teaching. For Petersen *et al.*, this reflected the semantic attributes of the task, an interpretation which clearly was at variance from predictions based on classical data (according to which semantic processes rather relate to functioning in the posterior temporal regions). Later on, at least two other interpretations of this finding were proposed : Frith *et al.* (1991) considered it to reflect the internal demand inherent to the task (as opposed to the most simpler reference task where subjects only have to repeat a heard word); Tulving *et al.* (1993) demonstrated that this activation was related to the effective learning of the same words, suggesting that left frontal activation might reflect the encoding processes in episodic memory.

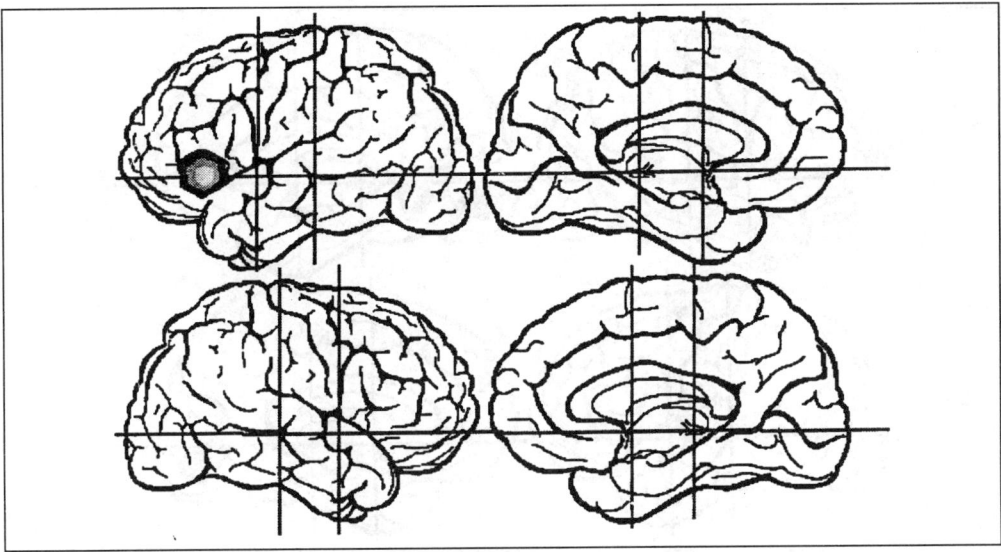

Figure 1. Petersen *et al.*, 1988. Generate uses minus repeat word = semantic activation?

Another quite unexpected result from the Saint-Louis studies was obtained on reading tasks. When a subject has to read words written in his own language, or pronounceable non-words which are phonologically plausible (such as «twifle» or «stoomy»), there is an activation in the primary visual areas bilaterally and a left unilateral activation in a more anterior mesial temporal (so-called extra-striate) region (Figure 2). These authors proposal was that this left extra-striate zone corresponds to the visual (or orthographic) lexicon postulated in cognitive psychology models. Another surprising result of this experiment was the lack of activation of Wernicke's area, since it was believed until then that reading processes involved a necessary step taking place in Wernicke's area, one allowing to transform word visual form into an auditory (phonological) representation in order to be read or understood (Geschwind, 1979). Moreover, the same model postulated that the brain center for «written images of words» (Dejerine, 1891) was located in the angular gyrus, at the lateral temporo-occipital junction, a region never activated by the presentation of written words. Finally, PET reading activation studies clearly contradicted the classical dogma on two points: the angular gyrus location of the visual word form and the necessity of transforming the written word into sound representation in Wernicke's area.

The proper role of Wernicke area was further detailed in several subsequent works. Zatorre *et al.* (1992) found, during listening of neutral sounds (Figure 3), a bilateral activation of primary auditory areas (Heschl's gyri) and a more anterior activation in the left superior temporal gyrus and Broca's area when subjects passively listened to phonemes, whereas when a active phonetic judgement task was required, activation was found in the upper part of Broca's area and in the left parietal region. Similar results were obtained by Demonet *et al.* (1992) using a more complex phoneme monitoring task (Figure 4). A common feature to both Zatorre and Demonet works was an activation of Broca's area in the absence of oral production (whereas this region was

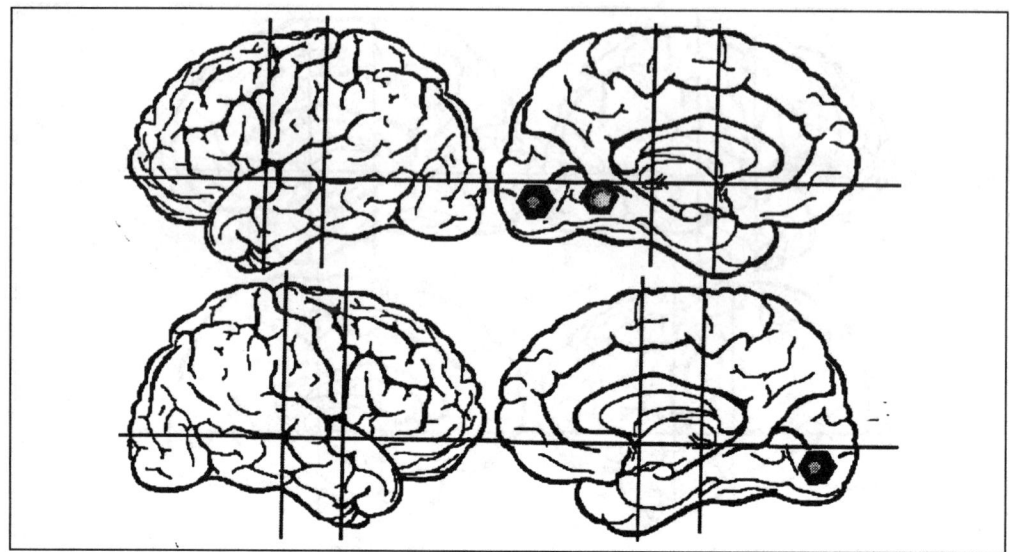

Figure 2. Petersen et al. (1988;1990). Reading words: visual word form?

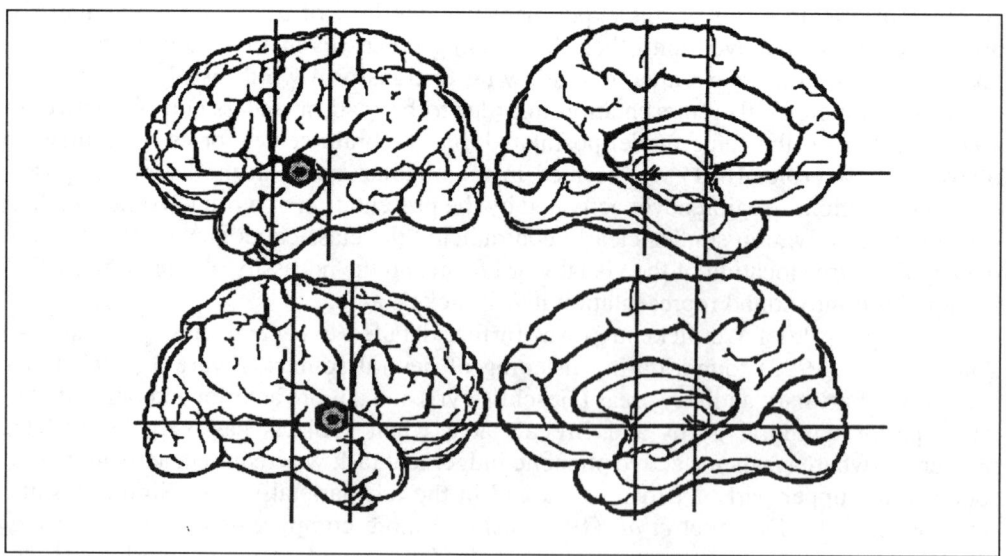

Figure 3. Zatorre et al., 1992. Passive speech: listening to syllables minus noise.

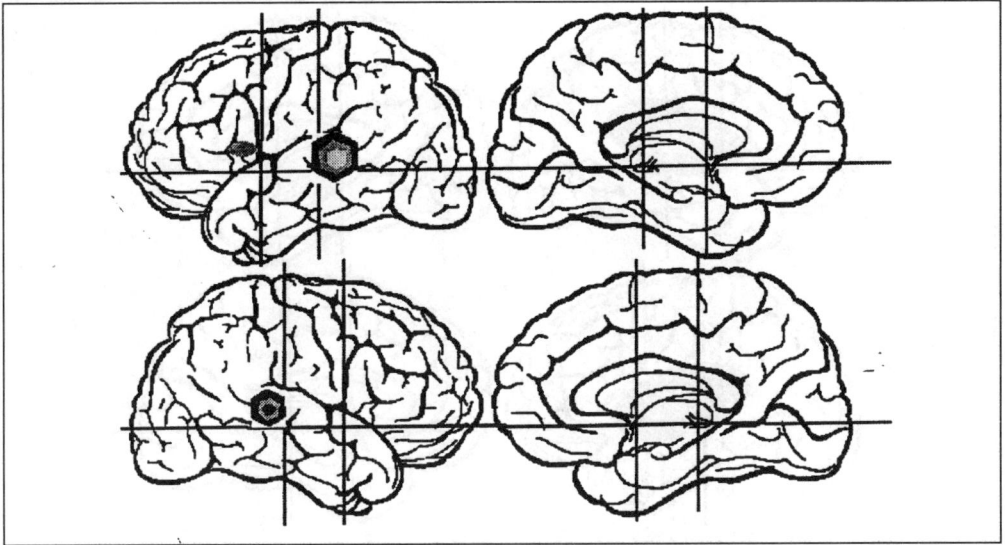

Figure 4. Démonet et al., 1992. Phonological processing: phonemes minus tones.

thought to be involved in articulatory aspects of oral language). Actually, both these studies argue in favor of broca's area playing a role not in effective vocalisation but in subvocal rehearsal of phonemic utterances.

This interpretation was strongly supported by a work by Paulesu et al. (1993) using a special task exploring the cognitive model of verbal working memory (Baddeley). According to this model, short term memorizing of verbal materials, so called articulatory loop, includes two different subsystems : the phonological loop, allowing mental rehearsal of verbal materials, and the phonological store in which this material is momentarily stored. Paulesu et al. asked their subjects to state whether one given letter was included among a sequence of six consonant letters previously appearing one by one on a computer monitor. In a second task, subjects had to state if letters from the same sequence «rhymed» with a target letter (T with B, not with A or H). The latter task was expected to only activate the phonological loop, whereas the former activated both subsystems. These authors were able to demonstrate that the whole process of verbal working memory relied on a large bilateral perisylvian area (Figure 5), whereas the phonological loop was restricted to a small left hemisphere region projecting on the supramarginal gyrus in the inferior parietal lobe (Figure 6).

A last work we will discuss here is that of Mazoyer et al. (1993). This study is somewhat different from all the above-mentioned studies in that subjects had to listen to sentences and continuous text rather than isolated words as in most previous studies. Unexpectedly, in an experimental paradigm comparing passive listening of a meaningful text (in French) and at text spoken in a foreign language unknown to subjects provided a bilateral activation of the temporal poles, a region not activated in other activation studies (Figure 7). The role of these regions in language is still unknown but could relate either to the continuous aspect of the heard material or to some kind of familiarity of emotional content of this material compared to an unknown language.

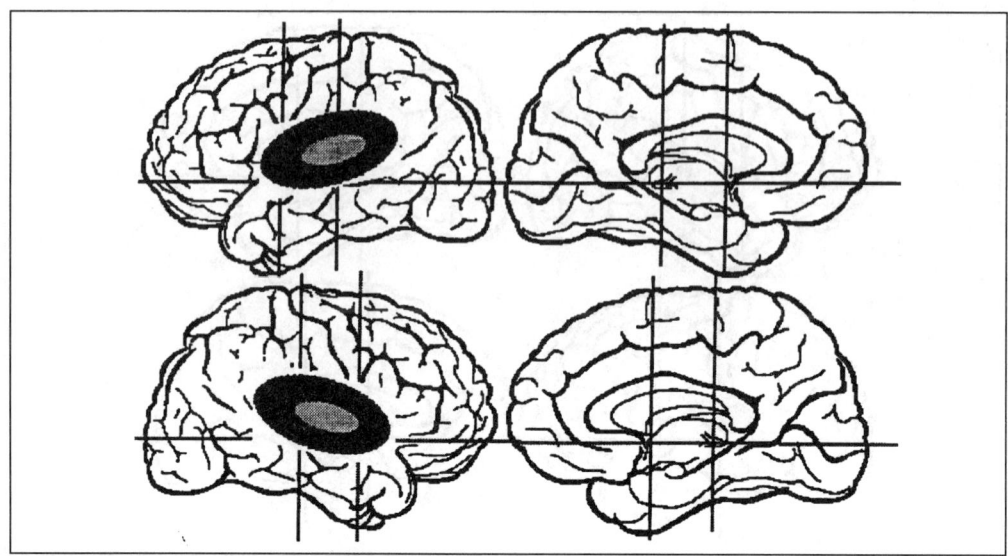

Figure 5. Paulesu *et al.*, 1993. Verbal working memory.

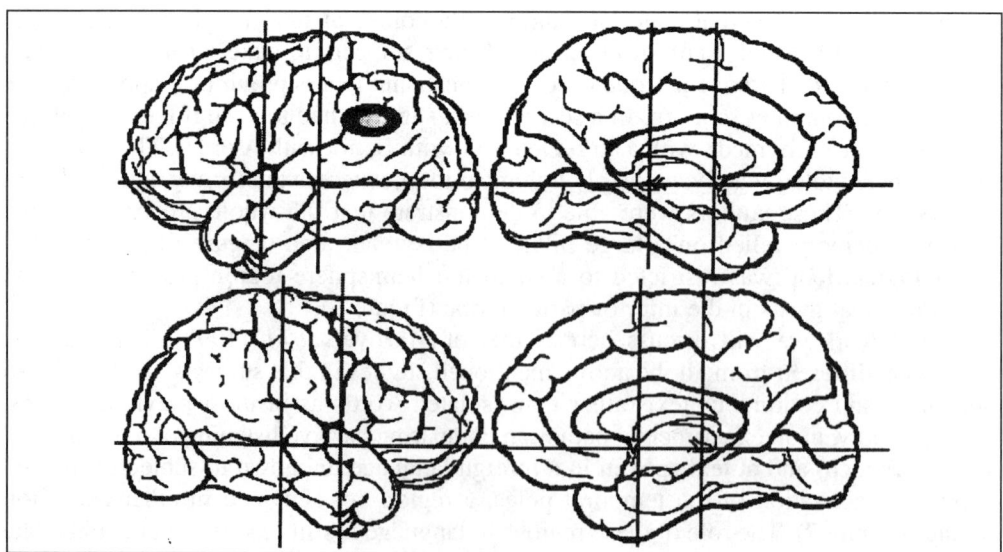

Figure 6. Paulesu *et al.*, 1993. Phonological store.

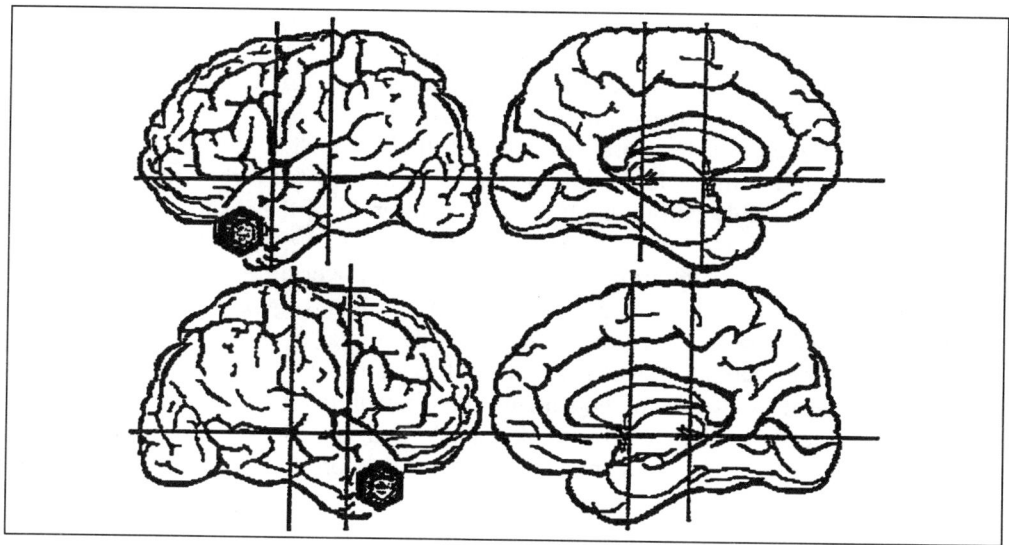

Figure 7. Mazoyer et al., 1993. Listening to story in French minus in Tamil.

Contributions of functional magnetic resonance imaging (fMRI) to the neuroanatomy of language functions

The advent of fMRI among modern means of functional neuroimaging has already allowed to replicate some of the PET results (McCarthy et al., 1993; Hinke et al., 1993; Lévrier et al., 1994; Binder et al., 1994). In this last section, we will summarize the potential advantages of the fMRI method over PET as applied to the functional anatomy of language.

One can grossly point out 3 main advantages of fMRI over PET scan.

First, fMRI is *totally innocuous*, since it is a technique without known biological risk (except claustrophobia), the signal being obtained directly, without contrast media, either radioactive or not. Second is *anatomical accuracy* : fMRI provides both anatomical and functional information for each individual with a spatial resolution of about 1-2 mm, which is clearly superior to PET.

Finally, *temporal resolution*, which theoretically is near to a few milliseconds, may allow much more precise exploration of neurofunctional events occurring «on line» during language processing.

Topics for fMIR research will thus try to take advantage of each of these characteristics.

For instance, taking advantage of the spatial resolution, it will be possible to define more accurately the actual boundaries of language areas: e.g. specificity of areas 44 and 22; involvement of the SMA; organization of « mediation areas » (Damasio) : differential locations for retrieving nouns of objects (animate and inanimate), colours, proper names, verbs... One of the objectives for future fMRI studies could also be to investigate the issue of interindividual variations in brain/language relationships: for instance, Bender *et al.* (1994) have shown large intra - and inter - hemispheric differences between subjects in degree of activation of the left superior temporal lobe when listening to various kinds of auditory stimuli.

Taking advantage of the temporal resolution will allow to study the effect of practice on brain activation : the role of hippocampal formation in verbal memory could probably be considerably enlightened, as well as the role of the insular cortex, which has been recently suspected in PET studies (Raichle *et al.*, 1994) : these authors, have studied changes in brain activation elicited by repetition over time of a verb generation task. The main result was a deactivation of the insular region when the subjects performed the task for the second time, whereas the initial pattern was recovered if a novel version of the same task was proposed subsequently.

The innocuousness of the method arises the possibility of longitudinal studies in some brain diseases such as recovery of aphasia and aphasic symptoms from focal lesions (role of the right hemisphere?, role of subcortical structures?) or some dementing conditions with predominant aphasic symptoms (so-called primary progressive aphasia).

Finally, fMRI may be used as a non-traumatic means of *in vivo* determination of cerebral dominance, an issue which, besides considerable theoretical importance, may have practical consequences if fMRI prove able to replace the much more invasive Wada test procedure.

To conclude, functional brain imaging of language is about to considerably modify our secular conceptions of brain language relationships: some concepts which were only based on inferences from brain-damaged subjects will probably be confirmed on the functioning brain itself, whereas others, even well-established and widely admitted, are already being modified. In return, functional studies of language may constitute one of the richest domains of application for future imaging studies as well as a good example of the complementarity between PET and fMRI.

References

1. Basso A, Lecours AR, Moraschini S, Vanier M. Anatomo-clinical correlations of the aphasias as defined through computerized tomography: on exceptions. *Brain Lang* 1985 ; 26, 201-229.
2. Binder JR, Rao SM, Hammeke TA, Yetkin FZ, Jesmanowicz A, *et al.* Functional magnetic resonance imaging of the human auditory cortex. *Ann. Neurol* 1994 ; 35, 662-672.
3. Damasio AR. Aphasia. New Engl. J. *Med* 1992 ; 326, 531-539.
4. Démonet JF, Chollet F, Ramsay S, Cardebat D, Nespoulous JL, Wise R, Rascol A, Frackowiak RSJ. The anatomy of phonological and semantic processing in normal subjects. *Brain* 1992 ; 115, 1753-1768.
5. Démonet JF, Wise R, Frackowiak RSJ. Language functions explored in normal subjects by positron emission tomography: a critical review. *Human Brain Mapping* 1993 ; 1, 39-47.
6. Frackowiak RSJ. Functional mapping of verbal memory and language. *TINS* 1994 ; 17 (3), 109-115.
7. Frith CD, Friston KJ, Liddle PF, Frackowiak RSJ. Willed action and the prefrontal cortex in man: a study with PET. *Proc. R. Soc. Lond. B* 1991 ; 244, 241-246.

8. Geschwind N. Specializations of the human brain. *Scientific American* 1979 ; 241 (3), 158-168.
9. Hinke RM, Hu X, Stillman AE, Kim SG, Merkle H, Saimi R, Ugurbil K. Functional magnetic resonance imaging of Broca's area during internal speech. *NeuroReport* 1993 ; 4, 675-678.
10. Joanette Y, Goulet P, Hannequin D. Right hemisphere and verbal communication. (Springer Verlag, New York) 1990.
11. Lévrier O, Sabbah P, Berry, I, Démonet JF, Habib M., Manelfe C, Salamon G. Functional magnetic resonance imaging of language. *Neuroradiology*, 36 (suppl. 1), 1994 ; 43-44.
12. McCarthy GM, Blamire AM, Rothman DL, Gruetter R, Shulman RG.Echo-planar magnetic resonance imaging studies of frontal cortex activation during word generation in humans. *Proc. Natl. Acad. Sci. USA* 1993 ; 90, 4952-4956.
13. Mazoyer BM, Tzourio N, Syrota A, Murayama N, Levrier O, Salamon G, Dehaene S, Cohen L, Mehler J. The cortical representation of speech. J. Cognitive *Neurosci* 1993 ; 5 (4), 467-479.
14. Paulesu E, Frith CD, Frackowiak RSJ.The neural correlates of the verbal component of working memory. *Nature* 1993 ; 362:342-344.
15. Petersen SE, Fox PT, Posner MI, Mintun M, Raichle ME. Positron emission tomographic studies of the cortical anatomy of single-word processing. *Nature* 1988 ; 331, 585-589.
16. Petersen SE, Fox PT, Posner MI, Mintun M, Raichle ME. Positron emission tomographic studies of the processing of single words. Journal of Cognitive *Neuroscience*s 1 1989 ; 153-170.
17. Petersen SE, Fox PT, Snyder AZ, Raichle ME. Activation of extrastriate and frontal cortical areas by visual words and word-like stimuli. *Science* 1990 ; 249, 1041-1044.
18. Sergent J. Brain-imaging studies of cognitive functions. *TINS* 1994 ; 17 (6), 221-227.
19. Tulving E, Kapur S, Markowitsch HJ, Craik FIM, Habib R, Houle S. Neuroanatomic correlates of retrieval in episodic memory: auditory sentence recognition. *Proc. Natl. Acad. Sci. USA* 1994 ; 91, 2012-2015.
20. Zatorre RJ, Evans AC, Meyer E, Gjedde A. Lateralization of phonetic and pitch discrimination in speech processing. *Science* 1992 ; 256, 846-849.

35

Proton MR spectroscopy in Parkinsonism

A. HEERSCHAP[1], J. C.M. ZIJLMANS[2], H.O.M. THIJSSEN[1],
A de KOSTER[1], M.W.I.M. HORSTINK[2]

*Departments of Diagnostic Radiology[1] and Neurology[2],
Faculty of Medical Sciences, University of Nijmegen,
Nijmegen, The Netherlands.*

In parkinsonism Idiopathic Parkinsons Disease (IPD) is recognized as the most frequent variant, but it also includes less frequent variants (parkinsonism plus) such as Multiple System Atrophy (MSA) [1]. Parkinsonism manifests itself clinically by akinesia, rigidity and tremor. Distinction between IPD and parkinsonism plus variants may not be trivial.

Usually IPD patients strongly respond to treatment with L-Dopa, while others respond less or not. Central in the progressive development of IPD is degeneration of the dopaminergic nigrostriatal tract [1,2]. Neuronal loss in the substantia nigra (mostly the pars compacta) leads to decreased dopamine content, mainly in the putamen, which is supposed to underlay defective motor performance in IPD patients.

With the increasing application of proton MR spectroscopy (^{1}H MRS) for metabolic monitoring in several human brain pathologies the question arises whether this approach might also be useful in the identification and characterization of Parkinsonian patients. In particular the affected brain areas listed above may show abnormal metabolic contents.

^{1}H MRS of parkinsonian patients have only recently been initiated and up till now in the literature just one study has been published [3] with another one in press [4]. Obviously, because of the small size of the substantia nigra ^{1}H MRS of this brain component is not as easy as it is has proven to be for other brain regions such as the basal ganglia, which therefore has been the target region in most MRS examinations of IPD patients. As yet studies have focused on the signals of 4 compounds in the brain that are relatively easy to observe by ^{1}H MRS : i.e the methylprotons of N-acetylaspartate (NAA), of creatine (Cr), of choline (Cho) and of lactate if this compound is sufficiently elevated.

In this report we will present some initial results of ^{1}H MRS of parkinsonian patients and briefly review (preliminary) results of others. Our aims were:

1. To identify possible spectral abnormalities in the basal ganglia and, because of occasional WM lesions, also in the deep white matter (centrum semiovale) of IPD patients.

2. Employing the results thus obtained as a basis to investigate whether ^{1}H MRS of patients suspected to suffer of Vascular Parkinsonism (VP) would show distinctive abnormalities such as lactate elevations [4]

3. Explore the feasibility of ^{1}H MRS of the substantia nigra area in IPD patients.

Materials and methods

MR examinations were performed on a Siemens MR system at 1.5 T - employing the standard circular polarized headcoil. For delineation of the volume of interest T2 weighted images were obtained in the coronal and transversal direction. Single volume MR spectra were acquired with a slice selective 90^0-180^0-180^0 pulse sequence (PRESS).

Experimental conditions for the striatum were : 8 cc nominal volume (2*2*2 mm) , Te = 135 ms, Tr = 2.5 s ; for the deep white matter (centrum semiovale) : 16 cc nominal volume (4*2*2 mm), Te = 135 ms , Tr = 2.5 s ; for the substantia nigra area : 3.4 cc nominal volume (1.5*1.5*1.5 mm), Te = 75 ms, Tr = 1.6 s. Spectroscopic imaging was performed within a 50 * 50 mm transversal slice of 15 mm thickness. This volume was also selected by PRESS at a Te of 135 ms to which phase encoding gradients were added for further spatial resolution to voxels of 1.5 - 2.0 cc.

Peak areas of MRS signals were obtained by fitting to a mixed Lorentzian-Gaussian model function. Data was further evaluated as metabolite signal ratios. For absolute quantification of MRS observed metabolites in the striatum and centrum semiovale the water signal was used as an internal standard and corrected for T2 weighting with available T2 values for metabolite and water signals for these areas.

Results

For the investigation of possible metabolic defects detectable by ^{1}H MRS in the basal ganglia a spectrum was obtained from an 8 cc volume centred on the putamen and globus pallidus. The ages of the IPD patients investigated in these areas ranged from 45 to 85 years (mean 64). Controls were selected in the same age range (mean 57 years). Evaluation of the ratios of the methylproton signals of NAA, Cr and Cho did not reveal a significant difference between IPD patients and controls for the lentiform nucleus. E.g. the average NAA/Cr ratio in controls was 1.70 ± 0.33 (n=14) and in IPD patients

1.55 ±0.30 (n=13). In addition no significant differences could be detected for metabolite contents estimated from the water content and MR signal from the same region. Although the population of patients and controls examined in the centrum semiovale was less (n= 6 and 4 respectively) also no obvious spectral abnormalities were detectable for this area in IPD patients. Furthermore, within the patient population investigated in this study, no significant relations between (relative) metabolite content and other particular conditions such as age and treatment was found.

Figure 1 shows an MR image of a transversal slice through the brain of a patient with VP together with the volume located at the centrum semiovale and spectra obtained from this volume. The top spectrum shows an inverted signal at 1.3 - 1.4 ppm typical for the methylprotons of lactate. This patient happened to have suffered from a transient ischemic attack about one week before the examination. The bottom spectrum was obtained 5 weeks later and shows a further reduced level of lactate. Upon examinations of more patients with VP (6 in the lentiform nucleus and 7 in the deep white matter) the presence of a lactate peak turned out to be an incidental finding. Also an evaluation of other MRS observable metabolite levels in these patients showed no clear abnormalities [4].

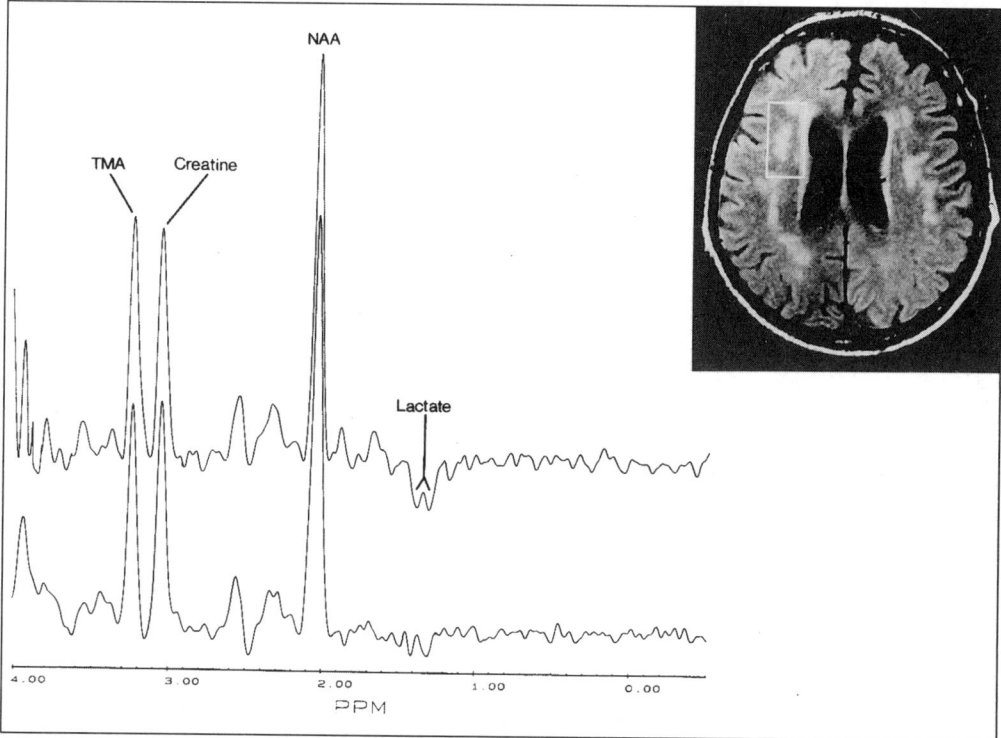

Figure 1. The MR image is obtained from a patient suspected to suffer from vascular parkinsonism. Two ^{1}H MRS spectra have been obtained from the volume shown on this image. The top spectrum was recorded one week after a transient ischemic attack and the lower spectrum 5 weeks later. Indicated are signals for TMA (= trimethylamines, mainly cholines), Creatine and NAA (N-Acetylaspartate) and Lactate. (Reproduced with permission from J. Zijlmans et al., Acta Neur Scan, 1994.)

Selection of a volume to obtain an MR spectrum of the substantia nigra is very difficult without a partial volume effect. To ensure that the whole substantia nigra was measured a cubic volume of 1.5*1.5*1.5 cm was selected in which the substantia nigra roughly had a diagonal orientation. Approximately 50 % of this volume was estimated to be occupied by surrounding tissue, mainly the red nucleus. In general shimming of this area was not a problem despite the assumed presence of accumulated iron in this region. Shimming failures (about 20 %, both for controls and patients) more likely seemed to be related to other factors such as movement. The evaluation of control and patient spectra with sufficient spectral quality (i.e. those with distinct signals for Cr and Cho) reveals a significant relative decrease of the methylproton signal of NAA. This is shown in Figure 2 for the average ratio of NAA/(Cr + Cho).

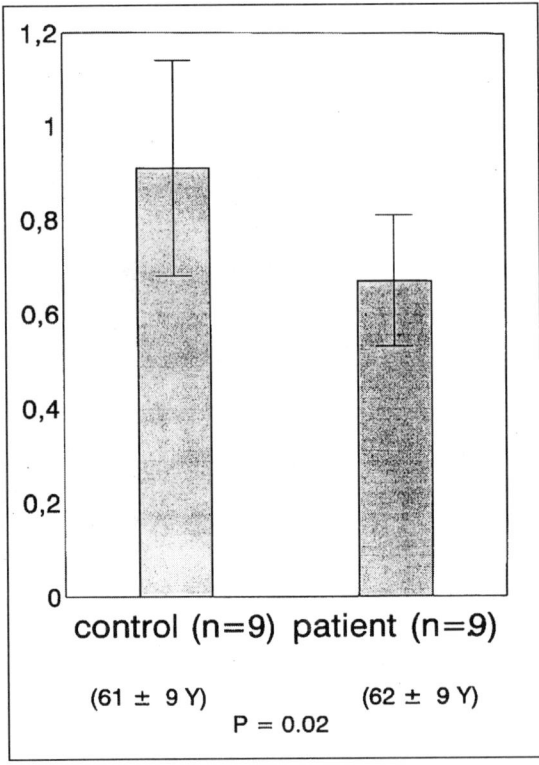

Figure 2. Ratio of NAA/(Cr + Cho) obtained from single voxel ^{1}H MRS measurements of the substantia nigra area. Standard deviations are indicated by bars.

In an attempt to obtain spectra with less partial volume effect we recently started to apply proton spectroscopic imaging techniques to the substantia nigra area with nominal volumes equal to or less than 2 cc. This approach has the additional advantage that matching of the MRS voxels with MR images can be optimized after the measurement. Figure 3 shows two spectra obtained of volumes centred on the substantia nigra area in a volunteer. In Figure 4 spectra are displayed of an IPD patient. The top two spectra, which are from the same regions as selected in the volunteer, show a relative reduced NAA methylproton signal and substantial linebroadening. Because most spectra from other locations in the preselected volume show no linebroadening (*see* the bottom spectrum which originates from a volume located more posteriorly) we assume this broadening is not due to movement artifacts.

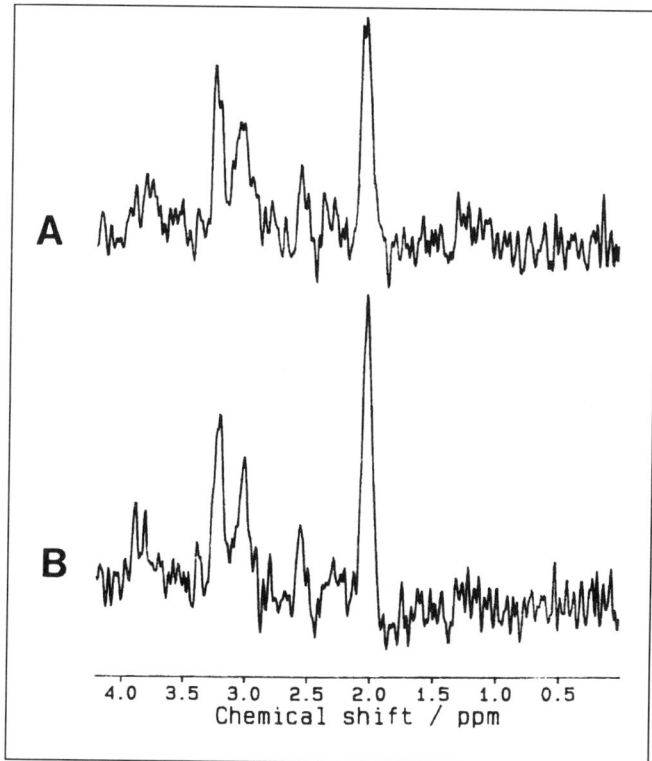

Figure 3. ¹H MRS spectra of 2 voxels (nominal volume 1.8 cc) of a spectroscopic imaging data set of a volunteer of 45 years old, one centred on the cerebral peduncle (A) and one on the pars compacta (B).

Discussion

In a number of studies it was found that IPD patients were not significantly different in their ¹H MRS detectable metabolic profiles of the basal ganglia compared to age matched controls [3 - 7]. This result was best documented in a multi-centre study of a large IPD patient and control population [5], although a tendency for a lower NAA/Cr and NAA/Cho is seen for IPD patients. This large data set may lend itself to analysis of more subtle relations between MRS detectable metabolites and for instance age, onset of symptoms, treatment and duration of treatment. In a recent study, investigating the striatum by ¹H MRS, again no significant difference was found between a group of IPD patients and controls with the exception of an elevated lactate level for severe IPD patients [6]. This latter finding is in contrast to most other studies in which no clear lactate signals were observable for this region.

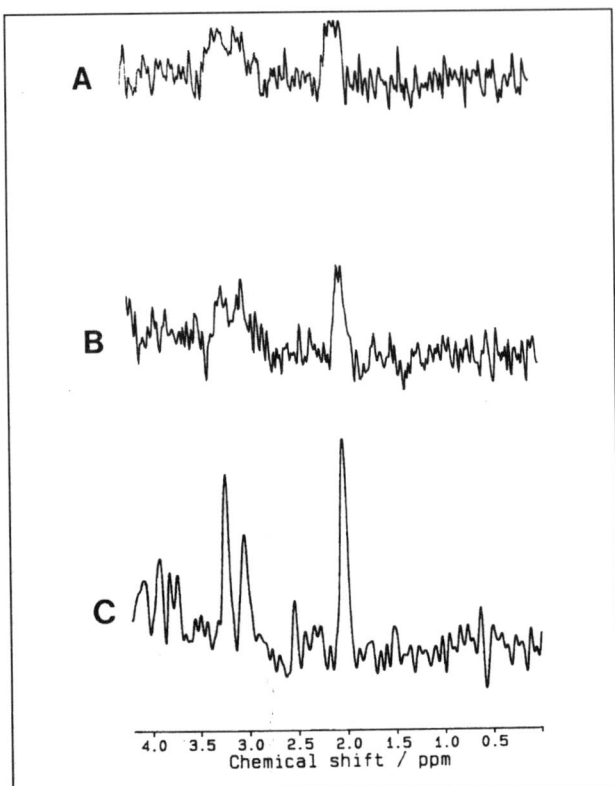

Figure 4. ¹H MRS spectra of 3 voxels (nominal volume 1.5 cc) of a spectroscopic imaging data set of an IPD patient of 74 years. The top 2 spectra have been obtained from volumes centred on the cerebral peduncle (A) and pars compacta (B) and the bottom spectrum (C) arises from a location more posteriorly (tectum).

Davie *et al* [3] find a significant reduction in the NAA to Cr signal ratio for MSA patients in the basal ganglia compared to controls and IPD patients. As NAA is assumed to be confined to neurons the authors suggest that this is due to neuronal cell loss in MSA, preferentially in the putamen. In our study of patients with VP (Zijlmans *et al.* [4]) no metabolic deviations were evident in ¹H MRS of the basal ganglia and deep white matter. Apparently, ischemia, if occurring in these patients in suspected brain regions, is not reflected in metabolic signs monitored by MRS (e.g. increased lactate).

To study the substantia nigra by MRS is more demanding because this brainstem component only occupies a volume of about 1.5 cc. Our single volume measurements of a brain area encompassing the substantia nigra revealed a significant reduction in the average relative NAA signal level for a group of IPD patients compared to age matched controls [7]. It seems most straightforward to explain this relative reduction as due to the well-known gross neuronal cell loss (and gliosis) in the substantia nigra of IPD patients [2]. Because of the large partial volume effect it cannot be excluded that this reduction is also related to a possibly more wide-spread relative decrease in NAA signal intensity in IPD brain such as (faintly) seen in some studies of the basal ganglia (*see above*). At this moment the large overlap of patient and control data precludes the clinical usefulness of this finding as far as diagnosis is concerned.

The proton spectroscopic imaging study of the substantia nigra area seems promising. The local line broadening observed in spectra of this area may be related to iron accumulation. This may have gone unnoticed in the single volume measurements due to a larger partial volume effect. Up till now we have been able to reproduce this result in one other patient; however, two younger IPD patients investigated in this way showed rather normal spectra in the substantia nigra area so that more studies are needed to establish the real meaning of these observations.

Conclusion

Proton MR spectroscopy of the brain in Parkinsonism has not yet brought readily discriminating markers to be used clinically, possibly with the exception of NAA reduction in the basal ganglia for MSA distinction. Obviously with the few investigations performed up till now it is much too early to come to a definitive conclusion about the value of this new approach.

References

1. Marsden. C. Parkinson's disease. *Lancet* 1990 ; 335, 948-955
2. Fearnley J, Lees A. Ageing and Parkinson's disease: Substantia nigra regional selectivity. *Brain* 1991 ; 114, 2283- 2301.
3. Davie C, Wenning G, Barker G, Brennan A, Quinn N, Miller D. MRS to differentiate multiple system atrophy from idiopathic Parkinson's disease. *Lancet* 1994 ; 342, 681-682.
4. Zijlmans J, Koster A de, Hof M van 't , Thijssen H, Horstink M, Heerschap A. Proton Magnetic Resonance spectroscopy in suspected vascular ischemic Parkinsonism. *Acta Neur Scan* 1994, in press
5. Holshouser B, Komu M, Möller H, Zijlmans J, Tosk J, Sonninen P, Marten, P van, Heerschap A, Kolem H. Single volume proton MR spectroscopy on patients with Parkinson's disease. A multicenter pilot study. *Proceedings SMRM* 1993, Abstract 235
6. Chen Y, Jenkins B, Fink S, Rosen. Evidence for impairment of energy metabolism in Parkinson's disease using in vivo localized MR spectroscopy. *Proceedings SMR* 1994, Abstract 194
7. Heerschap A, Zijlmans J, Koster A de, Thijssen H, Horstink M. Metabolite levels at three brain locations in Parkinsonism as viewed by proton MRS. *Proceedings SMRM* 1993, Abstract 234.

36

Functional imaging at 3 Tesla using interleaved EPI

F. HENNEL, N. BOLO, G. CROS, F. GIRARD, F. HODE, J.F. NEDELEC, J.P. MACHER

FORENAP, Centre Hospitalier, Rouffach, France.

Magnetic resonance imaging of brain function requires a measurement method providing images of moderate spatial resolution in a sub-second time and being sensitive to a parameter related to the cortical activity such as the blood oxygenation level. These requirements are fulfilled by interleaved echo-planar imaging (EPI). We present an application of a variant of this method, interleaved asymmetric EPI, to functional imaging of the motor cortex in the magnetic field of 3 Tesla and using a standard whole-body gradient system.

Functional magnetic resonance imaging (FMRI) of the brain employs the phenomenon of the increase of local blood oxygenation in the activated areas of the cortex [1]. The variation of blood oxygenation, i.e. the variation of the concentration ratio of oxygenated haemoglobin to deoxygenated haemoglobin can be detected by magnetic resonance imaging methods sensitive to local homogeneity of the static magnetic field i.e. to the apparent transverse relaxation time $T2^*$ [2]. Such methods require a long evolution time, 30 to 40 ms, between the excitation and the gradient echo. This limits the minimal repetition time of an experiment with single gradient echo acquisition, like FLASH [3] so that the entire experiment lasts several seconds, longer than the time constant of the haemodynamic response to cortex activity. The measurement can be accelerated by shifting the gradient echo beyond the next excitation (ES-FLASH, [4]) but this solution reduces the signal amplitude. A different strategy is used in echo-planar imaging (EPI) where the entire 2-dimensional data matrix is acquired using a single excitation and a train of gradient echoes [5]. The $T2^*$ contrast of the image is determined by the time between the excitation and the scan of the central data line, which contains most of the signal power. The drawback of EPI is that an inhomogeneity of the static magnetic field causes a distortion of the image. Especially at high fields, where strong inhomogeneities are produced by the shape of the head, such distortions are severe unless the EPI sequence is executed extremely fast using very strong gradients. For example at the field of 3T a gradient strength of 40 mT/m with a switching time of 200 microseconds is necessary to acquire an acceptable image with 2 mm resolution. The acquisition time of such image is about 50 milliseconds, much faster than really necessary for an FMRI experiment.

A good compromise between the measurement speed and the sensitivity to magnetic field homogeneity can be reached by dividing the EPI sequence to several shots, each scanning one interleaf of the data matrix [6]. Interleaved EPI (IEPI) does not require high gradient amplitudes nor the short switching times and can be performed using standard clinical systems, which are usually equipped with 10 mT/m gradients with 1 ms switching [7]. We describe the application of a variant of this technique, called interleaved asymmetric EPI [8] to functional imaging of human motor cortex.

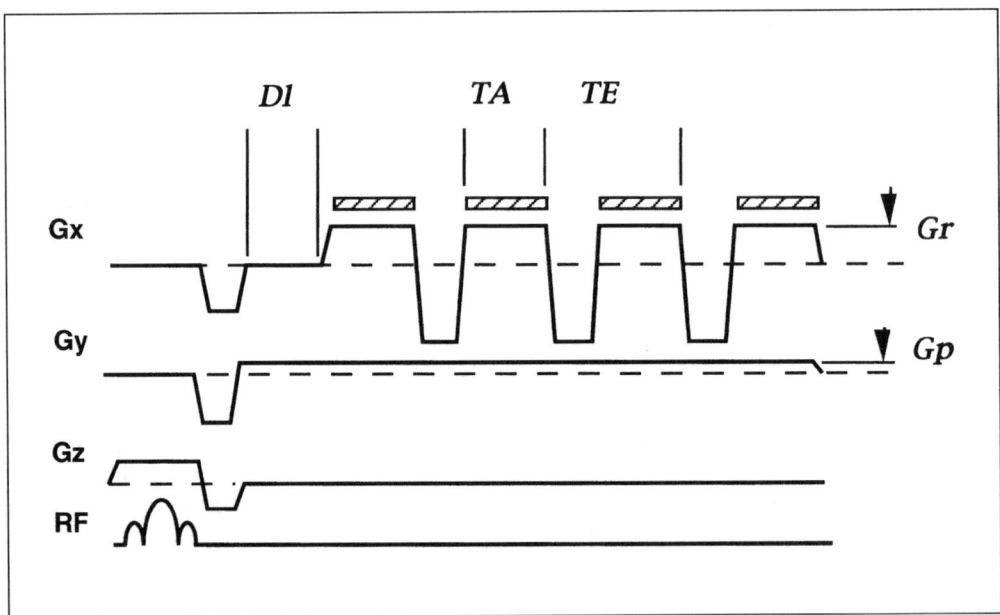

Figure 1. Gradient and radio frequency (RF) pulse sequence used in the interleaved asymmetric echo-planar imaging method.

Methods

The imaging sequence

The sequence involves a slice selective excitation followed by the typical EPI gradient wave form: the readout gradient (G_x) is oscillating and the phase encoding gradient (G_y) is constant (Figure 1). Analogically to ABEST [9], the signal acquisition takes place during the positive gradient pulses. Their amplitude depends on the field of view and sampling rate. The negative amplitude of the readout gradient is set to maximum to reduce the distance between gradient echoes, T_E. The length of the negative pulses is adjusted for a zero integral in each period. In each scan R gradient echoes are recorded. The experiment consists of $n = N_y / R$ scans where N_y is the size of the data matrix in the phase encoding direction. A variable delay D_l is placed between the excitation and the gradient echo train, the value of which in the l-th scan is

$$D_l = l \frac{T_E}{n} \qquad (1)$$

The role of this delay in the blipped IEPI was to smooth the off-resonance modulation of the data matrix, and thus to reduce ghosting artifacts [10]. In the present sequence, additionally, Dl controls the interleaving of partial scans. The Fourier domain trajectory of each scan, defined by [11]

$$\mathbf{k}(t) = \frac{\gamma}{2\pi} \int_0^t \mathbf{G}(\tau) \, d\tau, \qquad (2)$$

where $\mathbf{G}$ is the magnetic field gradient and γ the gyromagnetic ratio, is a zigzag line with a period of $\gamma G_p T_E / 2\pi$. Since the phase encoding gradient G_p is on during the incremented delay D_l, the trajectories of consecutive scans are shifted by the step

$$\Delta k_y = \frac{\gamma \, G_p T_E}{2\pi \, n} \qquad (3)$$

In this way, the parts of the trajectories on which the acquisition takes place become interleaved and form a «shear grid» tilted with respect to the k_x axis by the angle $\alpha = \arctan (G_p / G_r)$.

An application of the discrete 2D Fourier transform to a data set obtained on such a grid would give an image distorted by a shear in the phase encoding direction whereby neighbouring lines are shifted by T_A/RT_E pixels [8]. To avoid this effect the Fourier transformation must be performed first in the phase encoding direction (columns), then each row has to be modulated by the frequency corresponding to its shift and finally the transformation of rows can be executed.

Experimental parameters

The method of interleaved echo-planar imaging with asymmetric readout gradient waveform and the acquisition of odd gradient echoes was implemented on a whole body MR imager (Bruker S300) with a 3 Tesla magnet and an actively shielded gradient system capable of producing 10 mT/m with the switching time of 1 ms.

The method was used with the following parameters: a 128 x 128 matrix, 25 cm x 25 cm field of view, 5 mm slice thickness, 25° excitation tip angle, 8 gradient echoes per shot, and 50 kHz sampling frequency, repetition time of 64 ms. The acquisition time of one image was 1 second. The effective gradient echo time was 30 ms.

The functional paradigm involved periods of 16 seconds, each divided to the resting state part (8 sec) and the active state (8 sec). One image per second was acquired. The activation task was sequential tapping of the thumb to the opposing fingers of the left or right hand. A healthy right handed volunteer was examined. The slice containing active cortex zones was chosen based on preliminary functional measurements, measurements with two periods in which the average resting state image was subtracted from the average active state image to check whether a signal increase is present. The final measurement on the selected slice was performed twice, for the left and for the right hand finger movement, with 18 periods (2 minutes, 128 images). The activation maps were calculated by taking the magnitude of the Fourier transform of each pixel's intensity course at the frequency of the stimulus (1/16 Hz). This procedure is suitable for paradigms with repetitive tasks because it is not sensitive to a phase shift of the response [12].

Figure 2. Image obtained in 1 second using interleaved asymmetric EPI (A) and maps of brain activation during a finger movement of the left hand (B) and right hand (C).

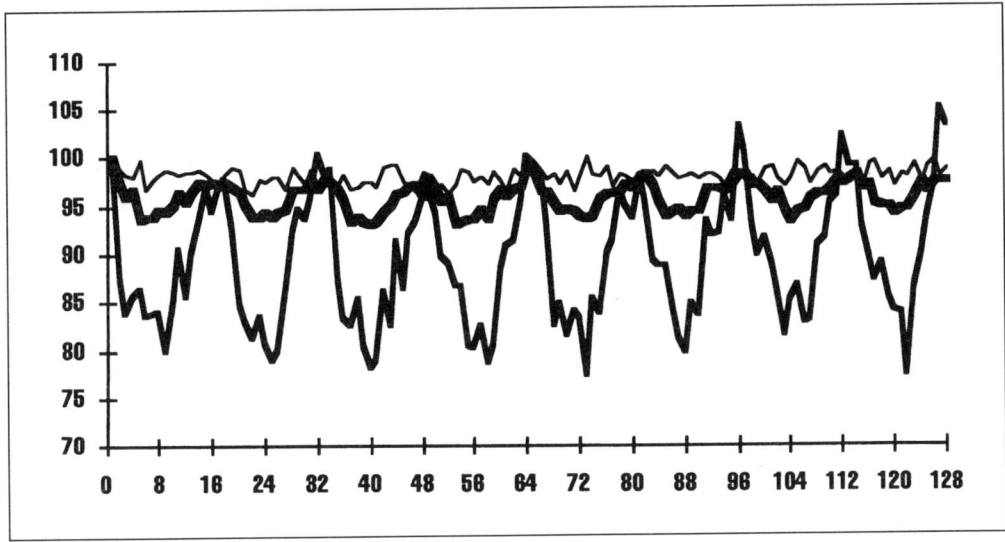

Figure 3. Pixel intensity variation during the experiment with the left hand finger movement: average of an arbitrarily chosen zone in the white matter (thin line), average of the active zone (thick line) and the pixel of strongest response in the active zone (medium line).

Results and discussion

Figure 2.A shows one interleaved EPI image of the selected slice. The image is mainly T2* weighted which is visible from the dark appearance of veins. No ghosting artefacts are visible. The signal-to-noise ration for the brain tissue is 40. The activation maps obtained for the right and the left hand are presented in figs. 2.B and 2.C, respectively. No artefacts are visible. In agreement with many previous studies of the same activation task [13] the contralateral arrangement of active sensory-motor zones is visible. However, it has not been verified to what extend the effect is related to pial veins and to the capillary bed. Within the clearly distinguishable zone in the right hemisphere a small group of pixels shows an intensity variation of 20%. This is higher than predicted by the capillary model [14] and should be attributed to a presence of a vein. The remaining pixels vary at a 5% level and may therefore represent capillary regions.

The method of interleaved asymmetric EPI proves to be a useful tool for functional imaging of the human head. Because only odd gradient echoes are sampled, the images are artefact-free without the necessity of tedious adjustments or calibration scans as in the standard EPI. The use of the asymmetric readout allows to improve the duty cycle of the sequence and to keep a reasonable signal to noise ratio. The method is sensitive enough to detect 1% signal intensity variations over a time of two minutes, which is the condition to see the functional response related to capillaries. It can be implemented on clinical imagers equipped with standard gradient systems. With the installation of an

EPI gradient insert the interleaved method should provide 1 mm resolution images in less than a second while still keeping a very low level of image distortion.

References

1. Kwong KK *et al. Proc. Natl. Acad. Sci. USA* 1992 ; 89 : 5675-9.
2. Ogawa *et al. Magn Reson Med* 1990 ; 14 : 68.
3. Haase A *et al. J Magn Reson* 1986 ; 67 : 258.
4. Liu G *et al. Magn Reson Med* 1993 ; 30 : 68.
5. 1. Mansfield P, *J Phys C: Solid State Phys* 1977 ; 10 : L55-8.
6. McKinnon GC, *Magn Reson Med* 1993 ; 30 : 609-16.
7. Butts K *et al. Magn Reson Med* 1994 ; 31 : 67-72.
8. Hennel F, Nédélec JF, *Magn Reson Med* 1995 in press
9. Feinberg DA *et al. Magn Reson Med* 1990 ; 13 : 162-9.
10. Feinberg DA, Oshio K, *Magn Reson Med* 1994 ; 32 : 535-9.
11. Liunggren S, *J Magn Reson* 1983 ; 54 : 338-43.
12. Lee AT *et al. Magn Reson Med* 1995 ; 33 : 745.
13. Kim SG *et al. Science* 1993 ; 26 : 615-7.
14. Ogawa S *et al. Biophys J*; 1993 ; 64 : 803-12.

37

How to improve fast imaging?

J. HENNIG

Klinikum der Albert-Ludwigs-Universität Freiburg,
Abt. Röntgendiagnostik,
MR-Tomographie,
Hugstetterstrasse 55,
79106 Freiburg,
Germany.

The basic problem of fast MR-imaging is the fact that the MR image, a two-dimensional entity, has to be reconstructed from the intrinsically one-dimensional MR signal. Even if all hardware restrictions are neglected, the sampling of data for a n x n image matrix then requires consecutive sampling of n x n time domain data. A well-known theorem of signal theory states that the noise of the signal is inversely proportional to the square root of the sampling frequency. The ultimate speed of MR-imaging is thus limited by signal-to-noise considerations even with infinitely fast gradients.

Practical limits are of course set by the speed, with which the magnetic field gradients necessary to encode spatial information into the MR signal, can be switched. Practically all imaging techniques used for clinical MR today use two-dimensional image reconstruction (2DFT) techniques. The domain in which the time domain data are sampled is called k-space. Reconstruction for a n x n image matrix thus requires sampling nxn time domain data points, which cover the whole area of the corresponding k-space.

Basically there are two possibilities by which spins can be moved across k-space: the application of a magnetic field gradient will lead to a monotonous path across k-space. A constant gradient will lead to motion along a straight line along the direction of the gradient, a gradient reversal will reverse the motion.

The second possibility is the application of a refocussing pulse. This will lead to a jump of the k-space trajectory to the mirror point at the origin. All imaging techniques use combinations of these two principles in order to generate their respective k-space trajectories.

Conventional 2DFT-imaging uses a gradient prewinder pulse in the read direction in order to bring magnetization to its starting point. A phase encoding pulse is used to select a certain line. Data are then read out line by line under a constant read gradient while the phase encoding gradient is varied from one acquisition step to the next. Depending on whether the signal is generated as a spin echo or a gradient echo and whether the various phase encoding lines are read out after successive excitations or by repeating the echo generation process after a single excitation pulse, all fast imaging sequences in use today can be sorted into four categories shown in Figure 1, where the Burst sequence, which generates n echoes after a pulse burst is added as a fifth possibility.

	multishot sequences		single shot sequences		
	spin echo	gradient echo	RARE (FSE, TSE)	EPI	Burst
RF-pulses (in deg) gradients (m = # of proj)	m (90 + 180) 5 m	mα (α<10) 4 m	90 + mα (30<α<180) 2 + 4 m	90 m + 3	mα (α<10) 3
limitations	**SAR** **Grad**	**SAR** **Grad**	**SAR** **Grad**	**Grad**	**SAR**
intrinsic timescale	T1, T2	T1, T2, T2*	T2	T2*	T1, T2

Figure 1. Table of fast imaging techniques and their performance parameters. a corresponds to the flip angle, SAR refers to limitations with respect to RF absorption, Grad to gradient power requirements.

Figure 1 lists the relevant parameters of these sequences, which determine the acquisition speed and also the image contrast. It is clearly seen, that multishot spin echo sequences are unlikely candidates for fast imaging due to the number of gradients used and the high degree of RF irradiation. Single shot RARE or hybrid RARE, which uses n/ne excitations with ne differently phase encoded echoes each, offers the possibility to reduce the acquisition time to 1/ne of the corresponding conventional spin echo sequence while maintaining the extremely good imaging properties of the basic spin echo sequence. It is extremely robust and stable and insensitive to artefacts due to magnetic field inhomogeneity; chemical shift, etc. The image contrast thus is determined by the relaxation times T1, T2 and the experimental parameters tr (recovery time) and te (echo time) alone. This extremely stable contrast behaviour at a reasonable overall examination time of several seconds to 1-4 minutes has made RARE (Fast Spin Echo, turbo Spin Echo...) the most commonly used imaging sequence for clinical diagnosis today.

Single shot RARE with conventional gradients lead to images, which due to their very heavy T2-contrast display liquid-filled structures alone. The scarcity of such structures allows the application without slice selection gradient to generate projection images of CSF-filled spaces (MR-myelography and MR-ventriculography), the urinary system (MR-urography) and - most recently - the biliary ducts (MR-cholangiography).

Fast gradient systems available today also allow the generation of single shot images of soft tissue structures. The most important clinical application of these techniques is likely to be breathhold imaging of the abdomen, where 20 slices can be acquired within one breathhold.

Multishot gradient echo yields much higher signal-to-noise at short recovery times compared to spin echo sequences. Fast imaging using this technique (Snapshot FLASH, turbo FLASH) is thus feasible. In contrast-based diagnostic imaging this sequence has, however, found only limited applications due to the fact that the image contrast is influenced by many and sometimes unpredictable parameters like fat/water-composition, susceptibility effects, etc. Much more pronounced are applications of gradient echo imaging techniques in examinations related to function. The possibility to use these techniques to look at flowing spins has led to the application in MR angiography. Of increasing importance are also examinations of the first pass effect after bolus injection of contrast agent for measuring tissue perfusion.

The single shot variant of gradient echo is echo planar imaging, which in fact is the oldest of all fast imaging techniques. Due to the very strong chemical-shift and susceptibility sensitivity of this sequence its use for diagnostic imaging is practically precluded. It has, however, began in recent years to find applications in parametric imaging to generate diffusion and perfusion images and - probably most important - for studies in brain activation. The Burst-sequence finally is intrinsically the fastest of all techniques due to the very low number of gradient switching steps required. The basic sequence and also its offsprings DUFIS, OUFIS, QUEST, etc., suffer, however, from low signal-to-noise and have only recently been introduced to clinical use to study perfusion using three-dimensional data acquisition.

Apart from these pure sequences a number of hybrids have been introduced with mixed success. Multishot gradient echo techniques with two or more gradient echoes have been used for chemical shift - and susceptibility - imaging. GRASE (gradient and spin echo) - imaging is a hybrid between RARE and EPI and leads to acquisition times in the range between the two generic sequences (100-400 ms).

Even with hypothetical improvements in gradient performance in the future it is unlikely that the acquisition time for a 256x256 high resolution image for diagnostic application can be brought much below the current limit of 200-500 ms. Although the pure imaging speed of i.e. EPI allows already faster scanning even today, the physical resolution for such scans is much lower than the nominal resolution due to T2*-dependent image blurring.

If faster acquisition times are acquired, other strategies have to be applied. The basic tenet of such strategies is the fact that not all that much changes in an image, if the image repetition time is sufficiently short. This allows the use of prior knowledge to reduce the amount of data necessary to update consecutive images. One such approach, which is already in clinical use today is keyhole imaging, which is based on the fact that the data relevant for image contrast are located at the center of k-space whereas its outer portions encode for edge information. If a series of measurements is made, where only the signal intensity is expected to vary, while the image plane remains the same, it is thus sufficient to update only the data at the center of k-space and to use the data from a reference scan acquired prior to the time-resolved acquisition for reconstruction of high-resolution images at short imaging times. One such typical example is the use of keyhole gradient echo imaging for first pass measurements of perfusion. For other applications other strategies for updating k.-space data are more appropriate. If changes are known to occur only at a previously known discrete area within an image, sampling of regularly spaced k-space lines, is much more appropriate and leads to an update of the relevant stripe of the image. Further improvements of this technique are possible, if more elaborate models of the un-sampled data are used.

All these techniques till are based on the concept of k-space data. Radically different approaches are possible, if data are encoded using approaches different from Fourier techniques. Wavelet encoding offers the possibility to acquire images with anisotropic resolution and thus allows focusing the acquisition to a particular area of interest. It suffers, however, from a low sampling efficiency compared to Fourier techniques. Singular value decomposition (SVD) allows the reconstruction of sharp images from only 16-32 projections. Its main problem is the development of feasible imaging techniques, which allow top bring the theoretical advantages of this approach into practice.

For functional imaging - the topic of this workshop - their are currently two methods it use, both of which reely on the BOLD (= blood oxygen level dependent) contrast to study activation effects. One uses gradient echo planar imaging (EPI), a fast imaging technique which still requires dedicated and expensive MR systems. On routine scanners such experiments can be performed using gradient echo sequences with long echo times. The nature of the contrast mechanism requires systems with a minimum of 1,5T field strength in order to measure reliable effects.

The advantage of EPI is of course its short acquisition time of 60-100 ms per image. Disadvantages are the high cost and the limited spatial resolution, which can even theoretically only be improved at the cost of lowering signal-to-noise.

Advantages of gradient echo techniques are the widespread availability and the high spatial resolution. Disadvantages are the sensitivity to motion artefacts and to false positive results from vascular signals. Effects higher than 6 % and results obtained with flipangles above 30 degrees should thus be strongly distrusted.

Improvements to make volumetric activation studies available with routine systems are the MUSIC (= multislice interleaced acquisition) - sequence and modifications of singe shot RARE-techniques.

To conclude, improvements in fast imaging are currently achieved by new developments in hardware and software. The basic sequences are known, but advances in gradient hardware bring them to reality on state-of-the-art system. Computers forn image reconstruction approach the demand for real-time imaging. Software developments, which incorporate new ideas based on the use of previous knowledge are still lacking as well as efficient implementations of totally new reconstruction techniques like wavelet encoding or SVD-based approaches.

38

Enhanced brain structure delineation in the rodent by diffusion weighted imaging

P.D. Hockings[1], D.C. Harrison[2], D.A. Middleton[3], D.G. Reid[3], D.M. Doddrell[1]

[1] Centre for Magnetic Resonance, University of Queensland, 4072, Australia.
[2] Biophysical Sciences, SmithKline Beecham Pharmaceuticals, New Frontiers Science Park, 3rd Avenue, Harlow, Essex CM19 5AW, UK.
[3] Analitycal Sciences, SmithKline Beecham Pharmaceuticals, The Frythe, Welwyn, Herts.

In the rodent brain it is comparatively difficult to discriminate between white and grey matter using MRI. Thus, while spin-echo images are excellent for delineating the major brain structures much of the fine structure is MRI invisible. Recently, a number of groups have shown that anisotropic diffusion of water in normal brain white matter of cats and humans can be used to determine the orientation in space of myelin fibres [1,2,3]. We have made use of the anistoropy of white matter in diffusion weighted images of gerbil brain to visualise white fibre tracts. The primary purpose of this work was to improve the MRI representation of rodent neuroanatomy.

Materials and methods

MR images were acquired on a Bruker AMX 300 spectrometer interfaced to a 89 mm 7 T vertical magnet system. A gradient strenght of up to 5 G/cm was available by pulsing the room temperature shims. A Bruker Image Directed Spectroscopy RF probe was employed. It consisted of a birdcage resonator (id 42 mm) for excitation and a decoupled surface coil (diameter 12 mm) acting as receiver. A set of 4 multi-slice diffusion weighted images were acquired simultaneously using a modified T_2 weighted, D2 FT sequence with TE 82 ms and a recycle time of 2 s. Diffusion gradients (5 G/cm) interpulse delay, b value 1860 s/mm^2). Images were acquired with 256x256 resolution and zero-filled to 512x512 pixels. A 2 cm field of view and 1.0 mm slice thickness was used. Thus, the in-plane resolution was 78 µm. For the T_2 weighted images one average per phase increment was collected and for the diffusion weighted images 4 averages per phase increment were collected.

Results

A horizontal spin-echo image was first acquired to act as a scout for the positioning of slices in the transverse plane. This is shown in Figure 1 together with the localion of the 4 contiguous slices in the transverse plane. In the scout image only gross structures such as ventricles and to some extent the corpus callosum is visible. Figures 2 et 3 contrast the structures visible in the standard T_2 weighted images with those visible in diffusion weighted images. There is also a marked change in contrast depending on the direction of the diffusion weighting. With the diffusion gradient in the phase direction, signal attenuation will be greatest for fibres running horizontally across the page, i.e. the same direction as the diffusion gradient. Similarly, with the diffusion gradient in the slice direction attenuation will be greatest for fibres running orthogonal to the place of the image.

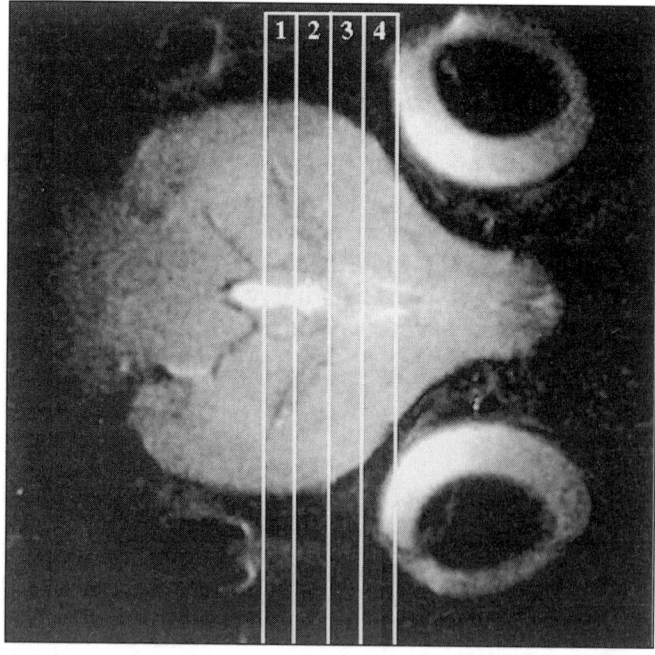

Figure 1. Spin echo scout image of the gerbil brain. TE 60 ms and TR 600 ms.

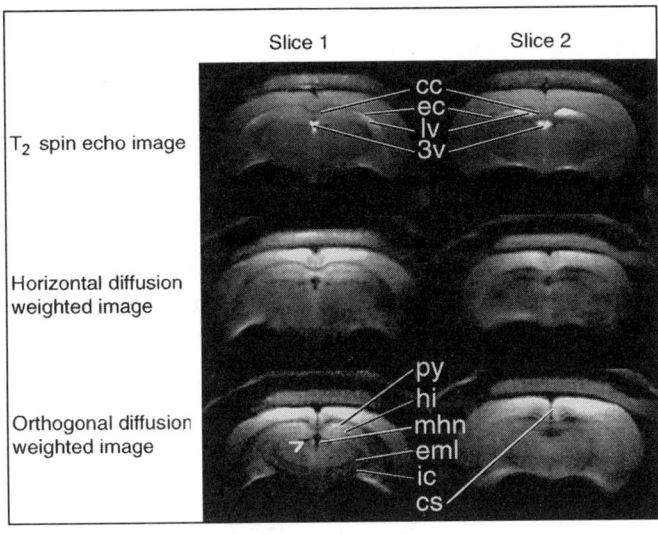

Figure 2. MR images of slices 1 and 2 through a gerbil brain.

Figure 3. MR images of slices 3 and 4 through a gerbil brain. < blood vessels, **3v** : third ventricle, **ac** : anterior commissure, **bnst** : bed nucleus of the stria terminalis, **cc** : corpus callosum **cs** : central sulcus, **ec** : external capsule, **eml** : external medullary lamina, **hi** : hippocampus, **ic** : internal capsule, **lv** : lateral ventricles, **mhn** : medial habenular nucleus, **oc** : optic hiasm, **on** : optic nerve, **poa** : pre-optic area, **py** : pyramidal layer.

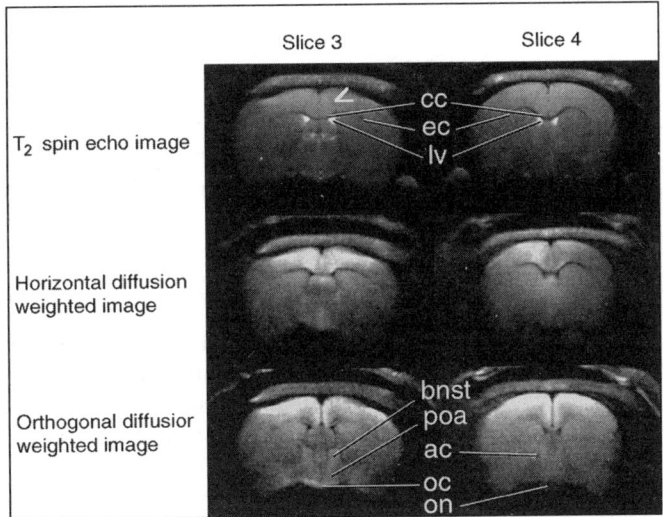

Corpus callosum and external capsule

This structure can be seen running through all 4 transverse slices in the standard T_2 weighted images. Contrast in enhanced in the horizontal diffusion weighting image as neurons in the **corpus callosum** run primarily in the transverse plane of the brain causing signal attenuation. For the same reason in the images with orthogonal diffusion weighting the corpus callosum appears lighter than the surrounding tissue. The **external capsule** visible in slice 1 is hypointense in both of the diffusion weighted images.

Ventricles

These have an intense bright appearance in the T_2 weighted images and are dark in the diffusion weighted images.

Hippocampus

The **hippocampus** is more clearly delineated from the surrounding structures in both of the diffusion weighted images owing to the contrast with the external capsule dorsally, and ventrally by the discontinuity between the hippocampus and the thalamus. Some of the internal structure of the hippocampus can also be seen and the brighter areas may correspond to the pyramidal layer of **Ammons's Horn**.

Thalamus and hypothalamus

In the ortogonal diffusion weighted image, the fibres of the **internal capsule** and **external medullary lamina** can be distinguished, as can some nuclei such as the **medial habenular**, in slice 1, and the **pre-optic area** and **bed nucleus of the stria terminalis** in slice 3.

Anterior commissure

This fibre tract can be seen in the orthogonal diffusion weighted image of slice 4, where the fibres run rostro-caudally beneath the lateral ventricles.

Cranial nerve

The **optic nerve** and **optic chiasm** appear in both diffusion weighted images of slices 3 and 4. Anisotropy of the nerve fibre bundles is quite evident from the disparity of the signal intensity of the two diffusion weighted images. In addition, other fibre bundles are visible on the ventral surface of the brain, corresponding to **cranial nerves** that have not been identified.

Cortex

The only structure visible in the cortex is a layer located bilateraly, close to the midline and immediatley above the corpus collosum that appears dark in the orthogonal diffusion weighted images and light in the horizontal diffusion weighted images. The **central sulcus** dividing the cortical hemispheres is not visible in T_2 weighted images, light in the horizontal diffusion weighted images and dark in the in orthogonal diffusion weighted images in all slices.

Blood vessels

In the T_2 weighted images of slices 1 and 2 there are clearly two small blood vessels running rostro-caudally on either side of the third ventricle. There are also visible in the diffusion weighted images. In the cortex a number of small blood vessels are also apparent in slices 3 and 4.

Discussion

The improved anatomical definition provided by diffusion weighted imaging will allow better identification of areas or structures within the brain. This will enable more precise characterisation of damage in models of brain disorders, such as the gerbil bilateral carotid artery occlusion model of global ischeamia, where damage may be diffuse and the lesion lacks a clear boundary of its own.

39

Fluorine MRS in human brain

R. A. KOMOROSKI [1,2] J. E. NEWTON [2,3] C. HEIMBERG [2,4] C. N. KARSON [2,4]

[1] *Departments of Radiology, Pathology, Biochemistry,*
[2] *Department of Psychiatry,*
[3] *Department of Pediatrics*
University of Arkansas for Medical Sciences, 4301 West Markham
St. John L. McClellan Memorial VA Hospital,
[4] *Little Rock, AR 72205, USA.*

Rationale

Drug response and side effects depend, in part, on the concentration at the receptor sites in the cells of the target organ. Measuring blood levels is an easy and inexpensive method to determine drug concentration. However, the plasma concentration of a drug may not reflect the concentration at the active site and there can be large variations in plasma pharmacokinetics arising from individual differences in physiologic function, disease state, diet, and other factors [1].

It is possible to measure drug concentrations *in vivo* in the target organ using NMR spectroscopy. Drug metabolism can be probed if metabolite resonances are resolved. Because it is noninvasive, repeat measurements in the same individual may permit testing of pharmacokinetic and pharmacodynamic models of drug response.

19F NMR of drugs

Fluorine-19 is a sensitive, spin-1/2 isotope which is advantageous for *in vivo* studies of drugs because of the absence of background signal, relatively narrow lines, short spin-lattice relaxation times (T_1), and high sensitivity (83% that of ^1H). Many drugs, including numerous psychoactive agents, have fluorine as a part of their molecular structure (Table I). Some of these drugs, particularly those containing trifluoromethyl groups, have both a low fluorine equivalent weight (Table I) and can reach sufficient concentration in the brain to be detectable *in vivo* by ^{19}F MRS. It is not possible to give a definitive minimum tissue concentration which can be detected by in vivo ^{19}F NMR spectroscopy. Several factors, including magnetic field strength, line width, T_1, and volume of tissue sampled will determine the minimum detectable concentration [2]. The typical *in vivo* concentration will be about 10 times that necessary *in vitro*, and for ^{19}F will be about 0.05-0.1 mM [2].

Table 1. Psychoactive drugs containing fluorine.

Generic Name	Trade Name	No. F Atoms	F Equiv. Wt.*
ANTIDEPRESSANTS			
Fluoxetine	Prozac	3	115
Fluvoxamine	Floxyfral, Faverin	3	145
Paroxetine	Paxil	1	366
ANTIPSYCHOTICS			
Penfluridol	Semap	5	
Trifluperidol	Triperidol, Trisedyl	4	149
Flupenthixol	Fluanxol, Depixol	3	
Fluphenazine	Prolixin, Permitil	3	170
Oxaflumazine	Oxaflumine	3	
Trifluoperazine	Stelazine	3	160
Triflupromazine	Vesprin	3	130
Pimozide	Orap	2	231
Fluspiriline	Imap, Redeptin	2	
Droperidol	Fentanyl, Innovar	1	
Fluperlapine		1	
Haloperidol	Haldol	1	376
Sertindole		1	
HYPNOTICS			
Quazepam	Doral	4	
Halazepam	Paxipam	3	118
Flunitrazepam	Rohypnol	1	
Flurazepam	Dalmane	1	461
Midazolam	Versed	1	
ANORECTICS			
Fenfluramine	Pondimine	3	
Flutiorex		3	

* Molecular weight/No. equivalent F atoms.

^{19}F NMR of psychoactive drugs *in vivo*

Trifluoperazine

In most cases, plasma concentrations of drugs used in the treatment of mental illnesses provide little useful information concerning clinical response and side effects [3]. Animal studies first pointed to NMR spectroscopy for the *in vivo* measurement of antipsychotic agents such as trifluoperazine (TFP) and fluphenazine [4-8]. Fluorinated drugs were subsequently detected in human brain by us [9,10] and others [8,11,12]. The initial human studies were typically limited by very low signal-to-noise (S/N) ratio *in vivo*, even at very high oral doses. Precise quantitation, accurate spatial localization (even to whole brain), and spin relaxation measurements were not possible. Nevertheless, in unlocalized studies we observed signal for six responding patients on a range of doses of TFP (10-120 mg/day) [13]. A good correlation between head concentration and daily dose was found. On four attempts we could not observe a signal from a nonresponder on a very high dose (120 mg/day) of TFP [13]. This preliminary result suggests that *in vivo* ^{19}F NMR may have a role in assessing response.

Fluoxetine

We later found that fluoxetine, a widely prescribed antidepressant, was easier to detect in human brain because of higher tissue concentration and lower fluorine equivalent weight [10,13-15]. This stronger signal permitted studies at normal clinical doses and additional experiments described below. In brain, fluoxetine metabolizes primarily to the pharmacologically active compound norfluoxetine, which we confirmed by *in vitro* analysis of postmortem brain tissue in one case [15]. Unfortunately, the chemical shifts of fluoxetine and norfluoxetine are very close, and cannot be resolved *in vivo* [15]. Estimates of brain concentration of fluoxetine/norfluoxetine (F/NF) in 22 patients receiving 20 or 40 mg/day ranged from about 1-11 mg/ml [14]. As expected, brain concentration rose after initiating treatment, but seemed to level off after about 6-8 months of treatment. For 6 subjects who also had plasma levels of F/NF measured, the brain concentration was about 20 times that in plasma [14]. Renshaw *et al.* [12] also found significantly higher levels of fluoxetine in brain than in plasma. For 2 subjects with multiple measurements during treatment, both brain and plasma concentration rose with time, and correlated reasonably well with each other [14].

Spatial localization

Of necessity, the above studies were performed without spatial localization techniques beyond the use of a surface coil (TFP and fluoxetine) [10,13] or small volume coil (fluoxetine) [14,15]. Thus nonbrain tissue such as muscle and fat could contribute substantially to the observed signal, particularly for the lipophilic TFP. Figure 1 shows the *in vivo* ^{19}F signal from the leg of a patient who had been on a high dose of TFP for several years. This signal was comparable to that typically seen for head in this patient [10]. In the TFP study, nonbrain signal was minimized by acquiring signal from the front of the head with a surface coil [13].

The situation is less severe for fluoxetine because of its higher accumulation in brain. We performed low resolution, 4-dimensional spectroscopic imaging to confirm that at least 80% of the signal seen in our *unlocalized* studies (with a 22-cm long volume coil) originated from brain [15].

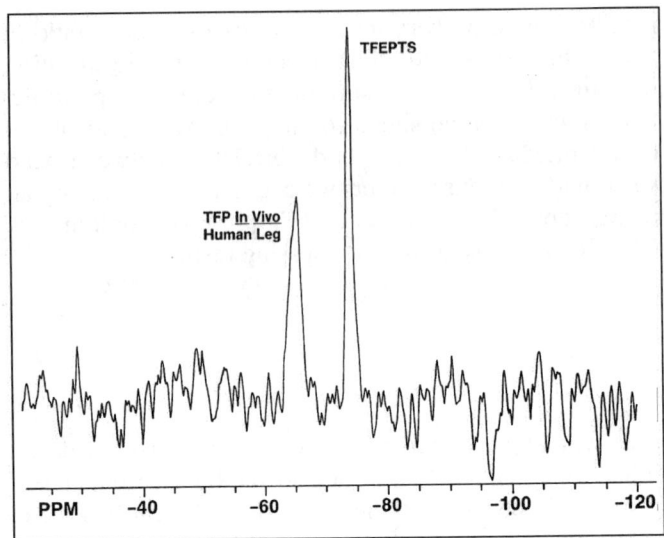

Figure 1. The 60.1 MHz ^{19}F spectrum of trifluoperazine (TFP) in human leg, taken *in vivo* with a surface coil. The peak labeled TFEPTS is from an external vial containing a $CDCl_3$ solution of 12 mM 2,2,2-(trifluoroethyl)-*p*-toluene sulfonate. The chemical shift scale is relative to CCl_3F.

Relaxation times

Knowledge of spin relaxation times is essential for optimization of NMR experiments. It is usually assumed that T_1 does not vary *in vivo* among individuals or in the same individual for a given isotope in a given environment. However, we found [15] that the ^{19}F T_1 of fluoxetine varied by about a factor of 4 among the individuals we studied. Figure 2 shows a plot of T_1 vs. brain concentration for 10 measurements on 5 patients. The T_1

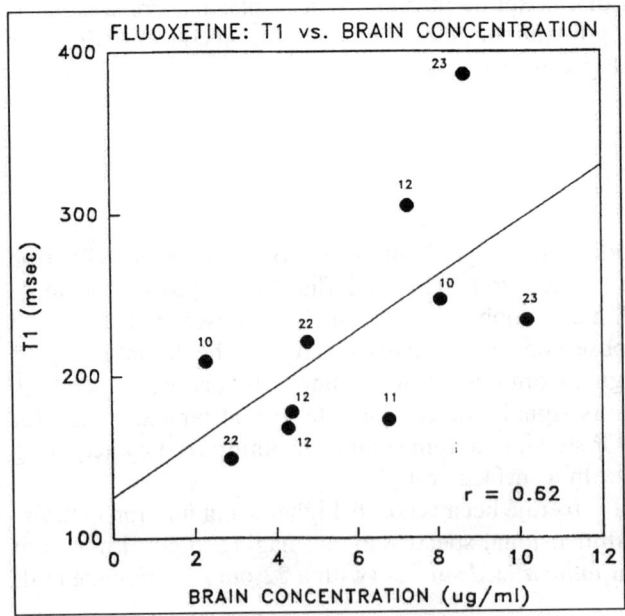

Figure 2. Plot of the *in vivo* ^{19}F T1 of F/NF vs. concentration in brain. Except for subject 23, subject numbers correspond to those in reference [14].

correlated weakly with brain concentration (r = 0.62, p=0.055). Phantom studies and a repeat measurement confirmed that the variation was not primarily experimental error [15]. The T_1 behavior with concentration can be rationalized on the basis of a simple model of fast exchange between bound and unbound fluoxetine. In brain the drug will undoubtedly bind to a variety of relatively immobile sites, which may or may not have pharmacologic significance. Such binding will restrict the mobility of the fluoxetine molecule and lower T_1 relative to unbound fluoxetine. For fast exchange,

$$1/T_{1obs} = f/T_{1b} + (1-f)/T_{1u}$$

where T_{1obs}, T_{1b}, and T_{1u} are the T_{1s} observed and in the bound and unbound states, respectively, and f is the fraction bound. With increasing drug concentration and an approximately fixed number of sites, a greater fraction will be unbound, and T_{1obs} will increase.

Metabolites

Psychoactive drugs typically metabolize in brain to compounds which may also have pharmacologic activity. Thus it would be valuable to observe independently the drug metabolites. As mentioned above, fluoxetine and norfluoxetine cannot be resolved *in vivo*. This is probably the case for most of the trifluoromethyl-containing psychoactive drugs. However, for a monofluorinated drug such as haloperidol, it may be possible to resolve metabolite signals. Figure 3 shows the high resolution, *in vitro* [19]F spectrum of a mixture of haloperidol and its major metabolites, one of which is reduced haloperidol. The chemical shift separation is adequate for *in vivo* resolution in this case. Unfortunately, because of inadequate sensitivity we have not been able to detect haloperidol in human brain [13]. However, Günther and Albert [16] have detected the chemically related neuroleptic melperone in the rat.

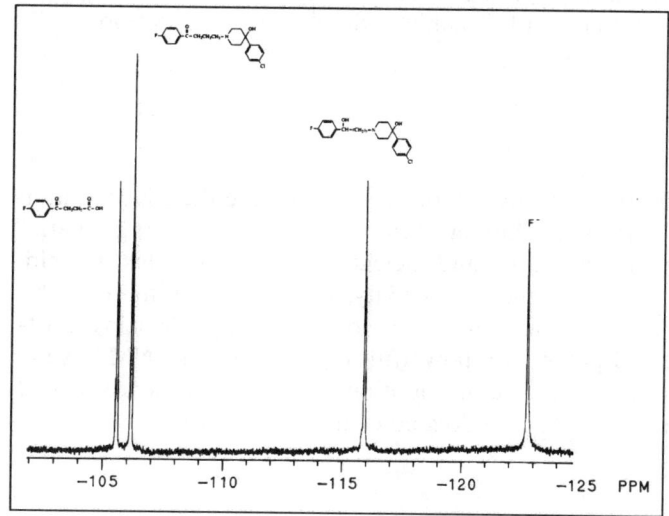

Figure 3. High resolution ^{19}F NMR spectrum at 282 MHz of a mixture of haloperidol and the metabolites reduced haloperidol, 3-(4-fluorobenzoyl)propionic acid, and fluoride ion, in aqueous solution at pH 5.7.

In vivo **concentrations**

Absolute concentrations are difficult to measure *in vivo*. Endogenous metabolites in ^{1}H or ^{31}P spectra *in vivo* are often measured relative to an internal standard for which the concentration may be known. This is usually not possible for drugs. Hence we used an external standard of known concentration in both *in vivo* and phantom measurements combined in a «dual-ratio» method [15]. Although not ideal, the method is acceptable for the single-peak spectra of relatively low S/N ratio we typically encounter.

The measurement of *in vivo* concentrations in brain by NMR spectroscopy is also complicated by the heterogeneous nature of biological tissue, which can contain a variety of cell types (neurons, glia) and compartments [intracellular, extracellular, cerebrospinal fluid (CSF)]. NMR will sample all liquid-state spins in the active volume. Without additional information on the compartmental distribution of a compound, only an average concentration over all cells and compartments can be given. For drugs, the compartmental distribution is important because the pertinent receptors probably reside in one compartment alone. However, overall tissue concentration of a drug should be an acceptable alternative to true active site concentration, and should be superior to plasma concentration.

It is also assumed that all of the drug in the active volume is contributing to the detected signal. However, some fraction may be strongly bound to macromolecules or membranes, have a very broad NMR resonance, and be invisible under high-resolution conditions. What fraction of the total amount of drug is represented by the *in vivo* NMR signal remains an open question, and can only be answered definitively by *in vivo* measurement followed by *in vitro* analysis of the same tissue. Although we have not yet had the opportunity to perform such a measurement, we did measure the combined F/NF concentration by *in vitro* ^{19}F NMR in the postmortem brain of a subject who had received fluoxetine for 19 weeks. In several brain regions we found values ranging from 12.3-18.6 mg/ml, which is higher than the maximum concentration of about 11 mg/ml determined by us in other subjects *in vivo* [14]. This result suggests, but does not prove, that a substantial fraction of F/NF may not be visible in the ^{19}F *in vivo* spectrum.

Future prospects

In favorable cases, ^{19}F NMR spectroscopy can be used to measure the concentration of fluorinated psychoactive drugs in human brain. Issues concerning spatial localization, signal visibility, quantitation, and detection of metabolites remain. Currently the greatest limitation is inadequate sensitivity, which may be improved by higher magnetic fields, better detection coils, and the use of sensitivity-enhancing, post-processing methods. A unique and potentially powerful feature of *in vivo* NMR is the ability to measure simultaneously the tissue concentration of a drug and the associated metabolic changes using ^{1}H or ^{31}P NMR of endogenous metabolites [17].

References

1. Shargel L, Yu ABC, *Applied biopharmaceutics and pharmacokinetics*, 2nd Edition, Norwalk, CT Appleton-Century-Crofts 1985.
2. Komoroski RA, In vivo NMR of drugs, *Anal Chem* ; 1994; **66** : xxxA-yyyA.
3. Komoroski RA, Measurement of Psychoactive Drugs in the Human Brain In Vivo by MR Spectroscopy, *Am J Neuroradiol* 1993 ; **14** : 1038-1042.
4. Bartels M, Albert K, Kruppa G, Mann K, Schroth G, Tabarelli S, Zabel M. Fluorinated psychopharmacological agents: noninvasive observation by fluorine-19 nuclear magnetic resonance *Psychiatry Res* 1986 ; **18** : 197-201.
5. Arndt DC, Ratner AV, Faull KF, Barchas JD, Young W. [19]F magnetic resoance imaging and spectroscopy of a fluorinated neuroleptic ligand: *in vivo* and *in vitro* Studies *Psychiatry Res* 1988 ; **25** : 73-79.
6. Nakada T, Kwee IL, One-dimensional chemical shift imaging of fluorinated neuroleptics in rat brain *in vivo* by ^{19}F NMR rotating frame zeugmatography *Magn Reson Imaging* 1989 ; **7** : 543-545.
7. Albert K, Rembold H, Kruppa G, Bayer E, Bartels M, Schmalzing G. *in vivo* [19]F Nuclear Magnetic Resonance Spectroscopy of Trifluorinated Neuroleptics in the rat. *NMR Biomed* 1990 ; **3** : 120-123.
8. Bartels M, Günther U, Albert K, Mann K, Schuff N, Stuckstedte H. [19]F nuclear magnetic resonance spectroscopy of neuroleptics: the first *in vivo* pharmacokinetics of trifluoperazine in the rat brain and the first *in vivo* spectrum of fluphenazine in the human brain *Biol Psychiatry* 1991 ; **30** : 656-662.
9. Komoroski RA, Newton J, Karson C, Walker E, Cardwell D, Ramaprasad S. *In vivo* NMR spectroscopy of psychoactive drugs in humans, *Magn Reson Imaging* 1989 ; **7** : Suppl. ; 132.
10. Komoroski R, Newton JEO, Karson C, Cardwell D, Sprigg J. Detection of psychoactive drugs *in vivo* in humans using ^{19}F NMR spectroscopy *Biol Psychiatry* 1991 ; **29** : 711-4.
11. Durst P, Schuff N, Crocq MA, Mokrani MC, Macher JP, Noninvasive *in vivo* detection of a fluorinated neuroleptic in the human brain by ^{19}F nuclear magnetic resonance spectroscopy *Psychiatry Res : Neuroimaging* 1990 ; **35** : 107-14.
12. Renshaw PF, Guimaraes AR, Fava M, Rosenbaum JF, Pearlman JD, Flood JG, Puopolo PR, Clancy K, Gonzalez RG. Accumulation of fluoxetine and norfluoxetine in human brain during therapeutic administration *Am J Psychiatry* 1992 ; **149** : 1592-4.
13. Karson CN, Newton JEO, Mohanakrishnan P, Sprigg J, Komoroski RA. Fluoxetine and trifluoperazine in human brain: a ^{19}F nuclear magnetic resonance spectroscopy study. *Psychiatry Res : Neuroimaging* 1992 ; **45** : 95-104.
14. Karson CN, Newton JEO, Livingston R, Jolly JB, Cooper TB, Sprigg J, Komoroski RA. Human brain fluoxetine concentrations, *J NeuropsychiatryClin Neurosci* 1993 ; **5** : 322-329.
15. Komoroski RA, Newton JEO, Cardwell D, Sprigg J, Pearce J, Karson CN. In vivo ^{19}F spin relaxation and localized spectroscopy of fluoxetine in human brain. *Magn Reson Med* 1994 ; **31** : 204-211.
16. Günther U, Albert K, *In vivo* [19]F nuclear magnetic resonance of a monofluorinated neuroleptic in the rat ; *NMR Biomed* 1993 ; **6** : 27-31.
17. Kato T, Takahashi S, Shioiri T, Inubushi T. Alterations in brain phosphorus metabolism in bipolar disorder detected by *in vivo* [31]P and [7]Li magnetic resonance. *J Affective Disorders* 1993 ; **27** : 53-60.

40

Hippocampal metabolite depletion in schizophrenia detected by proton magnetic resonance spectroscopy

M. MAIER, M.A. RON

Institute of Neurology, Queen Square, London WC1N 3 BG, UK.

Diffuse loss of cortical volume and ventricular enlargement have been demonstrated in schizophrenia using imaging. In addition histological studies have provided compelling evidence that the number of neurons in the medial temporal lobe structures is reduced and that the cytoarchitecture is abnormal, and Scheibel [25] and Altschuler [1] have reported these changes in brains of schizophrenics collected before the introduction of neuroleptic. In an attempt to correlate these histological findings with *in vivo* estimates of neuronal integrity, we have studied the concentration of the neuronal marker N-acetyl aspartate (NAA) in the hippocampi of schizophrenics using *in vivo* magnetic resonance spectroscopy (MRS).

Recent hypotheses have proposed a neurodevelopmental model to explain the genesis of schizophrenia [24,25,28]. Evidence to support this model comes from imaging studies that fail to show a correlation between the duration of the illness progression of structural changes over time [20]. Histological studies support the neurodevelopmental hypothesis by failing to show glial proliferation in those cortical areas where there is cell loss and cytoarchitectural disruption.

Proton magnetic resonance spectroscopy (MRS) is able to detect chemicals in the brain that contain hydrogen and that have concentrations of at least millimolar levels. The peak due to NAA is the largest signal in the proton spectrum, with creatine and choline also showing strong signals. NAA is an intra-neuronal chemical whose role in neuronal function is not fully understood [4,19,22]. However it has been shown that it is not present in non-neuronal tumours such as gliomas [15], and animal experiments have shown NAA to decline following selective neuronal death after kainate injection [19].

Reduced levels of NAA *in vivo* have been reported in a variety of conditions leading to neuronal or axonal loss such as in acute and chronic multiple sclerosis [2,22], acute cerebral infarction [6,11], hypoxic-ischaemic encephalopathy [16], Creutzfeld-Jakob disease [7], HIV [9], and seizure disorders [5]. Conversely, raised levels of NAA have been reported in Canavan's disease [3,17], a rare demyelinating autosomal recessive disorder linked with abnormally high concentrations of NAA in the brain as a result of aspartoacylase deficiency.

The aim of our study was to determine whether there was a detectable loss of NAA in the medial temporal structures and whether hemisphere asymmetries in NAA could be detected in normals and schizophrenics.

Methods

Subjects

25 right handed schizophrenic patients (mean age 36.3 +/- 8.7 years) fulfilling RDC diagnostic criteria and 32 right handed healthy controls (mean age 25.8 +/- 8.7 years) in the age range of 18 to 55 years were studied. Subjects with a history of alcohol use of more than 50 units a week, or a history of head injury that led to unconsciousness were excluded. Controls with past or present neurological or psychiatric disorder were also excluded.

Magnetic resonance imaging and spectroscopy were performed on a GE Signa 1.5T scanner using a standard quadrature head coil. T2 weighted fast spin echo images were used to obtain sagittal and coronal views of the brain. Both the left and the right hippocampi were studied on each subject. A volume of interest (typically 5-7 cm^3) in the anterior hippocampus was prescribed from the coronal series. Spectroscopy was done using stimulated echo acquisition mode (STEAM) sequence for water (TR/TE 6 000/10 msec.) and metabolites (TR/TE 2 350/135 msec.) [12,14]. 1 024 points were collected with a spectral width of 750 Hz. Water suppression and shimming, to a line width of ~3Hz, were reoptimized for each side of the brain. Analysis of the spectra was done using software provided by GE (spectroscopic application for GE) on a SUN SparcStation 10. After spectral processing the peaks were fitted to gaussian functions. Concentrations of NAA, creatine and choline were calculated from the ratio of the metabolite to water signals, using the water peak as an internal standard and assuming the concentration of protons due to water to be 94.4 M, a value measured for insular grey matter [13]. The water and metabolite signals were corrected for T1 and T2 relaxation times, and for water the correction was negligible because of the long repetition time and short echo time used in acquisition.

Results

The concentrations of NAA, creatine and choline obtained are plotted as a bar graph in Figure 1.

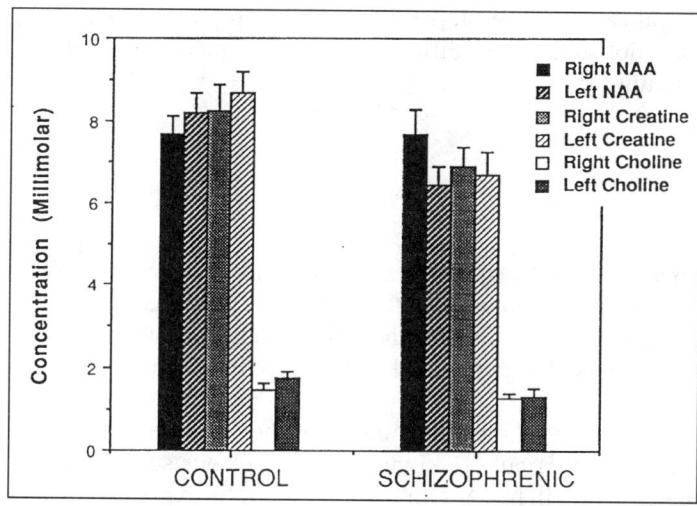

Figure 1. Bar graph showing concentrations of NAA, creatine and choline (Millimolar) for controls and schizophrenics, together with error bars showing standard error. Left sided NAA p=0.009, creatine p=0.012, and choline p=0.045.

In the schizophrenic group there is a significant left sided reduction in NAA of 22%, creatine 23% and choline 25%. The reductions on the right side do not achieve statistical significance. In order to study hemisphere asymmetries in the distribution of NAA, creatine and choline, the group differences in right minus left concentrations of these chemicals are compared and the results shown in Figure 2.

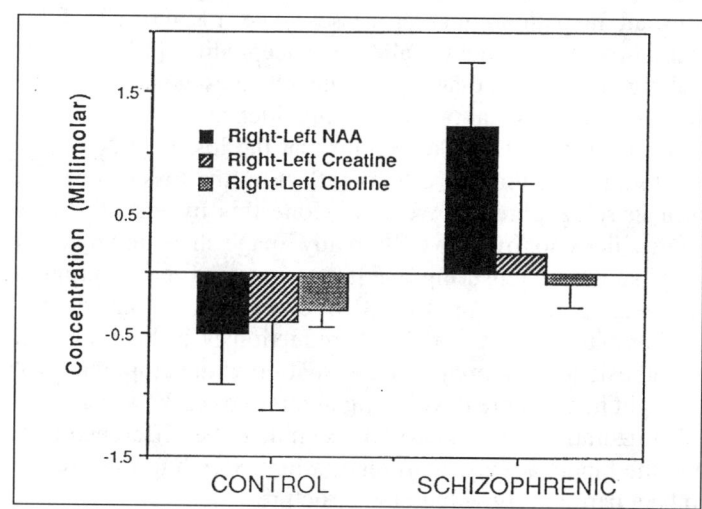

Figure 2. Bar graph showing right-left concentrations for NAA, creatine and choline (Millimolar) for controls and schizophrenics. Error bars show standard errors. NAA reversal p=0.014.

In controls the values of NAA, creatine and choline are greater in the left hippocampus. The asymmetry observed in controls for the three chemicals is reduced in schizophrenia and reversed for NAA and creatine. The reversal is statistically significant for NAA ($p<0.014$).

To exclude the effects of age we performed linear regression on scatter plots of the various metabolites plotted against age. The slopes of the fitted regression lines for controls and schizophrenics are not statistically different, and consequently age related changes are not significant in either group.

Discussion

The results show that compared to controls, in schizophrenia there is a loss of NAA, creatine and choline in the left hippocampus and that this loss achieves statistical significance. We have measured a 22% NAA loss in the left hippocampus and this is in striking agreement with the loss in pyramidal cell population reported in neuropathological studies [10].

In the normal brain NAA concentrations are found to be relatively constant throughout [21] and it is, therefore, particularly significant that in our schizophrenic group we find such strong lateralisation in NAA. Our results cannot be explained by the use of neuroleptic medication, as drug effects are unlikely to lead to a left sided NAA loss whilst leaving the right side of the brain unaffected. Moreover, animal studies show that chronic neuroleptic treatment does not alter levels of NAA [23,27]. Choline abnormalities detected in red cell membranes of schizophrenics have also been found to be independent of drug treatment [26].

Before accepting the results of this study, some methodological points, that may contribute to the findings, need to be considered.

Evidence exists from other studies to suggest that relaxation times remain relatively constant in pathological processes. The T1 and T2 of NAA are known to remain constant in experimental allergic encephalitis [18], an active inflammatory process, making it unlikely that significant changes would occur in schizophrenia where no «active» pathological process is in evidence.

We have tried to make certain that the losses in NAA, creatine and choline are not due to a partial volume effects reflecting the loss of cortical and white matter volume seen in schizophrenia. We have done this by visually inspecting that the volume of interest does not overlap CSF in any image slice, and by inspecting the volume adjusted water signal and ensuring that it was constant in each hippocampus studied. This would not be the case if signal from CSF contaminated our volume of interest. Our finding of predominantly left sided NAA reduction is in keeping with the neurodevelopmental hypothesis of schizophrenia. Normal brain development proceeds asymmetrically with the right hemisphere developing about two weeks ahead of the left [8]. An insult during this maturational period could accentuate the difference between the two hemispheres, and the hippocampus, with maturation extending into the post-partum period, is likely to be a particularly vulnerable structure.

It remains to be determined whether variation in the concentration of NAA and other chemicals is dependent on remissions and exacerbations of symptoms, and to what extent these abnormalities are specific to schizophrenia when compared to other psychoses.

Acknowledgements

Dr Maier is a welcome training fellow. Pr Ron is partly funded by the scarfe trust. We would like to thank Pr I. MacDonald, Mrs Amanda Brennan and the multiple sclerosis NMR group for their help.

References

1   Altshuler LL. Hippocampal pyramidal cell orientation in schizophrenia. *Arch Gen Psychiat* 1987 ; 44 : 1094-8.
2   Arnold DL, Mathews PM, Francis G, Antel J. Proton magnetic resonance spectroscopy of human brain in vivo in the evaluation of multiple sclerosis: assessment of the lad of the disease. *Magnetic Resonance in Medicine* 1990 ; 14 : 154-9.
3   Austin SJ, Connelly A, Gadian DG, Benton JS ,Brett EM. Localised 1H NMR spectroscopy in Canavan's disease: a report of two cases. *Magnetic Resonance in Medicine* 1991 ; 19 : 439-45.
4   Birken DL, Oldendorf WH. N-acetyl-l-aspartic acid: a literature review of a compound prominent in 1H-NMR spectroscopic studies of brain. *Neurosci Behav Rev* 1989 ; 13 : 23-31.
5   Breiter SN, Arroyo S, Mathews VP, Lesser RP, Bryan RN , Barker PB. Proton MR spectroscopy in patients with seizure disorders. *Am J Neuroradiol* 1994 ; 15 : 373-84.
6   Bruhn H., Frahm J, Gyngell ML, Merboldt KD, Haenicke W, Sauter R. Cerebral metabolism in man after acute stroke: new observations using localized proton NMR spectroscopy. *Magnetic Resonance in Medicine* 1989 ; 9 : 126-31.
7   Bruhn H, Weber T, Thorwirth V, Frahm J. *In vivo* monitoring of neuronal loss in Creutzfeldt-Jakob disease by proton magnetic resonance spectroscopy. *Lancet* 1991 ; 337 : 1610-1.
8   Chi JG, Dooling EC, Gilles FH. Gyral development of the human brain. *Ann Neurol* 1977 ; 1 : 86-93.
9. Chong WK, Sweeney B, Wilkinson ID, Paley M, Hall-Craggs MA, Kendall BE, Shepard JK, Beecham M, Miller RF, Weller IVD, Newman SP, Harrison MJ. Proton spectroscopy of the brain in HIV infection: correlation with clinical immunologic and MR imaging findings. *Radiology* 1993 ; 188 : 119-24.
10. Falkai P, Bogerts B. Cell loss in the hippocampus of schizophrenics. *European Archives of Psychiatry and Neurological Sciences* 1986 ; 236 : 154-61.
11. Fisher M, Sotak CH, Minematsu K, Li L. New magnetic resonance techniques for evaluating cerebrovascular disease. *Ann Neurol* 1992 ; 32 : 115-22.
12. Frahm J, Bruhn H, Gyngell ML, Merboldt KD, Hanicke W, Sauter R. Localized high-resolution proton NMR spectroscopy using stimulated echoes: initial applications to human brain in vivo. *Magnetic Resonance in Medicine* 1989a ; 9 : 79-93.
13. Frahm J, Bruhn H, Gyngell ML, Merboldt KD, Haenicke W, Sauter R. Localized proton NMR spectroscopy in different regions of the human brain in vivo. Relaxation times and concentrations of cerebral metabolites. *Magnetic Resonance in Medicine* 1989b ; 11 : 47-63.

14. Frahm J, Michaelis T, Merboldt KD, Bruhn H, Gyngell ML, Hanicke W. Improvements in localized proton NMR spectroscopy of human brain: water suppression, short echo times, and 1 ml resolution. *Journal of Magnetic Resonance* 1990 ; 90 : 464-73.
15. Gill SS, Thomas DGT, Van Bruggen N, Gadian DG, Peden CJ, Bell JD, Cox J, Menon DK, Iles RA, Bryant DJ, Coutts GA. Proton MR spectroscopy of intracranial tumours: *in vivo* and *in vitro* studies. Comput Assist Tomogr 1990 ; 14 : 497-504.
16. Graham SH, Meyerhoff DJ, Bayne L, Sharp FR, Weiner MW. Magnetic resonance spectroscopy of N-acetyl aspartate in hypoxic-ischaemic encephalopathy. *Ann Neurol* 1994 ; 35 : 490-4.
17. Grodd W, Kraegeloh-Mann I, Peterson D, Trefz FK, Harzer K. In vivo assessment of N-acetyl aspartate in brain in spongy degeneration (Canavan's disease) by proton spectroscopy. *Lancet* 1990 ; 336 : 437-438.
18. Inglis BA, Brenner RE, Munro PMG, Williams SCR, McDonald WI, Sales KD. Measurement of proton NMR relaxation times for NAA, Cr and Cho in acute EAE. society of magnetic resonance in medicine (book of abstracts) 1992 ; 2 : 2162.
19. Koller KJ, Zaczek R, Coyle JT. N-acetyl-aspartyl-glutamate: regional levels in rat brain and the effects of brain lesions as determined by a new HPLC method. *J Neuroch* 1994 ; 43 : 1136-42.
20. Marsh L, Suddath RL, Higgins N, Weinberger DR. (1994). Medial temporal lobe structures in schizophrenia: relationship of size to duration of illness. Schizophrenia Research 11, 225-238.
21. Michaelis T, Merboldt KD, Bruhn H, Haenicke W, Frahm J. Absolute concentrations of metabolites in the adult human brain in vivo: quantification of localized proton MR spectra. *Radiology* 1993 ; 197 : 219-227.
22. Miller BL. A review of chemical issues in 1H NMR spectroscopy: N-acetyl-L-aspartate, creatine and choline. *NMR in Biomedicine* 1991 ; 4 : 47-52.
23. Okumura N, Otsuki S, Nasu H. The influence of insulin hypoglycaemic coma, repeated electroshocks, and chlorpromazine or beta-phenylisopropylmethylamine administration on the free amino acids in the brain. *J Bioch* 1959 ; 46 : 247-52.
24. Roberts GW. Schizophrenia: A neuropathological perspective. *Br J Psychiatry* 1991 ; 158 : 8-17.
25. Scheibel AB, Conrad AS. Hippocampal dysgenesis in mutant mouse and schizophrenic man: is there a relationship ? *Schizophrenia Bulletin* 1993 ; 19 : 23-33.
26. Stevens JD. The distribution of phospholipid fractions in the red cell membranes of schizophrenics. *Schizophrenia Bulletin* 1972 ; 6 : 60-1.
27. Tews JK, Carter SH, Roa PD, Stone WE. Free amino acids and related compounds in dog brain: post-mortem and anoxic changes, effects of ammonium chloride infusion, and levels during seizures induced by picrotoxin and by pentylenetetrazol. *J Neuroch* 1963 ; 10 : 641-53.
28. Waddington JL. Schizophrenia: developmental neuroscience and pathobiology. *Lancet* 1993 ; 341 : 531-536.

41

Overcoming field inhomogeneities in MRI

D.J.O. McINTYRE [1], R.W. BOWTELL [2], M.-J COMMANDRE [2], F. HENNEL [3],
P. MANSFIELD [2], P.G. MORRIS [2]

[1] CRC Biomedical MR Group, St. George's Hospital, Tooting, London, UK
[2] Magnetic Resonance Centre, Department of Physics, University of Nottingham, UK
[3] FORENAP, Rouffach, France.

Magnetic resonance images are sensitive to distortions caused by inhomogeneities in the main magnetic field, which may be caused by poor shimming or by local field gradients at the interfaces of regions of different susceptibility. As magnetic resonance imaging is performed routinely at progressively higher field strengths, distortions due to susceptibility become more severe. Two techniques where this is a particularly acute problem are plant microscopy and clinical echo-planar imaging (EPI[1]). In the former case, the high fields (11.7T or higher) result in severe local gradients and hence distortions around air spaces in parenchymal tissue [2]. In the latter, the low frequency per point in the blipped gradient direction may lead to large distortions. This can be a significant problem for clinical applications where exact anatomical localization is necessary. At the other extreme of field strength, there is a potential market for a low-cost MRI system based on an inexpensive magnet of low field strength and low homogeneity, provided that undistorted images may be obtained.

Such distortions may be reduced either by sequence design or by post-processing of images. Multiples 180° pulses may be inserted in imaging sequences to refocus the effects of field inhomogeneities ; for instance, GRASE [3] is a modified version of EPI with a small number of refocusing pulses ; PEPI (π-EPI) includes a refocusing pulse at every switch of the read gradient, and has been used for fast imaging of oil-bearing rocks where extremely high susceptibility gradients must be overcome. RARE and techniques such as BURST and QUEST, which generate a train of echoes from a train of low flip-angle pulses under a gradient, do not accumulate phase shifts from inhomogeneity between one acquisition and the next. These sequences also reduce the loss of signal to phase randomization due to diffusion of water in steep susceptibility gradients. Other techniques for reducing the effects of susceptibility include the use of projection reconstruction to eliminate the delay for phase-encoding in conventional sequences (for instance, its application to lung imaging [4], enabling signal to be obtained from the large vessels in the lung before diffusion in the susceptibility gradients destroys all coherence); and the use of pulses which give rise to a non-linear phase shifts across the imaging slice, partially cancelling the phase shift due to susceptibility and improving the uniformity of the final image [5].

To eliminate distortion completely, a 180° pulse may be inserted between every point acquired in a line of k-space. We have studied such a sequence as part of a feasibility study for a low-field low-homogeneity magnet imaging system and present here images obtained on a 25 MHz small-bore permanent magnet system. This technique is applicable at low fields or for plant experiments, but would require dangerously high RF powers at higher fields.

Variants of EPI which include multiple 180° pulses are not appropriate for all experiments ; for example, in a Look-Locher experiment, where multiple EPI images with low excitation pulse flip angles are acquired over 1 to 3 seconds during recovery from an inversion pulse, the refocusing pulses would both alter the recovery curve and potentially exceed prescribed limits for RF heating. It is possible to correct distorted images if the form of the field distortion is known [6], but this technique is of limited use where the distortion is caused by the object being imaged, as is the case in high-field head imaging, especially close to the air spaces in the sinuses.

Imaging sequence

We present here a sequence which can produce images entirely undistorted by B_0 inhomogeneity or chemical shift artifacts. The imaging sequence is shown in Figure 1 and starts with a standard slice selection and phase encoding gradient. This is followed by a train of 180° refocusing pulses applied in the absence of field gradients and separated by an interecho time T_{ie}. A single point is sampled at the top of each spin echo when the phase shifts due to inhomogeneity and chemical shift are refocused and the only remaining phase shifts are those due to the cumulative effect of gradient pulses. Gradient blips are applied along an axis perpendicular to the phase-encoding gradient after every second refocusing pulse and before acquisition. The k-space trajectory for the first 8 points of one line of this sequence is shown in Figure 2. Dotted lines represent shifts due to RF pulses and solid lines shifts due to gradients. The phase-encoding gradient causes a shift along the k_y axis and the subsequent blips step the position in k-space along the k_x axis. Each RF pulse causes a reflection through the centre of k-space; for a full-Fourier experiment where every point in the train is acquired, the data must be reordered prior to Fourier transformation. An alternative implementation could apply

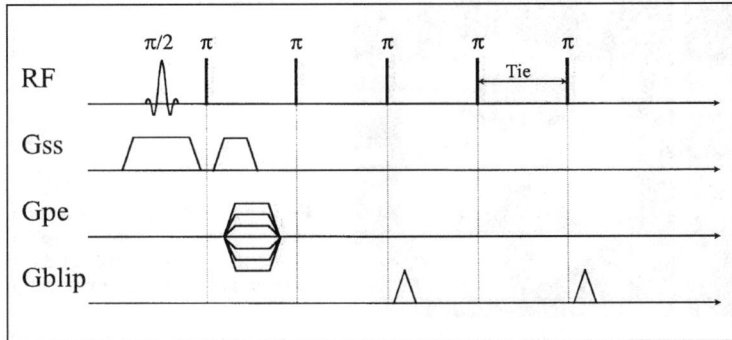

Figure 1. Single-point acquisition imaging sequence.

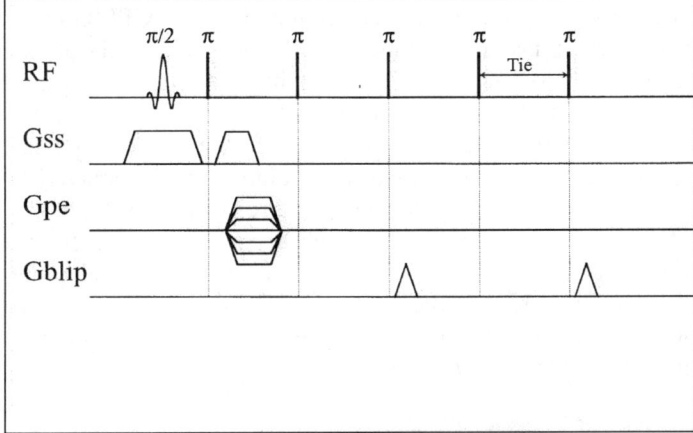

Figure 2. k-space trajectory for one echo train of the imaging sequence of Figure 1.

blips large enough to step from the k_y axis out to the point on the k_x axis and rewind the phase shift with a negative gradient blip after acquisition, as is done in RARE imaging. This would reduce the artifacts caused by imperfect refocusing of off-resonance spins, but would require very much higher gradient currents. The sequence illustrated requires relatively low peak currents; however, the gradient coils must have low inductance to allow fast switching as the gradient blips must last only a few hundred microseconds for T_{ie} to be reasonably short.

Figures 3a and 3b show computer simulations of this sequence to illustrate the characteristic artifacts. The simulations were run on an IBM RS6000 and took 20 minutes CPU time. For a given acceptable level of distortion, the permissible bandwidth due to field offsets is inversely proportional to the duration of the hard RF pulses, and therefore proportional to the square root of the available RF power. Here, the field distortion has a Gaussian profile reaching an offset equivalent to 460 Hz at the edge of the object. The bright horizontal streak across Figure 3a is caused by magnetization left unexcited by the initial 90° pulse but excited by the refocusing pulses. This is inaffected by the phase-encoding pulse and therefore appears only across the centre of the image.

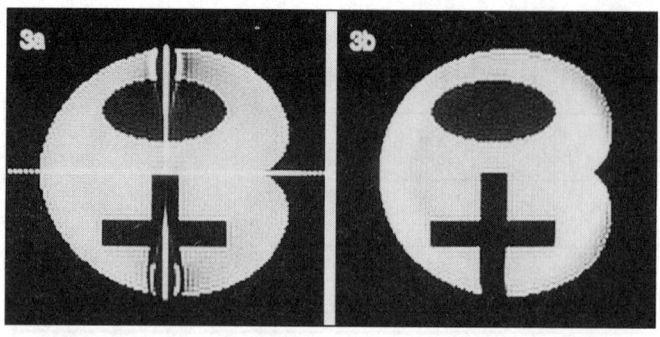

Figure 3. Computer simulations of the single point imaging sequence using (a) *xxxx* and (b) *xyxy* phasing of the refocusing pulses.

It may be eliminated by phase cycling of the 90° pulse, as he been done for Figure 3b. The distortion in the centre of the field of view in Figure 3a is caused by cumulative errors in refocusing off-resonance spins. Figure 3a was simulated with a CPMG echo train, where all pulses have the same phase (*yyy*) which is 90° away from that of the excitation pulse (*x*). The artifacts may be reduced by using alternative phasing sequences such as *yy-y-y* or *yxyx*; both of these shift the artifact to the edge of the field of view and reduce it. Figure 3b shows the result of using *yxyx* phasing with RF pulses of twice the duration used for Figure 3a. Symbolic matrix calculations using REDUCE show that with a CPMG train, off-resonance effects cause no error to first order at the edges of the field of view (where the blip gradient causes a phase shift of π) and maximum error in refocusing at the centre of the FOV. For the other two cycles the effect is reversed, with no error to first order at the centre of the FOV. If there are no spins close to the edge of the FOV, the majority of the magnetization will be correctly refocused and the artifacts are reduced as the simulation implies.

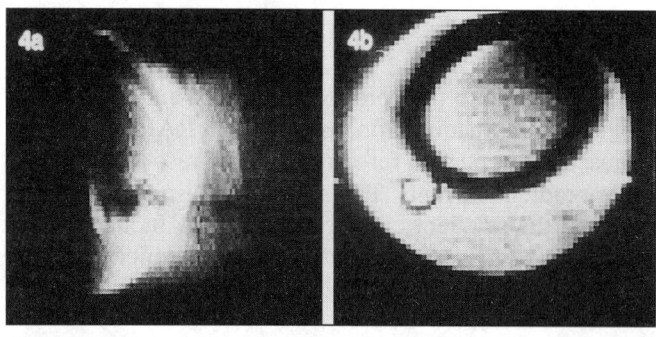

Figure 4. (a) 2DFT image demonstrating the inhomogeneity of the magnet used to produce image (b) using the inhomogeneity-resistant single-point imaging sequence.

Experiments to verify the simulations were performed on a home-built PC-based imaging system interfaced to a Bruker SXP4-100 console with a 25MHz permanent magnet of low homogeneity, sited at the Institute of Nuclear Physics in Krakow, Poland. The level of inhomogeneity is demonstrated in Figure 4a, which is a standard 2DFT image of the phantom used with an acquisition bandwidth of 1 kHz and no read gradient, showing the field spread to be several hundred Hz. Figure 4b shows a half-Fourier reconstruction of an image obtained using the inhomogeneity-resistant sequence with a T_{ie} of 1.4 ms, 700µs trapezoidal gradient blips, and a *yxyx* phase cycle on the refocusing pulses. The probe was a 10-turn solenoid and the sample a tube of water of inside diameter 25mm, containing two other tubes. No phase cycling was employed. The half-Fourier image shows signs of the artifacts seen in the simulations but is overall a good representations of the phantom. Full-Fourier reconstruction results in severe baseline distortion. This is due to phase errors in the odd-numbered echoes, partly to the uncalibrated analogue control over pulse phase provided by the Bruker console.

Software correction of epi images

Echo-planar imaging (EPI) is sensitive to distortion from main field inhomogeneities due to its relatively low frequency per point in the blipped direction. The problem becomes more acute at higher fields since the gradients due to susceptibility variation scale linearly with $B_\emptyset$ at the 3.0T field of the Nottingham EPI scanner, a 1 ppm variation in $B_\emptyset$ can cause a 16-pixel distortion in a 128^2 pixel image acquired in 128 ms. This is a problem where fast precise anatomical localization is required. We have adapted a technique published by Chang and Fitzpatrick [7] for correction of 2DFT images for use with EPI [8].

Figure 5 shows a standard EPI sequence. The switched read gradient used in EPI is so strong that no distortion appears in this direction at currently attainable values for $B_\emptyset$. Images may therefore be analysed as a series of independent one-dimensional profiles. The phase shift between echoes imparted by the blip gradient is gGDx, where x is the position in space, g the gyromagnetic ratio and G and Δ the amplitude and duration of the gradient blip as illustrated in Figure 5. If the inhomogeneity field has strength B_i at x, it causes a phase shift gBit between echoes. The magnetization at x will therefore appear in the image at

$$x_1 = x + \frac{B_i \tau}{G \Delta} \qquad (1)$$

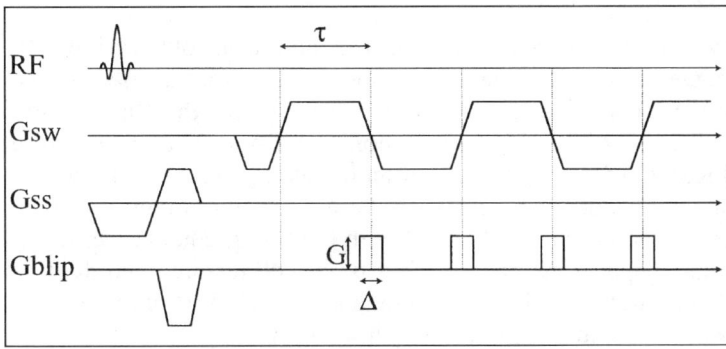

Figure 5. MBEST echo-planar imaging sequence.

If a second image is acquired with the blip gradient polarity reversed, this magnetization will appear at a point

$$x_2 = x - \frac{B_i \tau}{G \Delta} \qquad (2)$$

The correct position for the isochromat is therefore the average of $x1$ and $x2$. To identify which of the possible pairs of $x1$ and $x2$ correspond to a given x, the integrals of the magnitudes of the two profiles ($i1$ ($x1$ and $i2$ ($x2$) are compared. For a given x, $x1$ and $x2$ will satisfy Equations (1) and (2) and :

$$\int_{x_{10}}^{x_1} i_1(x') dx' = \int_{x_{20}}^{x_2} i_2(x') dx' = \int_{x_0}^{x} i(x') dx' \qquad (3)$$

where $x10$, $x20$ are the edges of the object in the two images. This results in correct reconstruction provided that the inhomogeneity field gradient dBi/dx is not so steep that $dx1/dx$ or $dx2/dx$ becomes negative. Then

$$i(x) = i_1(x_1) \frac{dx_1}{dx} = \frac{2 i_1(x_1) i_2(x_2)}{i_1(x_1) + i_2(x_2)} \qquad (4)$$

dx_1/dx may be calculated from a single pair of modulus images and used to correct subsequent single-shot images of the same region, provided that B_i does not change. The later images need not be modulus images. Linear interpolation between image points is used to calculate the integrals. Precise edge detection is necessary for accurate reconstruction; errors in the integrals from inaccurate location of the edges cause bright spots in the reconstruction of signal-free regions in the object. We have obtained the best results by using the output of a 3x3 gradient operator matrix [9] or, when the signal to noise ratio is sufficiently high, by integrating from the edge of the field of view.

Figures 6a and 6b show sample distorted and reconstructed images obtained by EPI at 3.0 T. The distorted images were 128^2 images acquired using a spin-echo sequence with a sinusoidal switched gradient. The echo duration T was 960 µs, the blip duration 60 µs, and the blip strength 2 mTm^{-1}, giving a resolution of 1.5 mm. The images were reconstructed on an IMB RS6000 5/30, each reconstruction taking 4 seconds. Figure 6a is a phantom image deliberately spoiled by offsetting the X^2-Y^2 shim. Figure 6b is the image reconstructed from 6a and an image obtained with the blip gradient reversed. It can be seen that the circular shape of the phantom has been well restored and the fine details generally retained, although there is some extraneous signal in the dark regions. Good results have also been obtained from human brain images.

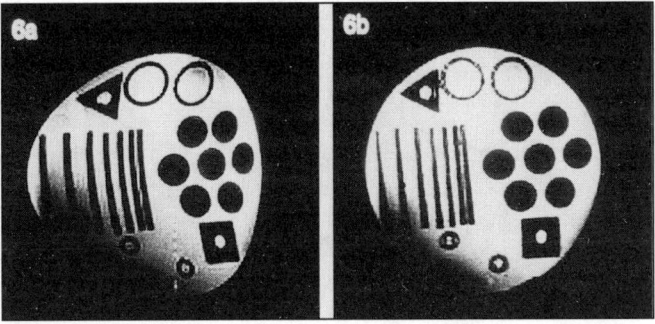

Figure 6. (a) EPI image distorted by offsetting the X2-Y2 shim. (b) Corrected EPI image obtained by software correction of (a) together with an image obtained using the reverse blip gradient.

Conclusion

The two techniques presented here are applicable to quite different imaging regimes. The software reconstruction is good for EPI at high field strengths, where the SNR is high, but would be difficult to apply at lower fields. It is also must useful at high fields where interfaces between regions of different susceptibilities give rise to large field offsets, and the increased RF power required limits the use of multiple refocusing pulses. It is sensitive to ghosting and can only correct over a limited range of inhomogeneity field gradients; for instance, it would not be capable of correcting rock images. For this a pulse-refocused sequence is necessary. For low-field or microscopic studies, the single-point imaging sequence is more useful; this allows the acquisition of undistorted images without the signal-to-noise penalty of very high read gradients. Additionally is reduces the loss of signal to diffusion in susceptibility gradients.

References

1. Mansfield P, *Phys J* 1977 ; C 10, L55 : 4.
2. Bowtell RW, Brown GD, Glover PM, McJury M, Mansfield P, *Phil Trans Roy Soc Lond* 1990 ; 333 : 457.
3. Feinberg DA Oshio K, *J Mag Res* 1992 ; 97 : 177.
4. Bergin C, Pauly J, Macovski A, *Abstracts SMRI-VIII* 1990 ; 132.
5. Ro YM, Cho ZH, *Mag Res Med* 1992 ; 28 : 237.
6. Sekihara K, Kuroda M, Kohno H, *Phys Med Biol* 1984 ; 29 : 15.
7. Chang H, Fitzpatrick JM, IEEE *Trans Med Imaging* 1992 ; 11 : 319.
8. Bowtell R, McIntyre DJO, Commandre MJ, Glover PM, Mansfield P, *Proceedings of the SMR Second Meeting* 1994 ; 411.
9. Gonzalez RC, Wintz P, Digital Image Processing, 2nd ed., *Addison Wesley* 1987.

Acknowledgements

D.J.O. McIntyre thanks the Medical Research Council for funding this research and the British Council for funding the link with the Institute of Nuclear Physics in Krakow.

42

In vivo metabolic study with NMR spectroscopy in Alzheimer's disease

G. MECHERI[1], M. MARIE-CARDINE[2]

[1]*Senior Resident, Hospital Assistant (Department of Pr. M. Marie-Cardine),*
[2]*University Professor, Hospital's Department Head University Hospital Department of Psychiatry, C.H.S. Le Vinatier, 95, boulevard. Pinel, 69677 Bron Cedex, France*

In vivo NMR spectroscopy allows metabolic exploration of the brain in ethically acceptable conditions (noninvasive, nonionizing examination).

Pettegrew's group (Pittsburgh, USA) reported alterations of membrane phospholipids observed with *in vitro* NMR spectroscopy. While some studies among a few *in vivo* examinations of patients did confirm *in vitro* results but others showed no phospholipid abnormalities.

We explored the *in vivo* metabolism of phospholipids in a parietal site, using an external NMR coil placed on the vertex and tuned to the resonance of phosphorus 31. Five patients over 65 years of age with probable Alzheimer's disease (DSM-III-R and NINCDS-ARDRA criteria) were selected. Other possible causes of dementia, including vascular causes, were excluded. A group of 4 age-matched normal subjects was used as a control. The patients were submitted to psychometric rating using Signoret's battery for the assessment of dementia (BED).

Although the number of subjects is small, appropriate statistical treatment was applied to the result (nonparametric Mann-Whitney U test): no statistically significant difference was noted in phospholipid metabolites in the volume of measurement (semisphere 60 mm in diameter, under the coil). No correlation was found between spectroscopic findings and psychometric scores, nor between spectroscopy and disease evolution time.

In state-of-the-art NMR spectroscopy, the volume in which all metabolic measurements are made has a geometric shape that does not adapt to the complex anatomical shapes of brain structures. The volume of measurement thus contains various tissues in which metabolism is probably different. This, along with methodological differences, may explain the contradictions between the first findings in this new field of investigation. Metabolic exploration with NRM spectroscopy provides both scientific assets (possibility of *in vivo* brain chemistry in man) and ethical benefits (noninvasive and nonionizing investigation).

The physiopathology of presenile dementia (Alzheimer's disease) seems to involve the phospholipidic membranes of neurons (Blusztajn *et al.*, 1984; Nitsch *et al.*, 1992). Intercellular communication requires a degree of membrane integrity (Samuel *et al.*, 1982; Traill *et al.*, 1984) that does not seems to be achieved in Alzheimer's disease (Suzuki *et al.*, 1965; Kanfer *et al.*, 1986; Miller *et al.*, 1986; Ellison *et al.*, 1987; Farooqui *et al.*, 1988).

The interest aroused by *in vivo* NMR spectroscopy (MRS) in Alzheimer's disease was produced by the first findings of abnormalities in phosphorus metabolites in *ex vivo* brain samples (*in vitro* MRS). In fact, abnormal phosphoester levels were initially described *in vitro* (Pettegrew *et al.*, 1984) and Pettegrew's group apparently explained the early rise in phosphomonoester (PME) levels (membrane anabolites) by a phase of adaptation to membrane catabolism that, failing to be compensated, may have a delayed expression in the accumulation of phosphodiesters (PDE) as membrane catabolites (Pettegrew, 1990).

However, the few studies using *in vivo* MRS are contradictory: some tend to demonstrate the same abnormalities as described *in vitro* (Brown *et al.*, 1989; Welch, 1990), while others do not observe them (Bottomley *et al.*, 1989; Murphy *et al.* 1993). We intended to contribute in this debate as we explored *the parietal metabolism of phosphorus 31* (^{31}P) using an *external NMR coil* (Figure 1) that could be applied only on the vertex of the skull (hence the parietal site of exploration) due to the *technical specifications of the device used* (described by Mehier *et al.*, 1988). *The volume of most sensitive measurement* located under the NMR coil (60 mm in diameter) *is a semisphere representing 0.6 times the diameter* where biomembranes metabolism is investigated (Figures 2 and 3 illustrate the principle of membranes' evaluation from ^{31}P spectrum).

Our series was small (5 patients aged 74 to 81 years and 4 normal controls in the same age group). The patients had a psychometric score indicating dementia on the Battery of tests of the Assessment of Dementia (Signoret *et al.*, 1989). The diagnosis of probable Alzheimer's disease was established both with the DSM-III-R (APA, 1987) and Tc-99m-SPECT criteria (Podreka *et al.* 1987). (The neurological and paraclinical assessment was aimed at ruling out other possible causes of dementia.)

Considering the small number of individuals in the series, *the statistical analysis* was carried out with *nonparametric methods* (Mann-Whitney U test and Spearman's rank correlation coefficient).

The protocol for this investigation was accepted by an ethics committee for biomedical research.

Spectrum peaks corresponded to the following metabolites: for phosphorus 31: PME, inorganic phosphate (Pi), PDE, phosphocreatine (PCr) and the gamma, alpha and beta forms of ATP (Figure 2).

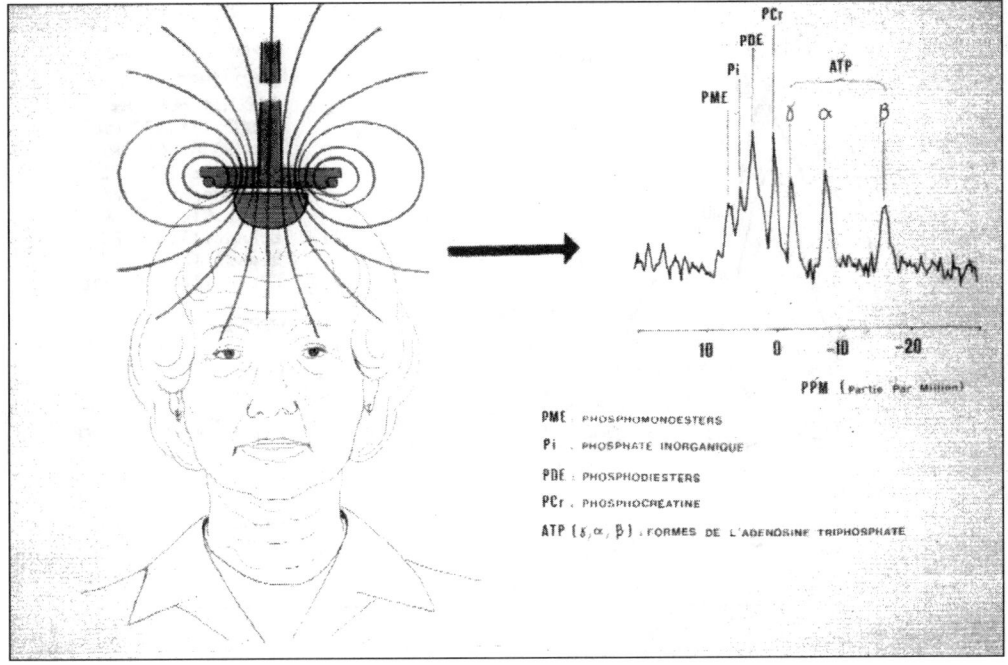

Figure 1.

No statistically significant difference was observed for phosphorus metabolites.

For patients, *no correlation* was found between the ranks of each of the homologous spectrum peaks (Table I) and (a) their psychometric scores on one hand and (b) the duration of disease evolution on the other hand (Table II).

Table I. (Mecheri *et al.*, 1994).

	PATIENTS	CONTROLS
n°1 =	2.2	1.9
n°2 =	1.8	4.2
n°3 =	19.0	8.0
n°4 =	25.3	9.2
n°5 =	26.6	

Table II. (Mecherie *et al.*, 1994)

	AGE (years)	duration of disease evolution (years)
n°1	74	2
n°2	81	3
n°3	79	4
n°4	80	2
n°5	77	5

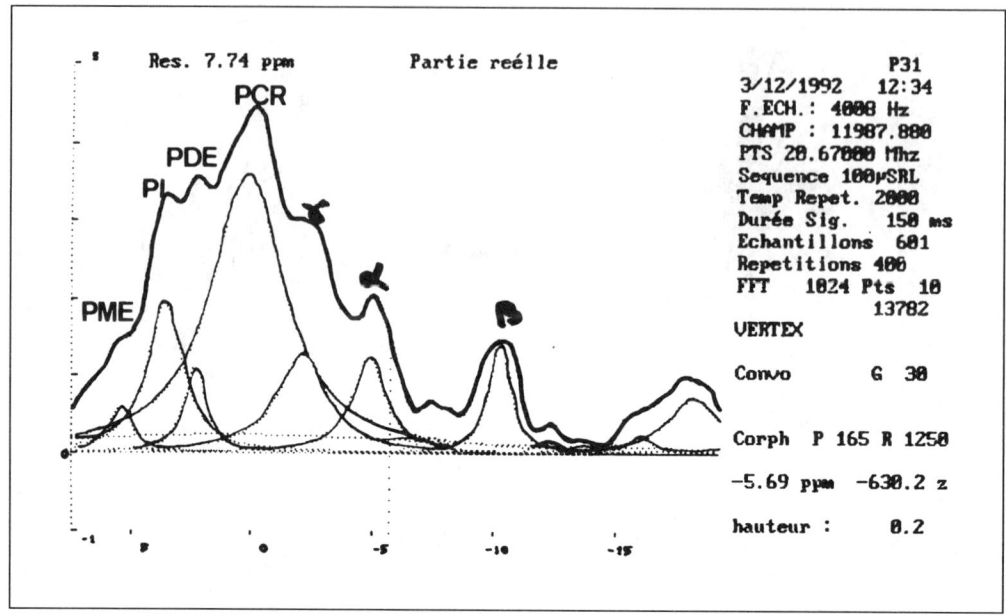

Figure 2.

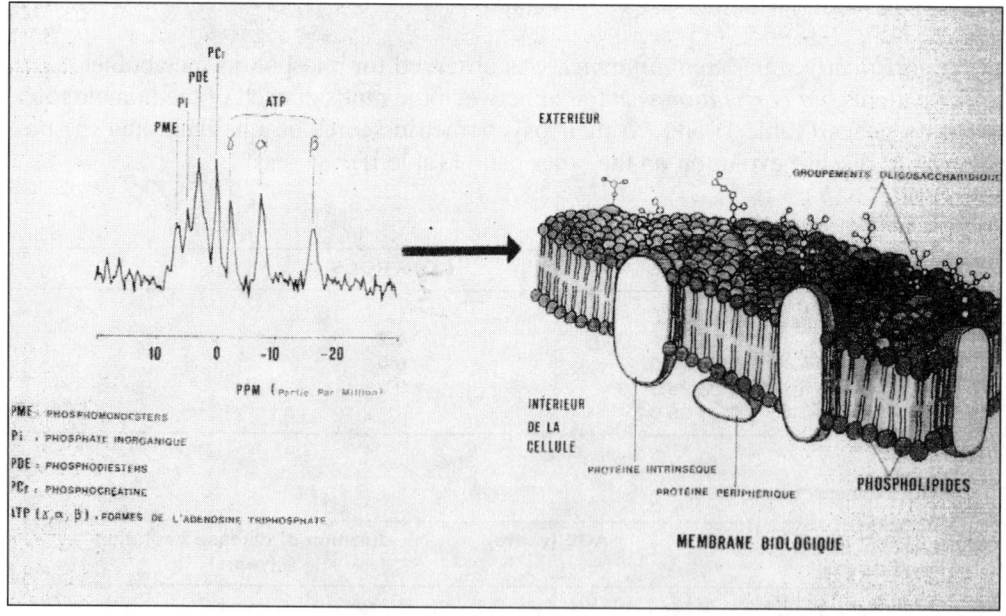

Figure 3.

Although a preliminary publication of results (without statistical analysis) reported what was thought to be a difference in PME percentages (relative to the total spectrum of ^{31}P) between patients and controls (Bissuel et al., 1993), nonparametric statistical processing has shown that there is no significant difference, and this result has been discussed in another paper (Mecheri et al., 1994). We shall not return to this discussion here, but it may be useful to add some supplemental comments.

The number of subjects in this study was too small (patients with Alzheimer's disease find it hard to remain as motionless as required for NMR spectroscopy). Other *major limitations* resulting from the localization method are worth emphasizing. (1) A first risk of methodological bias specific for MRS when it is not guided with imaging (as was the case for us) is that *miscellaneous anatomical tissues* (with a different metabolism) are included in the volume of measurement. (2) A second pitfall, which is not avoided by using an external NMR coil, nor by the other variants of localized NMR spectroscopy, is the risk that *metabolic abnormalities not located in the volume of interest may fail to be recognized:* hence the important help of NMR spectroscopic imaging (MRSI) that will allow an *anatomical mapping of each metabolite in the 31P spectrum* (Hugg et al., 1992). The possible absence of difference in vivo in some discrete brain structures that are typically involved in the disease remains to be demonstrated ; we are presently trying to perform such localized measurements in the hippocampus, on the basis of the great contribution of this structure to the physiopathology of this type of memory disorders in Alzheimer type's dementia (Ball et coll., 1985).

Results with *in vivo* ^{31}P NMR spectroscopy in SDAT are disparate. All technical and human sources of interindividual variability of *in vivo* studies do not allow drawing definite conclusions about membrane abnormalities that were demonstrated by *in vitro* studies. Thus the model of «autocannibalism» in SDAT is based on strong experimental evidence, but not yet on elements yielded by clinical research.

References

1. American Psychiatric Association DSM-III-R. APA Washington D.C. 1987.
2. Bissuel Y, Mecheri G, Mehier H et al. Intérêt de la spectroscopie RMN dans l'exploration du métabolisme cérébral de sujets atteints de maladie d'Alzheimer. *L'Encéphale* 1993 ; XIX, 29-35.
3. Blusztajn JK, Maire JC, Tacconi MT et al. The possible role of neuronal choline metabolism in the pathophysiology of Alzheimer's disease : a hypothesis. In : Alzheimer's disease : advances in basic research and therapies. RJ Wurtman et al. eds. Cambridge (USA) : Center for Brain Sciences and Metabolism. Charitable Trust. .1984 ; 183-98.
4. Bottomley PA, Cousins JP, Pendrey DL et al. Alzheimer dementia : quantification of energy metabolism and mobile phosphoesters with P-31 NMR spectroscopy. *Radiology* 1992 ; 183 : 695-699.
5. Brown CG, Levine SR, Gorell JM et al. In vivo P31 NMR profiles of Alzheimer's disease and multiple subcortical infarct dementia. *Neurology* 1989 ; 39 : 1423-27.
6. Ellison DW, Beal MF, Martin JB Phosphoethanolamine and ethanolamine are increased in Alzheimer's disease and Huntington disease. *Brain Res* 1987 ; 417 : 389-92.
7. Farooqui AA, Liss L, Horrocks LA. Neurochemical aspects of Alzheimer's disease : involvement of membrane phospholipids. *Met Brain Dis* 1988 ; 3 : 19-35.

8. Hugg JW, Matson GB, Twieg DB et al. Phosphorus-31 MR spectroscopic imaging (MRSI) of normal and pathological human brains. *Magn Reson Imag* 1992 ; 10 : 227-43.
9. Kanfer JN, Hattori H, Orihel D. Reduced phospholipase D activity in brain tissue samples from Alzheimer's disease patients. *Ann Neurol* 1986 ; 20 : 265-267.
10. Mecheri G, Bissuel Y, Dalery J et al. In vivo exploration of brain phosphorus 31 metabolism in patients with senile dementia of Alzheimer type. *European Psychiatry* 1994 ; 9 : 105-09.
11. Mehier H, Maurice M, Bonche JP et al. Spectrométrie RMN in vivo avec un aimant résistif à 1,2 T. *C.R. Acad Sci Paris* 1988 ; t. 306, Série III : 313-16.
12. Miatto O, Gonzalez RG, Buonanno F et al. In vitro 31P NMR spectroscopy detects altered phospholipid metabolism in Alzheimer's disease. *Can J Neurol Sci* 1986 ; 13 : 535-9.
13. Miller BL, Jenden DJ, Cummings JL et al. Abnormal erythrocyte choline and influx in Alzheimer's disease. *Life Sci* 1986 ; 38 : 485-90.
14. Murphy DGM, Bottomley PA, Salerno JA et al. An in vivo study of phosphorus and glucose metabolism in Alzheimer's disease using magnetic resonance spectroscopy and PET. *Arch Gen Psychiatry* 1993 ; 50 : 341-49.
15. Nitsch RM, Blusztajn JK, Pittas AG et al. Evidence for a membrane defect in Alzheimer disease brain. *Proc Natl Acad Sci USA* 1992 ; 89 : 1671-75.
16. Pettegrew JW, Minshew NJ, Cohen MM et al. 31P NMR changes in Alzheimer's and Huntington's disease brain *Neurology* 1984 ; 34 (Suppl. 1) : 281.
17. Pettegrew JW. NMR : *Principles and applications to biomedical research New York* 1990 ; Spinger-Verlag.
18. Podreka I, Suess E, Goldenberg G et al. Initial experience with Technetium-99m HM-PAO brain Spect. *J Nucl Med* 1987 ; 28 : 1657-66.
19. Samuel D, Heron DS, Herschkowitz M et al. Aging, receptor binding and membrane viscosity. In : *The aging brain : cellular and molecular mechanisms of aging in the nervous system*. E. Giacobini, A. Vernadakis eds. New York : Raven Press. 1982 ; 20 : 93-7.
20. Signoret JL, Bonvaret M, Benoit N et al. Batterie d'estimations des états démentiels : description et validation. In : La maladie d'Alzheimer et ses limites. Congrès de Psychiatrie et de Neurologie de langue française. LXXXVIe Session. Chambéry, 13-17 juin 1988. Compte rendu par JM Leger. Paris : Masson, 1989 ; 265-70.
21. Suzuki K, Katzman R, Korey SR. Chemical studies on Alzheimer's disease. *J Neuropathol Exp Neurol* 1965 ; 24 : 211-24.
22. Traill KN, WICK G. Lipids and lymphocyte function. *Immunol Today* 1984 ; 5 : 70-76.
23. Welch KMA. 31P in vivo spectroscopy of adult human brain. In : NMR : Principles and Applications to Biomedical research. JW Pettegrew New York, ed. Spinger-Verlag 1990 ; 429-67.

43

Effect of spatial resolution on activation ratio in echo-planar functional MRI

M.-E. MEYER, L. HERTZ-PANNIER, R.C. RISINGER*, S. POSSE, D. LE BIHAN

Radiology Department, Clinical Center and *Section on Clinical Pharmacology, NIMH, National Institutes of Health, Bethesda, MD, USA.

Unbalanced variations of cerebral blood flow and oxygen consumption during activation is assumed to decrease the amount of paramagnetic deoxyhemoglobin in the cerebral blood pool. The transient modulation of magnetic susceptibility, origin of the deoxyhemoglobin contrast in functional MRI (fMRI), may be monitored by using fast MRI acquisition schemes. This contrast allows to study brain function with use of both Echo Planar Imaging (EPI) and FLASH sequences.

The MR signal intensity changes that occur during cerebral activation are relatively small and, therefore, difficult to detect. Different groups have evaluated the effects of some acquisition parameters of conventional sequences in order to optimize the technique. Some of these parameters deal with voxel size, e.g. slice thickness, matrix size or field of view (FOV).

It has been shown, with FLASH type sequences, that the percent in signal change during activation was increased when the slice thickness was decreased, presumably due to reduced partial volume effects of small areas of activation with regions showing no signal change [1]. However, an increase in the matrix size did not affect the signal change. Other groups have found similar results but increased activation when increasing the FOV (2). These contradictory results do not allow to conclude clearly about the effect of spatial resolution in the case of conventional fast-imaging techniques, and this type of study has not been done with EPI.

EPI has a much better temporal resolution than conventional sequences. Although the spatial resolution is limited by gradient constraints, we have investigated its effect on the signal change during motor task by varying the in-plane resolution (slice thickness constant). Our goal was to evaluate the usefulness of higher spatial resolution in terms of signal changes and to ultimately better understand which structure is responsible for the MR signal increase in fMRI.

Materials and methods

Acquisition

The activation paradigm consisted of two periods of finger tapping alternated with rest conditions. Imaging was performed by gradient-echo BEST-EPI on a standard clinical 1.5T MRI system using a 5 inch surface coil. Acquisition parameters were TE=50msec, flip angle=90°, and, in the 64x64 matrix size's case, TR=3 sec. Slice thickness was 5mm in all cases. The different pixel sizes were obtained by changing the FOV (10, 12, 16, 20 and 24 cm) and the acquisition matrix. Two acquisition matrices (64x64 and 128x128) were used. 128x128 matrix was performed by two interleaved acquisitions, each of them allowing for one half of the required K-space to be acquired in TR period=1.5 sec [the odd rows are acquired during the first TR period and the even rows during the secong one, thus making the total scan time 2TR=3 sec]. This combination of FOVs and matrices resulted in pixel sizes ranging from 0.6 to 14 mm^2. The EPI images were superimposed on SPGR anatomical images (flip angle=70°, TR=0.1 sec, TE minimal, 2NEX, in a 192x256 matrix).

Processing

Pixels showing a significant cross-correlation of the MRI time-course signal with respect to a reference waveform following the paradigm were considered as activated. Cross-correlation was performed in the Fourier domain (time-course series), after eliminating the low frequency component. For each experiment and several regions of interest (ROI) in the sensorimotor cortex (e.g. one ROI in the depth of the sulcus, one ROI close to the brain surface and one large ROI covering the entire activated regions), the surface (volume) of the activated region (S) was measured. In each ROI, the mean activation ratio (AR) for the activated pixels was calculated (difference between the mean signal of the activated and rest condition images normalized by the mean signal of the rest condition images). Signal to noise ratio (SNR) was also determined for each experiment.

Results

• Typical data are represented in Figures 1 and 2. Figure 1 shows clear increase of AR when pixel size is decreased (5 fold increase between 10 and 0.9 mm^2 pixel size).

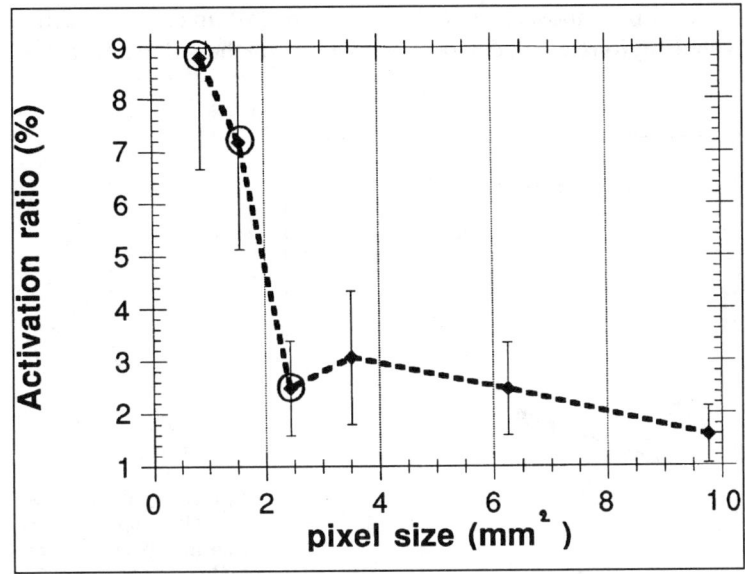

Figure 1. Typical plot of the AR versus pixel size (mm²). Acquisition matrix was 64x64 [for the 3 largest pixels, (•)] and 128x128 [for the 3 smallest pixels, (◎)].

Note that there seems to be two regimens in Figure 2a corresponding to 128² and 64² matrices respectively. In Figure 2, the size of the activated region (S) is plotted against the pixel size. S decreased while increasing the spatial resolution, the slope of the curve being higher for the biggest pixels.

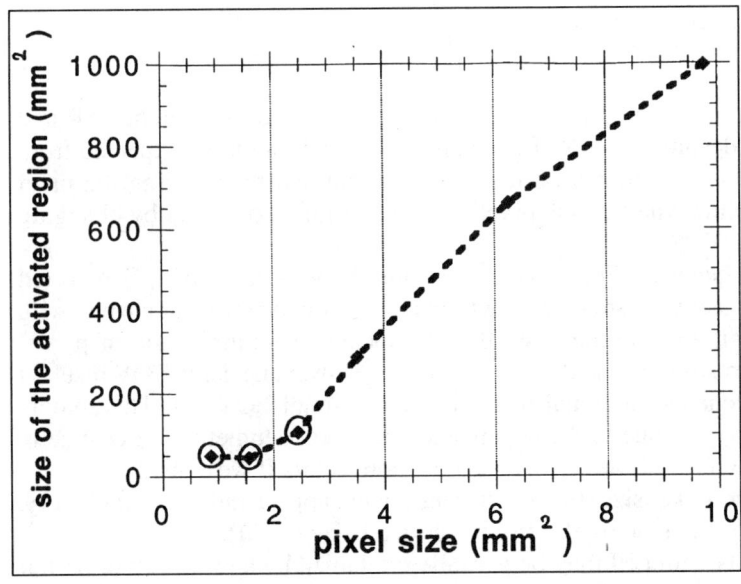

Figure 2. Typical plot of the size (mm²) of the activated region versus pixel size (mm²). Acquisition matrix was 64x64 [for the 3 largest pixels, (•)] and 128x128 [for the 3 smallest pixels (◎)].

- On the other hand, as expected, SNR dropped with voxel size (Figure 3).

• When EPI images are superimposed on SPGR anatomical images, it seems relatively clear that activated regions are located in the center of the sulcus, in areas close to vessels.

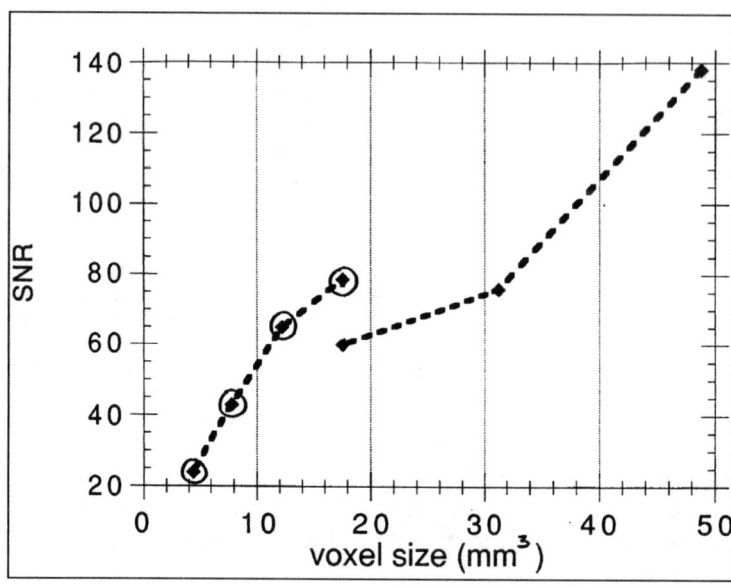

Figure 3. Typical plot of SNR versus voxel size (mm3). Acquisition matrix was 64x64 [one interleave, for the 3 largest voxels, (•)] and 128x128 [2 interleaves, for the 4 smallest voxels, (◉)].

Discussion

Our results show that increasing the spatial resolution in EPI leads to higher AR and smaller activated areas, despite lower SNR. In contrast to what might be expected from large susceptibility effects, AR increased rather than decreased by reducing the pixel size. This effect is the same whether this pixel size's variation is obtained by changing the matrix size or the FOV.

With conventional sequences, Frahm et al. [1] and Thompson et al. [2] reported greater change of MR signal with smaller slice thickness, but no significant change with matrix size. These authors explain the first effect by means of minimization of partial volume averaging of inert structures and activated cortex. However, a large FOV resulted in a greater percentage change in signal intensity than a small FOV [2]. The authors assume that this result may be due to the dependency on voxel geometry; the change in signal intensity would increase as the voxels become more cubic. If we consider all these parameters relative to the voxel size, these different results appear rather contradictory. It is therefore difficult to conclude on the effects of voxel size on AR.

In our study, the results with EPI may be partially explained by a reduction of partial volume effect of small activated areas with regions that are not activated. This hypothesis could be particularly valid for the biggest voxels where there is an important decrease of the size S of the activated region when the image resolution is increased.

However, our results also show that the smaller the pixel size, the higher his effect on AR, and the smaller the variation of S. This suggests that another kind of effect might also be involved, e.g. a greater dephasing in small pixels. Besides partial volume effect, it is likely that a difference in AR between two resolutions may be observed only when the size of an activated microregion is close to the pixel size of the highest resolution. Indeed, if these microregions are much smaller than the pixel size, or close to the largest pixel size, no gain in AR would be observed with resolution. In other words, this means that as long as we see this high AR variation, but few change of the size S of the activated region, the pixel size has not reached the minimal size of the activated microregions. Our results give therefore an upper limit of about 0.6 mm^2 to the size of at least some of these homogeneous microregions, which may correspond to large microvessels or to a portion of the cortical ribbon.

SNR dropped linearly with voxel size as expected from theory. The better SNR obtained with 128^2 matrix over 64^2 matrix with identical voxel size is explained by the two interleaves required to obtain 128^2 images on our system. Indeed, for a given voxel size,

$$SNR \sim \alpha \, (NEX.N_p.N_f/BW)^{1/2} \, [1-\exp(-TR/T1)]$$

where NEX is the number of excitations, Np and Nf the numbers of phase- and frequency-encoding samples and BW the bandwidth.

NEX and N_f are two times larger in 128x128 matrix, whereas BW and Np are the same in both matrices. The ratio between the two experiments (128x128 versus 64x64) should then be about 1.8 with $T_1 = 0.6$ sec.

Conclusion

Better AR can be obtained with EPI by improving spatial resolution. However, there could be a limit to this benefit, first when SNR becomes too low, increasing MRI signal fluctuations [3] and second, when the pixel size reaches the actual size of the microregion responsible for the MR signal increase.

References

1. Frahm J, Merboldt KD, Hanicke W. *Magn Reson Med* 1993 ; 29 : 139.
2. Thompson RM, Jack, Butts CR, K et al., *Radiology* 1994 ; 190 : 873.
3. Hertz-Pannier L, Cuenod CA, Jezzard P et al. *12th Annual SMRM Meeting, Book of Abstracts*, New-York 1993, 1429.

44

Metabolic alterations in Alzheimer's disease using *in vitro* ¹H NMR

P. MOHANAKRISHNAN[1], A.H. FOWLER[1], M.M. HUSAIN[1], J.P. VONSATTEL[2], P.R. JOLLES[1], P. LIEM[1], R.A. KOMOROSKI[1]

[1]*University of Arkansas for Medical Sciences, Little Rock, AR 72205,USA.*
[2]*Brain Tissue Resource Center,2 McLean Hospital, Belmont, MA, USA.*

The definitive diagnosis of Alzheimer's disease (AD) is made in terms of the relative number and regional distribution of senile plaques (SP) and neurofibrillary tangles (NFT) detected during the histopathologic examination of postmortem brains. It has not been clearly established if the roles of these hallmarks are causal. Other changes in AD brains include neuronal loss (NL) and alterations in metabolite levels. Radionuclide-based functional imaging modalities such as PET (positron emission tomography) and SPECT (single photon emission computed tomography) demonstrate characteristic metabolic and perfusion defects in AD brains, typically in bilateral posterior temporoparietal cortical areas, thereby aiding in the diagnosis of probable and possible AD in living patients.

The role of magnetic resonance imaging (MRI) in AD is mostly to rule out structural causes of dementia like tumors. However, MRI in combination with localized *in vivo* nuclear magnetic resonance (NMR) spectroscopy can noninvasively furnish simultaneous anatomic and metabolic information. With proton (^{1}H) as the probing nucleus, the latter can detect metabolites such as N-acetyl aspartate (NAA, a putative neuronal marker), creatine, choline, lactate and *myo*-inositol in various brain regions in vivo. At the low field strengths of clinical MR scanners (1.5 tesla), spectral resolution is poor due to overlap of signals, making peak assignment and metabolite quantitation difficult. On the other hand, high resolution ^{1}H NMR spectroscopic studies of the extracts of autopsy brains do not suffer from serious resolution limitations, can yield correlations with histopathologic parameters, and are complementary to *in vivo* NMR studies.

In this report we summarize the results of our high resolution ^{1}H NMR spectroscopic studies of AD [1-3]. The brain regions of interest were: 1) posterior temporoparietal cortex, 2) hippocampus/medial temporal cortex, 3) cerebellum and 4) frontal cortex. They were chosen because of the metabolic/perfusion deficits seen in PET/SPECT images (regions 1 & 4), the role in cognition (region 2), and the expectation that these regions would be differently affected by the disease.

Methods and materials

Samples (mostly gray matter) from the posterior temporoparietal cortex, hippocampus/medial temporal cortex, and cerebellum of thirteen AD and four nondemented autopsy brains (of individuals between the ages of 63 and 95) were extracted with 90% aqueous methanol in the manner of Koller et al. [4]. Samples of frontal cortex of six AD brains were studied to assess cortical variation in metabolic dysfunction. The solvent was removed first under dry nitrogen and then by freeze-drying, and the residue resuspended in a 50% mixture of H_2O and D_2O. The pH of the extract was 6.85-7.0. The ^{1}H NMR spectra of the extracts were recorded at 300.5 MHz on a General Electric GN-300WB FT NMR spectrometer using a 90° pulse of width 6 msec, a pulse delay of 20 sec, a spectral width 4000 Hz, 16K data points and 64 acquisitions/spectrum. The residual water signal was attenuated by the application of a 4-sec presaturation pulse. Spectral processing involved zero-filling and a simple exponential multiplication. Chemical shift referencing was relative to the NAA methyl signal at 2.02 ppm.

Figure 1 shows portions of a typical high resolution ^{1}H NMR spectrum of the hippocampus of a 76-year-old female AD patient [2]. The metabolites of primary interest in this study were NAA, creatine (Cre), GABA (4-aminobutyric acid), glutamate (Glu), and inositol. Their absolute concentrations (mM or mmoles/ml of tissue water) were estimated relative to a reference of known concentration in a capillary tube concentric to the NMR sample tube, assuming a tissue water content of 0.79 ml/g [1]. The concentrations for each group were provided as a mean ± standard error of the mean (SEM). Statistical analysis was performed using analysis of variance (MANOVA) or Student's t-test. All five metabolites could not be determined for the temporoparietal and hippocampal regions of one AD case, and hence it was omitted in the MANOVA treatment of those regions. Differences were considered significant where p£0.05.

The diagnosis of AD was confirmed by conventional neuropathologic examination [5,6] of the formalin-fixed contralateral side. Sections from 17 representative blocks were stained with Luxol fast blue for general survey and counter-stained with hemotoxylin and eosin for semiautomated sampling stage examination of neuronal density. Additionally, Bielshowsky silver stain was used for evaluating axons, plaques, and tangles. The histopathology was assumed to be bilaterally symmetric.

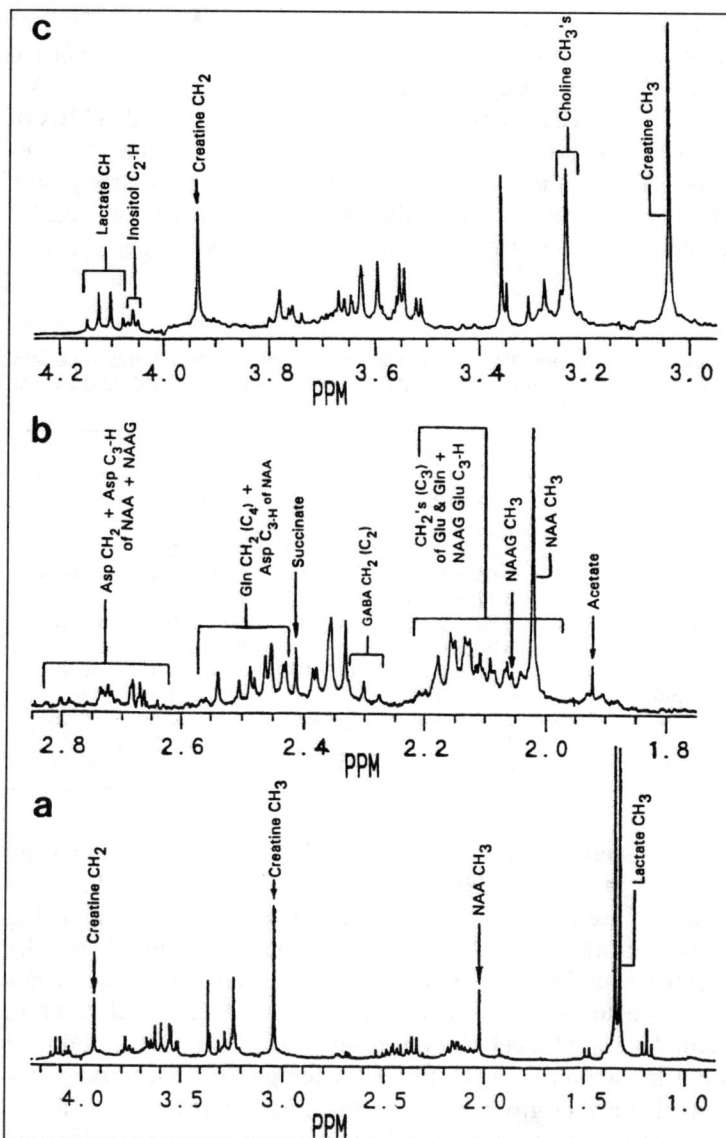

Figure 1. Portions of the 300-MHz proton NMR spectrum of the methanol-water extract of the hippocampus of a 76-year-old female AD patient. Spectrum a is the 0.8-4.2 ppm region; b is the 1.8-2.8 ppm region expanded (vertical gain of 4 ′ a); c is the 2.8-4.2 ppm region expanded (vertical gain of 2 ′ a).

Results and discussion

The postmortem interval (PMI) varied between 1.4 and 16.8 hours. The metabolite concentrations did not show any significant dependence on PMI. Table I summarizes the results for the five metabolites of interest in the cerebellum, the hippocampus, and the temporoparietal cortex. Due to extraction inefficiency, decreases in metabolites due to aging, and a possible underestimation of concentrations from adherent water (when frozen brains are used), the concentrations in Table I are expected to be about 70% of those in a normal, unaged adult brain in vivo. The average estimate of NAA in a normal adult human brain is 5-8 mM, with gray matter being ~2 mM higher in NAA concentration than white matter [7]. The average concentrations of NAA and GABA of the cerebellum, the temporoparietal cortex, and the hippocampal region of the AD cases were significantly lower ($p<0.05$) than the corresponding values for the control group. For comparison, the concentrations reported for other metabolites in cerebral cortex (biopsies) include 11-12 mM Cre, 11 mM glutamate, 8-11 mM inositol, and 2.2 mM GABA [8].

Table I. Concentrations (Mean ± SEM) of selected metabolites in cerebellum, posterior temporoparietal cortex (PTPC) and hippocampus/medial temporal cortex (HMTC) of AD (N=12 for PTPC and HMTC, N=13 for cerebellum) and control brains (N=4).

Metab.	Group	Concentrations (mM)					
		Cerebellum	p	PTPC	p	HMTC	p
NAA	Control	4.03 ± 0.61		4.30 ± 0.39		4.16 ± 0.54	
	AD	2.36 ± 0.22	<0.005	2.65 ± 0.21	<0.003	2.19 ± 0.14	<.0002
Cre	Control	8.12 ± 1.62		8.17 ± 0.23		7.39 ± 1.50	
	AD	7.08 ± 0.78	>0.05	5.53 ± 0.43	<0.005	5.87 ± 0.34	>0.05
Glu	Control	9.44 ± 1.91		8.38 ± 0.47		8.19 ± 1.10	
	AD	6.87 ± 0.71	>0.05	6.62 ± 0.53	0.0913	7.08 ± 0.47	>0.05
Inos	Control	3.88 ± 0.95		5.20 ± 0.86		5.52 ± 1.48	
	AD	3.08 ± 0.33	>0.05	3.79 ± 0.55	>0.05	4.61 ± 0.56	>0.05
GABA	Control	1.44 ± 0.27		1.48 ± 0.07		1.42 ± 0.28	
	AD	0.91 ± 0.11	<0.042	0.81 ± 0.07	<0.0002	0.89 ± 0.05	<0.01

The decrease in NAA is consistent with the occurrence of NL in the hippocampal and temporoparietal cortical regions in AD. The Glu estimates for the two cerebral regions of the AD group, though lower, are not significantly different from the corresponding estimates for the nondemented group. The GABA concentration of neurons is an order of magnitude higher than other neural cell types such as astrocytes or oligodendrocytes [9]. Thus a GABA decrease is also expected. Our results for NAA and GABA are in agreement with those of Klunk et al. [10,11]. But our results for Glu and inositol do not support some recent findings in the literature [11,12]. The average Cre concentration for the temporoparietal cortex of the AD group is lower than, and statistically different from, that for the control group, suggesting that Cre may not serve as a internal quantitation standard for in vivo NMR studies of AD.

The mean concentrations for NAA (2.36 ± 0.22 mM) and GABA (0.91 ± 0.11 mM) of the cerebella of the AD group (n = 13) are lower than those for the nondemented cases (4.03 ± 0.61 and 1.44 ± 0.27 mM, respectively). As cerebellum is considered unaffected in AD, it becomes necessary to invoke cerebellar dysmetabolism to account for the significant decreases in NAA and GABA of the AD group. Cerebellar dysmetabolism in the contralateral side may accompany supra-tentorial lesions [13]. Cerebellar atrophy and lesions (Alzheimer or non-Alzheimer type) in contralateral cerebrum may contribute to the metabolite decreases, in addition to age differences and perimortem factors. The mean ages of the AD and nondemented groups were 82 and 68 years, respectively. It was not possible to ascertain the contributions from each of these factors.

Arbitrary scores of 0, 1, 2, 3, and 4, were assigned respectively to the absence of, and mild, moderate, severe, and very severe presence of SP and NFT, to correlate the metabolite concentrations with histopathology in the hippocampal and temporoparietal regions. Figures 2a and 2b show typical fits for NAA in the temporoparietal cortex. The results for both regions are summarized in Table II. A significant correlation (r=-0.85, p=0.0001) was also obtained for NAA vs. NL in the hippocampus. Both NAA and GABA in both regions showed significant negative correlations with the amount of NFT or SP. In addition, for the temporoparietal cortex, Cre and Glu also showed such significant linear correlations.

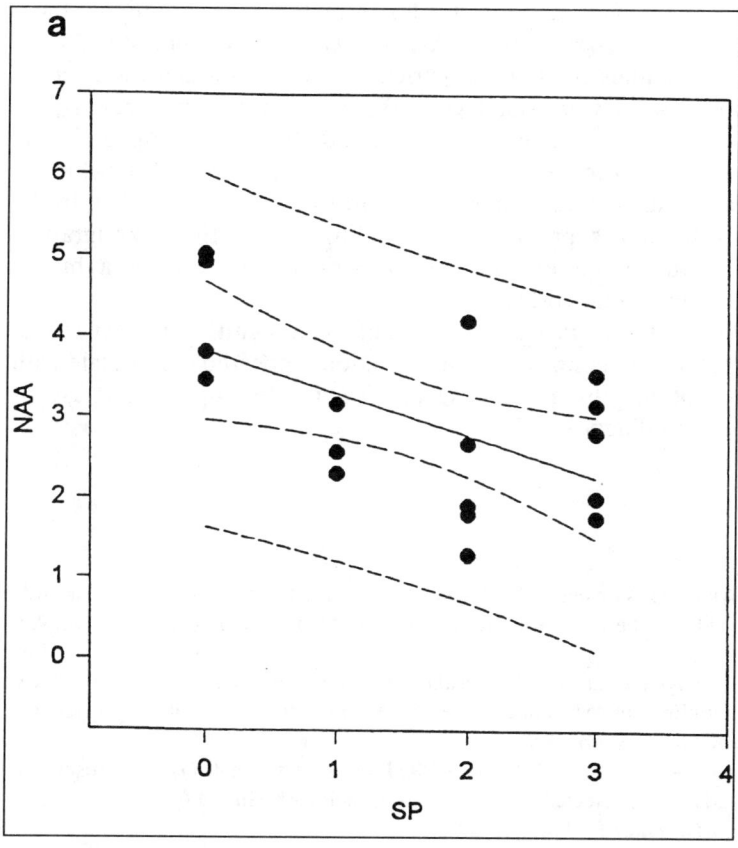

Figure 2. a) NAA concentration vs. semi-quantitative assessment of SP in temporoparietal cortex of AD patients; b) NAA concentration vs. semiquantitative assessment of NFT.

Table II. Correlations of metabolite concentrations with histopathologic parameters. For each case, the correlation coefficient and p-value (below) are listed.

SP, NFT or NL	Temporoparietal cortex				Hippocampal region	
	Cre	GABA	Glu	NAA	GABA	NAA
NFT	-0.67	-0.78	-0.55	-0.79	-0.57	-0.72
	<0.004	<0.003	<0.027	<0.0002	<0.025	<0.002
SP				-0.56	-0.54	-0.66
				<0.021	<0.031	<0.005
NL						-0.85
						0.0001

On the basis of *in vitro* and localized *in vivo* NMR results [7,14,15] in the literature, it is reasonable to assume that the concentrations of NAA, Cre, Glu, inositol, and GABA will be the same for both the frontal and temporal cortices. The average concentrations of these metabolites for the temporoparietal cortex of six AD brains were 2.27 ± 0.29, 5.08 ± 0.79, 6.39 ± 0.70, 3.94 ± 0.93 and 0.82 ± 0.02 mM, respectively. The corresponding values for the frontal cortex of the same brains were 3.13 ± 0.32, 6.46 ± 0.89, 8.84 ± 1.15, 4.69 ± 1.15 and 1.09 ± 0.18, respectively. The average concentrations of NAA, Glu, and inositol for frontal cortex were higher than, and statistically different from ($p<0.02$ for NAA, <0.05 for Glu, and <0.035 for inositol), the corresponding values for temporoparietal cortex. Although the average concentrations of Cre and GABA were statistically the same for the two regions, for five of the six cases the individual concentrations of Cre and GABA were higher for the frontal cortex than for the temporoparietal cortex. The lower average NAA value for temporoparietal cortex suggests a lower number of neurons in that region than in the frontal cortex. Our results are thus supportive of the finding from SPECT scintigraphic analysis [16] that the perfusion deficits in temporoparietal cortex have a higher predictive value than those in frontal cortex.

In summary, high resolution, *in vitro* 1H NMR confirmed significant biochemical alterations in AD brains relative to controls. These alterations appeared to correlate with histopathologic measures of the disease. These *in vitro* results support the use of localized, in vivo 1H NMR to diagnose AD.

References

1. Mohanakrishnan P, Fowler AH, Vonsattel JP, Husain MM, Jolles, P. Liem PR, Komoroski RA, An *In vitro* 1H NMR study of the temporoparietal cortex of Alzheimer brains, *Exp Brain Res* submitted.
2. Mohanakrishnan P, Fowler AH, Vonsattel JP, Husain MM, Jolles PR, Liem P, Komoroski RA. Regional metabolic alterations in Alzheimer disease. An *In vitro* 1H NMR Study of the Hippocampus and Cerebellum, *J Neurol Sci* submitted.
3. Mohanakrishnan P, Fowler AH, Husain MM, Jolles PR, Liem P, Newton JEO, Komoroski RA, Vonsattel JP. Cortical variation of selected metabolites in Alzheimer brains using High resolution 1H NMR Spectroscopy, *J Gerontol Biol Sci* submitted.

4. Koller KJ, Zaczek R, Coyle JT. N-acetyl-aspartyl-glutamate: regional levels in rat brain and the effects of brain lesions as determined by a new HPLC method *J Neurochem* 1984 ; **43** : 1136-42.
5. Tomlinson BE. Aging and Dementias, in *Greenfield's Neuropathology* (J. H. Adams and L. W. Duchen, Eds.), 5th Ed., New York Oxford University Press 1992 ; 1284-410.
6. Mirra SS, Heyman A, McKeel D *et al.*, The Consortium to Establish Registry for Alzheimer's Disease (CERAD), Part II. Standardization of the Neuropathalogic Assessment of Alzheimer's Disease *Neurology* 1991 ; **41** : 479-86.
7. Bilken DL, Oldendorf. WH, N-acetyl-L-aspartic acid: a literature review of a compound prominent in ^{1}H NMR spectroscopic studies of brain. *Neurosci Biobehav Rev* 1989 ; **13** : 23-31.
8. Petroff OAC, Spencer DD, Alger JR, Pritchard JW. High resolution proton magnetic resonance spectroscopy of human cerebrum obtained during surgery during epilepsy. *Neurology* 1989 ; **39** : 1197-202.
9. Urenjak J, Williams SR, Gadian DG, Noble M. Proton nuclear magnetic resonance spectroscopy identifies different neural cell types. *J Neurosci* 1993 ; **13** : 981-9.
10. Klunk WE, Xu CJ, Panchalingam K, Pettegrew JW. Quantitative *in vitro* NMR analysis of Alzheimer's and non-Alzheimer's demented and control brain. *Biol Psychiatry* 1994 ; **35** : 627.
11. Klunk WE, Panchalingam K, Moosy J, McClure RJ, Pettegrew JW. N-acetyl-L-aspartate and other amino acid metabolites in Alzheimer's disease brain: a preliminary nuclear magnetic resonance study. *Neurology* 1992 ; **42** : 81-93.
12. Miller BL, Moats RA, Shonk T, Ernst T, Woolley S, Ross BD. Alzheimer's disease: depiction of increased *myo*-inositol with proton MR spectroscopy. *Radiology* 1993 ; **187** : 433-7.
13. Kushner M, Tobin M, Alavi A, Chawlik J, Rosen M, Fazekas F, Alavi J, Reivich M. Cerebellar glucose consumption and pathologic states using fluorine-FDG and PET. *J Nucl Med* 1987 ; **28** : 1667-80.
14. Christiansen P, Henriksen O, Stubgard M, Gideon P, Larsson HBW. *In vivo* quantification of brain metabolites by ^{1}H-MRS using water as an internal standard. *Magn Reson Imaging* 1993 ; **11** : 107-18.
15. Hennig J, Pfister H, Ernst T, Ott D. Direct quantification of metabolites in the human brain with *in vivo* localized proton spectroscopy, *NMR Biomed* 1992 ; **5** : 193-9.
16. Holman BL, Johnson KA, Gerada B, Carvalho PA, Satlin A. The scintigraphic appearance of Alzheimer's disease: the prospective study of technitium-99-m-HMPAO SPECT. *J Nucl Med* 1992 ; **33** : 181-5.

45

Advances in brain MRI and MRS

P. MORRIS[1], H. BACHELARD[1], K. BINGHAM[1], R. COXON[1], P. GLOVER[1],
M. HUMBERSTONE[1], J. HYKIN[1], D. McINTYRE[1], G. SAWLE[3], N. THATCHER[1]

[1]*Magnetic Resonance Centre, Department of Physics University of Nottingham, University Park, Nottingham, NG7 2RD, UK.*
[2]*Division of Biochemistry, Department of Cellular and Molecular Sciences, St. George's Hospital Medical School, Cranmer Terrace, London, SW17 ORE, UK.*
[3]*Division of Clinical Neurology, Department of Medicine, University Hospital, Queen's Medical Centre, Nottingham, NG7 2UH, UK.*

This article discusses some of the approaches to brain MRI/S that are under development at the Magnetic Resonance Centre in Nottingham. A major neurospectroscopy programme has been underway there for several years now. Based on a superfused slice model, it is providing valuable new insights into cerebral metabolism under a variety of clinically relevant conditions. We regard these basic studies as an essential prelude to the human MRS studies that we are beginning to undertake on the newly completed whole body 3T system. Our main interest is in ^{13}C neurospectroscopy. However, our first human ^{13}C MRS studies, described below, have been of glycogen metabolism in muscle and liver. These have the advantage that they can be undertaken at natural abundance, and so are relatively inexpensive. Cerebral studies using ^{13}C-labelled material will follow shortly.

We have also been active in developing functional MRI, as detailed below, and see the combination of this with ^{13}C measurements of regional metabolic rates as being particularly powerful.

Functional magnetic resonance imaging (fMRI)

In the last few years, the feasibility of mapping changes in regional cerebral blood flow in response to task activation has been established. The first studies in man (Belliveau et al., 1991) were based on measurements of local blood volume. They aroused considerable excitement, but were of limited application because they required the intravenous administration of the exogenous contrast agent, Gd(DTPA). However, it had previously been shown in animal studies, that deoxyhaemoglobin is an effective endogenous contrast agent that reports changes in oxygenation state (Ogawa et al., 1990). Subsequently, it was shown that this provides the basis for completely non-invasive studies of brain activation. (Belliveau et al., 1992; Menon et al., 1992). This resulted in an explosion of interest, both within the magnetic resonance community, and more especially in the fields of psychology and psychiatry.

The contrast mechanism is not fully understood, but seems to involve an overcompensation of cerebral blood flow in response to brain activation, leading to an increase in the proportion of oxy- relative to deoxyhaemoglobin. Deoxyhaemoglobin is paramagnetic, and in MRI techniques sensitive to magnetic susceptibility (T_2^* effects), its presence in the microvasculature will cause signal attenuation. Conversely, an increase in the fraction of oxyhaemoglobin causes the signal intensity to increase. Hence task activation, for example by photic stimulation, causes the relevant areas of the brain to «light up». Although initially surprising, an increase in blood oxygen level can be rationalized in terms of the need for increased oxygen delivery to support the increased metabolic rate that must accompany activation. Some controversy remains concerning possible motion artefacts, and the less specific contributions to the activation signal from «draining veins» (Menon et al., 1993). Certainly, great care is needed, and some techniques will be more prone to artefacts than others, but the phenomenon now seems well established.

High speed imaging techniques are required if task activation (or at least the response of regional blood flow to it) is to be followed in real time. Such methods also help to minimise motional artefacts, suppressing those that arise within a single image: they do not suppress errors due to misregistration of the two images (control and stimulated) whose difference yields the activation map. However, reregistration, or more sophisticated methods of analysis (see below) can be used to alleviate this problem. At the Magnetic Resonance Centre, we are using the echo-planar imaging (EPI) techniques, originally developed in Nottingham by Mansfield (1977). In the past, technical difficulties have restricted EPI to relatively low resolution, typically with image matrices of 64 * 64 or 64 * 128. A combination of improved gradient design and better magnetic field homogeneity (0.5 ppm over a 35 cm diameter sphere) has recently enabled high quality EPI images of the human head to be recorded at 3T, using image matrices of 256 * 256, corresponding to an in-plane resolution of 0.75 mm (Mansfield et al., 1994).

This system, developed in house, around an Oxford Magnet Technology 3T magnet, is being applied to brain activation studies. Preliminary results on visual stimulation (Hykin *et al.*, 1995) have concentrated on controling for potential artefacts. Thus, a comparison between gradient echo and spin echo experiments reveals a much larger signal from the former, suggesting, on the basis of mathematical modeling, a significant contribution from larger vessels (draining veins). However, the pattern of activation is similar for the two methods, suggesting that these larger vessels are located at the activation site, rather than remote from it. Potential motion artefacts have been eliminated by using a Fourier analysis of a cyclical activation sequence. Such techniques, originally developed for studying periodic motion, such as the cardiac cycle (Doyle and Mansfield, 1986), allow activation events to be extracted that are synchronous with the activation sequence, eliminating the random effects of motion. They also allow the phase of the response to be determined relative to the stimulatory event, and offer the possibility of being able to derive the temporal sequence of brain activation, when several centres are involved.

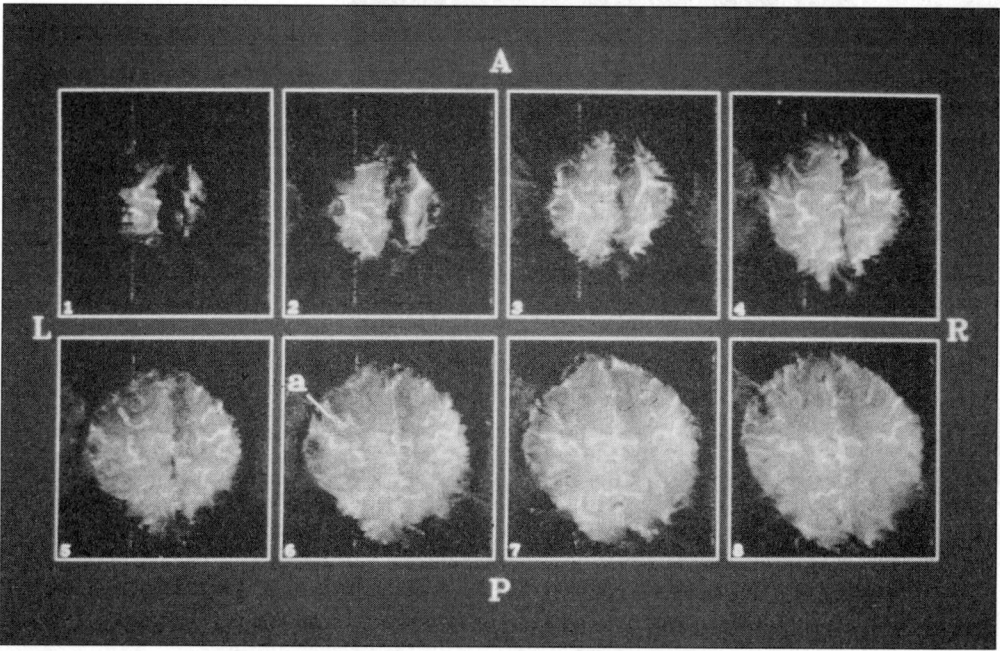

Figure 1. Set of 8 contiguous axial brain slices recorded using a 3T MR system using half Fourier EPI. Activation in response to a cued finger tapping protocol is overlaid in red. The region that correlates most strongly with the periods of activity is labelled «a». (See text for details.)

Figure 1 shows a set of 8 contiguous axial brain slices, acquired during a motor activation paradigm on the Nottingham 3T system, using half Fourier EPI (Mansfield *et al.*, 1994). The subject extended and relaxed the index finger of his right hand, paced at 3Hz by a single digit LED display. Finger movement was continued for 32 s, followed by a 32 s rest period. Data were acquired over 6 full activation cycles at the rate of 4 images per «on» or «off» period. Saturation effects were minimised by preceding the measurements with 16 «warm-up» scans. The data were analysed by calculating, for each pixel, the correlation coefficient to a square wave corresponding to the activation epochs. A threshold value for the correlation coefficient of 0.48 was chosen ($p < 0.01$) and the activation data superimposed on the base image. Figure 2 shows the variation in pixel intensity in the region of highest correlation, labelled «a» in slice 6 of Figure 1. This region is located within a sulcus in the left fronto-parietal cortex. It is reproducible between subjects, shows increasing activity with rate of movement and we believe represents the primary motor cortex.

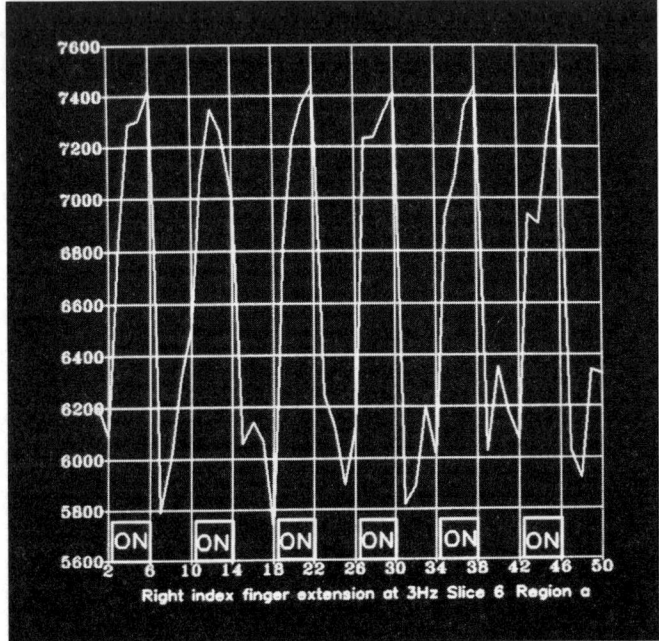

Figure 2. Variation in signal intensity for the region of highest correlation, labelled «a» in slice 6 of Figure 1.

^{13}C studies of glycogen metabolism in human muscle and liver

Pioneering ^{13}C NMR studies by Shulman and colleagues at Yale have contributed significantly to our understanding of glycogen metabolism in man. In particular, these studies have demonstrated unequivocally that muscle glycogen synthesis is the principal pathway of glucose disposal in normal and diabetic subjects (Shulman et al., 1990). Recently, we have studied the post exercise repletion of liver and muscle glycogen. Healthy volunteers were positioned inside the bore of the 3T whole-body superconducting magnet, and natural abundance ^{13}C NMR spectra were recorded at 32 MHz, without proton decoupling. The data were collected in blocks of 30,000 free induction decays, accumulated over periods of 5.5 min. For the liver, a circular surface coil of radius 6 cm, mounted on a plastic spacer, was taped to the skin of the volunteer;

for the muscle measurements, an elliptical surface coil of major axis 12 cm and minor axis 7 cm was attached to a thermoplastic cast, previously moulded to the upper leg of the subject. A small vial, containing a solution of doped sodium acetate, labelled in the C_1 position (carboxyl group), was attached to the reverse side of each coil at roughly the same height as the depth of tissue from which maximum signal was expected, and served as a reference standard.

The most prominent resonances arise from mobile lipids. A small but clear doublet at approximately 100 ppm (relative to TMS = 0), corresponds to the natural abundance signal from the C_1 position of glycogen. Resonances from the other glycogen carbons (C_2 - C_6) are hidden under the lipid peaks (mostly the triacylglycerol quartet). The glycogen contents of liver and muscle were determined from the integral of the doublet peak area and expressed as a percentage of the lipid peak. We believe that the measurements represent total glycogen (rather than a more mobile subfraction) on the basis of previous ^{13}C studies of glycogen in rat liver (Stevens et al., 1982).

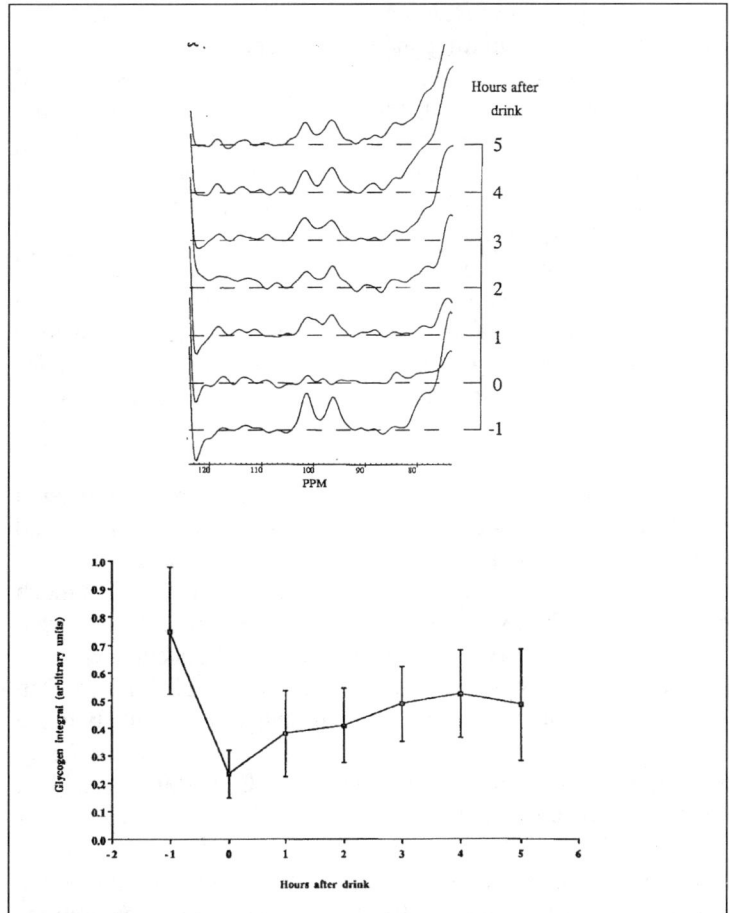

Figure 3. (a) ^{13}C MRS spectrum (70 - 120 ppm region) showing the depletion of muscle glycogen (doublet at 100 ppm) after intensive exercise and its subsequent recovery. Beginning from the bottom, spectra represent: 1h prior to exercise (control), immediately post exercise, 1, 2, 3, 4 and 5h post sucrose drink.
(b) Time course of relative muscle glycogen levels obtained by integration of the doublet peaks in (a).

After recording resting spectra from liver and muscle, the subject was exercised to voluntary exhaustion on an electrically-braked cycle at 75% of maximal O_2 uptake (VO_2max). (This was measured under medical supervision prior to the study.) Further ^{13}C spectra were recorded immediately post exercise and the subject then consumed a drink containing 192 g of (unlabelled) sucrose. Subsequently, ^{13}C time courses were recorded in an interleaved fashion from liver and thigh muscle. Muscle glycogen, severely depleted following exercise, recovers monotonically with a time constant of some hours (Figure 3). In contrast, the liver glycogen rises rapidly after the glucose intake and thereafter appears to decline slowly.

Neurospectroscopy

The brain has no substantial carbohydrate store, and ^{13}C studies of brain metabolism normally require labelled substrates 1-^{13}C glucose (Morris *et al.*, 1986). ^{13}C label from this source «flows» through glycolysis to pyruvate and thence to lactate, or else enters the tricarboxylic acid (TCA) cycle, accumulating in the C4 carbon of glutamate, and redistributing to the C2 and C3 positions in subsequent turns of the TCA cycle, as well as to other key cerebral metabolites. The rate of appearance of label in C3 lactate and C4 glutamate gives a measure of the cerebral glycolytic and TCA cycle fluxes, respectively. Under hypoxic conditions, we find in our studies on superfused cerebral cortical slices, that glycolysis is accelerated and the TCA cycle suppressed, whereas under depolarizing conditions, both are stimulated (Badar-Goffer *et al.*, 1992). Less predictably, in severe hypoxia, we also observe significant accumulation of alanine and glycerol 3-phosphate, reflecting, we believe, the inability of the brain to regenerate sufficient NAD (from NADH) by conversion of pyruvate to lactate: instead dihydroxyacetone phosphate is converted to glycerol 3-phosphate which accumulates (Ben-Yoseph *et al.*, 1993). The latter compound appears, therefore, to be a useful marker of severe hypoxia.

Cerebral metabolism is compartmented and acetate is thought to be metabolized exclusively by glial cells. ^{13}C label, supplied as 2-^{13}C acetate is incorporated into glutamine and citrate, which we take to be indicative of glial metabolism (Badar-Goffer *et al.*, 1990). Under depolarizing conditions, 1-^{13}C glucose labels these two metabolites much more strongly than under control conditions, suggesting a selective stimulation of glial metabolism. By using the combined precursors 1-^{13}C glucose and 1,2-^{13}C acetate, we have shown in preliminary experiments that it is possible to study neuronal and glial metabolism simultaneously. Essentially, the doubly-labelled acetate is always incorporated into both the C_4 and C_5 positions of glutamate whereas the former is (initially) incorporated only into the C_4 position. These labelling patterns can be distinguished in the C_4 multiplet, enabling the origin of the labelled material to be discerned.

^{13}C studies of the human brain are possible, but very large quantities of labelled material (up to 60 g) are required (Gruetter *et al.*, 1992), making these investigations extremely expensive. If such studies are to be more widely applied, indirect detection methods in which the ^{13}C label is detected *via* its coupling to attached protons, will be essential. Such methods give a potential gain in sensitivity over the direct method of a factor of 64. Unfortunately, the noise also increases with NMR operating frequency, a fact often ignored when estimating the potential benefits of inverse detection, but, assuming that the sample itself is the dominant source of this noise, the improvement in signal-to-noise ratio that we can reasonably expect is still about 16.

Current theories concerning the mechanism of ischaemic brain injury suggest that it is mediated by a rise in intracellular free calcium concentration, [Ca^{2+}]i, leading to stimulation of the ATP-consuming ion pumps and, at high levels, to the activation of cellular proteases and lipases. We have developed methods to measure cerebral [Ca^{2+}]i using the ^{19}F NMR indicator 5FBAPTA (Bachelard *et al.*, 1988; Badar-Goffer *et al.*, 1990), and have used them to study cortical brain slices under various combinations of hypoxia and hypoglycaemia (the major factors in ischaemia). In hypoxia, we find an initial decrease in [Ca^{2+}]i, followed by a return to control values. Only when it is followed or preceded by hypoglycaemia, is there a significant increase. This increase, to about 100% above control values, is much less than that which occurred during a combined simultaneous insult (350% above control values), suggesting an adaptive mechanism, protecting against the second insult. Although intact animal studies are possible using 5FBAPTA, difficulties in loading, and, more importantly, concerns over possible side effects, are likely to preclude the use of such techniques in human studies. Nevertheless, these novel observations are of high inherent interest and relevance and indicate that some revision may be necessary to the «excitotoxic hypothesis» - the current rationale for much of the neuroprotective drug design programme.

Acknowledgements

We thank the Medical Research Council for support of the neurospectroscopy studies in the form of a Programme Grant, the Parkinsons Disease Society for support of the functional imaging, and SmithKline Beecham for their support of the human liver and muscle studies.

References

1. Bachelard HS, Badar-Goffer RS, Brooks KJ, Dolin SJ, Morris PG. Measurement of free intracellular calcium in the brain by 19F-NMR spectroscopy. *J Neurochem* 1988 ; 51 : 1311-3.
2. Badar-Goffer RS, Bachelard HS, Morris PG. Cerebral metabolism of acetate and glucose studied by ^{13}C NMR spectroscopy. *Biochem J* 1990 ; 266 : 133-9.
3. Badar-Goffer RS, Ben-Yoseph O, Dolin SJ, Morris PG, Smith GA, Bachelard HS. Use of 1,2-bis(2-amino-5-fluorophenoxy)ethane-N,N,N',N'-tetraacetic acid (5FBAPTA) in the measurement of free intracellular calcium in the brain by 19F-nuclear magnetic resonance spectroscopy. *J Neurochem* 1990 ; 55 : 878-84.

4. Badar-Goffer RS, Ben-Yoseph O, Bachelard HS, Morris PG. Neuronal-glial metabolism under depolarizing conditions: a ^{13}C NMR study. *Biochem J* 1992 ; 282 : 225-30.
5. Belliveau JW, Kennedy DN, McKintry RC *et al.* Functional mapping of the human cortex by magnetic resonance imaging. *Science* 1991 ; 254 : 716-9.
6. Belliveau, J.W., Kwong, K.K. Kennedy, D.N, et al. (1992). Magnetic resonance imaging mapping of brain functionn: human visual cortex. Invest. Radiol. 27, S59-S65.
7. Ben-Yoseph O, Badar-Goffer RS, Morris PG, Bachelard HS. Glycerol 3-phosphate and lactate as indicators of the cerebral cytoplasmic redox state in severe and mild hypoxia respectively: a 13C and ^{31}P-NMR study. *Biochem J* 1993 ; 291 : 915-9.
8. Doyle M, Mansfield P. Real-time movie image enhancement in NMR. *J Phys (E)* 1986 ; 19 : 439-44.
9. Gruetter R, Novotny EJ, Boulware SD, Rothman DL, Mason GF, Shulman GI, Shulman RG, Tamborlane WV. Direct measurement of brain glucose in humans by ^{13}C NMR spectroscopy. *Proc Nat Acad Sci* 1992 ; 89 : 1109-12.
10. Hykin J, Bowtwll R, Mansfield P, Glover P, Coxon R, Worhington B, Blumhardt L. Functional brain imaging using EPI at 3T. *MAGMA* 1995 (in press).
11. Mansfield P. Multi-planar image formation using NMR spin echoes. *J Phys C* 1977 ; 10 : L55-8.
12. Mansfield P, Coxon R, Glover P. Echo-planar imaging of the brain at 3T: first normal volunteer results. *J CAT* 1994 ; 18(3), 339-43.
13. Menon RS, Ogawa S, Kim SG, *et al.* Functional brain mapping using magnetic resonance imaging: Signal changes accompanying visual stimulation. *Invest Radiol* 1992 ; 27 : S47-53.
14. Menon RS, Ogawa S, Tank DW, Ugurbil K. 4 Tesla gradient recalled echo characteristics of photic stimulation-induced signal changes in the human primary visual cortex. *Magn Reson Med* 1993 ; 30(3) : 380-6.
15. Morris PG, Bachelard HS, Cox DWG, Cooper JC. ^{13}C nuclear magnetic resonance studies of glucose metabolism in guinea-pig brain slices. *Biochem Soc Trans* 1986 ; 14 : 1270-1.
16. Ogawa S, Lee T, Nayak A, Glynn P. Oxygenation-sensitive contrast in magnetic resonance image of rodent brain at high magnetic fields. *Magn Reson Med* 1990 ; 14 : 68-78.
17. Shulman GI, Rothman DL, Shulman RG. ^{13}C NMR studies of glucose disposal in normal and non-insulin-dependent diabetic humans. *Philos Trans R Soc A* 1990 ; 333 : 525-9.
18. Stevens AN, Iles RA, Morris PG., Griffiths JR. Detection of glycogen in glycogen storage disease by ^{13}C NMR. *FEBS Lett* 1982 ; 150 : 489-93.

46

High temporal and spatial resolution in functional MRI

E. MOSER [1,2], R. BEISTEINER [3], E. MÜLLER [4], C. TEICHTMEISTER [1], V. EDWARD [3]

[1]*NMR Group, Institute for Medical Physics,* [2]*Magnetic Resonance Institute,* [3]*Neurological University Clinic, University of Vienna, Austria,* [4]*Siemens AG, Erlangen, Germany.*

We present a novel method to improve time resolution of functional magnetic resonance imaging (fMRI) below 100 ms without reducing spatial resolution. This approach does not require dedicated hardware and thus may be easily installed on regular clinical imagers. Based on this method monitoring of event related blood flow changes with functional MRI in the millisecond range becomes feasible. This may open new perspectives for neurophysiologists and neurologists for measuring the relationship between neuronal activation and blood flow changes.

Following the work of Belliveau *et al.* 1991 [1] there is increasing international interest in fMRI for monitoring regional brain activity. The first publication was based on the use of intravenous Gd-DTPA, however, fMRI is now possible without the use of contrast agents [2,3]. The method is an important extension of the possibilities currently available for location of brain activity since it allows simultaneous recording of functional and anatomic images of the brain with high spatial resolution [4,7]. The underlying mechanism is believed to be the increase of blood flow in activated brain areas. This increase has 2 effects : an in-flow effect producing a signal increase on gradient echo images [8] and a relative decrease of deoxyhemoglobin producing a signal increase also on spin echo images [9]. Both effects depend on field strength and the design of the measurement sequence. Currently one of the main drawbacks of fMRI is the poor time resolution compared to electrophysiological methods such as electroencephalography (EEG) or magnetoencephalography (MEG). These provide time resolutions in the range of milliseconds, while in fMRI time resolution is in the range of 5 - 10 seconds with the typical clinical systems and 1 - 2 seconds with echo planar (EPI) imagers [10] or 4 T [11] systems.

A combination of high time and spatial resolution is of great interest to neuroscientists because it enables event related recording during short stimuli. This means recording of brain responses triggered to the start of a short event (e.g. one short light pulse, one finger movement) which allows insight into the coupling process between brain stimulation and blood flow response.

We present an approach which combines the high spatial resolution of clinical imagers with a good time resolution. The time resolution is increased about 100 fold compared to conventional gradient echo methods. A main advantage of the new method is that it does not need EPI hardware [12] or high magnetic field (e.g. 4 T) systems and is suitable for use on most clinical systems.

Material and methods

The basic idea is to implement event related recording by synchronisation of the stimulus with the recording process combined with a high time resolution. Similar to electrophysiological methods, the underlying principle is coupling of repetitive stimulation and recording. When necessary, a decrease of the signal to noise ratio due to the increased time resolution can be counterbalanced by averaging.

Recording procedure

Measurements were performed on a commercial 1.5 T system (Siemens Magnetom SP) using the regular circular polarized head coil. Parameters of the flow compensated gradient echo sequence (*see* Figure 1) were as follows: T_E=60 ms, T_R=91 ms, flip angle=40°, FOV=230 mm, 128*128 matrix. Slice selection (d = 3 mm) was achieved by a 8 mT/m gradient and data were accumulated during a long read out gradient of 51.2 ms duration (0.3 mT/m) to improve signal-to-noise ratio. Between 50 to 55 images were recorded per experiment. After global shimming of the volunteers head a single parasagital slice running through the primary visual cortex of the left hemisphere was chosen for the functional measurement. In the same location a T_1 - weighted image displaying anatomical details as well as a flow sensitive «MR angiogram» displaying major vessels were taken. Time locking of the visual stimulation with the data recording was achieved by using a homebuilt quartz based (10 MHz) electronic timing unit which triggered the GRASS - goggles and defined the length of the stimulation as well as the inter-stimulation period. Recording of the first Fourier line of the first image is followed by recording of the first Fourier line of the second image and so on (*see* Figure 2). After finishing the first line of the last image the second Fourier line of the first image is sampled followed by the second Fourier line of the second image, etc., until all lines of all images are obtained. Thus, the stimulus is always given at the same phase during the recordings of corresponding Fourier lines of the images, i.e. the time period for recording one series of Fourier lines in all images must exactly match the interval between stimuli.

HIGH TEMPORAL AND SPATIAL RESOLUTION IN FUNCTIONAL MRI

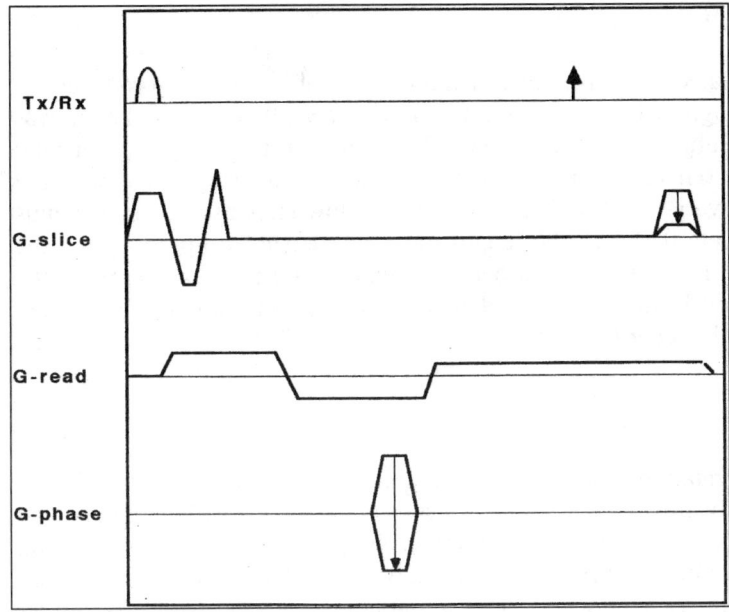

Figure 1. Schematic representation of the timing of RF - pulses and gradient switching in the gradient echo sequence used for data sampling. (Tx/Rx = RE channel, G-slice = slice selection gradient, G-read = readout gradient, G-phase = phase encode gradient, the arrow shows the position of the echo maximum.) Note the long sampling period to improve signal to noise ratio.

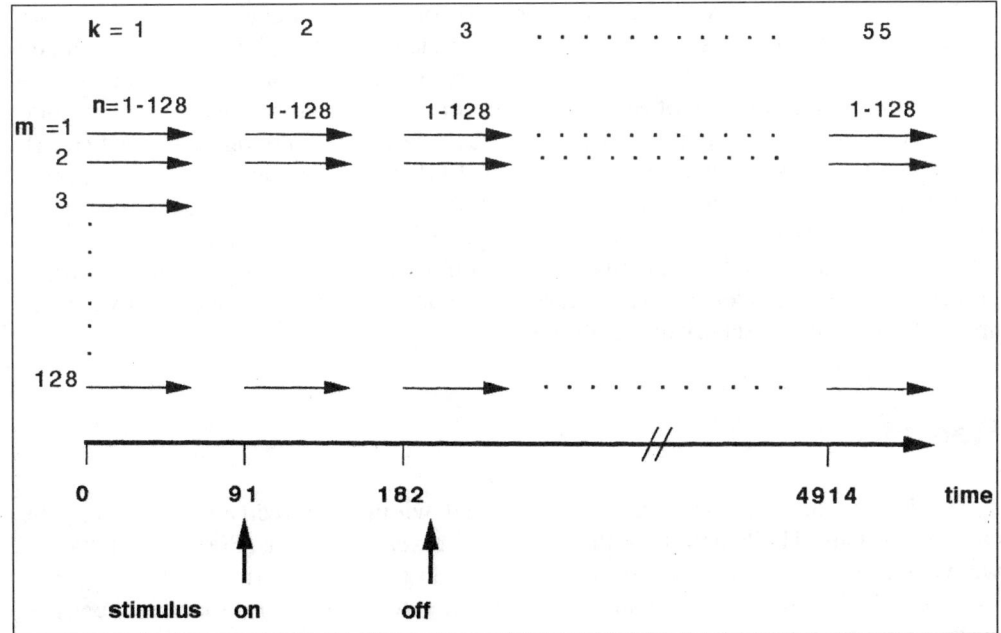

Figure 2. Schematic representation of the recording procedure. The first Fourier line of all k images is sampled first, thereafter the second Fourier line of all images and so on. As an example, a 100 ms stimulus is shown, starting with the second image. (k = number of images recorded (up to 55), m = number of Fourier lines per image recorded, n = number of sampling steps per Fourier line.)

Experimental Paradigm

Subjects were stimulated by pulses of red light of variable duration produced by goggles designed for high risk environments (GRASS SV10): the stimulation was presented binocularly. Subjects were stimulated three times in the same experimental session using 100 ms, 300 ms and 700 ms stimulus duration to investigate the potential of the method to detect very small differences in blood flow response. Every stimulus was followed by complete darkness the length of which depended upon T_R and the number of images used. In order to avoid head movements during measurements, the head was fixed with an evacuation pillow and all subjects were instructed to lie relaxed without moving during the recording.

Data analysis

For data analysis correlation images and mean signal courses were produced. The first step was to visually inspect the signal courses of all pixel of the primary and secondary visual cortices. A reference pixel was then chosen according to the following criteria: best correlation with the stimulation course, best signal to noise ratio, not lying in a visible vessel in the MR angiogram. The signal course of that pixel was further processed by IDL software (Interactive Data Language Corp., USA). The signal course of the reference pixel was used as a reference to correlate the signal courses of all other pixel by using the sum of squared differences for each time step. All pixel with summed squared differences below a threshold value were colour coded and overlayed on the T_1 weighted (anatomic) image of the same slice. Since the signal to noise ratio was good enough (about 50), no averaging procedure was employed. A region-of-interest (ROI), of the same size as the selected «stimulated» ROI, in the frontal lobe was chosen as control time course. Motion artefacts, from head movements were screened for by two procedures, (a) careful inspection of all images recorded and (b) analysis of various difference pictures made by subtraction of different phases of the whole recording process. If a head movement had occurred, artefacts would have appeared over large areas of the head, especially along all margins.

Results

The best result pixel were most often found within or directly neighbouring the calcarine sulcus. The locations of the best result pixel for 100 ms, 300 ms and 700 ms were found to lay within 1 cm from each other on the visual cortex of the individual subjects. The best correlations with the best result pixel were always found in the visual cortex. However, we found that when increasing the threshold value (allowing lower correlations) all subjects had additional brain areas correlating, especially in the frontal lobe, the parietal lobe and the cerebellum. This indicates that stimulus correlated signals may be found in various brain areas. This may be due to neuronal activity, draining veins or chance. Thus, for a topographic analysis random effects have to be reduced as far as possible by using at least 3 stimulations and 4 rest periods [13]. Since only two signal minima and one signal maximum were used in our study, topographic analysis is not feasible. Therefore, we can only state that the very best signal courses and accordingly the very best correlations were found in areas corresponding to the primary and secondary visual cortex. As a typical physiological blood flow response, an increase of the signal amplitude was observed in the visual cortex starting 2-3 sec post stimulation start. The maximum was reached after about 1.5 to 2 seconds and the signal decrease usually took the same time. The maximum signal amplitude was between 5 % and 10 % of the baseline level. As expected, the latency of the maximum of the signal course was found to correlate with the delay between stimulus onset and data collection onset. When the stimulus started closer to the recording onset, the signal maximum appeared some time (images) later and vice versa. The control ROI located in cortical grey matter of the frontal lobe did not show the above described activation pattern. Screening for head movements as described in the methods section showed no head movements with any subject included in the study.

Discussion

We present the first non-invasive high spatio-temporal resolution (<10 μl, <100 ms) data of cerebral blood flow response modulation. As is demonstrated by variation of the stimulus durations, time and shape modulations of the signal courses can be very small. Nevertheless, they may provide important clues for the future study of a stimulus specific blood flow response.

An important feature of the new method is the relatively good signal to noise ratio (about 50) which renders averaging in most subjects superfluous. However, if the repetition time used (91 ms) is further decreased to something below 30 ms (depending on the read-out bandwidth and the amount of T_2^* weighting chosen), averaging may become necessary.

One aspect of high resolution fMRI (HRFI) seems especially important to us. It is the feasibility of combining this method with classical electrophysiological methods such as EEG or MEG [14]. Both are complementary to FMRI since they measure the neuronal activity which triggers the blood flow response. What investigations is high resolution fMRI best suited for ? Flow response differences of the magnitude observed could not have been detected by any other non-invasive imaging method currently available. Thus HRFI promises much for future investigations of short and ultrashort effects. However, an obvious problem of HRFI when compared with Echo Planar Imaging is the sensitivity for motion artefacts. This can partly be counterbalanced by reduction of the field of view and minimizing T_R x number of images. Furthermore, analysis of physiological motion by fourier analysis of the data and retrospective elimination also can be of help. Since movements of internal organs or muscles may hardly be avoided over minutes of recording, HRFI is predominantly suited for brain measurements. Here, a sufficient fixation of the head is possible and cooperative subjects will not move for a considerable amount of time, additionally allowing fourier line averaging which may facilitate answering two questions of great interest with functional brain experiments; first, what is the spatial relationship of activated brain tissue and second, what is the latency between activated areas? This is especially important when investigating cognitive may be blurred by the continuing response of the primary areas, especially if subcomponents originate from spatially closely related brain areas. It is not yet clear, what the physiological limit of the brains blood flow response is (i.e. whether there is a minimum limit of the stimulation length that will still produce a vascular response). To explore this physiological limit, however, the methodological limitations have to be reduced.

Acknowledgements

We are grateful for support and stimulating discussions to Pr. L. Deecke, Pr. H. Imhof and Pr. A. F. Fercher. This work was financially supported by the Austrian Science Foundation (grant P 10091 Med), the «Jubiläumsfonds der OeNB» and the «L. Boltzmanninstitut für radiologisch - physikalische Tumordiagnostik».

References

1. Belliveau JW, Kennedy DN, McKinstry RC, Buchbinder GR, Weisskoff RM, Cohen MS, Vevea JM, Brady TJ, Rosen BR. *Science* 1991 ; 254 : 716-9.
2. Ogawa S, Tank DW, Menon R, Ellerman JM, Kim S, Merkle H, Ugurbil K, *Proc Natl Acad Sci USA* 1992 ; 89 : 5951-5.
3. Kwong KK, Belliveau JW, Chesler DA, Goldberg IA, Weisskoff RM, Poncelet BP, Kennedy DM, Hoppel BE, Cohen MS, Turner R, Cheng H, M Brady TJ, Rosen BR. *Proc Natl Acad Sci USA* 1992 ; 89 : 5675-9.
4. Belliveau JW. In Book of Abstracts, 11th Meeting SMRM (Berlin) : 1992 ; 203.
5. Bandettini PA, Wong EC, Hinks RS, Tikofsky RS, Hyde JS. *Magn Res Med* 1992 ; 25 : 390.
6. Frahm J, Merboldt KD, Hänicke W. *Magn Res Med* 1993 ; 29 : 139-44.
7. Constable RT, McCarthy G, Allison T, Anderson AW, Gore JC. *Magn Res Imag* 1993 ; 11 : 451-9.
8. Gomiscek G, Beisteiner R, Hittmair K, Mueller E, Moser E. *MAGMA* 1993 ; 1 : 109-13.
9. Ogawa S, Lee TM, Kay AR, Tank DW. *Proc Natl Acad Sci USA* 1990 ; 87 : 9868-9872.
10. McCarthy G, Blamire AM, Rothman DL, Gruetter R, Shulman RG. *Proc Natl Acad Sci USA* 1993 ; 90 : 4952-6.
11. Hu X, Kim SG. *Magn Res Med* 1993 ; 30 : 512-517.
12. Cohen MS, Weisskoff RM. *Magn Res Imag* 1991 ; 9 : 1-37.
13. Teichtmeister C, Gomiscek G, Beisteiner R, Moser E. In Book of abstracts, «The international seventh Swiss brain mapping meeting» (Zürich, CH) 1994.
14. Beisteiner R, Gomiscek G, Erdler M, Teichtmeister C, Moser E. In Book of abstracts, «First meeting of the SMR» (Dallas, USA), works-in-progress S16 1994.

47

Methods to improve EEG spatial resolution with implications for medical and cognitive science

P.L. NUNEZ

*Brain Physics Group,
Department of Biomedical Engineering,
Tulane University,
New Orleans, LA 70118 USA.*

Limitations of conventional EEG

It is widely appreciated that electroencephalography (EEG) is a direct measure, albeit often a crude measure, of conscious experience. Many distinct spatio-temporal patterns are now recognized and correlated with physiological, clinical, or cognitive states [1-3]. While several new imaging methods (CT, MRI, PET) have partly eclipsed some of EEG's former clinical applications (such as location or cortical tumors), EEG remains the primary tool for the study of neocortical dynamic function at the millisecond time scale at which information is processed.

The general field of electroencephalography spans about five orders of magnitude of spatial scale ranging from scalp recordings to micro-EEG studies at minicolumn (~~0.03 mm) and smaller scales. The actual practice of EEG spans about nine orders of magnitude of temporal scale. For example, peaks in the brainstem auditory evoked potential, separated by about 1 ms, are sufficiently robust for use in standard clinical studies of peripheral auditory dysfunction or brainstem integrity. At the other extreme of temporal scale, scalp EEG is routinely recorded in all-night clinical studies (e.g., neuropsychiatric patients). In another example, candidates for epilepsy surgery are implanted with depth electrodes that typically stay in place for at least several days in order to monitor seizure onset.

Because of its unique ability to view neocortical dynamic function at very short time scales, EEG would appear to have substantial potential value in the study of neuropsychiatric illness and cognitive disorders, in addition to its traditional role in the epilepsies. However, conventional scalp recordings have been very severely limited by poor spatial resolution. A reasonable conjecture is that application of the high resolution EEG methods described here will greatly extend the EEG as a tool in both the clinical and cognitive sciences.

In order that the reader fully appreciate high resolution EEG, a review of the severe limitations of conventional EEG seems appropriate. The resolution available with conventional EEG is limited by :
1. Spatial sampling.
2. Reference electrode contamination.
3. «Smearing» of cortical potentials by the head volume conductor.
4. Failure to exploit information about the physics of volume conduction. This issue partly overlaps #3, but includes additional effects.

High resolution EEG involves a critical synergy in which all four of these issues are addressed simultaneously. Experienced electroencephalographers are often skeptical that adding additional electrodes beyond the standard 10/20 montage (~ 20 electrodes) adds useful information. This skepticism is perhaps justified for unprocessed data. However, when data obtained from dense electrode arrays (for example, 64 channels over the entire scalp) is processed with high resolution EEG algorithms, potential information content increases by at least several orders of magnitude over that available with conventional EEG. The question of how to make use of this vast amount of new information remains mostly open.

In order to illustrate the reference electrode (#2), and smearing issues (#3), consider the following idea, which has long been part of the EEG folklore (sometimes made explicit, but more often implicit in conclusions drawn from the data):

If a «quiet reference» is used, scalp potential is mainly due to sources under the «recording electrode».

The inaccuracy of this idea has been illustrated using simulations with 4200 dipole sources at the macrocolumn scale [6,7].

These studies also illustrate the problem of volume conductor smearing (#3), even in the idealized, but unrealistic case of potentials measured with respect to infinity. For example, suppose we assume sources are distributed uniformly in the cortex, and wish to obtain a rough idea of the following ratio at a particular electrode location :

$$\frac{\text{contribution to the recorded potential from sources within a surface distance d}}{\text{total contribution to recorded potential}}$$

When d ~ 3 or 4 cm, the above ratio is about 0.5 [7] That is, about half the contribution comes from sources within 3 or 4 cm; the other half comes from the entire cortex. Of course, sources are not normally uniformly distributed in neocortex and sub-cortical sources may contribute, but the above ratio provides a general idea of EEG spatial resolution.

Other simulations show that even with a very large number of spatial samples (660), the surface potential (with respect to infinity) map does not reveal patterns of cortical source activity at moderate scales [6,7]. This inaccuracy occurs even with no reference electrode distortions. By contrast, the surface Laplacian (involving spatial derivatives in the two surface tangent coordinates) converges to the pattern of cortical sources at scales greater than about 1-3 cm as the number of electrodes is increased above about 50. Also, the addition of 20% random (i.e., spatially uncorrelated) noise to 64 or 118 sample potentials or setting one of the potentials to zero (simulating a «bad» electrode contact) have almost no effect on the Laplacian estimate obtained with a 3-dimensional spline function. Finally, artefact generated outside the electrode array (for example, eye movements) causes much less contamination of the surface Laplacian than the raw potential map.

A partial appreciation of the potential significance of high resolution EEG can be obtained from the following argument (admittedly very crude): Suppose conventional EEG allows us to monitor independent activity over M cortical regions (with minimal overlap), for example, anterior and posterior regions of both hemispheres. Let each region produce S possible «states» (i.e., some general measure like amplitude, phase, coherency, etc.). Then the number of different patterns that can be resolved is S^M. When spatial resolution is increased by the factor R, the number of regions that can be separately monitored increases by R^2, and the number of distinct spatial patterns (related to information content) is increased by the factor $S^{M(R-1)}$ with high resolution EEG. For example, if M=4, R=3, and S=2 (binary states), the number of possible patterns that can be observed is increased from 16 in the case of four distinct scalp regions to $2^{36} \sim 6.9 \times 10^{10}$ in the case of 36 regions. High resolution EEG methods that do increase spatial resolution by a factor of R=3 or more are now available as shown here. While the resulting spatial resolution is, by itself, quite modest compared to other brain imaging methods, the combined spatial-temporal resolution is excellent for the observation of relatively large scale (~1 to 3 cm) dynamic patterns of neocortical activity. The primary goal of these methods generally not «source localization» per se since at any given time, sources associated with a clinical or cognitive event may be widely distributed. Rather, it is the measurement and quantification of neocortical dynamics and the relationship of such measures to clinical and cognitive states of the brain for which high resolution EEG is best suited.

High resolution EEG

Two general methods have been proposed to improve the spatial resolution of scalp recorded potentials:

1. The surface Laplacian (e.g., «current source density»). These methods provide estimates of local current density flowing perpendicular to the skull into the scalp. This is not generally true of surface Laplacians, rather it applies specifically to the skull-scalp region. The close physical relationship between scalp Laplacian and skull current density is a direct consequence of the law of current conservation and the fact that skull resistivity is much higher than that of brain tissue [1,8] The latter condition implies that skull current is mostly normal to its surface. Cortical surface potential may also be estimated using estimated skull current and Ohm's law if desired [7]. Estimation of

source nature or location (radial/tangential, cortical/noncortical) may be obtained as a separate step based on knowledge of the underlying physiology and anatomy. However, since the Laplacian is much more sensitive to local sources (both tangentially and in depth), most significant contributions to Laplacian maps are believed to be due to cortical sources.

Actually, there are many versions of the Laplacian estimate, [1,9,10] ranging from the use of groups of five or more local electrodes [1,11-14] to global measures based on spline fits to recorded potentials [6,7,9,10,15-19]. These methods act to band pass data. In the spline-based methods, spatial filter characteristics are chosen to match head volume conductor properties as closely as possible, by choosing the «best» spline type and order.

2. Cortical imaging («spatial deconvolution»). These methods make use of a volume conductor model of the head (usually a three-concentric sphere model) to predict cortical surface potential from scalp potential [20-26] In theory, more accurate estimates of cortical potential can be obtained using finite elements models [23,26] however, our limited knowledge of tissue boundaries and resistivities results in significant uncertainty in the accuracy of these methods when applied to unknown sources.

One partial solution to this problem is the development of cortical imaging methods with explicit criteria for choosing the optimum trade-off between smoothness and error for a given signal [27]. This approach involves the use of a smoothing function. When smoothing is large, predicted cortical potential is similar to measured scalp potential. As smoothing is decreased, more and more detail is evident in the predicted cortical potential. However, at some intermediate value of the smoothing parameter, this detail becomes unreliable because of errors in the head model and/or noise in the signal. Thus, an optimum smoothing parameter may be chosen based on estimated uncertainty in the head model and signal-to-noise ratio. In summary, one tries to display just the right amount of detail in the spatial structure of the estimated cortical potential map, consistent with the limitations of the procedure.

Other approaches include magnetoencephalography (MEG) and dipole localization (with either MEG or EEG). Dipole localization depends on the constraint that sources consist of a single (or perhaps several) isolated regions of tissue. For this reason, it is apparently applicable to only a small subset of brain states for which this constraint is reasonably accurate (refer to references 10 and 28 for discussions of this topic). Of course, some of these applications are quite important (for example, in epilepsy surgery patients).

With either Laplacian or cortical imaging methods and additional prediction of cortical source density can be obtained; however, this step requires critical assumptions about the location (e.g., in the cortex) and nature (e.g., mix of radial and tangential dipoles) of the sources. Such assumptions must be based on additional physiological and anatomical information which may be much less reliable than the estimate of cortical surface potential. Thus, such source estimates should be considered separate from the high resolution methods, which are then independent of any assumptions about the nature and location of sources. High resolution methods are viewed here as simply estimates of cortical surface potential and/or perpendicular skull current.

An important advantage of Laplacian methods is their reference-independence. On the other hand, cortical imaging methods have more potential to make use of information about the volume conductor to improve the accuracy of cortical potential estimates. Actually, one may think of high resolution EEG methods on a continuous scale with local Laplacians as entirely model-independent, spline-Laplacians as minimally model-dependent, smoothed cortical imaging methods as moderately model-dependent, and unsmoothed cortical imaging as strongly model-dependent. At this stage of our understanding of brain sources and head volume conductors, it makes sense to apply methods from different parts of this spectrum to the same data. Only those conclusions about brain function which are robust to choice of method can be considered reliable.

Comparaison of Laplacian and cortical imaging methods

Direct comparisons between our spline-Laplacian method [6,18,19,29,30] and a spline-based cortical imaging estimate [27] for both simulated and actual EEG data have recently been obtained [7]. The Laplacian methods carry out interpolation in three-dimensions. In most illustrations, spherical head surfaces are used, although extension to general ellipsoidal surfaces has been obtained [19,29]. The Laplacian approach is an extension of earlier spline-Laplacian methods which use interpolation in a plane [9,15,16,18] or on a spherical surface [17]. However, we have found the three dimensional interpolation to be more robust for a wide variety of source distributions, when applied to either spherical or ellipsoidal head surfaces.

The cortical imaging estimates are predictions of cortical surface potential, given a known scalp distribution and volume conductor [27]. The new methods involve the same physical principles as earlier, crude deconvolution methods (for example, [20]). However, the new cortical imaging methods are more sophisticated and robust in that they include an explicit smoothness criterion t allow for noisy data and an imperfect volume conductor model. Thus, the relationship of the new cortical imaging methods to earlier spatial deconvolution is somewhat analogous to the relationship of then new spline-Laplacian method to earlier nearest-neighbor Laplacians as described by Hjorth [11] and Nunez [1], for example. Recently, finite element based cortical imaging methods have been applied to isolated cortical sources [23].

In the case of simple cortical source patterns, both the Laplacian and cortical imaging methods based on the three-concentric spheres model yield nearly identical patterns. In the case of the moderately complicated source distributions, there are relatively minor differences in predicted patterns a scales greater than about 1-3 cm (depending on electrode density). For example, correlation coefficients between the two typically vary between 0.8 and 0.95 for both simulated and real EEG data. These illustrations suggest the practical equivalence to two resolution methods based on quite different theoretical approaches, at least in selective applications involving distributed neocortical sources.

References

1. Nunez PL, *Electric fields of the brain : the neurophysics of EEG*. New York : Oxford University Press, 1981.
2. Gevins AS, Remond, A, *Methods of analysis of brain electric and magnetic signals, handbook of electroencephalography and clinical neurophysiology,* Vol.1. Amsterdam : Elsevier, 1987.
3. Regan D, *Human brain electrophysiology, evoked potentials and evoked magnetic fields in science and medicine.* Elsevier : New York, 1989.
4. Rush, S, Driscoll, DA. EEG electrode sensitivity: an application of reciprocity. *IEEE Trans Biomed Eng,* 1969 ; 16 : 15-22.
5. Ary JP, Klein SA, Fender DH. Location of sources of evoked scalp potentials : corrections for skull and scalp thickness. *IEEE Trans Biomed Eng,* 1981 ; 28 : 447-52.
6. Nunez PL, Pilgreen KL, Westdorp AF, Law SK, Nelson AV. A visual study of surface potentials and Laplacians due to distributed neocortical sources: computer simulations and evoked potentials. *Brain Topography,* 1991 ; 4 : 151-68.
7. Nunez PL, Silberstein RB, Cadusch PJ, Wijesinghe R. Theoretical and experimental bases for high resolution EEG based on surface Laplacians and cortical imaging. Electroencelphalogr Clin Neurophysiol, 1994 ; 90 : 40-57.
8. Katznelson RD, Chapter 6 In Nunez PL : *Electric fields of the brain : the neurophysics of EEG.* New York : Oxford University Press, 1981.
9. Nunez PL. Estimation of large scale neocortical source activity with EEG surface Laplacians. *Brain Topography,* 1989 ; 2 : 141-54.
10. Nunez PL. Localization of brain activity with electroencephalography. In: S Sato, ed., *Advances in Neurology.* Vol. 54 : Magnetoencephalography, New York : Raven Press, 1990 ; 39-65.
11. Hjorth B. An on-line transformation of EEG scalp potentials into orthogonal source derivations, Electroencephalogr *Clin Neurophysiol,* 1975 ; 39 : 526-30.
12. Gevins AS, Cutillo BA. Signals of cognition. In : FA Lopes da Silva, W Strom van Leeuwen, A Remond eds. *Handbook of Electroencephal. clin. Neurophysiol.* Revised series. Vol. 2. New York : Elsevier, 1986 ; 335-81.
13. Gevins AS. Obstacles to progress. In : AS Gevins, and A Remond, eds. *Handbook of electroencephalography and clinical neurophysiology.* Revised Series, Vol. 1. New York : Elsevier, 1987 ; 665-73.
14. Nunez PL, Pilgreen KL. The spline-Laplacian in clinical neurophysiology: a method to improve EEG spatial resolution. *J Clin Neurophysiol,* 1991 ; 8 : 397-413.
15. Perrin F, Bertrand O, Pernier J. Scalp current density mapping: value and estimation from potential data. *IEEE Trans. Biomed. Eng.,* 1987 ; 34 : 283-8.
16. Perrin F, Pernier J, Bertrand O, Giard MH, Enchallier JF. Mapping of scalp potentials by surface spline interpolation. *Electroencephal. Clin. Neurophysiol.,* 1987 ; 66 : 75-81.
17. Perrin F, Pernier J, Bertrand O, Enchallier JF. Spherical splines for scalp potential and current density mapping. *ElectroencephalClin Neurophysiol,* 1989 ; 72 : 184-7.
18. Nunez PL. Spatial filtering and experimental strategies in EEG. In : Samson-Dollfus ed. *Statistics and topography in quantitative EEG,* Paris : Elsevier, 1988 ; 196-209.
19. Law SK. *Spline generated surface Laplacian estimates for improving spatial resolution in electroencephalography.* Ph.D.Dissertation, Tulane University, 1991.
20. Nunez PL. Removal of reference electrode and volume conduction effects by spatial deconvolution of evoked potentials using a three-concentric sphere model of the head. The London Symposium. *Electroencephal Clin Neurophysiol,* 1987 ; [Suppl], 39:143-8.

21. Gevins AS, Brickette P, Costales B, Le J, Reutter B. Beyond topographical mapping: towards functional-anatomical imaging with 124 channel EEG and 3-D MRIs. *Brain Topography,* 1990 ; 3 : 53-4
22. Gevins AS.Analysis of multiple lead data. In: JW Rohbraugh, R Parasuraman, JR Johnson eds. *Event-related brain potentials.* New York : Oxford University Press, 1990 ; 44-56.
23. Gevins AS, Le J, Brickett P, Reutter B, Desmond J. Seeing through the skull: advanced EEG's accurately measure cortical activity from the scalp. *Brain Topography,* 1991 ; 4 : 125-32.
24. Kearfott RB, Sidman RD, Major DJ, Hill CD. Numerical tests of a method for simulating electrical potentials on the cortical surface. *IEEE trans. biomed. eng.,* 1991 ; 38 : 294-9.
25. Sidman RD. A method for simulating intracerebral potential fields : the cortical imaging technique. *J Clin Neurophysiol,* 1991 ; 8 : 432-41.
26. Yan Y, Nunez PL, Hart RT. A finite element model of the human head: scalp potentials due to diploe sources. *Med Biol Eng and Compu,* 1991 ; 29 : 475-81.
27. Cadusch PJ, Breckon W, Silberstein RB. Spherical splines and the interpolation, deblurring and transformation of topographic EEG. Melbourne, Australia, *Pan Pacific Workshop on Brain Electric and Magnetic Topography,* Feb. 1992 ; 17-18.
28. Scherg M. Fundamentals of dipole source potential analysis,. In : M Hoke, F Grandori, GL Romani, eds. *Auditory evoked magnetic fields and potentials. Advances in neurology,* Vol. 6. Basel : Karger, 1989.
29. Law SK, Nunez PL, Wijesinghe RS. High resolution EEG using spline generated surface Laplacians on spherical and ellipsoidal surfaces. *IEEE Trans Biomed Eng,* 1992 ; 40 :1 45-53.
30. Nunez PL. Neocortical dynamics and human EEG rhythms, New York : Oxford University Press, 1995, in press.

48

Localizing sources within the human brain by means of MEG and EEG

M. J. PETERS, S. P. VAN DEN BROEK, T. KNÖSCHE, F. ZANOW

Twente University
Faculty of Applied Physic
P.O. Box 217
7500 AE Enschede, Pays-Bas

Using arrays of superconducting magnetic field detectors, it is possible to measure the extracranial magnetic field distribution. Such a measurement is called a magnetoencephalogram (MEG) (see for an overview Hämäläinen et al., 1993). MEGs and EEGs are used to localize neuronal activity within the human brain with a time resolution of 1 ms. MEG measurement technology has moved on from single channel detectors, which had to be moved across the head to produce a map, to whole-cortex systems with up to 140 detection sites. The current state of EEG instrumentation includes techniques to record EEG data utilizing up to 124 channels (Gevins et al., 1994). EEG records both radial and tangential sources, the MEG records only tangential sources, that is, those in the fissures of the brain. The MEG and EEG data should preferably be integrated with anatomical data obtained from magnetic resonance images (MRI) of the same subject to produce a coherent system for functional brain imaging. Firstly, the MRI can be used to derive a model of the head, which is necessary for the calculation of the location of electrical activity. Secondly, the MRI can be used to indicate the location of the sources within the head. Thirdly, the cortex can be extracted from the MRI, which is important if the localization procedure is based on the assumption that the sources are confined to a segment of the cortex. Finally, the position of a source depicted in the MRI enables us to validate the physiological significance of the result and, if necessary, to correct the estimated position within the error estimate.

The computation of the electric potential and/or the magnetic field generated by given sources within the brain is called the forward problem. The computation of the location and the strength of sources from MEG and/or EEG measurements is called the inverse problem. Unfortunately, it can be proved that, even if we measure the EEG and/or MEG in an excessive number of points, there is not enough information to create a unique picture of the source distribution. In order to localize electrically active populations of neurons within the brain using MEG and/or EEG, it is necessary that the sources and the head are properly modelled. The sources of EEG and MEG are caused by the activity of neuronal membranes. Membrane currents occur at sites where a change in membrane conductance is caused by synaptic activity. This results in an active current source or sink. Since the currents form closed loops, a passive source or sink at other sites of the membrane and Ohmic currents both in the cell and in the surrounding tissue will occur. At least 10^4 neurons have to be active synchronously in order to generate potentials and magnetic fields which are measurable at points at the scalp or near the scalp. The membrane currents do not produce a measurable magnetic field, since the membranes are very thin, and tend to mutually cancel their magnetic fields. Therefore it is convenient to split the currents into two parts: the Ohmic currents and the currents in the source regions. The sources are either modelled by current dipoles (i.e., a source and a sink, connected by a small current element), current dipole layers or a combination of dipoles and quadrupoles. The Ohmic currents are dependent on the distribution of the electric conductivity within the head. Till now, compartment models of the head are used representing different tissues, where each compartment is assumed to have a homogeneous conductivity. Several strategies for the solution of the inverse problem, such as the non-linear dipole localization, linear estimation techniques and the multiple signal classification (MUSIC) algorithm have been developed in the recent years (Hämäläinen and Ilmoniemi, 1994; Mosher *et al.*, 1992). The influence of various models and strategies will be discussed.

Modelling the sources

An adequate source model for neural activity in a region that is small compared to the distance to the observation points is an electric current dipole, the so-called equivalent dipole. A current dipole is completely characterized by six parameters, namely the three coordinates defining its location and three parameters describing its strength and orientation. The inverse problem is a parameter estimation problem. Because the measurements are noisy, the number of parameters to be estimated has to be less than the number of measurements used to calculate those parameters. Different assumptions are possible. One is to assume that the patch of active cortex moves as a function of time. This can be modelled by a single dipole that changes its position, orientation and strength in time. This model is the so-called moving dipole model. At sequential time instants the location, the strength, and the orientation of the dipole is estimated. Consequently, at each time instant six parameters are estimated from N_m measurements, where N_m is the number of points where a measurement is carried out. An other assumption is that several cortical areas are activated simultaneously. The activation of the small cortical areas is followed by a spread of activity to neighbouring areas. This can be modelled by an adaquate number of dipoles which are fixed in location during a certain time interval. This time interval may, for example, be a time window of 40 ms and if the measurements are sampled with a frequency of 1000 Hz, the number of time instants that a measurement is carried out is 40. Two different approaches exist: First, both the orientations and strengths of the dipoles are functions of time. Thus, if the number of dipoles to be estimated is n, the number of time instants is N_t (40 in our example), and the number of measurement points is N_m, we have to estimate $3n + 3nN_t$ parameters (i.e., once for each dipole the three parameters defining the location and for all time instants of interest the three parameters defining the strengths and orientations) from $N_t N_m$ measurements. Second, both the locations and orientations are fixed and only the strengths are a function of time. In this case we have to estimate $5n + nN_t$ parameters from $N_t N_m$ measurements. Comparing the measured values of the magnetic field and/or the electric potential to the values of the forward problem solution, the dipoles are iteratively moved into such a position, that the forward solution fits the measured data optimally. The localization procedure is only able to give the right position if the number of sources is known *a priori*, and if the number is not too high. The localization of discrete multiple dipoles can be simplified using the so-called multiple classification (MUSIC) approach. A measure is computed that represents how good a source at this location can explain the data. The result of the algorithm is a probability map showing certain extrema, which indicate where a dipole can be expected. It is also possible to assume that the sources will be found in a certain region. An obvious choice for this region would be the cortex itself. No *a priori* assumptions on the number of dipoles have to be made. In elements of the source region dipole strengths are computed by means of linear estimation. The result of this procedure is always an extended source.

Modelling the head

Usually the head is described by a set of four concentric spheres, where the various regions represent the brain, the cerebro-spinal fluid, the skull and the scalp. The reason to use this model is that it is easy to handle since an analytical expression is known for the potential and magnetic field generated by a current dipole. Within the context of this model, the MEG is independent of the conductivities involved and radially orientated dipoles do not generate any magnetic field outside of the head.

However, a spherical model has some serious disadvantages. The geometry is often obtained by taking the best-fitting sphere with respect to the electrodes used to measure the EEGs or with respect to a segment of the scalp. The choice of this geometrical reference is subjective. Since a sphere is a poor approximation of the shape of the head, the localization errors may be substantial. An other problem is that the source space is limited to the innermost sphere, which does not necessarily include the entire brain. Futhermore, the projection of the electrode positions onto the outer sphere may cause some errors because their distance to the sphere surface can be several centimeters, *see* Figure 1. To avoid the problems mentioned above, inverse solutions based on a realisti-

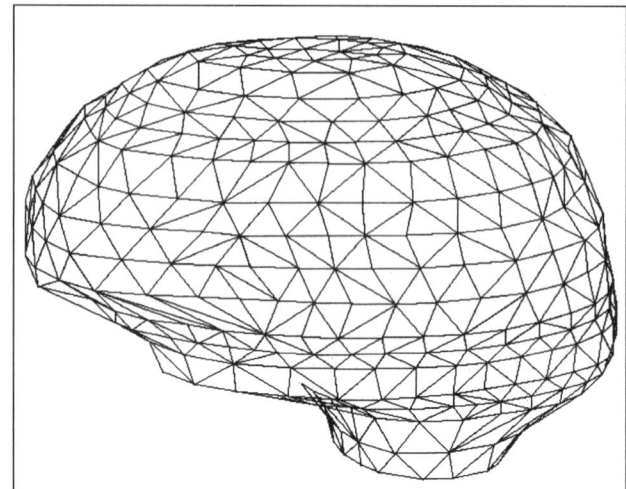

Figure 1. Three-sphere model fitted to the scalp surface with 52 electrodes projected onto the sphere surface. The contour of the scalp is additionally shown to illustrate that some of the projected electrodes lie at a considerable distance from the actual scalp surface.

cally shaped model, describing the brain, the skull, and the scalp have been developed. The conductivity of the various regions is assumed to be homogeneous. The numerical procedure to solve the inverse problem is based on the boundary element method. A piecewise homogeneous conductor can be considered equivalent to a uniform conducting medium of infinite extent in which fictitious sources (the so-called secondary sources) lie at the interfaces between regions of different conductivities. The strengths of these secondary sources are proportional to the local potential. The boundary surfaces are approximated by means of triangles. The potential is considered to vary linearly over a triangle.

Since the skull is poorly conducting the main contribution to the magnetic field outside the head originates from currents flowing within the brain tissue. From simulation studies it can indeed be concluded that a homogeneous model with the shape of the inner surface of the skull will give within a range of 1 to 3 mm the same magnetic field distribution as a realistically shaped three-compartment model. Using a realistically shaped homogeneous model instead of a sphere to localize a current dipole from MEG, it is found that the differences in location obtained with the two types of models, depend on the region of the brain where the dipole is localized. From these simulation studies it can be concluded that a sphere can be used to calculate the sources of visual evoked magnetic fields. However, a homogeneous realistically shaped model should preferably be used to localize a source from MEG which is in the frontal region. Using a realistically shaped three-compartment model instead of a spherical one to localize a source from EEG leads to differences which are in the range of 5 to 11 mm. However, the presence of noise in the data remarkably decreases the localization accuracy obtained if a realistically shaped compartment model is used.

In order to assess the importance of anisotropy in the conductivity, to study the effect of boneless areas in the skull such as the fontanelle in neonatal brain research, and to estimate the effect of complex-shaped fluid-occupied volumes such as the ventricles, the finite element method can be used. The head is subdivided in three-dimensional

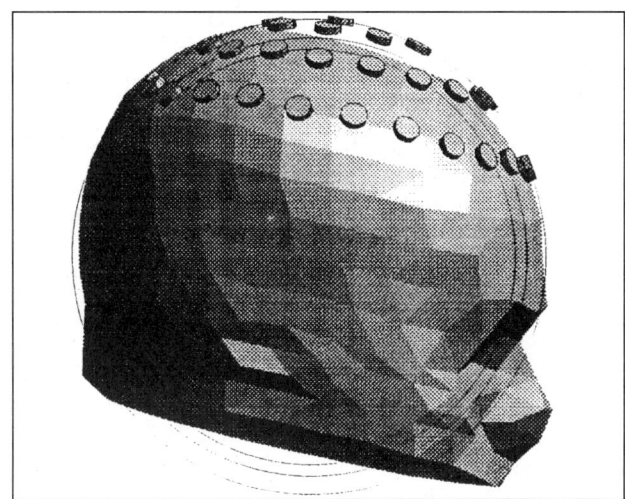

Figure 2. Realistically shaped model with the geometry of the inside of the skull. The number of nodes is 1098.

finite elements e.g., tetrahedrons. Each element is allowed to have its own (anisotropic) conductivity. An impression of a finite-element model of the brain is given in Figure 2. From simulation studies it can be concluded that an opening in the skull shell has a strong influence on the potential distribution (Bertrand *et al.*, 1992) and not on the magnetic field distribution.

Simulations show that the strengths of dipoles deduced from EEG are very dependent on the conductivity model used to describe the head. Unfortunately, the values of the conductivities in the various tissues are not known precisely. However, the orientation of the dipoles deduced from EEG is hardly influenced by the conductivity distribution in the head. Hence, the EEG can be used to deduce the location and orientation of the dipoles. The MEG can be used to estimate the location and tangential component. A combination of these findings gives us the locations, orientations and strengths of the dipoles. Using values for the neuron density of an active segment of cortex, the combination of MEG and EEG can give us an estimate of the spatial extent of the source.

The information about the anatomy of the subject's head is obtained from MR images (Wieringa and Peters, 1993). The data set consists of 256 transversal slices. A segmentation procedure is developed in order to determine automatically which voxels are part of the head and which are not. When an MRI scan is performed, little V-shaped Gadolinium filled markers are attached to the nasion and preauricular points of the subject. The positions of the electrodes and/or pick-up coils used to measure the magnetic field with respect to the head are determined using a 3D tracker system.

Discussion

When analyzing EEG and/or MEG data, we have to deal with the non-uniqueness of the inverse problem. However, the three-dimensional localization of a current generator within the brain can be inferred quite accurately from MEG/EEG measurements when enough a priori information is available. This so-called functional brain imaging is used for medical diagnosis (e.g., the localization of an epileptic focus, the functional mapping of the sensory cortex before surgery). However, for late evoked responses the functional imaging is not such a straightforward procedure, the results obtained are dependent on the constraints e.g., the model of the head or the number of dipolar sources. Different inverse solutions may explain the measured data with a comparable goodness of fit. They are therefore equally good in a mathematical sense but provide different interpretations of the measurements. The ambiguity can be reduced by the incorporation of electrophysiological and anatomical a priori information. A common assumption is that the EEG and MEG are generated by electrical activity of the pyramidal cells in the cortex. These cells are perpendicular to the cortical surface. Consequently, the dipoles obtained have to have an orientation which is perpendicular to this surface. The orientation of this surface can be obtained from MRI. However, errors in the localization procedure and in the MRI may be in the order of one centimeter and the direction of the normal on the cortical surface in gyri and sulci is very variable. Consequently, within the error estimate many solutions will be found which have the correct orientation. Comparison of the results obtained from MEG with those obtained with EEG is important because the sources have to coincide within the error estimates. Findings obtained with PET, SPECT or functional MRI may provide information which can be incorporated in strategies to calculate the sources from MEG and EEG. It may be concluded that in order to develop functional imaging based on MEG and/or EEG for cognitive science, it is a prerequisite to use neurophysiologically adequate *a priori* information and more than one imaging method.

References

1. Bertrand O, Thevenet M, Perrin F, Pernier J. Effects of skull holes on the scalp potential distribution evaluated with a finite element model. Satelite Symp. on Neuroscience and Technology, 14th An. Int. Conf. of the *IEEE Engin in Medicine* and Biology Soc, Lyon, 1992 ; 42-5.
2. Gevins A, Le J, Martin NK, Brickett P, Desmond J, Reutter B. High resolution EEG: 124-channel recording, spatial deblurring and MRI integration methods. *Electroenceph Clin Neurophys*, 1994 ; 90 : 213-337.
3. Hämäläinen MS, Hari R, Ilmoniemi RJ, Knuutila J, Lounasmaa OV. Magnetoencephalography - theory, instrumentation and applications to noninvasive studies of the working brain. *Rev Mod Phys*, 1993 ; 654 : 203-13.
4. Hämäläinen MS, Ilmoniemi RJ. Interpreting magnetic fields of the brain: minimum norm estimates. *Med Biol Eng Comput*, 1994 ; 32 : 35-42.
5. Mosher JC, Lewis PS, Leahy RM. Multiple dipole modeling and localization from spatio-temporal MEG data. *IEEE Trans Biomed Engin*, 1992 ; 39 : 541-57.
6. Wieringa HJ, Peters MJ. Processing MRI data for electromagnetic source imaging. *Med Biol Eng Comput*, 1993 ; 31 : 600-6.

49

Automated estimation of metabolite concentrations from localized proton MRS

S. W. PROVENCHER

*Max Planck Institute for Biophysical Chemistry,
Postfach 2841, D-37018 Göttingen, Germany.*

Recently, there have been significant improvements in the quality and localization of NMR spectra *in vivo*. This could open up important new possibilities for clinical diagnoses and biochemical studies, but only if there are corresponding developments of data-analysis methods for the objective and reliable determination of the metabolites and their concentrations.

The usual approaches of estimating concentrations from amplitudes or areas of resonances in the frequency - or time domain - are unreliable with localized *in vivo* spectra for many reasons, but five major problems are:

(a) *peak overlap*, e.g., due to field inhomogeneities, invalidates peak areas as measures of metabolite concentrations;

(b) *baseline distortions* due to incomplete water suppression and the large background signal also contributing to the peak;

(c) *multiplets*, which cannot be properly resolved or quantified as single peaks;

(d) *unpredictable forms* for the lineshape and baseline invalidate parameterized fits to fixed functional forms (e.g., Gaussian-Lorentzian lineshapes) right from the start;

(e) *subjectivity and bias* in the interactive graphical selection of the baseline and peak boundaries for integration, or in the choice of a parameterized model for quantitation.

Method

The LCModel method [1] analyzes an *in vivo* spectrum as a linear combination of complete model spectra of the individual metabolites *in vitro*. By using complete spectra, rather than just single peaks, the complexities of the metabolite spectra now become and advantage, since two metabolites with overlapping peaks at one chemical shift can still be resolved if they have different structures at other chemical shifts. Thus, problem (a) is optimally reduced. By using the same protocol for the model *in vitro* spectra as for the *in vivo* spectra, complications with multiplets (e.g., due to spin-spin couplings) are automatically accounted for, thus eliminating problem (c).

Problem (d) has been particularly serious with parameterized quantitation. A model with too few parameters introduces bias. Too many parameters produce artifact and instabilities in the analysis. Both situations produce errors in the estimates. LCModel uses a nearly model-free constrained regularization method [2] that attempts to find the best compromise between these two situations by finding the smoothest lineshape and baseline consistent with the *data*, thus reducing problems (b), (d), and (e). With this regularization technique, the data determine the complexity of the model; no subjective *a priori* parameterized model is required. Only complexity *demanded* by the data is allowed into the lineshape or baseline. This permits flexibility, but at the same time suppresses artifacts.

Problem (e) must be reduced if results are to be exchanged with confidence and credibility within and between laboratories. LCModel is fully automatic in that the only necessary input is the time-domain data; there is no user interaction. Phasing, referencing, and quantitation are done automatically. Approximately maximum-likelihood estimates of the metabolite concentrations and their uncertainties are obtained.

Results and discussion

The group of J. Frahm have automatically analyzed all of their 2500 rat - and 7000 human brain *in vivo* STEAM spectra with LCModel. Analyses of typical spectra and of poor-quality spectra have been illustrated elsewhere [3,1]. Field strengths of 2.0 and 2.35 T were used. The echo time, *TE*, was usually 20 ms, but there were also series with *TE* = 120 ms and 270 ms.

AUTOMATED ESTIMATION OF BRAIN METABOLITE USING ¹H. MRS

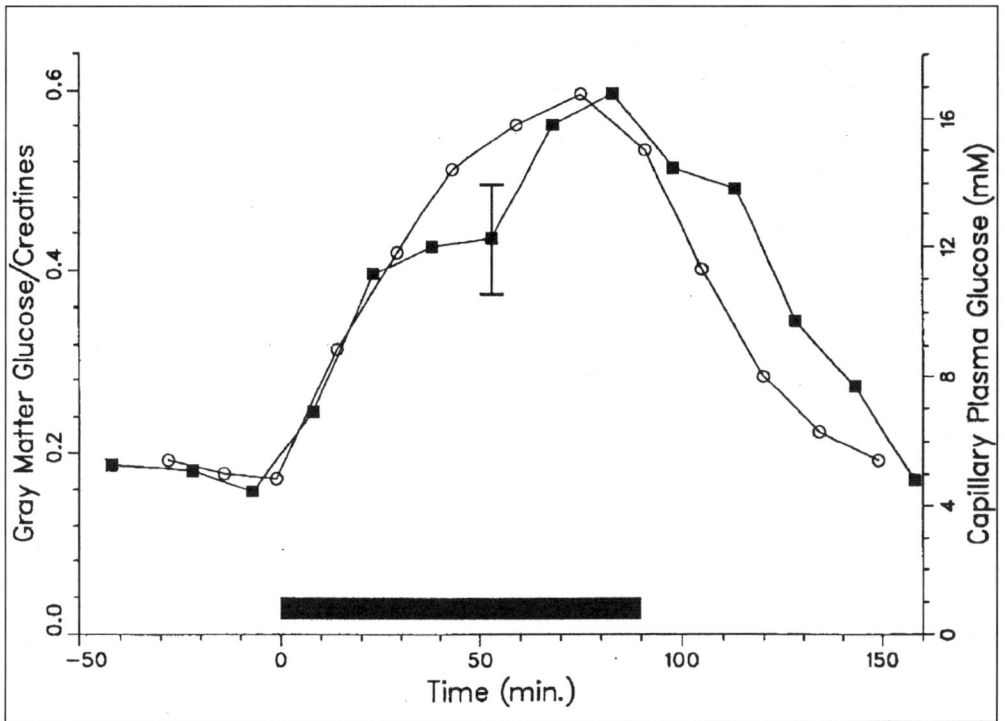

Figure 1. Fully automatic quantitation. Capillary plasma Glc measured directly (circles, right scale) and the ratio of glucose to total creatines (Glc/Cr) in human gray matter estimated with LCModel (squares, left scale). The horizontal bar shows the time during which Glc was infused (10 mg/kg/min) into a healthy volunteer. The brain Glc is nearly proportional to the plasma Glc, with a delay beyond the initial stage. The error bar is the Cramer-Rao lower bound for the standard deviation and is about the same for all points.

Capabilities with typical spectra

To more rigorously test the accuracy of the method, spectra from a glucose (Glc) infusion experiment [4], were analyzed with LCModel (Figure 1). Figure 2 shows that, even at the maximum brain Glc concentration, peak overlap would cause peak integration methods to fail. Only by simultaneously using the full information in the complete spectra of the metabolites can reliable estimates be made. Table I of [1] shows the precision with which the other metabolites could be estimated during this infusion experiment, which was done at 2.0 T with *TE/TM/TR* = 20/30/3000 ms, 128 scans, and an 18 mL localized volume.

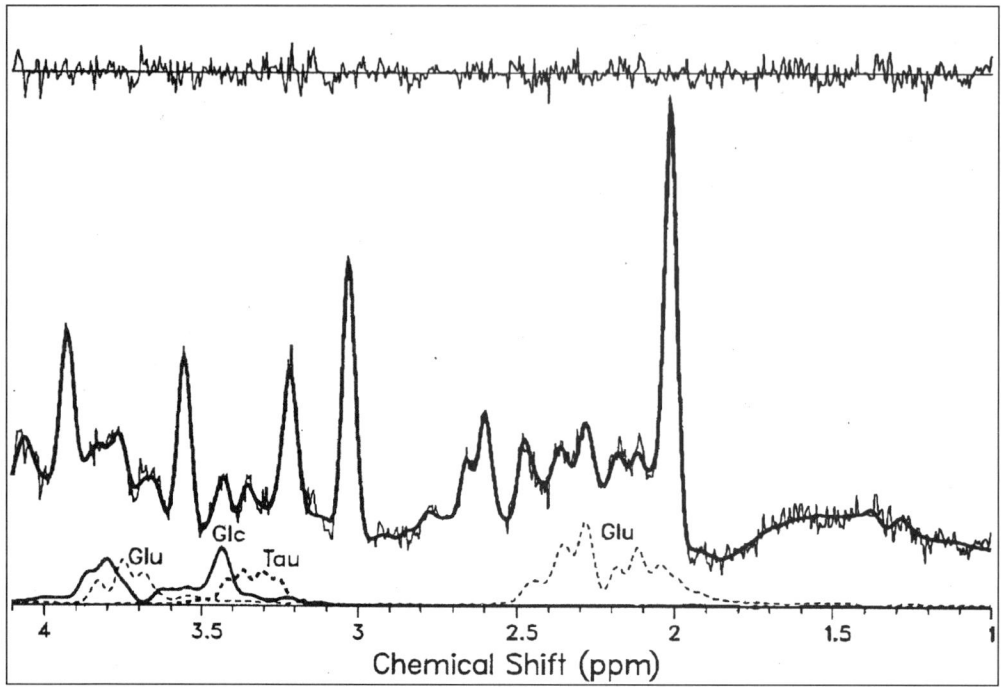

Figure 2. Contributions of the Glc, glutamate (Glu), and taurine (Tau) model spectra to the LCModel analysis of the spectrum corresponding to the maximum Glc/Cr value in Figure 1. Baseline distortion and peak overlap of Glc with Tau and Glu (and other metabolites not shown) make it impossible to reliably estimate concentrations using peak integration. Also shown are the unsmoothed spectrum (thin curve) and the fit to this data (thick curve), with the differences (residuals) between these two plotted above.

Capabilities and limitations with poor-quality spectra

Lineshape distortions

Figure 3 in Ref. [1] illustrates the ability of LCModel to automatically account for extreme lineshape distortions, e.g., due to eddy-current effects. This is possible because all the data in the frequency window are simultaneously used to determine the lineshape. However, it is much better to reduce these distortions from the start by using the Klose eddy-current correction [5]. This is now an integral option in LCModel. This not only reduces the well-known high-frequency oscillations in the lineshape, but also often results in a much smoother baseline.

Baseline distortions

Figure 3 illustrates the ability of LCModel to automatically account for extreme baseline distortions. As with lineshape distortions, the constrained regularization method imposes no subjective prior parameterized form for the baseline and is therefore

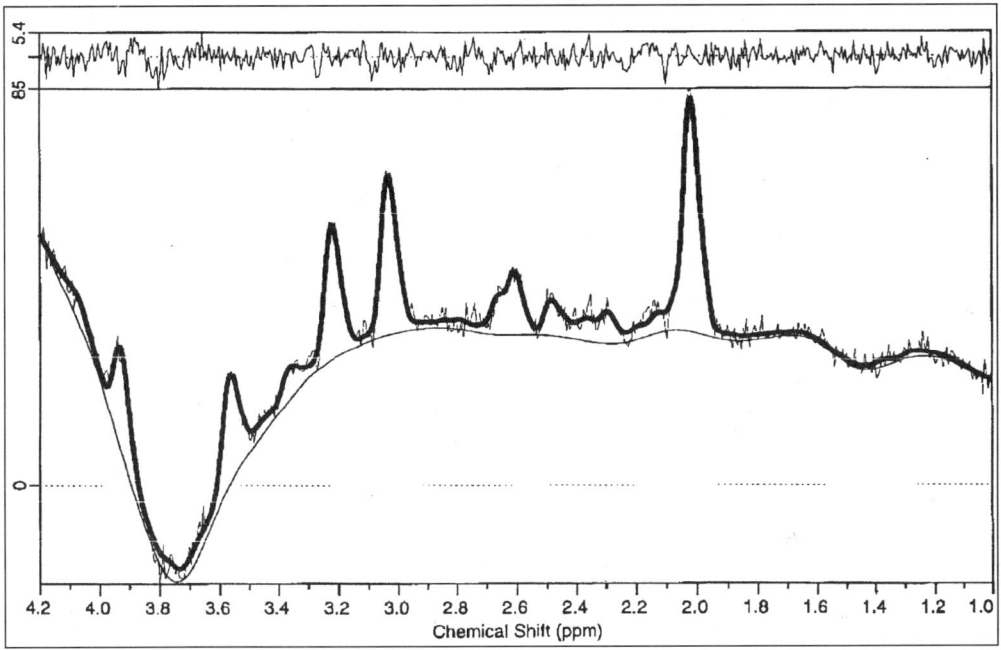

Figure 3. LCModel can automatically account for extreme baseline distortions (in this case due to a strong artifact in the data). Curve conventions are as in Figure 2; in addition, the baseline is plotted as a thin curve.

flexible when the data require this. Of course, in this extreme example, the data would be rejected, because the distortion is clearly due to a serious artifact in the data, which probably distorts the whole analysis. Figure 4 illustrates a more typical case, with a completely reasonable baseline gradually climbing toward the residual water peak.

Noise

Figure 5 illustrates the stability of LCModel to noise. Cerebrospinal fluid (CSF) is particularly difficult, because the useful landmarks, N-acetylaspartate (NAA), Cr, and choline-containing compounds (Cho), are practically missing. It is nevertheless possible to consistently detect and quantify Glc and lactate (Lac) in CSF, because the complete, detail-rich, spectra are used, and not just single peaks. This can be seen in the upper table in Figure 5, where the Cramer-Rao lower bounds (expressed in the second column as percent of the concentration estimates) correctly warn that all metabolites, except Glc and Lac, have very large percent uncertainties.

Figure 5 is the standard one-page output from LCModel. The second table, in this example, simply informs that landmark peaks are weak and that the spectral resolution is unusually good. The last table shows input changes to the default settings (in this example to proportion and simplify the tables and plot for reproduction). Figures 3, 4, and 6 are also the one-page output, but with the size specification for the tables input vanishingly small. All 9500 spectra were fully automatically analyzed with only objective input, such as filenames, field strength, dwell time, etc.

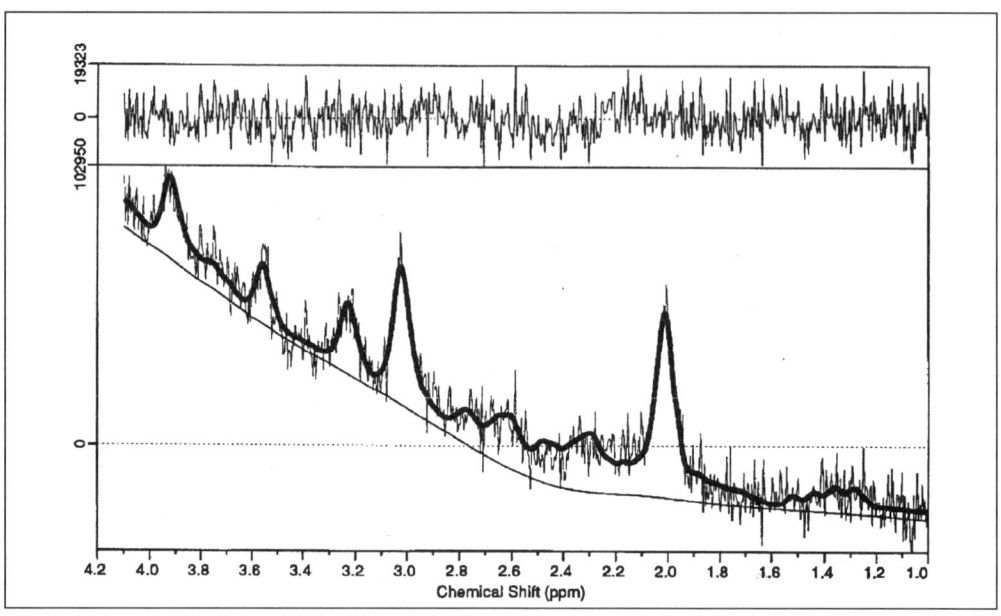

Figure 4. LCModel analysis with a moderately climbing baseline. Curve conventions are as in Figure 3.

Spectral resolution

It is the most important factor in NMR quantitation *in vivo*. Poor resolution combined with the large baselines of spectra with short echo times can lead to a range of significantly different metabolite concentrations that all fit the data to within experimental error. Without more data or prior knowledge to restrict the model, no data analysis method can resolve this fundamental nonuniqueness.

With short echo times (e.g., 20 ms), the linewidth should no exceed 0.1 ppm FWHM [1]. With long echo times (e.g., 120 ms) the baseline is greatly reduced, and lower resolution is much less of a problem, as illustrated in Figure 6. This was part of a diffusional study (with low resolution and S/N), and LCModel analyses with basis spectra of only five metabolites (NAA, Cho, Cr, myo-inositol, and Lac) seem to adequately fit the data. Thus, there is obviously much less information in these long-echo-time spectra. Nevertheless, if the linewidth exceeds 0.1 ppm, then the advantages of short echo times are lost, and a long echo time would generally be better. More than five metabolites might be able to be estimated with these long echo times if the S/N were better.

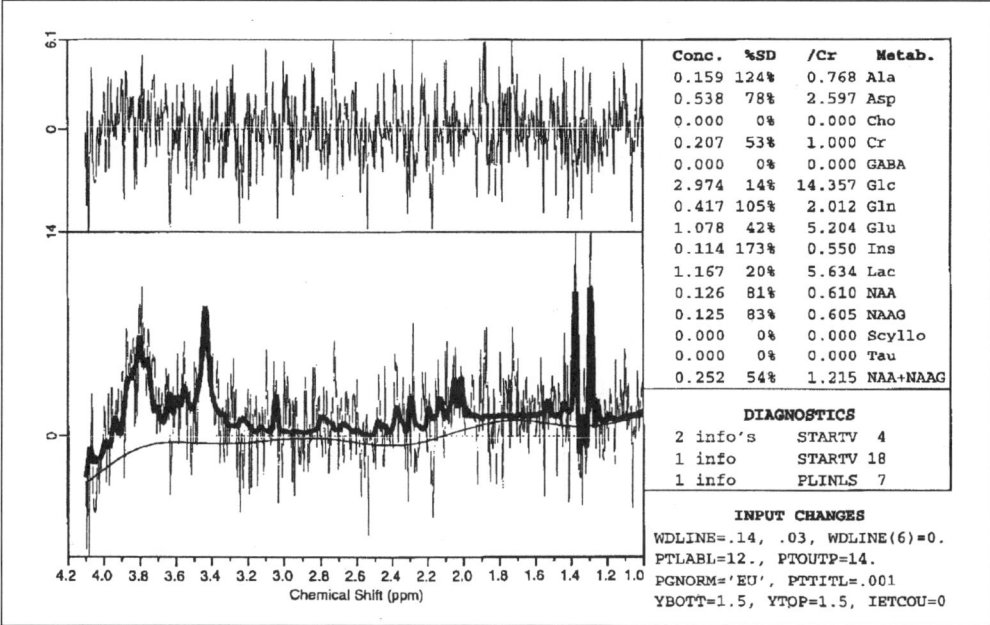

Figure 5. Standard one-page output from LCModel illustrating its stability to a low signal-to-noise ratio (S/N). Despite the lack of strong landmarks (such as NAA, Cr, Cho), Glc and Lac can still be detected and quantified in CSF. Curve conventions are as in Figure 3.

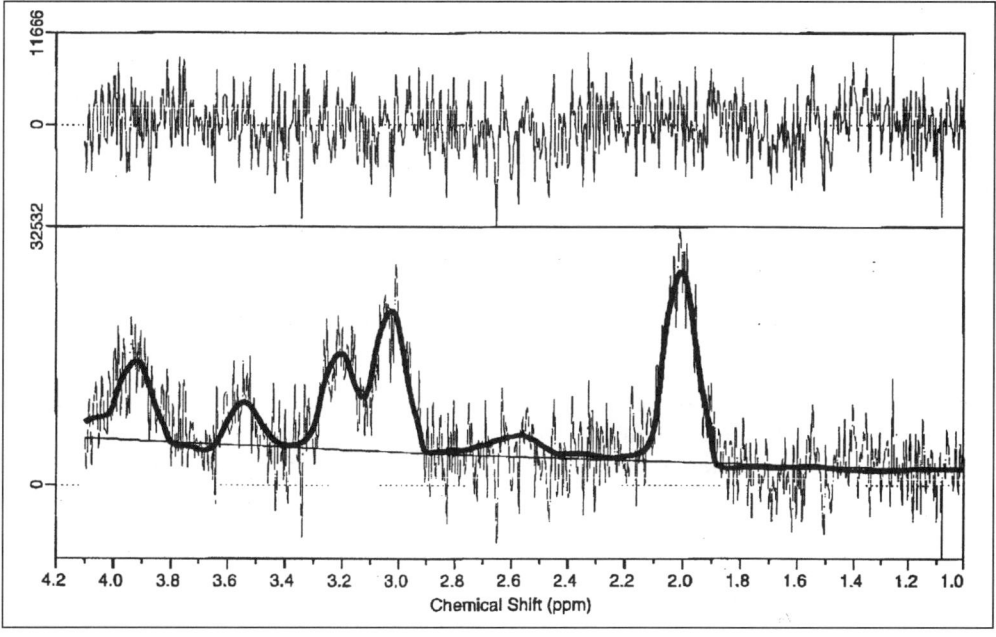

Figure 6. Low resolution (0.12 ppm linewidth, FWHM) is much less of a problem with long echo times (120 ms). Curve conventions are as in Figure 3.

Conclusions

With TE = 20 ms, NAA, Cho, Cr, myo-inositol (Ins), and Glu can be reliably determined, and abnormal levels of these or elevated levels of Lac, alanine (Ala), *scyllo*-inositol (Scyllo), glutamine (Gln), or Glc clearly indicate numerous pathologies. The 14 metabolites used in these analyses can be roughly ranked in order of decreasing reliability of their estimated concentrations as follows:

(A) total NAA +NAAG (N-acetylaspartylglutamate), Cr, NAA, Cho;
(B) Lac, Ala, Ins, Glu, Scyllo;
(C) Gln, NAAG;
(D) Aspartate, Glc, γ-Aminobutyric Acid (GABA), Tau.

Quantitative data are given in Table I of [1]. However, we can make the following qualitative generalizations: The metabolites in Class A can be reliably estimated even with poor-quality spectra. With normal-quality spectra, Class A metabolites can be very accurately estimated and Class B metabolites reliably.

Class C metabolites can be estimated semi-quantitatively. For example, the Gln/Glu ratio can be very reliably and reproducibly seen in certain pathologies to be about twice that of normal controls. This factor of two increase is easily seen, but not a 20 % increase, which is about the minimum uncertainty in Gln estimates. Similarly, it can be reproducibly determined that the NAAG/NAA ratio in adult white matter is several times that in gray matter.

Class D metabolites are generally difficult to reliably quantify. However, under conditions where sources of variability are removed, as in the Glc infusion experiment in Figure 1, even these weak metabolites can be reliably estimated. Also, very high resolution, a s is often attainable in CSF and with children (in Figure 5), can yield significant improvements in accuracy. Conversely, spectra of the cerebellum are often very poor. Resolution and good shimming seem to be the most important factors in localized NMR spectroscopy with one short echo time.

Acknowledgments

All spectra have been acquired and were run with LCModel buy the Biomedizinische NMR Group in Göttingen. I thank J. Frahm for permission to use the examples, and W. Hänicke, M. Wick, F. Prielmeier, and K.D. Merboldt for helpful comments.

References

1. Provencher SW, Estimation of metabolite concentrations from localized in vivo proton NMR spectra, *Magn Reson Med* 1993 ; 30 : 672-9.

2. Provencher SW. A constrained regularization method for inverting data represented by linear algebraic or integral equations. *Comput Phys Commun* 1982 ; 27 : 213-27.
3. Hänicke W, Michaelis T, Merboldt KD, Frahm J. On the use of a fully automatic data analysis method for in vivo MRS. Metabolite concentrations and relaxation times from proton spectra of human brain, In: *Proceedings of the Society of Magnetic Resonance in Medicine Twelfth Annual Meeting* Berkeley Society of Magnetic Resonance 1993 ; 977.
4. Frahm J. Nuclear magnetic resonance studies of human brain in vivo: anatomy, function, and metabolism. In: Firnagl U, Villringer A, Einhäupl KM, eds. Optical imaging of brain function and metabolism New York (Plenum) 1993 ; 257-71.
5. Klose U. *In vivo* proton spectroscopy in presence of eddy currents. *Magn Reson Med* 1990 ; 14 : 26-30.

50

Perils and pitfalls of fMRI: photic stimulation in subjects with schizophrenia

P.F. RENSHAW, D.A. YURGELUN-TODD, B.M. COHEN

Brain Imaging Center, McLean Hospital, Belmont, MA, USA.
Department of Psychiatry, Harvard Medical School, Boston, MA, USA.

Functional magnetic resonance imaging (fMRI) has opened a new window for studies of cerebral activation. Most fMRI studies reported to date have studied primary sensory stimulation in normal subjects. Results derived from normal subjects may differ form those with clinical brain disorders.

Patients with schizophrenia are known to have substantial anomalies of brain structure and function. In this study we have investigated fMRI signal intensity changes caused by photic stimulation [1] in patients with schizophrenia. Additionally, dynamic susceptibility contrast MRI (DSCI; 2) was employed to determine whether patients with schizophrenia have alterations in their vascular distribution.

Methods

Eight schizophrenic subjects (mean age 33 +/- 6 years, 7 right handed and 1 left handed, 1 female and 7 males) and nine normal control subjects (mean age 34 +/- 9 years, 8 right handed and 1 left handed, 4 female and 5 males) underwent fMRI during photic stimulation. Each subject received a structured clinical interview (SCID-P;3) and diagnosis was made blind to scanning results according to DSM-III-R criteria. Subjects with a history of organic brain syndrome, head injury, or substance abuse were excluded.

Echo planar images were collected every second from an oblique plane running parallel to the calcarine fissure using a gradient echo pulse sequence (TE = 40 msec, flip angle = 66 deg, 3 mm x 3 mm in plane resolution, slice thickness = 7 mm). Data were obtained over a four minute period consisting of four 30 second cycles of darkness alternating with four 30 second cycles of binocular, 8 Hz patterned flash photic stimulation produced by goggles with light-emitting diodes. The signal intensity for both the right and left primary visual cortex (V1) was measured using a 6 mm x 6 mm region in the occipital lobe.

In a second experiment we performed DSCI in six subjects with DSM-III-R schizophrenia and six normal control subjects. Images were acquired from 6 oblique planes running parallel to the calcarine cortex every second before and after the intravenous injection of 0.200 mEq/kg of the paramagnetic contrast agent gadoteridol infused as a bolus over 5-7 seconds. A spin echo EPI sequence was used to acquire images with TR=1sec, TE=100 msec, 3 mm x 3 mm in-plane resolution, and 7 mm slice thickness with a 1 mm skip.

The change in image intensity during infusion of contrast, $S(t)$, was calculated for a 1 cm^3 region within the left and right posterior occipital lobes corresponding to the location of V1. The fixed dose of paramagnetic contrast agent is related to the regional cerebral brain volume (CBV) as:

$$CBV \sim Integral\ [-\ln(S(t)/s(t0)]$$

where $S(t0)$ is the precontrast image intensity [2]. To estimate the relative size of the CBV within the occipital regions the integral of $-\ln(S(t)/S(t0))$ was calculated for each subject by numerical integration over a ten second period.

Results

Figure 1 displays the averaged MR signal intensities by group for schizophrenics and control subjects across the period of data collection for the photic stimulation experiment. Differences in mean signal intensity change between patients and controls are statistically significant for right V1 ($p=.05$) and for the average of right and left V1 ($p=.03$) (Table I).

The results of the DSCI MRI study are shown in Figure 2 (2a and 2b). The CBV was higher in the schizophrenic subjects in both occipital regions with a statistically significant increase in CBV evident for the right occipital region ($p=.01$). Of note, mapping of T1 and T2* in these brain regions did not reveal any significant differences in the tissue relaxation times between patients and controls (data not presented).

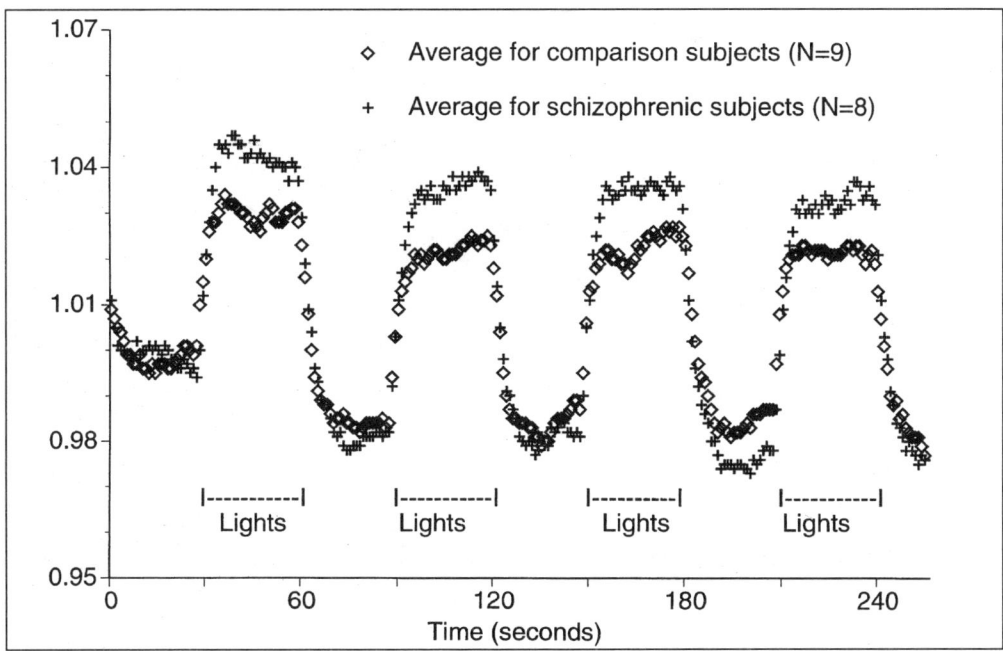

Figure 1. Normalized signal intensity change during photic stimulation in patients with schizophrenia and control subjects.

Table I. Mean Signal Intensity Changes During Photic Stimulation (1).

	Normal controls	Schizophrenic patients
Left V1	3.3 +/- 1.9 %	5.0 +/- 2.1 % (2)
Right V1	3.0 +/- 1.1 %	4.3 +/- 1.2 % (3)
Average	3.1 +/- 1.3 %	4.6 +/- 1.5 % (4)

(1) Mean change +/- standard deviation in percent.
(2) $p = .12$ (Mann-Whitney U Test, DF = 15, Z = - 1.54).
(3) $p = .05$ (Mann-Whitney U Test, DF = 15, Z = - 1.93).
(4) $p = .03$ (Mann-Whitney U Test, DF = 15, Z = - 2.18).

Discussion

We have used echo planar MRI to document an increased signal intensity change within primary visual cortex in response to photic stimulation in subjects with schizophrenia relative to normal controls. Since the signal intensity changes seen during activation are thought to result from a washout of deoxyhemoglobin, one explanation for this result would be an alteration in the vascular distribution in the brain of schizophrenics. Using DSCI we have observed abnormalities of occipital CBV in patients with schizophrenia which may contribute to the observed increase in signal intensity.

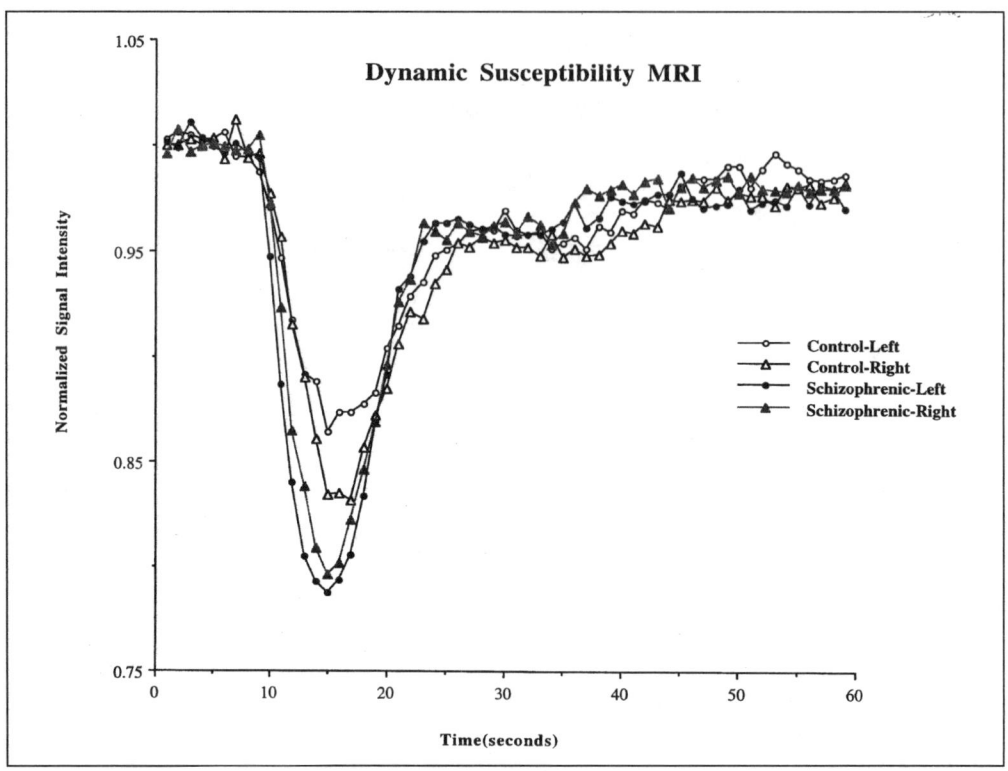

Figure 2 a. Normalized signal intensity change during the first pass of gadoteridol through the occipital cortex.

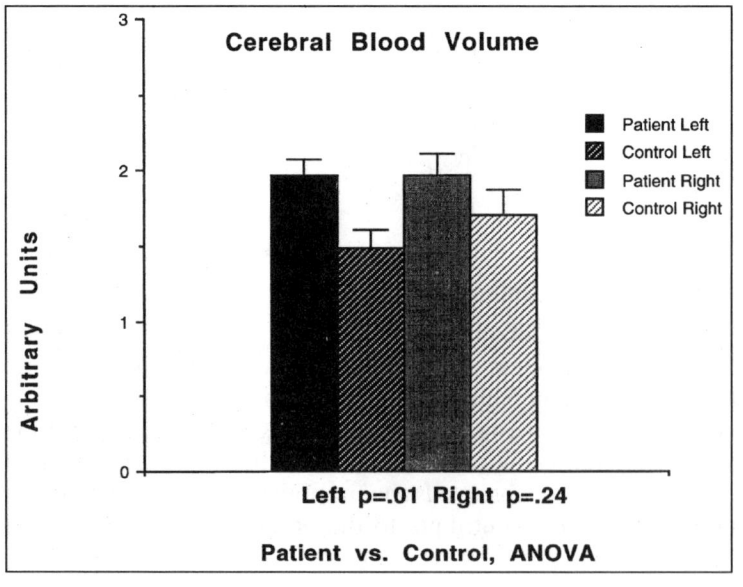

Figure 2 b. Relative occipital lobe CBV measures.

The extent to which abnormalities of vascular distribution exist in other brain regions of schizophrenic subjects is uncertain. However, there has been a preliminary report that the cortical fMRI signal intensity change associated with motor tasks is decreased in patients with schizophrenia [4]. Similarly, we have found both decreased frontal lobe signal intensity changes and increased temporal lobe signal intensity changes in schizophrenic subjects relative to normal comparison subjects during a verbal fluency paradigm [5].

These results suggest that caution is required in the direct extension of fMRI techniques from normal populations to subjects with clinical brain disorders.

References

1. Kwong KK, Belliveau JW, Chesler DA, *et al. PNAS* 1992 ; 89 : 5672.
2. Belliveau JW, Rosen BR, Kantor HL, *et al. Magn Res Med* 1990 ; 14 : 538-46.
3. Spitzer RL, Williams JBW, Gibbon M. *Structured clinical interview for DSM-III-R (SCID)*. New York State : Psychiatric Institute, Biometrics Research Department, 1989.
4. Wenz F, Schad LR, Baudendistel K, *et al. Proc Soc Magn Reson Med* 1993 ; 1419.
5. Yurgelun-Todd DA, Renshaw PF, Gruber SA *et al. Proc Soc Magn Reson* 1994 ; 686.

51

¹H MR spectroscopy in multiple sclerosis

W. ROSER[1], G. HAGBERG[1], I. MADER[2], E.W. RADÜ[2],
H. BRUUNSCHWEILER[3], L. KAPPOS[3], J. SEELIG[1]

[1]MR-Center and Biocenter, [2]Department of Medical Radiology and [3]Department of Neurology
of the University Hospital, University of Basel, CH-4031, Switzerland.

Multiple sclerosis (MS is an inflammatory demyelinating disease of the central nervous system. In T_1-weighted images lesions are iso- or hypointense. Some plaques may show Gadolinium contrast agent enhancement over several weeks [1]. Gd-enhancement, due to a disturbance of the blood-brain-barrier, is thought to be correlated with disease activity. However, MRI cannot make a prediction of the clinical and morphological course. Clinical proton MRS is able to reveal some biochemical aspects of MS-plaques. But existing reports on acute mS-plaques defined by GD-enhancement are based on small numbers of patients, and their results are controversial [2-8].

Most studies found a decrease of the N-acetylated metabolites compared to creatine and phosphocreatine (NA-to-Cr-ratio, NA/Cr), either with [2,6-8] or without [4,6] and increase in the ratio of the choline-containing compounds (Cho) to Cr. No significant metabolic changes were found in another study [3]. An increase of lactate [2,6,8], *myo*-inositol [8], or 'marker peaks' in the region of 2.1 to 2.6 ppm [5] was also reported.

There exist only a few reports on serial MRS of MS plaques. But also here, the reported metabolic changes are contradictory. For instance, a persistent decrease of the NA/Cr [9] or of NA/Cho [10] with time was reported, whereas others did not find any changes of these metabolites during the investigated time period [11,12]. A recovery of NA/Cr 4-8 months after the initial measurement was also reported [13].

The purpose of the present study was therefore to investigate and to follow up Gd enhancing acute plaques in a large number of carefully selected patients.

Material and methods

Twenty-two patients participating in a 2 year, double-blind controlled trial on the effect of the new immuno-modulating drug in active MS [14] were included in the present study. They were carefully selected and had to fulfil special inclusion criteria [15].

One or two days after appearance of Gadolinium-enhancing lesions in diagnostic MRI, consisting of contiguous axial T_2-weighted (TE=90 ms, TR=2500 ms) and T_1-weighted (TE=15 ms, TR=700 ms) images without and with Gadolinium contrast agent, one of the enhancing lesions was examined by proton MRS. Medical treatment was begun after the first spectroscopy session.

The measurements were performed on a Siemens Magnetom Helicon GBS II, whole body system operating at 2.0 T using the standard circularly polarized head coil. Spectra were acquired after image-guided localization using a STEAM sequence with TE=20 ms and TM=30 ms and, to control the presence of lactate, a PRESS sequence with TE=135 ms. The repetition time was set to 3000 ms, and the cubic voxel size was 8 ml in all measurements. Post-processing consisted of an eddy current correction [16], zero-filling to 4096 data points, exponential line broadening, and, if necessary, phase correction in zero and first order after Fourier transformation. Peak areas were calculated after a square spline baseline correction using the standard equipment software.

Serial ^{1}H MRS of the chosen plaque could be performed in 16 of the 22 patients. Until now, each selected plaque was investigated in 8 patients every month during the first half year and once after one year. In another 8 patients each plaque was investigated 0, 1, 3, 6 and 12 months after primary Gd-enhancement. Follow-up MRS will be performed in the 24th month. Nine healthy volunteers were once investigated as controls.

Results

Acute, Gd-enhancing MS-plaques (month 0).

The spectra of 18 patients were of sufficient quality to be evaluated. The relative plaque size within the voxel, determined from the T2-weighted images, ranged from 3 to 75 % with a mean of 21 %. The average plaque was therefore 1.5 cm in diameter. 9 healthy volunteers were investigated as controls.

Figure 1 shows a STEAM spectrum of an acute, Gd-enhancing MS plaque. No baseline correction was applied. The NA is clearly reduced, whereas Cho is increased compared to Cr. We also evaluated the peak of myo-inositol and glycine (Ino). It showed no significant changes. Resonances in the region of 2.1 to 2.6 ppm, previously described as marker peaks [5], are not significantly elevated. An inverted doublet of lactate was not visible in any PRESS-spectrum of the acute plaques.

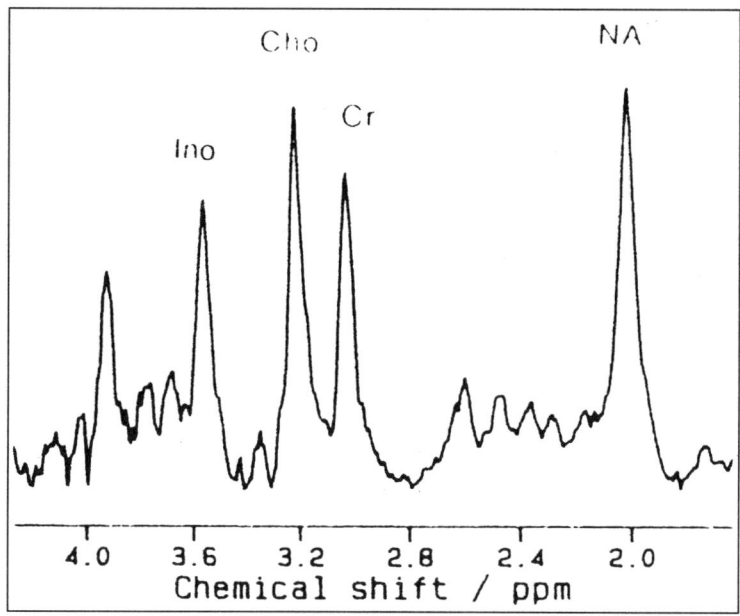

Figure 1. STEAM 1H spectrum (TE/TM/TR = 20/30/3000 ms) of a Gd-enhancing MS plaque.

Table I summarizes the obtained metabolic ratios and their standard deviations for patients and healthy controls. No corrections were applied for finite T_1 or T_2-relaxation.

Table I. Metabolic ratios and standard deviations (in brackets) for the groups of MS patients and healthy controls.

	Ino/Cr	Cho/Cr	NA/Cr	NA/Cho
MS patients	0.78 (0.31)	0.97 (0.17)	1.41 (0.35)	1.48 (0.38)
Healthy volunteers	0.87 (0.26)	0.81 (0.15)	1.98 (0.55)	2.53 (0.83)
Significance	n. s.	$p < 0.05$	$p < 0.05$	$p < 0.001$

In order to investigate partial volume effects, the variation of the ^{1}H NMR spectra with the plaque size was also analyzed. As an example, the NA-to-choline ratio of all patients is plotted against the relative plaque size within the VOI in Figure 2. The bars indicate the average of the healthy volunteers ± one standard deviation. The difference between both groups is evident. Even in the case, when the plaque occupied only a small percentage of the VOI, the same spectral changes were observed.

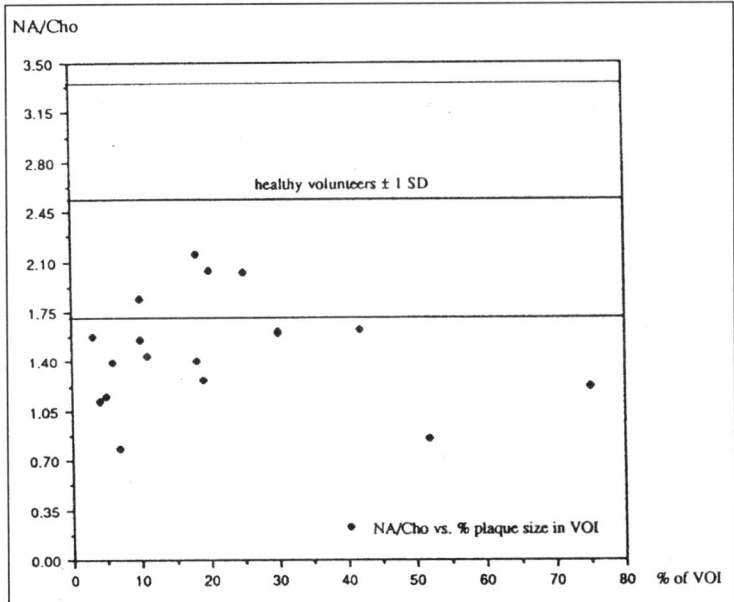

Figure 2. NA/Cho as function of the % plaque size within the VOI of 8 ml. The average of the healthy volunteers ± one standard deviation is indicated by the horizontal bars.

The other metabolite ratios exhibit a similar behaviour. This slide demonstrates no unequivocal dependence of the metabolic ratios upon the plaque size. It is not important whether we use the relative plaque size as estimated in the T_2-weighted images or as that estimated from the typically much smaller Gd-enhancing region in the T_1-weighted images.

Serial MRS of the acute, Gd-enhancing MS-plaques

A complete series of spectra from one patient using the TE = 20 ms STEAM sequence is displayed in Figure 3. No baseline correction was applied to these spectra. Some transient changes of *myo*-Inositol, the choline containing compounds, creatine and phosphocreatine, and the N-acetylated metabolites are visible. An interesting finding in this patient was the clear appearance of a resonance at 3.35 ppm in all spectra, probably due to *scyllo*-Inositol [17].

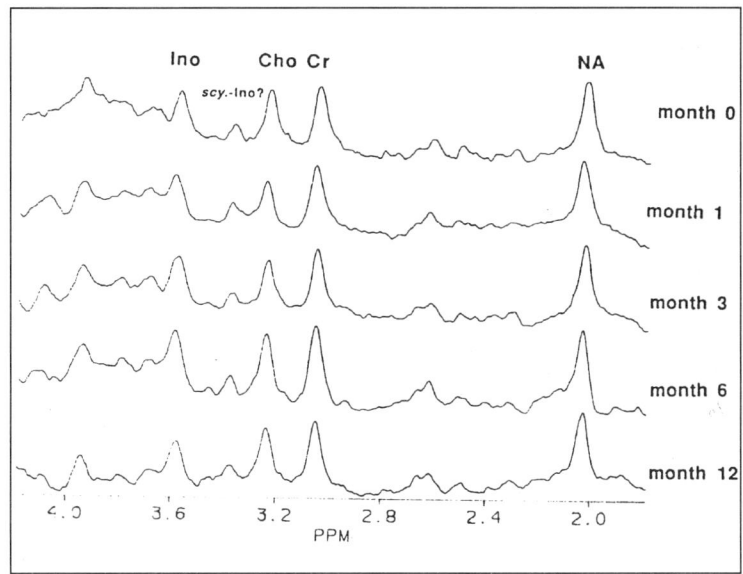

Figure 3. Spectral series of one patient. (STEAM, TE/TM/TR = 20/30/3000 ms).

The time course of the investigated metabolites (values ± SEM) relative to PCr/cr is displayed in Figure 4 (a). As mentioned above, Cho/cr was initially (month 0) increased, NA/Cr decreased, and Ino/Cr was unchanged relative to healthy volunteers. No lactate was found in any PRESS spectrum of the Gd-enhancing plaques in month 0. During the observation period only minor changes were visible. The linear regression lines indicate a trend towards decreased levels of all ratios. In 2 patients an increase of lactate was detected after 12 months.

Figure 4 (b) displays the individual time course of the investigated metabolites. Absolute concentration values were created by correcting the metabolite area of each spectrum for different coil loading by multiplication with the transmitter amplitude necessary for a non-selective 90° pulse [18], and comparing the peak areas to investigations of metabolite solutions of known concentrations, measured on another occasion. A small increase of Cr over time is indicated by the regression line, whereas the other metabolite ratios show no definite trend.

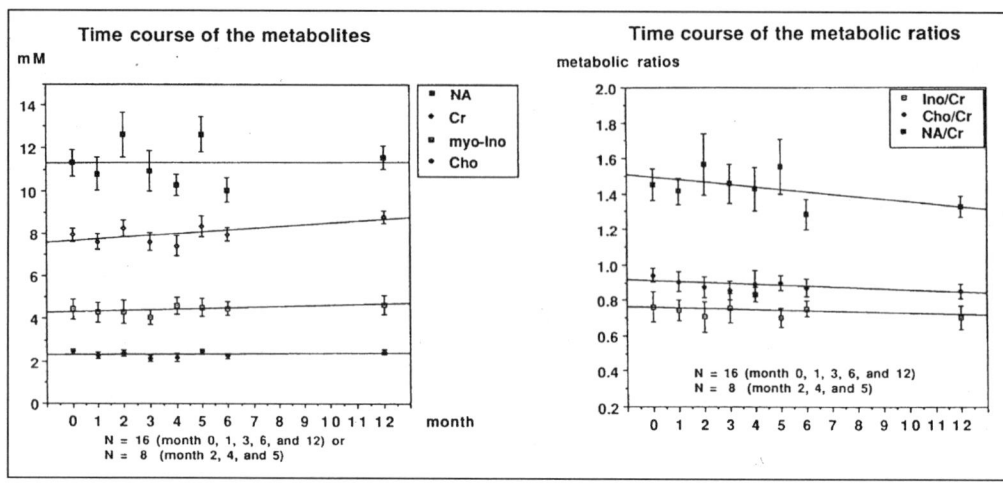

Figure 4. Metabolic ratios (a) and absolute metabolite concentrations (b) of the investigated plaques as a function of time after initial Gd-enhancement.

Discussion

The findings in Figure 2 indicate that the metabolic changes measured with proton MRS are not only confined to the are depicted by MRI, but must be also present in the surrounding normal appearing tissue. This result would support previous reports describing areas of relaxational abnormalities in regions of the brain of MS patients which appeared normal in MRI [19-24]. Such changes of the normal appearing matter might be due to microscopic plaques which are not visible in clinical standard MRI.

The decreased ratios of NA/Cr and NA/Cho indicate a loss of NA which has been discussed to be due to gliosis, neuronal or axonal loss, signal contribution from non-neuronal tissue or oedema, or an increase in Cr.

In agreement with most previous works we see a small, but significant increase in the Cho/Cr-ratio. The suspected increase in choline may be due to demyelination or the imflammatory myelin breakdown and/or increased turnover of membrane constituents in proliferative oligodendrocytes and astrozytes, resulting in fibrillary gliosis.

In this double blinded follow up study some patients are treated whereas others receive placebo. A differential effect of the treatment on the measured values should lead to an increase of the standard errors. Until now such an effect could not be confirmed.

The trend of the metabolite ratios, NA/Cr, Cho/Cr, and Ino/Cr is a slight decrease with time, mainly due to an increase of Cr. However, these small changes were not significant. Interestingly enough, the patient in whom an intense resonance at 3.35 ppm was present, probably from scyllo-Inositol, he had an unexpected positive evolution of his clinical symptoms. On the other hand both patients having increased levels of lactate in month 12, both had significant clinical deterioration at that time.

Conclusion

Acute, Gd-enhancing MS plaques show significant spectral changes compared to healthy volunteers. NA/Cr and NA/Cho are decreased, Cho/Cr is increased, Ino/Cr not significantly altered. The metabolic changes seem to be independent of the plaque size within a VOI of 8 ml. Therefore in MRI normal appearing matter also contributes to the metabolic changes.

During follow up investigations of these plaques during a medical trial, the trend of the metabolic ratios, NA/Cr, Cho/Cr, and Ino/Cr was a slight decrease with time, mainly due to an increase of Cr. However, these small changes were not significant.

The results of this work in progress may be further elucidated at the end of the study, when the blinding has been broken and each of the 16 patients has been investigated for 2 years.

References

1. Miller DH *et al. Brain* 1988 ; 111 : 927-39.
2. Miller DH *et al. Lancet* 1991 ; 337 : 58-9.
3. Narayana PA *et al. JMRI* 1992 ; 2 : 263-70.
4. Bruhn H *et al. Ann. Neurol* 32, 140-150.
5. Grossman RI *et al. AJNR* 1992 ; 13 : 1535-43.
6. Yousry T *et al.* Works in Progr. of the 11 th SMRM 1992 ; 1964.
7. Roser W *et al.* Proc. of the 12th SMRM, 1993 ; 278.
8. Davie CA *et al. Brain* 1994 ; 117, 49-58.
9. Matthews PM *et al. Neurology* 1991 ; 41 : 1251-6.
10. Larsson HBW *et al. Mag Reson Med* 1991 ; 22 : 23-31.
11. Yousry T *et al.* Works in Progr of the 11th SMRM 1992 ; 1964.
12. Bruhn H *et al. Ann Neurol* 1992 ; 32 : 140-50.
13. Davie CA *et al. Brain* 1994 ; 117 : 49-58.
14. Kappos L *et al. Nervenarzt* 1992 ; 63 : 768-71.
15. Roser W *et al. to Magn Reson Med* 1994.
16. Klose U. *Magn Reson Med* 1990 ; 14 : 26-30.
17. Michaelis T *et al. NMR Biomed* 1993 ; 6 : 105-9.
18. Michaelis T *et al. Radiology* 1993 ; 187 : 219-27.
19. Lacomis D *et al. Magn Reson Med* 1986 ; 3 : 194-202.
20. Larsson HBW *et al. Magn Reson Med* 1988 ; 7 : 43-55.
21. Feinstein A *et al. J Neurol Neurosurg Psychiatry* 1992 ; 55 : 869-76.
22. Haughton VM *et al. Magn Reson Med* 1992 ; 26 : 71-8.
23. Barbosa S *et al. Magn Reson Imaging* 1994 ; 12 : 33-42.

52

Quality control in volume selective spectroscopy

K.V. SCHENKER

Bruker/Spectrospin, Fällanden, Switzerland.

A «high quality» volume selective spectrum shows a good signal-to-noise ratio, narrow lines, signal intensities and signal-to-noise ratio, narrow lines, signal intensities and signal positions according to expectations. Obviously, this are very vague quality criteria. Nevertheless, for lack of unbiased and easy to measure parameters this is what many spectroscopists know about the quality of their spectra. On the other hand, it is not too difficult to produce a list of relevant quality criteria which can include properties like e.g.
- quality of voxel shape and positioning
- volume selectivity
- detection sensitivity
- quality of water suppression
- eddy current effects
- reliability/reproducibility.

The problem is much more how to measure parameters that give us information about the performance of the «spectroscopy system» with regard to such criteria. Meaningful test spectra must be measured under absolute reproducible conditions and partly evaluated in a quantitative way. Thus, measurements on appropriate phantoms have usually a higher information content and are faster and easier to obtain.

In this presentation quality aspects for volume selective spectroscopy are discussed on the example of the double spin echo sequence PRESS applied to protons. Most of it is valid for other techniques and applications to other nuclei, too.

The pulse sequence press

A profound analysis of quality aspects of any method requires a detailed understanding of the mechanism of a pulse sequence. PRESS (Pulse REsolved volume Selective Spectroscopy) is one of the classical spectroscopy methods for localized spectroscopy producing a three-dimensional volume selection in a single shot. The technique is mainly used for ^{1}H spectroscopy but can be applied to other nuclei (e.g. ^{31}P, ^{19}F, ^{13}C etc.) as well. The PRESS scheme consists of three slice selective rf pulses which act on three orthogonal slices (Figure 1). The volume common to these three slices is the VOI (Volume Of Interests). In principal each rf three-pulse sequence produces 3 FID signals, 3 single refocused spin echoes, a stimulated echo, and a double refocused spin echo (Figure 2). The crucial point in volume selective spectroscopy now is to detect solely the double refocused spin echo in case of PRESS (SE2) or the stimulated echo (STE) in case of STEAM. The suppression of the unwanted signal is done by means of spoiling gradients, rf pulse phase cycling and proper timing of the sequence. Note that spins of a full slice contribute to the FID signals FID1, FID2, and FID3, spins of the common volume of two intersecting slices will give rise to the single refocused spin echoes SE1, SE3, and SE4, and finally the spins common to all three slices experience all three rf pulses and keep result in the occurrence of the double refocused spin echo SE2 and the stimulated echo STE. Thus, the total signal to be suppressed is typically hundreds of times more intense compared to the desired signal of the VOI.

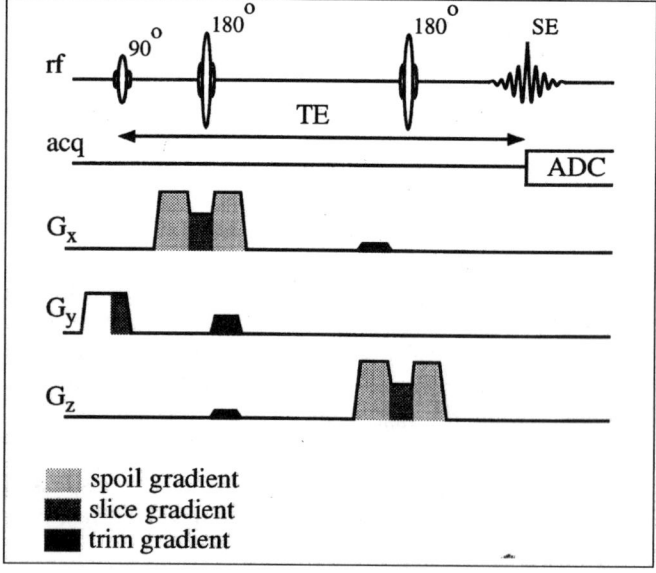

Figure 1. The PRESS rf pulse and gradient sequence. Other gradient patterns may be used as well.

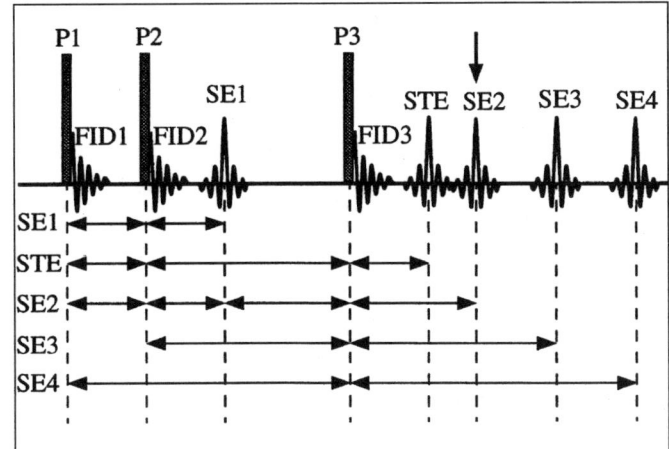

Figure 2. The rf three-pulse sequence and the signals it produces. The double refocused spin echo signal SE2 is the one selected by PRESS.

The advantages of PRESS are that the sequence is volume selective in a single shot (unlike e.g. ISIS) which allows to do shimming, rf pulse gain, and water suppression adjustments on the VOI. PRESS produces the full signal inherently available from the spins inside the VOI (unlike e.g. STEAM).

The disadvantages of PRESS are that it uses two 180° refocusing rf pulses (unlike e.g. STEAM) which increases the rf power requirements considerably if a proper bandwidth should be maintained. Moreover, refocusing pulses are usually more critical in terms of their slice profile (voxel shape) and gain adjustments. PRESS gives somewhat longer minimum TE times compared to STEAM which may be critical for applications where short T_2 values or relatively large J couplings occur.

The voxel shape and position

A good voxel shape requires good slice profiles of the rf pulses, i.e. steep edges that guarantee a sharp transition from outside to inside the VOI and therefore give maximum signal and minimum contamination. It is very difficult to measure the voxel shape indirectly by moving the voxel around in a test phantom and look for contamination and other effects which may be related to the voxel shape. The best way is to detect the signal produced by e.g. PRESS in an experiment which resolves it in one, two or three spatial dimensions (Figure 3). This can be achieved by adding read and phase encoding gradients to the volume selective pulse sequence. This allows the control of the voxel position at the same time. The adjustment of the rf pulse gains is critical for the voxel shape, too. The slice profiles of the rf pulses may depend quite dramatically on the effective pulse angle of the excitation and refocusing pulse. It seems to be a good idea to adjust the rf pulse gains on the voxel profile and not on the time domain signal intensity. Adjusting for maximum time domain signal usually leads to considerable distortion of the voxel shape. The acquisition of a 2D image of the voxel typically requires about one minute (e.g. TR = 500 ms x 128 PE steps) and can be part of a routine spectroscopy protocol without a substantial lengthening of the procedure.

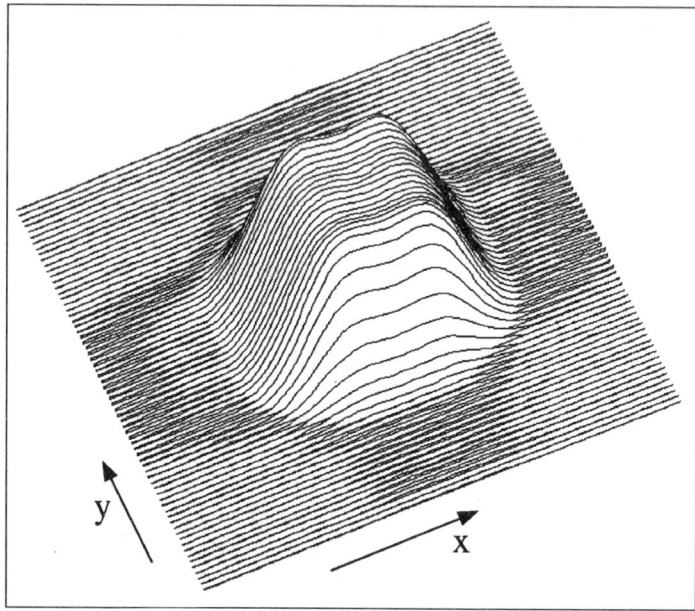

Figure 3. The voxel signal of PRESS resolved in the two spatial dimension x and y corresponding to the directions of the 90° and one 180° rf pulse. A relatively simple Hermite rf pulse shape of 1 ms duration was used for the 90° and 180° rf pulses resulting in 4.5 kHz and 2.8 kHz bandwidth, respectively.

Optimizing the voxel shape means optimizing the slice profiles of the rf pulses and their corresponding pulse shapes. An immense number of pulse shapes has been published giving us a great choice of combinations of properties of rf pulses. Clearly, there is no best rf pulse shape for all applications. The most important properties of rf pulses are a good slice profile for the best signal-to-noise and least contamination combined with a good bandwidth and acceptable rf power requirement. A compromise must be found between bandwidth and rf power requirements. In order to limit the chemical shift displacement (e.g. < 20 % of the total VOI over a spectral range of 3 ppm) a bandwidth of > 40 ppm is required. This is about 5 times more than what is typically used for imaging experiments. Longer rf pulses usually allow us to generate better slice profiles but in return increase the minimum TE time. Thus, another compromise must be found between voxel shape and minimum TE time.

Volume selectivity

The volume selectivity is naturally the most important quality criterion for a volume selective spectroscopy technique. There are different ways to quantify the volume selectivity or signal contamination, e.g. one can calculate ratios of signal originating from spins inside the VOI versus signal of spins from outside the voxel. Very often the problem is more complex, however. A typical case may be a brain spectrum which is contaminated by signal from fat tissue outside the voxel. The unspoiled (residual) fat signal is usually identifiable but may overlap with other signals. The phase of such a contaminating signal is often completely scrambled (Figure 5) which makes a quantification of this contamination difficult.

In this section the prevention of contamination rather than their quantification shall be discussed. The phantom which was used for the experiments together with the voxel position for the volume selective spectra is shown in Figure 4. This phantom represents an extreme model case to test for fat contamination in e.g. brain spectra. The voxel position indicated in Figure 4 used for all spectra in this section is in a critically close neighborhood to the oil compartment.

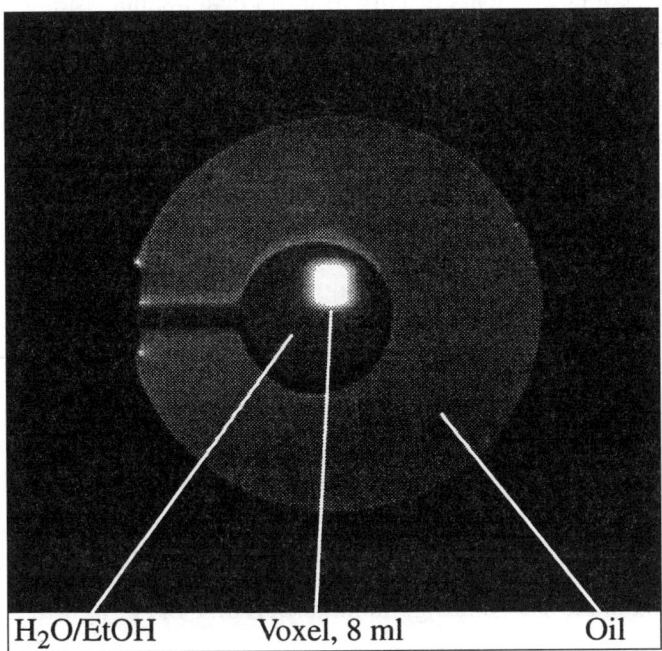

Figure 4. Sagittal image of the phantom used to test for signal contamination from outside the VOI. The image of the voxel is overlapped indicating its size (2 cm)^3 and position. The phantom consists of a large glass sphere containing silicon oil and a smaller inner glass sphere containing a water ethanol (~ 1:1) mixture.

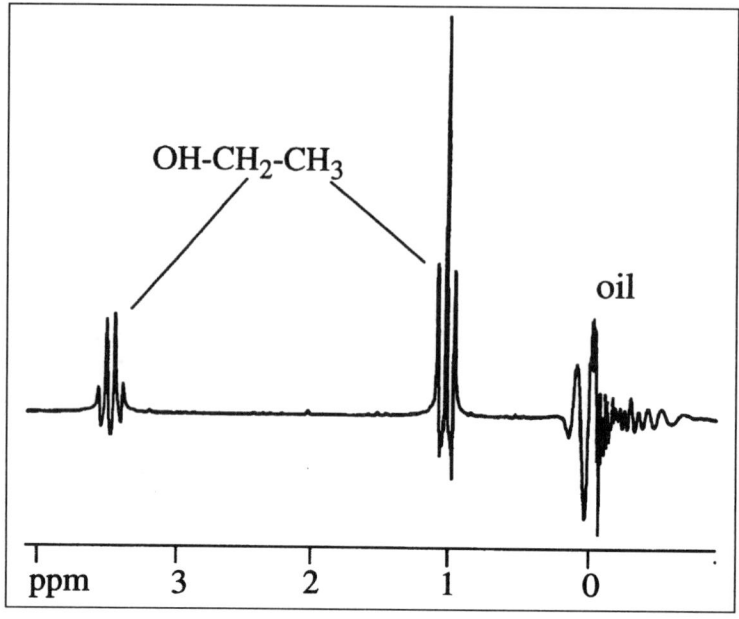

Figure 5. PRESS spectrum (TE=29 s, 1 average) from a (2 cm)3 voxel as indicated in Figure 4. The spoiler gradients were used as represented in Figure 1 with a duration of 3 ms each and a strength of 0.8 mT/m.

The most important tool to eliminate contamination is the application of spoiler gradients. Stronger and longer spoiler gradients usually result in better suppression of signals originating from spins outside the VOI. A long duration of spoiler gradients, however, increases the minimum TE time considerably, and strong spoiler gradients may produce stronger eddy currents than tolerable. Moreover, diffusion can lead to a substantial signal loss when spoiler gradients are misapplied. Setting the spoiler gradient strength to 0.8 mT/m with a duration of 3 ms (Figure 1) gives a spectrum with a strong contaminating oil signal (Figure 5). If the spoiler gradient strength is increased from 0.8 mT/m to 8.0 mT/m (Figure 6) the oil signal is almost completely suppressed. The mechanism of the contamination is mainly such that signal components other than SE2 (Figure 2) contribute to the spectrum. Instead of using spoiler gradients one could completely rely on phase cycling of the rf pulses and the receiver reference signal. This would give us a PRESS sequence which is no longer single shot volume selective but needs and add/subtract cycle of different spectra to achieve volume selectivity. Phase cycling is advantageous for other reasons, too, e.g. for the compensation of rf pulse and receiver imperfections. A spectrum which was acquired using a phase cycle over 32 averages is shown in Figure 7. Even so the spoiler gradient strength was only 0.8 mT/m like for the spectrum in Figure 5 the suppression of the oil signal is slightly better than the one in the spectrum of Figure 6 with a 8.0 mT/m spoiler gradient strength. It is essential to find a good compromise for the spoiler gradient switching pattern, their strength and switch-on duration on one side, and e.g. minimum TE time or eddy current impairment on the other side.

QUALITY CONTROL IN VOLUME SELECTIVE SPECTROSCOPY 435

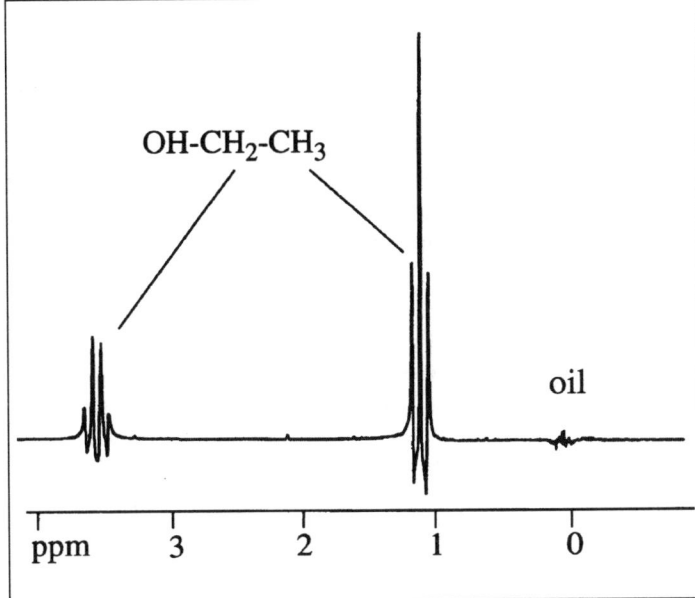

Figure 6. Same as Figure 5 except for the spoiler gradient strength which is increased by a factor of 10 from 0.8 mT/m to 8.0 mT/m.

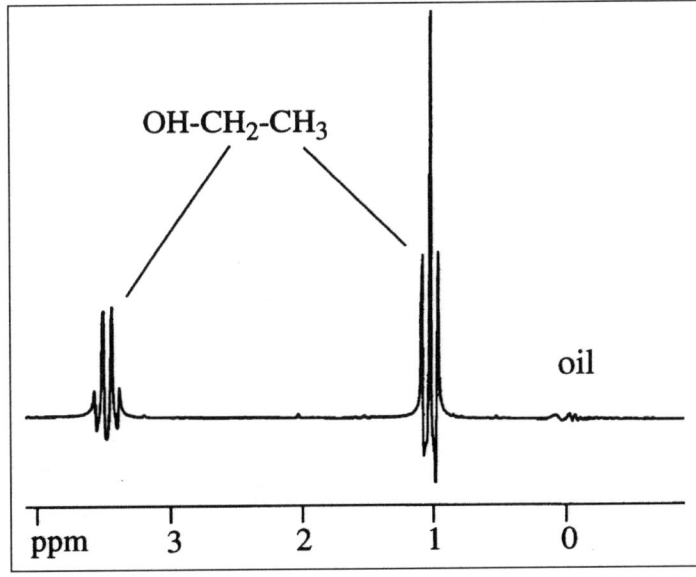

Figure 7. PRESS spectrum (TE = 29 ms, TR = 3000 ms) acquired with a phase cycle over 32 averages.

Detection sensitivity

Different factors play an important role for the detection sensitivity. Basic MR system properties like B_0 field strength or the fidelity of the rf hardware are most essential but not part of this presentation. The selection of the right rf coil for excitation and detection is another factor of great importance. Since in localized spectroscopy the signal source (VOI) is usually much smaller compared to the source of noise (all the tissue in the rf coil surrounding the voxel) the proper choice of the rf coil is extremely important. Thus, for many applications it may be advantageous to use two separate rf coils for excitation and detection.

To test the PRESS sequence itself for avoidable loss in sensitivity one can acquire a spectrum of a small phantom. The voxel shall be selected larger than the size of the phantom such that the signal with and without volume selection should be the same. Comparing now the PRESS spectrum with a simple one-pulse spectrum gives us an idea of the signal loss due to imperfections of the PRESS sequence. This loss should not be more than 10 %. To make sure that we finally obtain the best signal-to-noise ratio it is worth-while to test for additional «noise-like» signal contamination in the PRESS spectra which can originate from incomplete suppression of e.g. fat or water signals.

Table I. All possible rf pulse phase combinations of a three-pulse sequence and the resulting signal phases of the FIDs, spin echoes and stimulated echo (cf. Figure 2). If the receiver phase follows the phase of the PRESS signal SE2 all other signal components will be cancelled.

	1	2	3	4	5	6	7	8	9	10	11	12	13	14	15	16
phase pulse 1	0°	0°	0°	0°	0°	0°	0°	0°	0°	0°	0°	0°	0°	0°	0°	0°
phase pulse 2	0°	0°	0°	0°	90°	90°	90°	90°	180°	180°	180°	180°	270°	270°	270°	270°
phase pulse 3	0°	90°	180°	270°	0°	90°	180°	270°	0°	90°	180°	270°	0°	90°	180°	270°
FID 1	270°	270°	270°	270°	270°	270°	270°	270°	270°	270°	270°	270°	270°	270°	270°	270°
FID 2	270°	270°	270°	270°	0°	0°	0°	0°	90°	90°	90°	90°	180°	180°	180°	180°
FID 3	270°	0°	90°	180°	270°	0°	90°	180°	270°	0°	90°	180°	270°	0°	90°	180°
SE 1	90°	90°	90°	90°	270	270	270	270	90	90	90	90	270°	270°	270°	270°
SE 2	270°	90°	270°	90°	90°	270°	90°	270°	270°	90°	270°	90°	90°	270°	90°	270°
SE 3	90°	270°	90°	270°	0°	180°	0°	180°	270°	90°	270°	90°	180°	0°	180°	0°
SE 4	90°	270°	90°	270°	90°	270°	90°	270°	90°	270°	90°	270°	90°	270°	90°	270°
STE	270°	0°	90°	180°	0°	90°	180°	270°	90°	180°	270°	0°	180°	270°	0°	90°

Water suppression

The water suppression problem has two aspects : i) the saturation of the water signal inside the VOI and ii) the suppression (saturation and spoiling) of the water signal from outside the VOI. A residual water signal from inside the VOI is in most cases not posing a real problem. It is a well defined signal with a relative narrow linewidth not covering any of the interesting chemical shift ranges. The dynamic range of the receiver is usually good enough that we expect no problem from this side, too. On the other hand, the water signal from outside the VOI can easily be 3000 times larger and inhomogeneity and susceptibility effects can smear it over the full chemical shift range of interest. Therefore, it is extremely important that the suppression of this water signal is most complete.

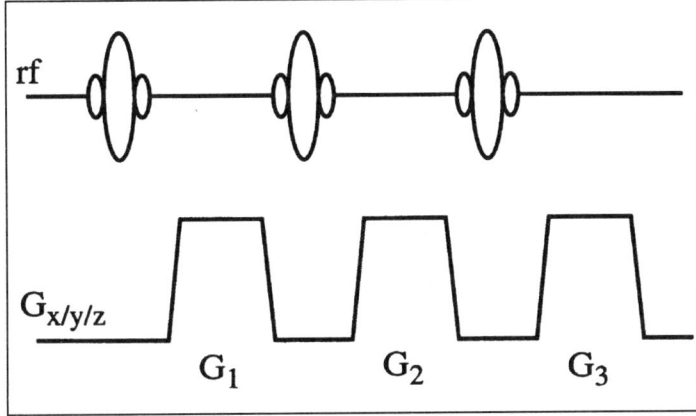

Figure 8. The water suppression scheme used consists of three narrow-band saturation rf pulses each followed by a spoiler gradient.

The water suppression scheme discussed here (Figure 8) applies three narrowband excitation (saturation) rf pulses. The immense transverse magnetization created is dephased by three spoiler gradients leave room for optimization, too. The spectra shown in this section have been measured on a 4.7 Tesla BIOSPEC equipped with a 20 cm free access active shielded gradient system. The phantom was a 10 cm sphere filled with water containing 1 % ethanol (~ 150 mM). A (1 cm)^3 voxel was selected. The strength and direction of the three spoiler gradients is important for the quality of the water suppression. In Figure 9 a spectrum with a water suppression applying three spoiler gradients in z direction of equal strength is shown. Using three identical spoiler gradients is obviously not a good idea since part of the water signal will be rephased. When the three spoiler gradients are applied in three different direction (G_1 in y, G_2 in x, and G_3 in z direction) the result improves a lot (Figure 10). Other combinations of spoiler gradient strengths and directions may have their own advantages and disadvantages. The water suppression always leaves a large amount of water unsaturated or water will partly recover before the last rf pulse of PRESS is applied. This can lead to a significant contamination by water signal from outside the voxel. Therefore, the spoiling scheme of the PRESS sequence itself is important for a good water suppression, too. Figure 11 shows two spectra WITH 12.5 mT/m and 50 mT/m spoiler gradient strength in the PRESS sequence, respectively. In the upper spectrum on can recognize a residual water signal from inside the voxel (arrow a) and unspoiled water signal from outside the VOI (arrow b). Unspoiled ethanol signal from outside the voxel is indicated by arrows c. The unspoiled water signal from outside the voxel is smeared over a considerable chemical shift range (4.0 - 4.7 ppm) due to inhomogeneity effects across the whole phantom. Even larger shift ranges can be covered since inhomogeneities of a few ppm across an object are not unusual. Like for the signal suppression discussed in the section «Volume selectivity» phase cycling does improve the overall performance of the water suppression, too.

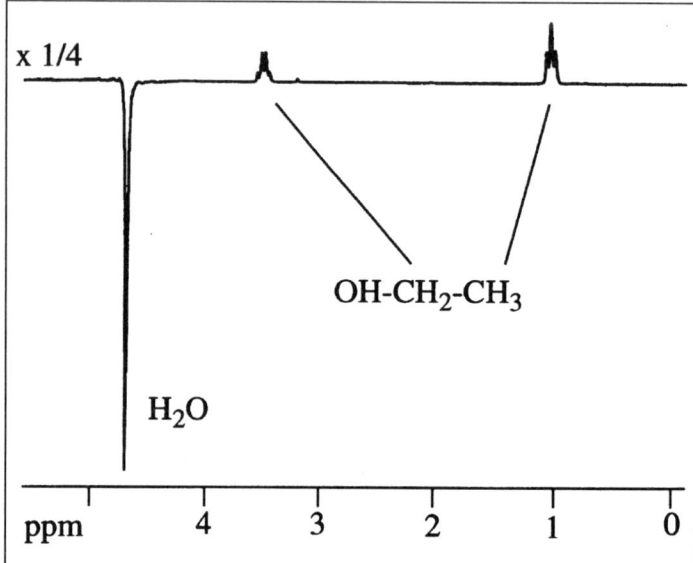

Figure 9. PRESS spectrum (TR=290 ms, 8 averages) of a (1 cm)³ voxel applying three spoiler gradients G_1, G_2, G_3 in the water suppression scheme, each 50 mT/m in z direction and of 15 ms duration. The vertical scales is 1/4 compared to all other spectra in this section.

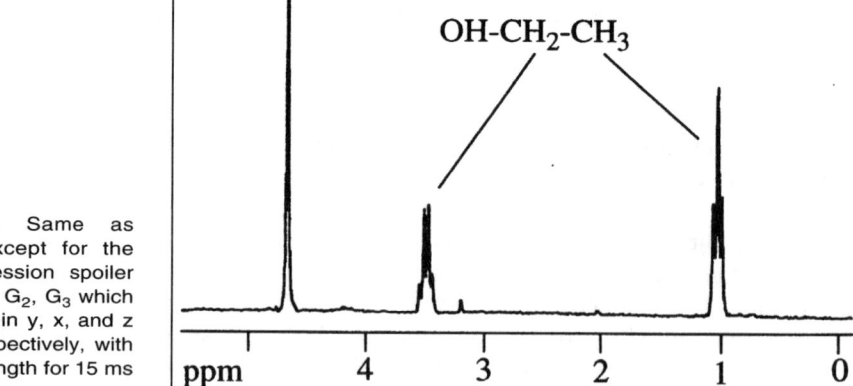

Figure 10. Same as Figure 9 except for the water suppression spoiler gradients G_1, G_2, G_3 which were applied in y, x, and z direction, respectively, with 50 mT/m strength for 15 ms each.

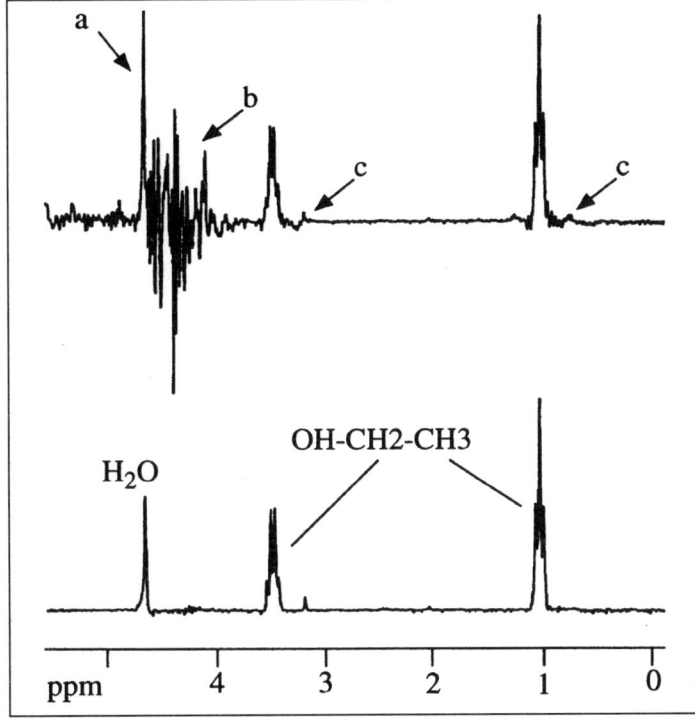

Figure 11. PRESS spectra (TE=290 ms, single shot) of a (1 cm)³ voxel. The spoiler gradients or water suppression (cf. Figure 8) were g1=y(12.5 mT/m), G2=x(25 mT/m), and G3=z(50 mT/m) switched on for 15 ms each for both spectra. The upper spectrum was acquired with a PRESS spoiler gradient (Figure 1) strength of 12.5 mT/m, the lower spectrum with 50 mT/m, each 4 ms duration.

Conclusions

A number of quality aspects in volume selective spectroscopy have been discussed emphasizing the connection between the mechanism leading to artifacts, how they can be recognized and what are the tools to avoid them. It is symptomatic that no in-vivo spectra are presented in this overview. Most quality aspects are related to the spectrometer or the spectroscopic technique used and not to the object under investigation. The use of proper phantoms make the analysis and optimization of the hardware or spectroscopy technique much easier. Of course one has to admit that what counts at the end is the outcome of the invivo experiments and therefore itself is the ultimate test case.

Also, this presentation should encourage to modify spectroscopy pulse sequences and to try to optimize the techniques for particular applications. There is plenty of room for variations and no simple way for clear predictions about the outcome. The practical experiment together with the understanding of the result and mechanisms producing it leads the way to the best spectroscopy technique for a certain application.

53

Sensorimotor cortex changes and neurological soft signs in schizophrenia : a study with functional magnetic resonance imaging

J. SCHRÖDER[1], F. WENZ[2], R. NIETHAMMER[1], L.R. SCHAD[3], K. BAUDENDISTEL[3], A. STOCKERT[1], M.V. KNOPP[3], H. SAUER[4]

[1]*Department of Psychiatry, University of Heidelberg, Voß-St. 4, 69115 Heidelberg, Germany.*
[2]*Department of Clinical Radiology, University of Heidelberg, INF 400, 69120 Heidelberg, Germany.*
[3]*German Cancer Research Centre, INF 280, 69120 Heidelberg, Germany.*
[4]*Department of Psychiatry, University of Jena, Philosphenweg 3, 07745 Jena, Germany.*

Kraepelin is among the first authors who recognized minor motoric and sensoric disturbances or neurological soft signs (NSS). In reviewing the literature he concluded that « severe and manifold psychomotor deficits » were frequently found in dementia praecox and mentioned adiadochokinesia, impaired balance, swaying, and shaking (Kraepelin, 1913). These early observations were confirmed by recent studies which found a higher prevalence of NSS in schizophrenia than in other psychiatric disorders or in healthy controls (for review, see: Heinrichs and Buchanan, 1988). Further studies demonstrate that NSS are significantly correlated with psychopathological symptoms, in particular formal thought disorders (Manschreck and Ames, 1984; Ticker *et al*, 1975), and neuropsychological deficits, such as attentional dysfunction or working memory impairment (Mohr *et al*, 1993).

Yet, the underlying cerebral changes have not been identified. Three computed tomography studies (Franz *et al*, 1992; Schröder *et al*, 1992; Weinberger, 1984) found a significant covariation between NSS and the size of the internal cerebral spinal fluid spaces, in particular width of the 3rd ventricle and the ventricle brain ratio. However, these findings were only partially confirmed in other studies (Stein *et al.*, 1993; King *et al*, 1991; Torrey, 1994).

Evidence indicating a relation between sensorimotor cortex changes and NSS comes from functional imaging studies: Günther et al. (1991) reported a bilateral overactivation in the precentral gyrus in the type I, but a decreased reactivity in the type II patients. An increased activity in the sensorimotor cortex was also reported in a positron emission tomography (PET) study under an attentional task (Schröder et al., in press[1]). These changes in the sensorimotor cortices were predominantly found in schizophrenic patients with persisting formal thought disorders who clinically showed the highest NSS-scores (Schröder et al., in press[1]).

While these studies agree in suggesting a relation between NSS and sensorimotor cortex changes, both share one major drawback: lateralization effects were not addressed. Among the NSS finger-to-thumb opposition is regarded as a particularly valid sign (Binkert, 1994) and may be executed in the fMRI environment. In the present study we therefore investigated sensorimotor cortex activation under finger-to-thumb opposition using functional magnetic resonance imaging (fMRI).

Methods

10 patients with a DSM-II-R (APA 1987) schizophrenia and 7 healthy volunteers were included. All subjects were right handed. Patients received 300-600 mg clozapine qd (mean: 287.5±177.5 mg) and were investigated after remission of the acute illness. Psychopathological symptoms and neurological soft signs were assessed on the Brief Psychiatric Rating Scale (BPRS/Overall and Gorham,1962) and Heidelberg NSS-scale[1] (Schröder et al. 1992), respectively. In addition, the Scale for the Assessment of Negative Symptoms (Andreasen, 1983) and the Strauss-Carpenter Prognostic Scale (Strauss and Carpenter, 1974) were applied. Particular care was taken to exclude any subject with a history of neurological disorders or substance abuse. A completer set of T1 weighted 3D MPRAGE images was acquired to exclude gross morphological changes.

fMRI

fMRi were taken on a standard Siemens 1.5 Tesla scanner using the technique described by Schad and coworkers (1993 and 1994). For slice selection, a sagital scout scan and a set of 16 contiguous T1 weighted axial images were acquired. Consequently, a single 3mm axial slice was selected covering the sensorimotor cortex. To optimize field homogeneity, interactive magnet shimming with all first order coils was performed on the selected slice.

A modified FLASH sequence was used for functional imaging. For each hand, three periods (10 images each) of rest and finger-to-thumb opposition were performed. During the fMRT, subjects were asked to held their hands in front of the abdomen so that the performance could be visually controlled. The performance was rated according to the Heidelberg NSS-scale (item no. 10). For further details, see Wenz et al. (in press).

---

[1]. A detailed manual and a video tape demonstrating the examination will be sent on request.

Data analysis

Image analysis was performed on a VAXstation 3100 and a cine mode used to detect significant head motion during the acquisition. Since the resolution capacity may be optimized by averaging a number of images, sets of rest and activation images were combined, resulting in 30 pairs of activation-rest images per hand (Figure 1). For each pixel, student's t-tests were calculated to compare the activities measured under activation and under rest for significant changes. On basis of the resulting t-values, statistical parametric maps (SPM/Friston *et al.,* 1991) were constructed. In contrast to subtracted images, SPM enhanced visibility of the activated areas (Figure 1). To minimize type I errors a significance level of $p<0.005\%$ was chosen and a neighborhood analysis performed. Following the latter any pixel which showed a significant activation was excluded unless it was adjacent to other pixels activated.

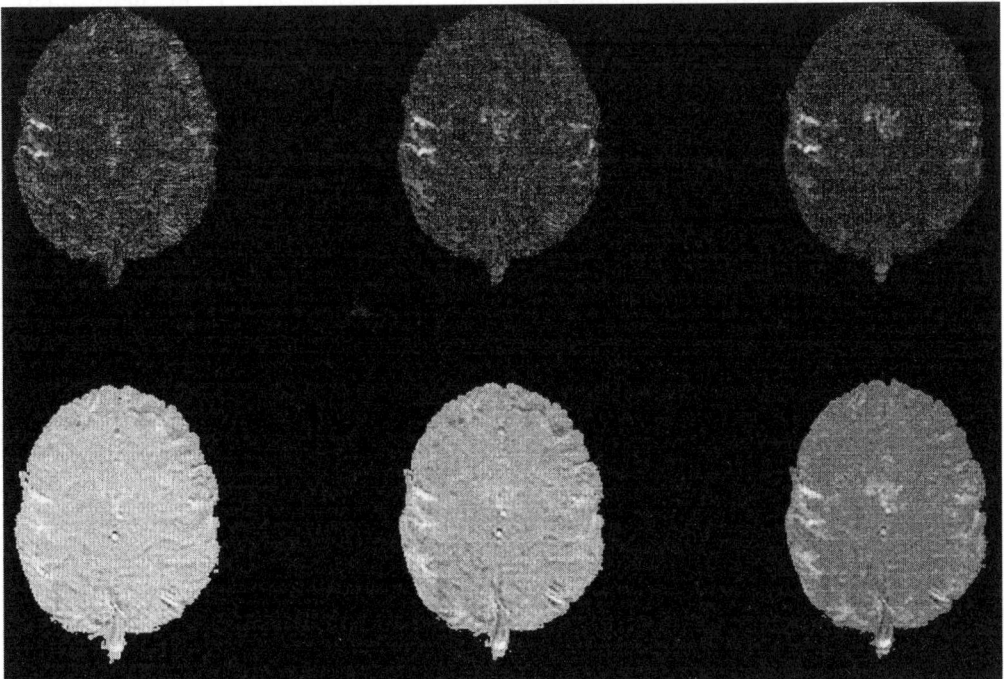

Figure 1. Images reconstructed according to statistical parametric maps (above) and subtracted images (below). The resolution capacity is a function of the number of images included (from left to right: 10, 20, 30), with more images allowing a better identification of cortical areas activated.

In a last step, a grid overlay consisting of 5 × 6 equally sized square regions of interest was superimposed. The grids were symmetrically placed over the functional images that the midline structures were fully included in the central and the sensorimotor cortex in the lateral column. For exact localisation the fMRI were superimposed on corresponding T1 weighted images.

In every region of interest, two variables: the activation strength and the percentage of pixels activated were measured. The activation strength was defined as the mean t-value of the corresponding region of interest corrected by the number of pixels. Analyses of variance were calculated to compare the activation strength and the number of pixels activated in patients versus controls and in right versus left regions of interest. The main effect « diagnosis » was used to represent patients versus controls, the main effect « hemisphere » to represent right versus left finger-to-thumb opposition.

Results

All subjects showed a significant activation of the sensorimotor cortices under both, ipsi-and contralateral finger-to-thumb opposition (Figure 1). In the healthy controls, ipsilateral finger-to-thumb opposition lead to greater left right hemispheric sensorimotor cortex coactivation (Figure 2). In contrast, the schizophrenic patients showed an overall diminished activation with a reversed activation pattern under ipsilateral finger-to-thumb opposition. These findings were confirmed by a multivariate analysis of variance which revealed a significant main effect « diagnosis » for both, ipsilateral (F=53.14; df=1; p<0,0001) and contralateral (F=19.77; df=1 ; p<0,0006) finger-to-thumb opposition. The main effect « hemisphere » was non-significant in both conditions (F=1.06; df=1; p=0,32, versus F=0.09; df=1; p=0,76; respectively), while the interaction « diagnosis*hemisphere » was significant for ipsilateral finger-to-thumb opposition only (F=7,65, df=16; p<0.01 versus F=0.30; df=16; p<0.59; respectively).

When analyzing the number of pixels activated, similar results were obtained: the main effect « diagnosis » was significant for contralateral (F=9.19, df=1, p<0.01) finger-to-thumb opposition (ipsilateral: F=2.17, df=1, p=0.16); the main effect « hemisphere » was non-significant in both conditions (F=0.50, df=1, p=0.49, versus F=0.72, df=1, p=0,41; respectively). Again, the interaction « diagnosis*hemisphere »

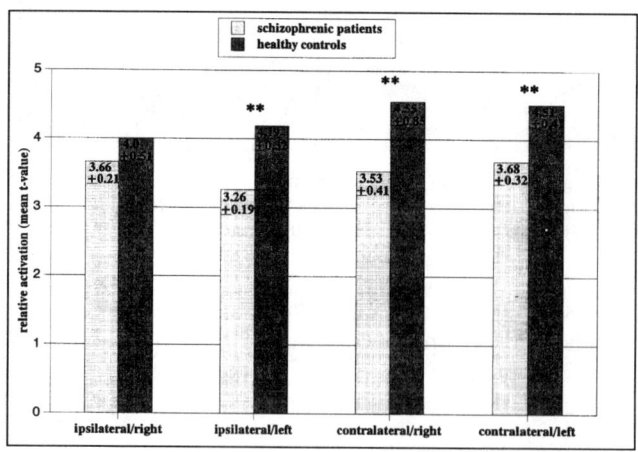

Figure 2. Activation of the sensorimotor cortices under ipsi- and contralateral finger-to-thumb opposition (results of an univariate of variance: **p<0.005).

was significant for ipsilateral finger-to-thumb opposition only (F=4.28, df=16, p<0.05; versus F=2.28, df=16, p<0.15; respectively).

Neither age, years of school education, duration of illness, daily clozapine dosage, severity of illness (total BPRS-score) nor negative symptoms was significantly correlated with any of the activation measures. The same applied for task performance during the fMRI.

Discussion

Our study provides three findings: 1. further evidence indicating a lateralization effect in healthy controls with a higher left than right hemispheric sensorimotor cortex activation under ipsilateral finger-to-thumb opposition; and 2. an indication that sensorimotor cortex dysfunction may contribute to NSS.

With respect to the healthy controls, our findings clearly replicate the results of Kim et al. (1993) who investigated 16 healthy volunteers (10 right-handed, 6 left handed) in a 4 Tesla scanner during finger-to-thumb opposition. For quantification, the absolute size of the cortical surface activated was measured. In the right-handed, Kim et al. (1993) observed a greater left than right hemispheric sensorimotor cortex coactivation during ipsilateral movements, whereas the left-handed did not present with a similar lateralization effect.

In interpreting their findings, Kim et al. (1993) suggest that the lateralisation effect with a predominantly left hemispheric sensorimotor cortex coactivation during ipsilateral movements may account for the significant deficits produced by left hemispheric lesions on motor performance of the ipsilateral hand. Furthermore, some activation of the ipsilateral sensorimotor cortex during hand movement could be expected since a small proportion of fibers in the pyramidal tract were uncrossed.

When compared with the healthy controls the schizophrenic patients showed a decreased activation in the sensorimotor cortex with a reversed lateralisation pattern under ipsilateral finger-to-thumb opposition. Using single photon emission computed tomography (SPECT) with Xenon-133 as tracer Günther and coworkers (1991) investigated unmedicated 31 DSM-III schizophrenics and 8 healthy controls in a resting condition and during repetitive movement (opening and closing the right hand against constant resistance at a frequency of 1/sec). When compared with the healthy controls, the schizophrenic patients showed different activation patterns with a bilateral overactivation in the acute type I patients, but a diminished activation in the type II patients. Further evidence suggesting sensorimotor cortex changes in schizophrenia comes from a PET study on 83 unmedicated schizophrenic patients and 47 healthy volunteers (Schröder et al., in press). Subjects were investigated while executing the continuous performance task. In contrast to the healthy controls, the schizophrenic patients showed a bilateral hyperactivation of the parietal cortex and motor strip. After subgrouping the patient's sample into four cluster with a chronic delusional, chronic negative, and chronic disorganized and remitted symptomatology, parietal cortex and motor strip changes were predominantly found in the disorganized subgroup. In addition, the disorganized were characterized by the highest NSS-scores and a decreased activity in the corpus callosum. These findings are confirmed by the present study and suggest that both, sensorimotor cortex changes and a disturbed interhemispheric balance may contribute to NSS.

While the studies discussed above agree in suggesting sensorimotor cortex changes in schizophrenia, they differ with respect to the direction of the particular changes. Obviously, methodological issues, such as the different imaging methods used and the different tasks applied may account for these differences. Following Günther et al. (1991), one may hypothesize that different patient's subgroups may correspond to different patterns of cortical changes with acute type I schizophrenia resulting into a hyperactivation, but type II schizophrenia into a hypoactivation of the sensorimotor cortices.

The activation changes found in the schizophrenic patients do not appear to be affected by age, duration and severity of illness, or clozapine dosage. Significant correlations between the activation changes and the respective variables were not found; moreover, while such overall effects may correspond to the overall activation decrease found in the sensorimotor cortices, it can not explain dissociated changes such as the reversed lateralisation pattern.

Therefore one may speculate that the activation changes in the sensorimotor cortices do not result from the disease process itself, but may reflect a premorbid dysfunction. In fact, clinical studies revealed a preponderance of NSS in first degree relatives of schizophrenic patients (Rossi et al., 1990) and high-risk children (Marcus et al., 1985). in an attempt to determine the onset of motor changes more precisely, Walker et al. (1994) investigated home-movies from children who latter developed schizophrenia and their healthy siblings. According to their findings, motor changes occurred as early as in first two years of life and primarily involved movements of the left hand which also lead to the most severe activation changes in our study.

Yet, methodological questions, in particular the potential impact of the neuroleptic medication and of the velocity of movement need to be further clarified. However, the results of our fMRI study support the hypothesis that both, sensorimotor cortex dysfunction may contribute to NSS.

References

1. American Psychiatric Association DSM-III-R *Diagnostic and statistical manual of mental disorders* (3rd edn). Washington, DC: American Psychiatric Press, 1987.
2. Andreasen NC. *The scale for the assessment of negative symptoms (SANS)*. Iowa City, Iowa: The University of Iowa, 1983.
3. Binkert M. Diskrete sensorische und motorische Störungen (neurologische soft signs) bei endogenen Psychosen. Inauguraldissertation zur Erlangung des medizinischen Doktorgrades der Ruprecht-Karls Universität Heidelberg, 1994.
4. Günther W, Petsch R, Steinberg R, et al. Brain dysfunction during motor activation and corpus callosum Iterations in schizophrenia measured by cerebral blood flow and magnetic resonance imaging. *Biol Psychiatry,* 1991 ; 29 : 535-55.

5. Franz U, Mohr F, Fratz S, *et al.* CCT-Befunde bei schizophrenen Patienten : Psychopathologische und neurologische Korrelate. *Fortschritte der Neurologie Psychiatrie 60 Sonderheft* 1992 ; 2 : 161.
6. Friston KJ, Frith CD, Liddle PF, *et al.* Comparing functional (PET) images: the assessment of significant change. *Journal of Cerebral Blood Flow and Metabolism,* 1991 ; 11 : 690-9.
7. Heinrichs DW, Buchanan RW. Significance and meaning of neurological signs in schizophrenia. *Am J Psychiatry,* 1988 ; 145 : 11-8.
8. Kim SG, Ashe J, Hendrich K, *et al.* Functional magnetic resonance imaging of motor cortex and handedness. *Science,* 1993 ; 261 : 615-8.
9. King DJ, Wilson A, Cooper SJ, *et al.* The clinical correlates of neurological soft signs in chronic schizophrenia. *Brit J of Psychiatry,* 1991 ; 158 : 770-5.
10. Kraepelin E. *Psychiatrie. Ein Lehrbuch für Studierende und Ärzte.* Band III, Teil 2.8. Auflage. Leipzig,Johann Ambrosius Barth Verlag, 1913.
11. Manschreck TC, Ames D. Neurologic features and psychopathology in schizophrenic disorders. *Biol Psychiatry,* 1984 ; 19 : 703-19.
12. Marcus J, Hans SL, Mednick SA, Schulsinger F, Michelsen N. Neurological dysfunctioning in offspring of schizophrenics in Israel and Denark. *Arch Gen Psychiatry,* 1985 ; 42 : 753-61.
13. Mohr F, Cohen R, Hubmann W *et al.* Neurologische soft signs: Gruppenunter-schiede und klinische Korrelate. In : *P Baumann ed.Biologische psychiatrie der Gegenwart.* Wien, Bukarest, Berlin, Heidelberg, New York: Springer-Verlag, 1993.
14. Overall JE, Gorham DR. The brief psychiatric rating scale. *Psychological reports,* 1962 ; 10 : 799-812.
15. Rossi A, de Cataldo S, Di Michele V, Manna V, Ceccolo S, Stratta P, Casacchia M. Neurological soft signs (NSS) in schizophrenia. *Brit J Psychiatry,* 1990 ; 157 : 735-9.
16. Schad L.R, Trost U, Knopp MV, *et al.* Motor cortex stimulation measured by magnetic resonance imaging on a standard 1.5T clinical scanner. *Magnetic Resonance Imaging,* 1993 ; 11 : 461-4.
17. Schad LR, Wenz F, Knopp MV, *et al.* Functional 2d and 3d magnetic resonance imaging of motor cortex stimulation at high spatial resolution using a standard 1,5 T-imager. *Magnetic Resonance Imaging,* 1994 ; 12 : 9-15.
18. Schröder J, Niethammer R, Geider FJ, *et al.* Neurological soft signs in schizophrenia. *Schizophrenia Research,* 1992 ; 6 : 25-30.
19. Schröder J, Buchsbaum MS, Siegel BV, *et al.* Patterns of cortical activity in schizophrenia. *Psychological Medicine,* in press.
20. Schröder J, Buchsbaum MS, Siegel BV, *et al.* Structural and functional correlates of subsyndromes in chronic schizophrenia. *Psychopathology,* in press.
21. Stein DJ, Hollander E, Chan S, *et al.* Computed tomography and neurological soft signs in obsessive-compulsive disorder. *Psychiatry Research, Neuroimaging,* 1993 ; 50 : 143-50.
22. Strauss JS, Carpenter WT, Jr. The prediction of outcome in schizophrenia. II. Relationship between predictor and outcome variables. Archives of General Psychiatry, 1974 ; 31 : 37-42.
23. Torrey EF. *Schizophrenia and manic-depressive disorder. The biological roots of mental illness as revealed by the landmark study of identical twins.* New York : BasicBooks, 1994.
24. Tucker GJ, Campion EW, Silberfarb PM. Sensorimotor functions and cognitive disturbance in psychiatric patients. *Am J of Psychiatry,* 1975 ; 132 : 17-21.
25. Volkow ND, Tancredi LR. Biological correlates of mental activity studied with PET. *Am J of Psychiatry,* 1991 ; 148 : 439-43.
26. Walker EF, Savoie T, Davis D. Neuromotor precursors of schizophrenia. *Schizophrenia Bulletin,* 1994 ; 20 : 441-51.
27. Weinberger DR. Computed tomography (CT) findings in schizophrenia: speculation on the meaning of it all. *J Psychiatr Res,* 1984 ; 18 : 477-90.

28. Wenz F, Schad LR, Knopp MV *et al.* Functional magnetic resonance imaging at 1.5 T: activation patterns in schizophrenic patients receiving neuroleptic medication. *Magnetic Resonance Imaging,* in press.

54

Vascular reponses in fMRI of motor activity

C. SEGEBARTH[1,3], C. DELON-MARTIN[1], V. BELLE[1],
R. MASSARELLI[1], J. DECETY[2], J.-F. LEBAS[1], M. DÉCORPS[1]

[1]*INSERM U 438, Centre Hospitalier Universitaire, Pavillon B, BP 217 X, 38043 Grenoble, France.*
[2]*INSERM U 94, 16 Av. du Doyen Lépine, 69500 Bron, France.*
[3]*Hôpital Erasme, Université Libre de Bruxelles, 808 Route de Lennik, B1070 Bruxelles, Belgique.*

Recent studies have shown that MRI can detect changes in cortical activity in the human brain. This detection relies upon the measurement of changes in certain haemodynamic parameters such as cerebral blood flow or cerebral blood volume, or in blood oxygenation. The changes in blood oxygenation result from the focal physiological uncoupling of cerebral blood flow and oxidative metabolism during cortical stimulation [1]. During stimulation, blood flow increases locally much more than oxidative metabolism, resulting in a decrease in the venous concentration of deoxyhaemoglobin. Thus, the magnetic susceptibility of the venous blood decreases, thereby reducing the magnetic field inhomogeneities around capillaries and larger size vessels draining venous blood from the activated cortical areas. Gradient-recalled echo (GRE) MR techniques are very sensitive for detecting these local changes in field homogeneity, and most of the functional MRI (fMRI) studies published sofar make use of these techniques. The fMRI contrasts obtained by means of GRE MR techniques have been called "BOLD" (Blood Oxygenation Level Dependent) [2].

The fMRI studies are very often characterized by a limited spatial resolution, either because of instrumental limitations such as when echo-planar techniques are used, or because of constraints determined by the temporal resolution required. Due to the latter constraints, the fMRI studies are also very often performed on single slices. The identification of the origin of the fMRI signals has been rendered difficult, as a consequence. Also, this identification has not been given very high priority in early fMRI studies. It has generally been considered that the signals observed arise from cortical areas. However, several recent papers have suggested a significant role of larger size veins in fMRI signal contrast [3-7].

We have concentrated on the role of the veins on signal contrast in fMRI of motor activity at 1.5 Tesla. Therefore, the fMRI responses were investigated following different approaches.

Functional MR angiography

In a first approach [8], the GRE "BOLD" fMRI response of the upper part of the brain was obtained. This was done by measuring the fMRI reponse on a large number of axially oriented, adjacent slices, in a sequential multi-slice (SMS) manner. These slices were measured first during a resting period and subsequently during performance of a particular hand motor task. The fMR images were then obtained by subtracting, slice-wise, the MR images obtained during the first from those acquired during the second period. Following regular practice in conventional MR angiography, maximum intensity projections (MIPs) were then derived from the set of fMR images.

In a second approach [9], the 2D GRE "BOLD" fMRI technique was equally applied. This time, fMR images were obtained following the measurement of single slices, one centered over the left and one centered over the right hemisphere. The image planes were carefully positioned so that they encompassed most of the pial veins of interest. Slice orientation was axial, with a double angulation around the left-right and antero-posterior axes. The veins responding to the motor task had been identified during preliminary fMRI examinations. The fMR images were obtained by the subtraction of an image measured during rest from one measured during task performance.

In a third approach [10], the fMRI response of the upper part of the brain was investigated by means of 3D GRE phase-contrast (PC) techniques. Two identical 3D PC MR scans were run in the axial orientation, the first during a resting period and the second during performance of a motor task. Functional MR images were obtained by subtracting, slice-wise, the PC MR images measured during the first from those measured during the second period. From the set of fMR images, MIPs were calculated, similarly as in the first approach.

In a fourth approach [9], SE rather than GRE MRI techniques were applied. The MR pulse sequence parameters of the SE MR sequence were carefully adjusted so that the sequence was sensitive to activity induced changes in venous flow velocity. The SE fMRI response from the upper part of the brain was then obtained similarly as the GRE fMRI response in the first approach. The brain was explored twice in a SMS manner, first during a resting period, subsequently during performance of a hand motor task. Functional SE MR images were obtained by subtracting, slice-wise, the SE MR images acquired during the first from those acquired during the second period. Maximum intensity projections were eventually derived from the set of fMR images.

In each of these 4 studies, regular MR angiograms were obtained from the volumes investigated functionally. They were compared with the MIPs derived from the sets of functional MR images (approaches 1, 3 and 4) and with the fMR images obtained following the mere subtraction of the MR images measured during rest and during task activation (approach 2).

Results

The comparison of the fMR MIPs (approaches 1, 3 and 4) and images (approach 2) with the regular MR angiograms has shown that the fMR signals detected arise predominatly from pial veins draining the cortical areas involved in the motor task. Thus, the fMR MIPs (approaches 1, 3 and 4) as well as the fMR images (approach 2) constitute examples of *functional MR angiograms*.

Figure 1 shows typical results obtained with approach 1.

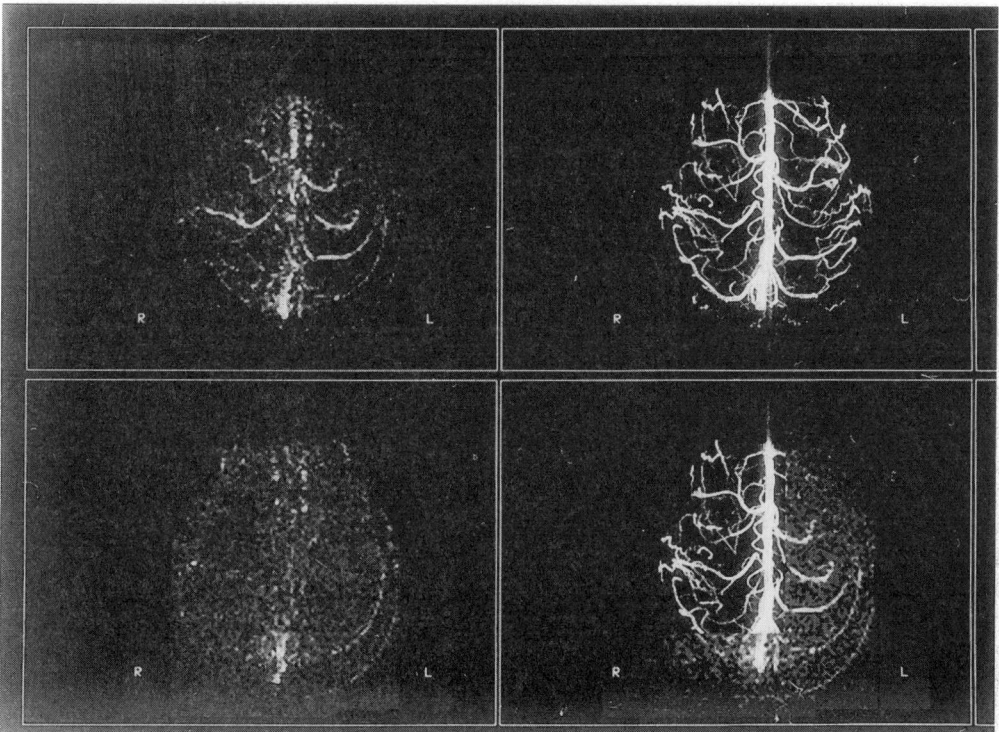

Figure 1. (a) Upper left: fMRI MIP image obtained with a GRE "BOLD" fMR sequence during bilateral finger tapping. (b) Lower left: Control fMRI MIP image. (c) Upper right: Corresponding MR angiogram. (d) Lower right: Combination of fMRI MIP image and MR angiogram.

Figure 1a (upper left) shows a fMR MIP image derived from 26 contiguous fMR images, covering the upper part of the brain. The fMR images were obtained by subtracting 2D GRE MR images measured during bilateral, sequential, finger tapping from those measured during a previous resting period. The image planes were axially oriented and slightly tilted around the left-right axis, so that the intersection of the angled transverse planes with the sagittal plane was parallel with the bicommissural axis. The MIP projection axis was perpendicular to the image planes. The major sequence parameters of the 2D GRE MR technique were the following: TR=59 ms, TE=40 ms, a=30°, FOV=154 mm*220mm, slice thickness=2mm, scan matrix=90*128, pixel bandwidth=35 Hz, acquisition time per image: 5.5 sec.

The fMR MIP image in Figure 1b (lower left) has been acquired in a manner technically identical to that of Figure 1a. However, rather than tapping his fingers, the volunteer remained at complete rest during the second MR measurement period.

Figure 1c (upper right) shows a regular MR angiogram of the volume covered by the set of fMRI images. The angiogram was derived from a 3D PC MR data set.

Figure 1d (lower right) is a combination of Figures 1a and 1c. It highlights the matching, in the left hemisphere, of the fMRI hyperintensities in the fMR MIPs and 3 venous structures in the regular MR angiogram.

Discussion

In this study, the venous signals in fMRI of motor activity have been detected following different approaches.

The results obtained with the first and second approaches demonstrate the predominance of signals from pial veins in GRE "BOLD" fMRI of motor activity, at 1.5 Tesla. This predominance has important implications. It suggests that number of signal intensities reported in 1.5 Tesla fMRI studies of motor activity may be due to veins intersecting the image planes. These venous signals constitute an indirect signature from changes in activity in cortical areas drained by the veins.Thus they may be detected at some distance from the activated cortical area.

The results obtained following the third and fourth approaches provide additional ground to the role of veins in fMRI of motor activity. Those obtained with the SE MR technique demonstrate that fMRI signals may be based only upon activity related changes in venous flow velocity. The latter changes may play an important role in GRE "BOLD" fMR imaging.

References

1. Fox PT, Raichle ME, Focal physiological uncoupling of cerebral blood flow and oxidative metabolism during somatosensory stimulation in human subjects. *Proc Natl Acad Sci USA* 1986 ; 83 : 1140-44.
2. Ogawa S, Lee TM, Kay AR, Tank DW. Brain magnetic resonance imaging with contrast dependent on blood oxygenation. *Proc Natl Acad Sci USA* 1990 ; 87 : 9868-72.
3. Lai S, Hopkins AL, Haacke EM, Li D, Wasserman BA, Buckley P, Friedman L, Meltzer H, Hedera P, Friedland R. Identification of vascular structures as a major source of signal contrast in high resolution 2D and 3D functional activation imaging of the motor cortex at 1.5 T: Preliminary results. *Magn Reson Med* 1993 ; 30 : 387-92.

4. Frahm J, Merboldt KD, Hänicke W, Kleinschmidt A, Boecker H. Brain or vein - Oxygenation or flow? On signal physiology in functional MRI of human brain activation. *NMR Biomed* 1994 ; 7 : 45-53.
5. Haacke EM, Hopkins A, Lai S, Buckley P, Friedman L, Meltzer H, Hedera P, Friedland R, Klein S, Thompson L, Detterman D, Tkach J, Lewin JS. 2D and 3D high resolution gradient echo functional imaging of the brain: Venous contributions to signal in motor cortex studies. *NMR Biomed* 1994 ; 7 : 54-62.
6. Kim SG, Hendrich K, Hu X, Merkle H, Ugurbil K. Potential pitfalls of functional MRI using conventional gradient-recalled echo techniques. *NMR Biomed* 1994 ; 7 : 69-74.
7. Duyn JH, Moonen CTW, de Boer RW, van Yperen GH, Luyten PR. Inflow versus deoxyhemoglobin effects in "BOLD" functional MRI using gradient echoes at 1.5 T.*Twelfth Annual Meeting of the Society of Magnetic Resonance in Medicine*. Abstr 1993 ; 168.
8. Segebarth C, Belle V, Delon C, Massarelli R, Decety J, Le Bas JF, Décorps M, Benabid AL Functional MRI of the human brain. Predominance of signals from extracerebral veins. *Neuro Report* 1994 ; 5(7) : 813-6.
9. Belle V, Delon-Martin C, Massarelli R, Decety J, Le Bas JF, Benabid AL, Segebarth C Intracranial gradient-echo and spin-echo functional MR angiography (fMRA) in humans. *Radiology*, 1995, in press.
10. Belle V, Delon-Martin C, Massarelli R, Decety R, Le Bas JF, Benabid AL, Segebarth C. Intracranial functional MR angiography (fMRA) in humans. *MAGMA* 1994 ; 2 : in press.

55

Combination of MRI and EEG data for realistic source localization

L. SOUFFLET, J-F. NEDELEC, N. BOLO, J-P. MACHER

FORENAP, Centre Hospitalier, 68250 Rouffach, France.

The aim of the Source Imaging Software developed at FORENAP, is to visualize EEG maps on the real head anatomy of the patients, and to localize and visualize the electrical generators (the sources) of the EEG inside the head using a realistic head model.

For this purpose, we use the Boundary Element Method, a numerical method used in source localization. This method only needs a modeling of the surfaces of separation (the interfaces) between media of the head with different electrical conductivities. We generally take into account four interfaces: Air - Scalp, Scalp - Skull, Skull - CSF, CSF - Brain. Magnetic Resonance Imaging gives us anatomical images, which are processed in order to extract the different volumes of the head (Brain, CSF, Skull, Scalp). Image processing is the first step of our work. Once the different volumes have been extracted, a three-dimensional meshing algorithm allows a modeling of the surfaces with triangular facets on which the Boundary Element Method is applied.

Problems appear when trying to reconstruct Scalp - Skull and Skull - CSF interfaces, because the skull is invisible on MR images, and because the boundaries between the different volumes are not always clear. MRI acquisition sequences, based on inversion recovery, are developed in order to highlight the different volumes.

Surface modeling of the interfaces

Our program allows to work on two kinds of data: 2-D-multislice or 3-D data sets. When using a set of slices, each volume has to be extracted for each slice. A contour modeling of the volume is performed for each slice, and the different contours are connected using a triangulation procedure. This procedure generates triangular facets between the upper and the lower contours. Algorithmic difficulties happen when one contour needs to be connected to more than one contour [1].

When using a 3-D data set, once the volume has been extracted (as a set of connected voxels), a predefined spherical mesh constituted by triangular facets is fitted onto the external surface of the volume. Such a procedure is much less time consuming than the reconstruction with contour modeling. With our Onyx Silicon Graphics station and our program, the head surface of the patients is reconstructed with about 10 000 facets within 10 to 20 seconds.

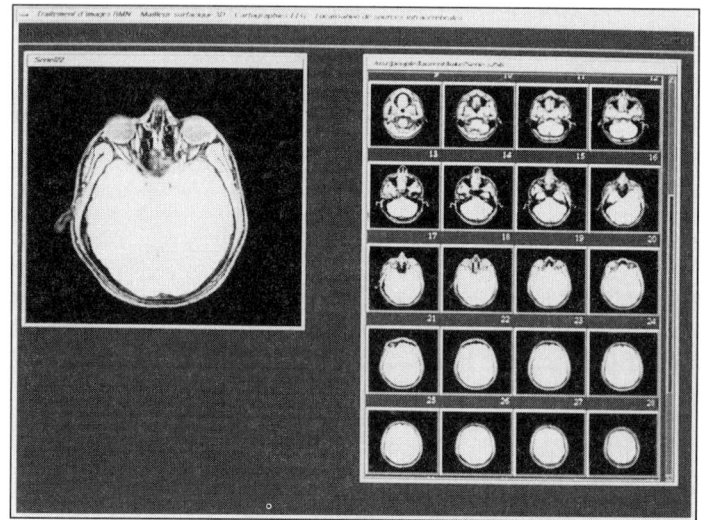

Figure 1. A 2-D multislice NMR image data set used for 3-D surface reconstructions. Extraction of Air - Scalp and CSF - Brain interfaces are easily performed using a thresholding procedure, with this type of contrast. Imaging using different parameters is necessary to extract the two other interfaces used in source localization.

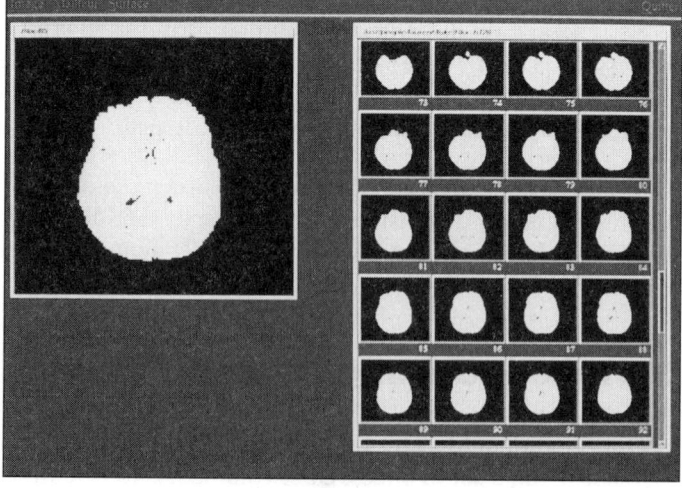

Figure 2. Extraction of brain structure using thresholding and mathematical morphology algorithms. The same processing algorithms are used for 2-D multislice and 3-D data sets.

Visualization of EEG maps onto real head anatomy

The goal of EEG mapping is to visualize the distribution of the electrical activity (EEG energies in different frequency bands, Evoked potentials), onto a representation of the head of the patient. Old EEG systems only used a two-dimensional representation: the head is symbolized by a circle or by an oval. The realism is poor.

Since 1988 we have been using a 3-D standard head model onto which electrical potential distributions or energy distributions are mapped. Recently, with the help of MRI, we have been able to use real head anatomy. The head surface is reconstructed from MRI data, the positions of the recording electrodes are precisely computed by means of four references positioned by the operator, a 3-D spline interpolation is used in order to estimate the potential distribution over the scalp surface at the vertices of the mesh, from the discrete values under the electrodes [2], and the map is visualized onto the head using a texture mapping.

Source localization with the boundary element method

The Boundary Element Method is one of the numerical methods the most commonly used for solving the forward problem (computing the distribution of the potentials over the scalp surface, knowing the electrical sources inside the brain).

Previously developed by Barr et al. [3] and Barnard et al. [4], the method has been recently improved by Hämäläinen et al. in [5] and Meijs et al. [6]. The improvements concern the accuracy and the errors generated by the method. A linear equation system is to be solved which is a discrete form of an integral equation. This discretization generates approximations and consequently errors. We use also a new approach for reducing the errors. This method allows to better estimate the matrix coefficients of the linear algebraic equations occuring in the discrete equation formulation of the Boundary Element Method. Instead of approximating the potentials by constants inside the triangular elements that model the surfaces, we use a linear potential approximation. This last method is more accurate than the classical one.

The Boundary Element Method is also limited in accuracy by the small number of triangular elements that can be used to model each interface. A great number of triangles generates large matrices which overflow the memory capabilities of the computers and increase dramatically the computation time. A powerful computer, with large memory, is thus needed for better accuracy.

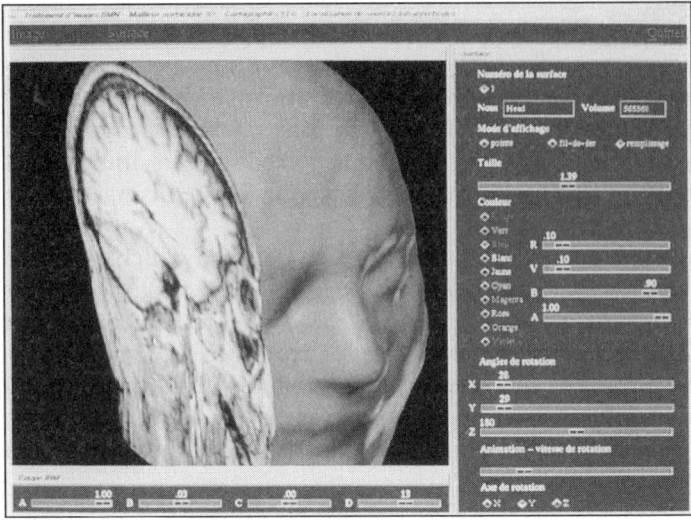

Figure 3. View of the NMR image inside the reconstructed surface of the head. The software allows to define any clipping plane. The NMR image is mapped using a texture mapping algorithm.

Figure 4. The ventricules and the brain seen by transparency inside the head.

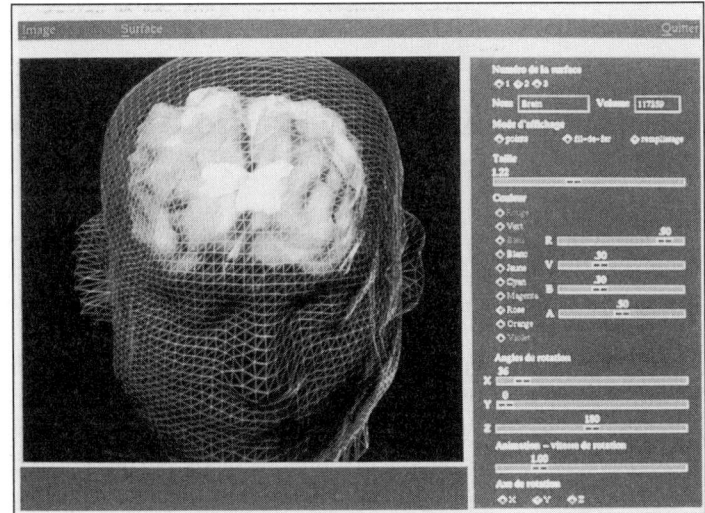

Source imaging

Finally, Source Imaging is a graphical way to vizualize the sources. Once the sources, generally assumed to be current dipoles, are localized, it is therefore possible to visualize them inside the reconstructed interfaces and in the 3-D MR images. These representations are useful for investigations in which knowledge of the position and time course of brain activation during sensory, motor or cognitive tasks is important.

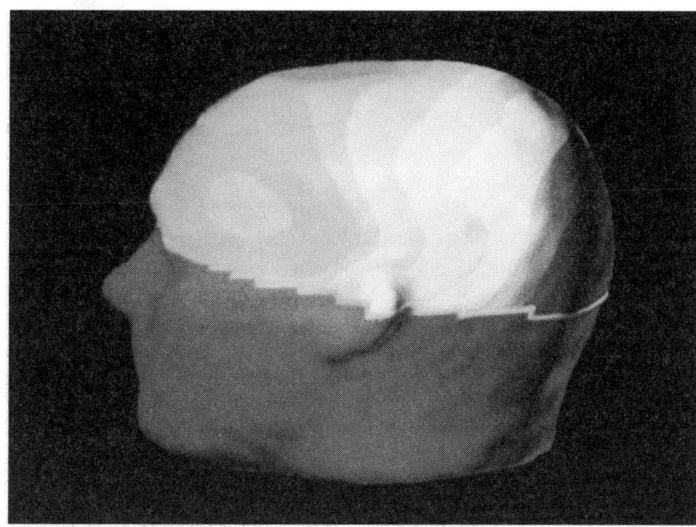

Figure 5. EEG mapping onto real head anatomy. SGI texture mapping reduces processing time by a factor of two by using potential values estimated at facet vertices instead of facet centers. Our Source Imaging Software allows too simutaneous anatomo-functional representation of EEG maps and underlying brain structures. Further developments include vizualization of generating sources inside brain reconstructions.

References

1. Soufflet L, Bolo N, Nédélec JF, Macher JP. *3-D reconstruction with facet representation of cerebral structures from MRI sections*, Proceedings of the Society of Magnetic Resonance in Medicine 1993 ; 680
2. Soufflet L, Toussaint M, Luthringer R, Gresser J, Minot R, Macher JP. A statistical evaluation of the main interpolation methods applied to 3-dimensional EEG mapping, *Electroenceph Clin Neurophysiol* 1991 ; vol. 79 : 393-402.
3. Barr RC, Pilkington TC, Boineau JP. Determining surface potentials from current dipoles with application to electrocardiography. *IEEE Trans Biomed Eng* 1966 ; vol. 13 : 88-97
4. Barnard AC, Duck JM, Lynn MS, Timlake WP. The application of electromagnetic theory to electrocardiography. II. Numerical solution of the integral equations. *Biophys J* 1967 ; vol. 7 : 433-62
5. Hämäläinen M, Sarvas J. Realistic conductivity geometry model of the human head for interpretation of neuromagnetic data. *IEEE Trans Biomed Eng* 1989 ; vol 36, 2 : 165-71
6. Meijs JWH. *The influence of head geometries on electroencephalograms*. University of Twente, The Netherlands Ph.D. dissertation, 1988.

56

MRS studies on excitotoxic cell damage in brain

N.M. THATCHER, R.S. BADAR-GOFFER, P.G. MORRIS, M.A. McLEAN,
A. TAYLOR, H.S. BACHELARD

M.R. Centre, Department of Physics, University of Nottingham, University Park, Nottingham, NG7 2RD, UK.

The 'excitotoxic hypothesis' has been proposed for the mechanisms of cell death in various neurodegenerative conditions such as those associated with Huntingdon's disease, Alzheimer's disease and ischaemic stroke. It is suggested that in disease states an excessive amount of the excitatory neurotransmitter, glutamate, is released which binds to the NMDA sub-type of glutamate receptor. In response to the sustained binding of glutamate the NMDA receptor allows an influx of abnormal amounts of calcium ions. The corresponding increase in free intracellular calcium ($[Ca^{2+}]i$) is thought to trigger metabolic events leading to cell death and the release of further amounts of glutamate causing a cascade of further cell death [1].

Attention has focused on the proposed glutamate cascade to understand the mechanisms underlying the spread of damage in the penumbral region of the brain surrounding an occluded artery in ischaemic stroke, and to indicate possible therapeutic interventions. Due to the proposed role of calcium ions in cell death it is obviously vital to be able to measure $[Ca^{2+}]i$ in intact cerebral tissue. Our use of the ^{19}F - MRS visable $[Ca^{2+}]i$ indicator 5,5'-F^2-1,2-bis (*o*-aminophenoxy)ethane-N,N,N',N',-tetraacetic acid (5FBAPTA) allows us to measure $[Ca^{2+}]i$ in actively metabolising guinea - pig cortical slices with interleaved ^{31}P - MRS to monitor the energy state. The mixed biochemical insult of ischaemia has been investigated using this technique by focussing on the effects of its two major components, low oxygen (hypoxia) and low glucose (hypoglycaemia), and also depolarisation (using 40 mM k^+_e) on $[Ca^{2+}]i$ and the energy state [2]. The effects of the proposed excitotoxins, glutamate and NMDA, have also been investigated [3].

In order to understand the metabolic effects of sustained glutamate binding to the NMDA receptor on cerebral metabolism ^{13}C metabolic tracer studies have been performed. Guinea - pig cortical slices were incubated with [1 - ^{13}C] - glucose and NMDLA (the racemic mixture containing NMDA), perchloric acid extracts taken and investigated using ^{13}C - MRS, ^{1}H-MRS, gas chromatography - mass spectroscopy (GC - MS) and automated amino acid analysis. Pool sizes, % ^{13}C enrichments and labelling patterns of metabolites were compared to those obtained under control conditions and on depolarisation.

Methods

Superfused cortical slice preparation

Slices of 0.35 mm thickness from one guinea - pig cerebral cortex were pre - incubated for 30 min in control media to restore normal levels of metabolites such as lactate, ATP and PCr. 5FBAPTA was then loaded into the cells in its acetoxymethyl ester form, which renders it membrane permeable. Once inside the cells it is de - esterified by cytoplasmic esterases leaving the carboxyl groups free to chelate calcium ions. After 30 minutes of loading the slices were rinsed, transferred to the superfusion apparatus and placed within the NMR magnet. The control superfusion medium contained (mM); NaCl (124), KCl (5), KH_2PO_4 (1.2), $MgSO_4$ (1.2), $CaCl_2$ (2.4), NaHCO3 (26) and glucose (10) gassed with O_2/CO_2 (95:5) at 37°C. After control ^{19}F and ^{31}P spectra had been obtained the superfusing medium was replaced to achieve the superfusing medium was replaced to achieve the metabolic insult under investigation; 0.5 mM glucose (mild hypoglycaemia) and/or N_2/CO_2 (95:5) (moderate hypoxia), 40 mM K+e (depolarisation), glutamate or NMDLA.

On binding to calcium inside the cell the ^{19}F resonance of 5FBAPTA shifts 5.7 ppm downfield. The system is in slow exchange so at non - saturating conditions of $[Ca^{2+}]i$ two resonances are observed in the $_{i9}$F spectrum corresponding to the free indicator and the calcium bound indicator. The ratios of the measured areas under the two peaks multiplied by the K_D of the bound indicator at 37°C (600 nM) gives a value for $[Ca^{2+}]i$.

MR spectra were obtained using an Bruker AMX - 500 spectrometer operating at 202.46 MHz for ^{31}P and 470.51 MHz for ^{19}F. The magnetic field was shimmed using the ^{1}H resonance of the superfusing media. ^{31}P data were accumulated as 360 transients using 60° radiofrequency pulses repeated every 2 seconds. ^{19}F data were accumulated in blocks of 5,000 transients using 44° radiofrequency pulses, a sweep width of 10 KHz and an interpulse interval of 0.2 seconds. ^{19}F spectra were obtained by Fourier transformation using a line - broadening (exponential weighting) of 70 KHz.

Cortical slice extract preparation and analysis

Slices of guinea - pig cerebral cortices were obtained and pre - incubated as above. They were then incubated for up to 6 hours in media containing 5 mM [1 - ^{13}C] -

glucose, NMDLA (20 - 200 µM), 1 µM glycine with or without extracellular magnesium. Slices were removed at set intervals and PCA extracts prepared for analysis by GC - MS and MRS. ^{13}C and ^{1}H MR spectra were obtained on a Bruker AMX - 500 spectrometer operating at 125.7 and 500.1 MHz respectively.

Pool sizes of N - acetyl aspartate (NAA), lactate and NMDLA were quantitated from the ^{1}H spectra using sodium 3(trimethylsilyl)propanionate (TSP) as the internal standard. To quantitate resonances in the ^{13}C spectra an internal dioxan standard is used and the areas of the peaks obtained using a Bruker software routine for integrating the areas under the peaks. Corrections were made for T1 of each resonance and also for 1.1% natural abundance in the metabolite pool. For GC - MS analysis samples adjusted to pH 2.8 and dried under nitrogen, resuspended in ethanol/benzene and again dried under nitrogen. The samples were then derivatised with MTBSTFA and ^{13}C% - excess (APE) was determined from the mass ratios according to the Biemann method. Total pool sizes of amino acids were determined by automated amino acid analysis.

Results and discussion

[Ca^{2+}]i and the energy state of superfused cortical slices using ^{31}P and ^{19}F MRS

Hypoxia and hypoglycaemia

Subjecting the slices to the single insults of moderate hypoxia or low glucose resulted in no increase in [Ca^{2+}]i from control. Moderate hypoxia and mild hypoglycaemia both resulted in a reversible decrease in PCr from control.

The combined insult of hypoxia and hypoglycaemia was investigated in two main ways; (a) sequentially, where the combined insult was preceded by a single insult of hypoxia or hypoglycaemia or (b) immediate, where the combined insult was introduced directly after control spectra had been recorded. [Ca^{2+}]i increased to a similar extent when the combined insult was preceded by either hypoxia or hypoglycaemia to a mean of 202 % of control values. PCr content fell to 25 - 30 % of control as a result of the combined sequential insult and recovered on return to control conditions. When the combined insult was introduced immediately after control spectra had been recorded the measured [Ca^{2+}]i rose within the first 15 minutes to 455 % of control and remained high thereafter. There was a marked decrease in PCr content to 20 - 25 % of control with ATP undetectable (Table I). These changes were irreversible.

The result of this study support the proposed involvement of an increase in [Ca^{2+}]i in cell death as suggested by the «excitotoxic hypothesis». The difference in [Ca^{2+}]i increase between the immediate combined insults (455 % of control) and the sequential combined insults (202 % of control) should be noted. This suggest that the tissue is adapting by some unknown mechanism to the single insult of hypoxia or hypoglycaemia rendering it less vulnerable to the combined insult.

Table I. Measurements of [Ca^{2+}]i and PCr content of guinea - pig cerebral cortical slices under conditions of low oxygen and/or low glucose, glutamate or NMDLA exposure and depolarisation.

Conditions	n	[Ca^{2+}]i	PCr
Combined sequential	7	202	27
Combined immediate	2	455	23
glutamate (1mM)	4	181	
glutamate (1mM)*	4	242	35
NMDLA (200 µM)	1	157	
NMDLA (200 µM)*	3	169	39
Depolarisation	1	190	35

Values of [Ca^{2+}]i and PCr are % control
* glutamate/NMDLA in the presence of extracellular magnesium

Proposed excitotoxins; glutamate and NMDLA

To assess the role of the proposed excitotxins on the [Ca^{2+}]i increase observed in the previous study the effects of glutamate and NMDLA (agonist of the NMDA - subtype of glutamate receptor) were investigated.

On exposure of actively metabolising cortical slices to 0.5 to 1.0 mM glutamate a new resonance was observed in the $_{19}$F spectra with a chemical shift specific to the zinc - 5FBAPTA complex (Figure 1). This peak appeared with or just following an increase in [Ca^{2+}]i and decrease in PCr, between 45 - 90 min after exposure to glutamate. These effects were independent of the presence of magnesium (Table I). Similar results were obtained with 200 µM NMDLA but the increase in [Ca^{2+}]i was slower at 2 - 3 hours after exposure. The zinc - 5FBAPTA resonance was again observed, also later, after 3 - 6 hours. The zinc - 5FBAPTA resonance disappeared when experiments were performed in the presence of TPEN, a cation chelator with a high affinity for Zn^{2+} and much lower affinities for Ca^{2+} and Mg^{2+}.

The zinc observed has been calculated from the ratio of the area of the zinc - 5FBAPTA resonance to the total area of 5FBAPTA resonances (assuming an intracellular concentration of 5FBAPTA of 100 µM) to range between 10 - 20 µM.

Histochemical studies have shown that zinc is enriched in various parts of the brain including the cerebral cortex. The zinc observed in this study has moved from a 5FBAPTA - inaccessible site to a 5FBAPTA - accessible site within the cell. This may be a movement from a 5FBAPTA - inaccessible site within the cell or release from a bound form e.g. on an intracellular protein. Histochemical studies have shown zinc in synaptic vesicles [4] and a movement of histochemically reactive zinc from nerve - endings to cell bodies after kainate - induced seizures and ischaemia in animal brains [5,6]. Zinc has, however, also been observed, using 5FBAPTA , in synaptosomes after methylmercury treatment suggesting protein - associated release [7]. Proposed roles for zinc include modulation of excitatory and inhibitory neurotransmission, enzyme activation, protection against excitotoxicity but also a possible cytotoxic effect at higher concentrations. Interestingly, zinc has been implicated in various brain disorders such as dementia, depression, schizophrenia and epilepsy.

It should be noted that no zinc resonances were observed with the combined insults of hypoxia and hypoglycaemia or with depolarisation (Figure 1).

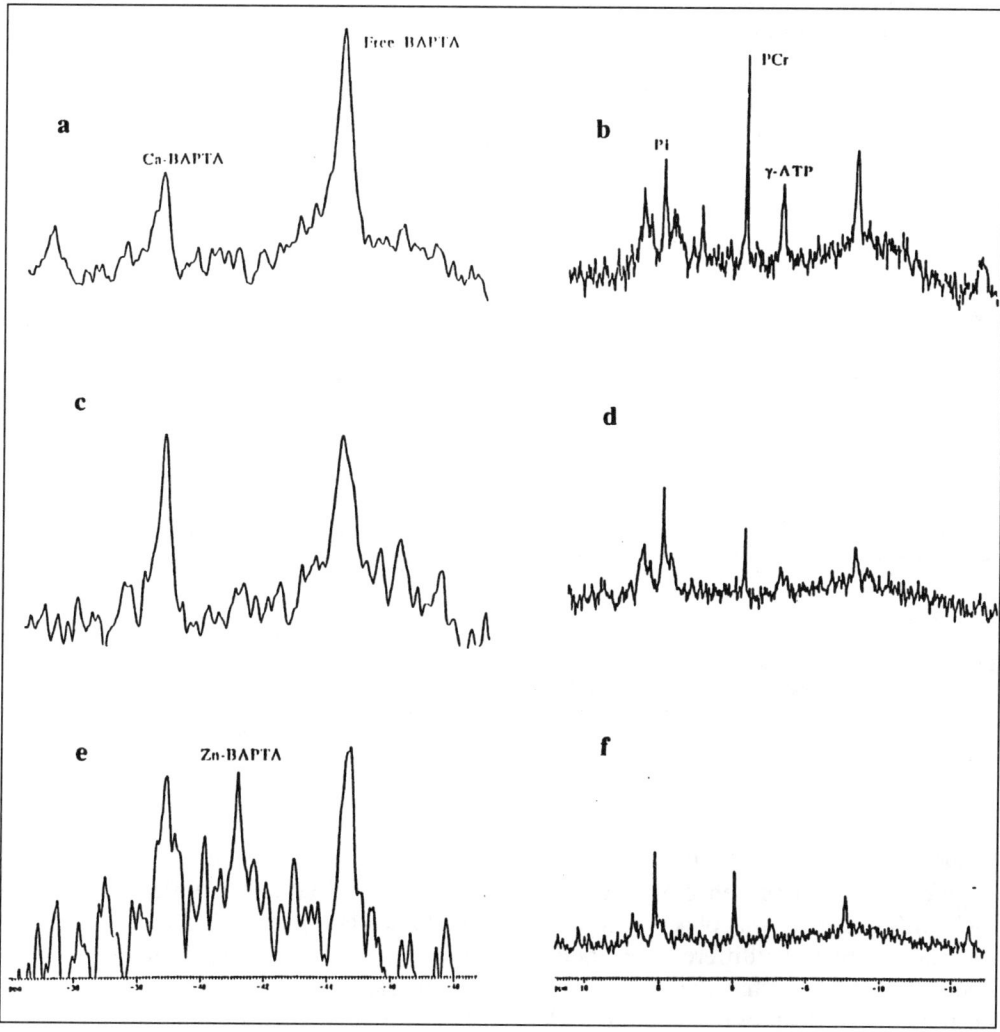

Figure 1. ^{19}F (a,c and e) and ^{31}P (b, d and f) MR spectra of guinea - pig cerebral cortical slices superfused in control media (a and b), in media containing 1.0 mM glutamate (c and d) and in media containing 40 mM k^+_e - depolarisation (e and f).

^{13}C MR, ^{1}H MRS and GC - MS studies of cerebral metabolism after exposure to NMDLA - a comparison with depolarisation

On depolarisation of guinea - pig cortical slices in the presence of [1-^{13}C] glucose the resonances of the metabolites citrate and glutamine are much higher than under control conditions (Figure 2.). This was explained by an increase in pool sizes of these metabolites compared to control and appear to reflect a stimulation of glial metabolism - since citrate and glutamine are associated with glia. No differences in final enrichments of metabolites with ^{13}C were observed under control and depolarising conditions although the steady state enrichments are thought to be reached more quickly with depolarisation [8].

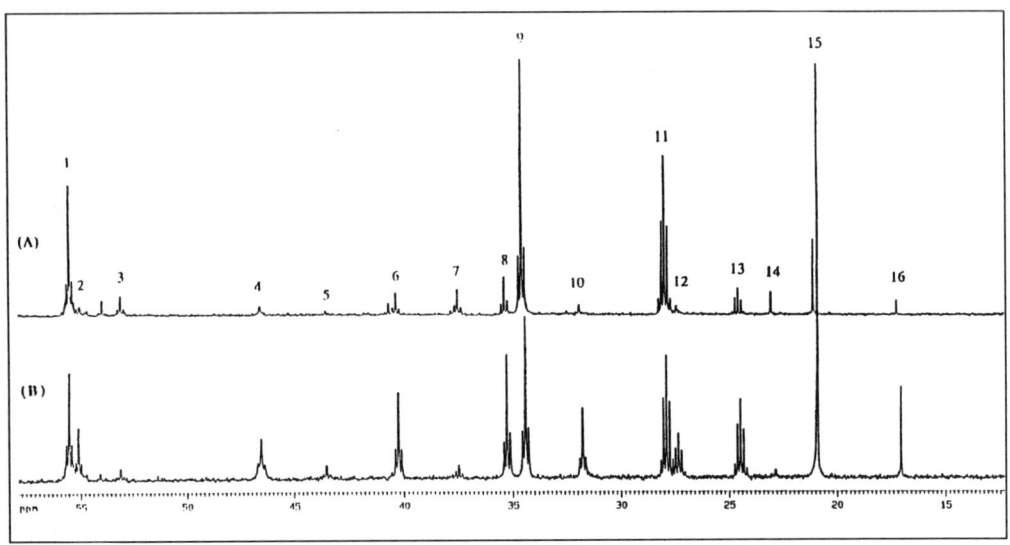

Figure 2. ^{13}C - MR spectra of extracts of guinea - pig cortical slices incubated with [1 - ^{13}C] - glucose, (A) for 4 hours under control conditions, (B) for three hours under depolarising conditions. Assignments: 1) C2 -Glu, 2) C2 - Gln, 3) C2 - Asp, 4) C2/C4 - citrate, 5) C3 - malate, 6) C4 - GABA, 7) C3 - Asp, 8) C2 - GABA, 9) C4 - Glu, 10) C4 - Gln, 11) C3 - Glu, 12) C3 - Gln, 13) C3 - GABA, 14) C6 - NAA, 15) C3 - Lac, 16) C3 - Ala [8].

On exposure to NMDLA (20 - 200 µM) in the presence of [1-^{13}C] glucose, independent of the presence of magnesium, no changes in final ^{13}C % enrichments (from GC - MS or MRS) was observed from controls (Table II). There was also no change in the rate at which the different metabolites became enriched. However, from ^{13}C MRS it could be observed that the amount of ^{13}C incorporated into metabolites (µmol) had decreased significantly from controls. Pool sizes of the amino acids glutamate, glutamine and aspartate all decreased on exposure to 20 - 200 µM NMDLA from control with the decrease significantly lower in the absence of magnesium (Table III). From ^{1}H spectra a significant increase in lactate from control was observed which was confirmed by enzymic analysis of tissue lactate (Table III). The NAA tissue pool sizes, also measured from the ^{1}H spectra, decreased from control (Table III) - this was thought to reflect neuronal loss since NAA is a putative neuronal marker. ^{1}H spectra also showed resonances for NMDLA which must therefore be taken up into the cells [9].

Table II. Atom percent enrichment of ^{13}C-labelled metabolites in extracts of guinea - pig cortical slices analysed by GC - MS.

Conditions	t (min)	Glu	Gln	Asp	GABA	Cit	Succ	Mal	Lac
control	360	39.4	33.0	41.4	41.8	36.1	26.3	38.9	37.6
200µM NMDLA	240	37.8	33.7	38.8	40.2	39.7	20.0	32.0	31.5
200µM NMDLA	360	37.4	34.7	39.0	41.9	38.6	16.8	37.5	30.6
200µM NMDLA*	240	38.2	—	39.2	40.1	—	20.0	34.4	30.9
200µM NMDLA*	360	38.0	—	—	41.0	—	17.4	—	34.8

1) * with 1.2 mM mg^{2+}$_e$; all expt with NMDLA with 1µM glycine.

Table III. Amino acid, NAA and lactate pool sizes from extracts of guinea - pig cortical slices determined by automated amino acid analysis and ^{1}H MRS.

Conditions	t	Glu	Gln	Ala	Asp	GABA	Lac	NAA
control	45' - 15hr	8.7±3.0	1.5±0.8	1.0±0.5	1.6±0.4	0.9±0.5	1.0±0.0	3.5±0.1
20µM NMDLA*	4hr - 6 hr	5.8±0.4	0.6±0.1	0.2±0.0	1.0±0.1	0.6±0.1	1.9±0.5	2.2±0.1
20µM NMDLA	4hr - 6hr	4.1±0.5	0.7±0.2	05±0.2	0.7±0.2	0.7±0.1	1.6±0.2	1.7±0.2
20µM NMDLA*	4hr - 6hr	4.4±0.8	0.8±0.2	05±.02	0.6±0.1	0.6±0.1	1.5±0.3	2.2±0.1
20µM NMDLA	4hr - 6hr	3.6±0.8	0.5±0.1	05±0.1	0.6±0.1	0.5±0.2	1.6±0.8	1.9±0.3

1) * with 1.2mM Mg2+e ; all expt with NMDLA with 1 µM glycine.
2) all pool sizes are expressed as µmole/100 mg protein.

Conclusions

[Ca^{2+}]i was observed to increase and PCr to decrease from control values with a combination of moderate hypoxia and mild hypoglycaemia as predicted by the «excitotoxic hypothesis». The effects of the proposed excitotoxins, glutamate and NMDLA, on [Ca^{2+}]i and the energy state were therefore investigated. A new resonance was observed in the ^{19}F spectra on exposure to glutamate and NMDLA, with the chemical shift specific to zinc - 5FBAPTA. This is an important observation in the light of a possible modulatory or protective role for zinc in excitotoxicity. This observation also highlighted the advantage that MRS has over fluorescent methods in its specific identification of the cations. The zinc - 5FBAPTA resonance was not observed in cortical slices exposed to low oxygen or low glucose or on depolarisation of the tissue slices (using 40 mM K$^+$e). This suggest that the mechanisms of damage in the latter insults can not be solely attributed to the release of excitotoxins.
^{13}C and ^{1}H MRS and GC - MS of extracts of cortical slices also demonstrated a difference in cerebral metabolism between depolarisation and NMDLA exposure. NMDLA exposure results in an increase in tissue lactate, decrease in NAA and

decreases in pool sizes of amino acids. ^{13}C MRS and GC - MS results suggest there was no change in % ^{13}C enrichment of metabolites but a significant decrease in the total amount of ^{13}C incorporated into the metabolites. These results suggest NMDLA exposure causes widespread damage to neurones and also possibly glia with the remainder of the cells metabolising normally. ^{1}H MRS also showed a significant build - up of NMDLA inside the cells and therefore it is not possible to distinguish effects to sustained binding to the NMDA receptor from effects to NMDLA accumulation inside the cells.

References

1. Olney JW. In Excitotoxins, (Fuxe K, Roberts P and Schwarts R, eds). London: *Macmillan* 1983 ; 82-96.
2. Badar - Goffer RS, Thatcher NM, Morris PG and Bachelard HS. *J Neurochem* 1993 ; 61 : 2207-14.
3. Badar - Goffer RS, Morris PG, Thatcher NM and Bachelard HS. *J Neurochem* 1994 ; 62: 2488-91.
4. Perez-Clausell J, Danscher G. *Brain Res* 1985 ; 337 : 91-8.
5. Howell GA, Welch M, Frederickson. *Nature* 1984 ; 308 : 736-8.
6. Tonder N, Johansen FF, Frederickson CJ, Zimmer J, Diemer JH. *Neurosci Letts* 1990 ; 109 : 247-52.
7. Denny MF, Atchison WD. *J Neurochem* 1994 ; 63 : 383-6.
8. McLean MA. PhD thesis, University of Cambridge, *Cambridge* (UK) 1993.
9. Thatcher N.M., Badar-Goffer R.S., Morris P.G., Bachelard H.S. Abstracts 12th. *SMRM Meeting* New York 1993 ; 1505.

These studies were supported by the M.R.C.

57

Functional MRI of the human cortex: effect of stimulus speed and handedness

S. VAN OOSTENDE, P. VAN HECKE, E. CORTHOUT, A.L. BAERT

Department of Radiology, University Hospitals, K.U. Leuven, Leuven, Belgium.

Since it was demonstrated that changes in blood flow and blood oxygenation affect the MR signal, numerous studies have shown that stimulation induced motor cortex activation could be detected with MR imaging. Our purpose was to investigate how the MR signal intensity changes when a subject performs a finger tapping exercise at various frequencies and to study the dependence of the MR signal on handedness and hemispheric dominance.

Methods

Imaging parameters

Images were acquired at 1.5 T (Magneton, Siemens, Erlangen) in a standard quadrature head coil. A 2-dimensional T_2^*-weighted FLASH gradient echo sequence, TR/TE/flip angle = 100 ms/60 ms/40°, was used to detect motor cortex activation. The FOV was 200 mm for a matrix size of 128 x 256. The slices intersected the central sulcus at near right angle. The receiver bandwidth was 4.8 kHz. Two averages were taken, which resulted in a scan time of 27 seconds per image. The anatomical images were recorded using a T_1-weighted spin echo sequence, TR/TE=680 ms/20ms, a FOV of 200 mm, a slice thickness of 8 mm and a 256 x 256 matrix.

Protocol 1

The finger tapping exercise consisted of a sequential finger-to-thumb opposition. In a first protocol, 5 right- and 5 left-handed subjects performed the finger tapping at frequencies of resp. 1, 2, 3 and 4 Hz. The tapping speed was paced by an acoustic signal. The finger exercise was continuously repeated during one image acquisition, followed by rest during the next one. The whole cycle was repeated 8 times, so that one experiment took up 7 minutes. Each experiment was performed successively with the right and the left hand at each of the 4 frequencies. The compliance of the finger tapping to the metronome was monitored by an observer.

Protocol 2

In this protocol, the tapping exercise was performed only at 1 and at 4 Hz. These frequencies were alternated during one experiment, which lead to a total of 16 ON/OFF cycles. Again, the exercise was performed with the right as well as the left hand. 7 right-handed and 10 left-handed subjects were included in this protocol.

Image processing and statistics

The images were processed with Advanced Visual Software (AVS, Waltham, MA, USA), an image processing and visualisation oriented software package. The difference in signal intensity between the activation and the rest image was calculated pixelwise and the result was subjected to a paired Student's t-tes. This t-value image was thresholded ($p<0.0025$) and processed with a 3-by-3 pixel spatial median filter to eliminate isolated pixels. Next, the image, representing the mean percent change in signal intensity between activation and rest image, was calculated and a logical «AND» operation was performed on this image and the thresholded t-value image. The result was overlaid on the anatomical image (Figure 1).

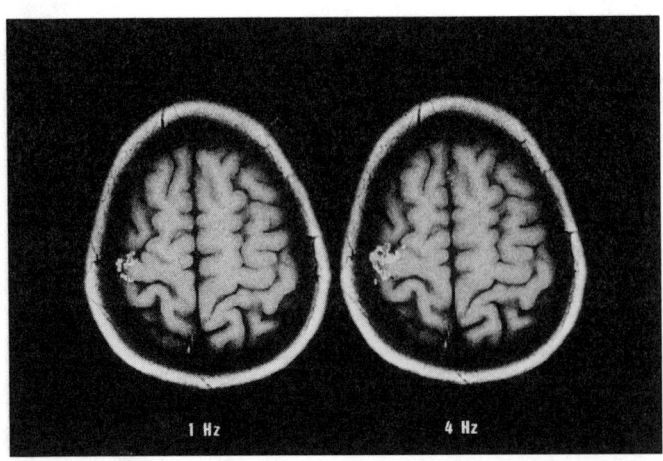

Figure 1. Overlay of the thresholded ($p<0.0025$) percent increase map on the anatomical T_1-image for the left hand of a right-handed volunteer at 1 Hz and 4 Hz. Note increased area at 4 Hz.

The «activation area» consists of the largest groups of connected, significant pixels in the precentral gyrus. The «activation signal» is the mean percent increase in signal intensity averaged over all the pixels in the activation area. The experiments were performed in 2 or 3 contiguous slices, maximally covering the total activated motor area. For each subject, the activation area and activation signal were averaged overt these slices. Only contralateral activation was taken into account in further statistical analysis, since the activation on the ipsilateral side was variable among subjects. Statistical analysis on these results was performed using non-parametric statistics, as indicated.

Results

Protocol 1

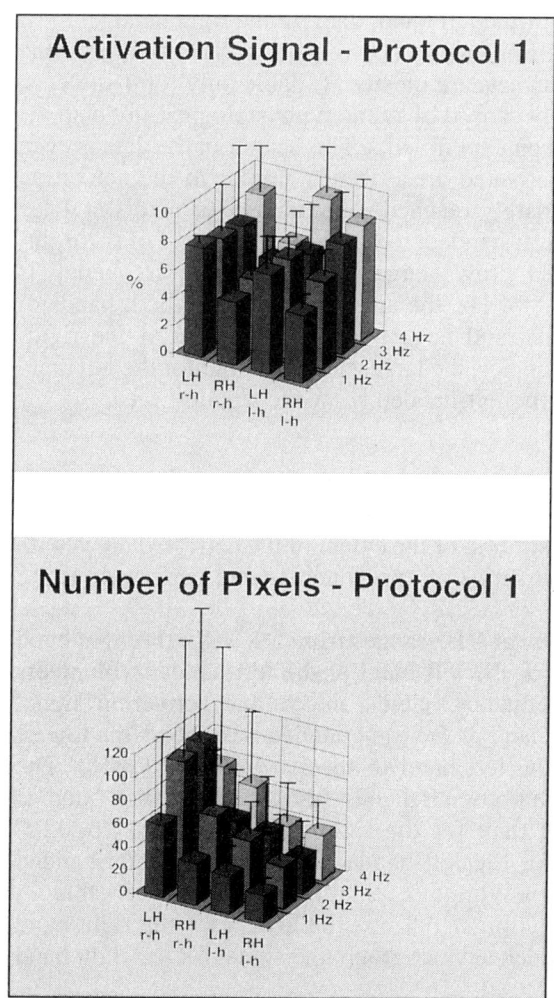

Figure 2. Protocol 1 : activation/rest alternations at a single activation frequency. (a) Percent increase of the MR signal in the contralateral activated area in the motor cortex upon stimulation at resp. 1, 2, 3 and 4 Hz, for the right hand (RH) and left hand (LH) of right-handed (r-h) and left-handed (l-h) volunteers. Error bars show the SD.
(b) Number of pixels in the activated area in the motor cortex upon stimulation at resp. 1, 2, 3 and 4 Hz, for the right and left hand of right- and left-handed volunteers.

At 1 Hz, the activation signal ranges from 4.5 % for the right hand of the right-handed to 7.8 % for the left hand of the left-handed (Figure 2a). The increase in finger tapping frequency from 1 to 4 Hz shows for both hands of both left-and right-handed volunteers a positive correlation with the increase of the activation signal. This correlation is significant ($p < 0.05$, Spearman Rank) for the right hand of the left- and right-handed volunteers. The frequency increase from 1 to 4 Hz yields an average signal increase ranging from 15 to 75 %, being the largest for the left-handed volunteers. This results in an activation signal at 4 Hz of 5.7 % for the right hand of the right-handed up to 9.6 % for the left hand of the left-handed. When comparing the activation signal for handedness and hemispheric dominance at each frequency separately, it is found that the activation signal for the right hand of the right-handed is smaller than that for the other hands at all frequencies. The difference in activation signal between the right hand of the right-handed and the left hand of the left-handed subjects is significant ($p<0.05$, Mann-Whitney) at each frequency, except at 3 Hz. Comparison within each subject group shows that the activation signal is larger for the left hand, than for the right hand, at most frequencies. Generally, the statistical significance is not very high. This is due to the limited number of subjects : complete data sets are mostly available only for 4 subjects, and to the large scatter on the data possibly caused by random physiological fluctuations or slight shifts of the head during or between experiments. This scatter of the data is even larger for the number of pixels in the activated area. Trends similar to the activation signal are observed, but significance is barely reached. The number of pixels at 1 Hz ranges from 23, for the right hand of the left-handed, to 62, for the left hand of the right-handed (Figure 2b). The activation area grows larger as the tapping frequency is increased, but not to a significant level. At 4 Hz, the area is smallest for both hands of the left-handed, extending over 39 pixels, and largest for the left hand of the right-handed, containing 77 pixels. At all frequencies, the largest area is found for the left hand of the right-handed, while both hands of the left-handed show the smallest area.

Protocol 2

In order to obtain a more accurate registration of the extent of the activated areas with increasing finger motion speed, a second series of experiments were performed using protocol 2, described above.

In this experiments, the activation signal at 1 Hz ranges from 5.1 % for the right hand of the right-handed subjects, to 6.7 %, for the left hand of the left-handed volunteers (Figure 3A). Increasing the tapping frequency, yields an average activation signal increase of 5 to 35 %. At 4 Hz, the right hand of the right handed still shows the lowest signal (5.4 %), while it is highest for the left hand of the left-handed (7.6 %). The increase in activation signal is significant for all hands ($p<0.05$, Wilcoxon) and is significantly higher for the left-handed, than for the right-handed subjects ($p<0.05$, Wilcoxon) and is significantly higher for the left-handed, than for the right-handed subjects ($p<0.05$, Kruskal-Wallis, Mann-Whitney), a trend already observable in protocol 1. At either frequency, the activation signal was the lowest for the right hand of the right-handed subjects and, within each subject group, the signal for the right hand remains below that of the left hand.

At 1 Hz, the number of pixels in the activation area ranges from 36 to 70, being the lowest for both hands of the left-handed subjects (Figure 3b). When increasing the frequency, the activation area on the average gains size by about 10 to 30 pixels, except for the right hand of the left-handed volunteers. The increase is only significant ($p<0.05$, Wilcoxon) for the left hand of both right- and left-handed volunteers. At 1 as well as at 4 Hz, the right-handed subjects show a larger activation area, similar to the first protocol. At the lowest frequency, the number of pixels for the left hand of the left-handed volunteers is significantly smaller ($p<0.05$, Mann-Whitney) than for both hands of the right-handed and the same conclusion can be made for the right hand of the left-handed at 4 Hz. Within each subject group, the left hand shows a larger activation area than the right at 4 Hz. Large interindividual variations in pixel area still remained in this second protocol, but more significant results could be obtained, due to the interleaved excitation and the larger number of subjects.

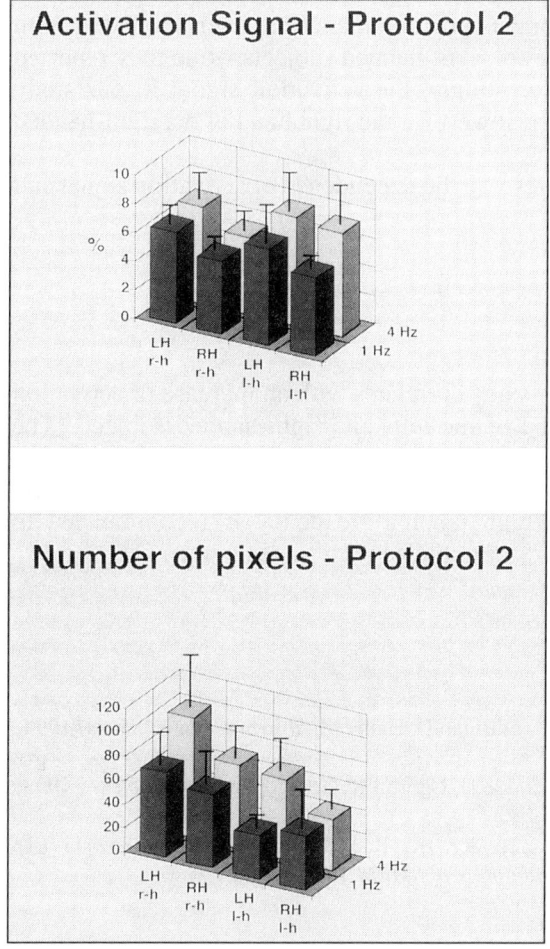

Figure 3. Protocol 2 : activation/rest alternations with interleaved activation frequencies of 1 Hz and 4 Hz.
(a) Percent increase of the MR signal in the contralateral activated area in the motor cortex upon stimulation at resp. 1 and 4 Hz, for the right hand (RH) and left hand (LH) of right-handed (r-h-) and left-handed (l-h) volunteers. Error bars show the SD.
(b) Number of pixels in the activated area in the motor cortex upon stimulation at resp. 1 and 4 Hz, for the right and left hand of right- and left-handed volunteers.

Since the results of the two protocols show the same tendencies for the activation area as well as for the activation signal, pooling of the data increases the significance of the results.

Discussion

Many PET studies have been performed on motor activation, but as far as we know, no results have been reported on finger exercise frequency. However, a few NMR studies have been performed at higher field strengths and with Echo Planar Imaging. The studies of Sadato et al. [1] and Bandettini *et al.* [2], using and EPI sequence, demonstrated an increase of the activation signal with increased repetition rate of finger tapping, for right-handed volunteers. This increase was larger than ours. Sadato further reported an initial increase of activation area up to 2 or 3 Hz, followed by a decrease at higher frequency, which was explained as a saturation of the blood flow increase upon stimulation. In our first protocol, we also noticed tendencies to a saturation at 3 Hz.

The dependence on handedness and hemispheric dominance has been studied by Kim *et al.* [3] at 3 T. We found the largest area for right-handed subjects while they reported the largest area for the left-handed. Interestingly, the activation signal in our study behaves as the area in their study, being the lowest for the right hand of the right-handed volunteers.

Obviously more studies are needed to resolve the dependence of activation signal and area on the MR sequence and field used.

Conclusions

The increase of the finger tapping frequency correlates with an increase of activation signal and activation area for either hand of the left- and right-handed subjects. The amount of activation signal and the extent of activation area and their change upon increase of the tapping frequency show significant asymmetries related to hemispheric dominance and handedness. Finally, a high tapping frequency is recommended to maximize the activation signal in motor cortex studies with finger movement.

References

1. Sadato N, Leonard M, Ibanez V, Deiber MP, LeBihan D, Hallet M. *abstract book of SMRM* 1994 ; 673.
2. Kim SG, Ashe J, Hendrich K, Ellerman J, Merkle H, Ugurbil K, Georgopoulos AP. *Science* 1993 ; 261 : 615-7.
3. Bandettini PA., Wong EC, DeYoe EA., Binder JR, Rao SM, Birzer D, Estkowski LD, Jesmanowicz A, Hinks RS, Hyde JS. *abstract book of SMRM* 1993 ; 1382.

58

Volumetric measurements of the temporal lobes in Alzheimer's disease

L.-O. WAHLUND, P. JULIN

*Karolinska Institute,
Department of Clinical Neuroscience and Family Medicine,
Section of Geriatric Medicine, Stockholm, Sweden.*

The diagnosis of Alzheimer's disease is currently based on a large number of clinical, neuro-radiological, neuro-physiological and neuro-psychological evaluations. The definite diagnosis can only be established at autopsy or via brain biopsy. The typical histopathological changes of senile plaques and neurofibrillary tangles form the diagnostic hallmarks of the disease. At present, there are no simple biological marker(s) to assess the disease process.

Modern neuroimaging techniques and new knowledge about the biochemical events leading to the formation of senile plaques and neurofibrillary tangles should provide promising future tools in the search for highly accurate biological markers.

The need for a simple and accurate diagnostic marker is increasing as new therapeutic drugs are emerging. In this article putative radiological markers such as volumetric mesurements of the temporal lobes will be discussed.

Alzheimer's disease represents an increasing financial and health care burden to society. The need for effective treatment is tremendous but until now pharmacological interventions have been mainly symptomatical. During recent years a number of putative drugs have been proposed to halt or reverse the progressive neuro degeneration in Alzheimer's disease. Increasing knowledge of the processes leading to ß-amyloid accumulation in senile plaques (SP) and the formation of neurofibrillary tangles (NFT) should make possible the development of pharmaceuticals to effectively reduce the disease progression. Such knowledge also gives great opportunities to search for simple blood and CSF tests that could serve as biological markers of the disease.

One problem in the search for suitable drugs is that the diagnosis of Alzheimer's disease is based purely on clinical data, with the definitive diagnosis only being established at autopsy. Furthermore, whether Alzheimer's disease is an unambiguous conception or a group of several different diseases has not been fully elucidated. To find a simple test or marker that unequivocally assesses the diagnosis of AD is therefore of greatest importance.

The use of modern brain imaging modalities has greatly improved the possibility to distinguish Alzheimer's disease patients from vascular demented subjects, as well as from demented due to expanding and infectious brain processes.

The possibillity to increase knowledge of the disease process itself has also been facilitated by the use of modern functional brain imaging methods.

Methods and results

CT and MRI

Computed tomography has been used in the investigation of demented patients for the last twenty years. This technique is now mandatory as a clinical procedure at dementia investigation centres. The structural changes found in dementia include global and regional atrophy of the brain and the presence of white matter changes known as leukoaraiosis. The advent of MRI has only came recently and this modality has not been used as extensively for studying demented patients. However, MRI is in many ways superior to CT, since the spatial and contrast resolution is much higher. Also the possibility to image in arbitrary planes, as well as the lack of bone artifacts, makes the modality excellent for studying small bone near structures in the center of the brain such as the hippocampal formation. Several attempts to find a simple linear or areal measurement that can unequivocaly distinguish Alzheimer's disease from normal aging or and from vascular dementia have been undertaken. For instance, Dahlbeck et al. suggested that the interunctal distance (the minimal distance between unci measured on transaxial slices at the level of the supracellar cistern), as estimated with MRI, distinguished Alzheimer patients from healthy controls [1]. In another study, Early et al. reported a great overlap in interunctal distance between Alzheimer's disease patients and healthy vounteers [2]. The patient population in the latter study was less severely affected, than in the former, which might explain the different results between the two studies. Investigations of the hippocampal formation with other linear or volume measurements have given more positive results and de Leon et al. reported that dilatation of the perihippocampal fissures measured on CT scans might serve as a radiologic marker for identifying early Alzheimer disease [3]. The baseline measure of the perihippocampal fissure made by de Leon et al. predicted cognitive decline of minimally impaired Alzheimer's disease patients with a sensitivity of 91% and a specificity of 89%.

The CT scans, obtained in this and other studies, for measuring structures in the hippocampal formation are usually obtained with so called «negative angulation», that is using a transaxial imaging plane 20°-30° negative to the cantho-meatal plane. This permits good visualization of the hippocampal formation. In another CT study, Jobst et al. reported that a simple estimation of temporal lob atrophy namely the minimum width of the medial temporal lobe as measured by temporal-lobe-oriented-CT, could almost completely separate Alzheimer's disease patients from controls [4]. The patients diagnoses were histopathologically verified and the CT scans obtained 1-2 years before death.

CT and linear measurements are relatively easy to use and require only different angulation of the imaging plane as compared to standard procedures.

Obtaining volume measurements is more complicated. The most convenient method for the latter is to use MRI with 3D acquisition. This permits calculation of volumes without leaving gaps between the slices. There are many methods for volume measurements of the hippocampal formation all of them reqire imaging computers with specially developed software. Also, carefully analysed error calculations are necessary, since the MR image generation is complicated the risk for low reliability is high if the method errors are not controlled.

As mentioned previously one great problem in assessing Alzheimer's disease diagnoses concerns the possible heterogeneity of the disease. To avoid this problem one might use «models» of the disease. A familial form of Alzheimer's with a mutation in the APP gene on chromosome 21 has recently been identified at the Alzheimer Research Center at Huddinge Hospital [5]. It is proposed that this APP gene mutation leads to abnormal deposition of ß-amyloid in senile plaques in the brain. In this family the cause of Alzheimer's disease is known and the family therefore represents a unique research model for Alzheimer's disease. In a recent study, we calculated the hippocampal volumes in 13 of the family members including subjects with manifest disease, healthy subjects with the mutation and subjects without the mutation. The brains of the family members were investigated using a 1.5 Tesla Magnetom™ from Siemens, Germany. For volume measurements a T1w, 3D acquisition sequence (MPRAGE) was used. The slice thickness was 2.8 mm and 64 coronal contiguous slices were obtained. All images used for volume calculations were then transferred to an computer (SUN) and the volume calculations were undertaken with x3D image processing software from Context Vision, Sweden. Volumes of the grey matter in the hippocampal formation, between the anterior and posterior commisures were calculated. The measurements were done by one operator (PJ) and the intra-operator error was <10%.

The study showed a clear relation between the grey matter volumes in the hippocampal formation and age (r=0.96, p<0.03) in mutation carriers regardless of whether they had manifest symptoms or not (Figure 1). This result suggested that the hippocampal grey matter undergoes abnormal atrophy with age in those subjects with the APP gene mutation. A significant relation between recent memory and the volumes of the hippocampal grey matter (r=0.997, p<0.0002) was also seen for the APP mutation carriers. (Figure 2.) Although these findings are based on a limited number of subjects, they provide promise that hippocampal volume measurements can serve as a radiological marker for Alzheimer's disease.

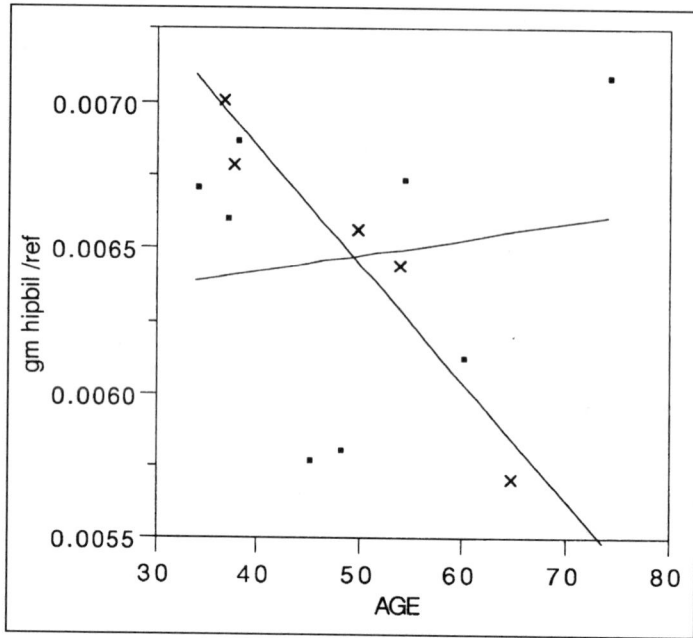

Figure 1. Relative volumes of grey matter in the medial temporal lobes (y-axis) related to age in carriers (n = 5) and non-carriers (n = 8). In the carriers there is a negative correlation between the grey matter volumes and age.
r = -0.96, p < 0.05.
Crosses = carriers. Squares = non-carriers.

Figure 2. Test of immediate memory (CorUD=Corsi's up and down) related to relative volumes of grey matter in medial temporal lobes (x-axis) in carriers (n = 5) and non-carriers (n = 8). In the carriers there is a strong positive correlation between immediate memory and the relative volumes of medial temporal grey matter.
r = 0.997, p < 0.001.
Crosses = carriers. Squares = non-carriers.

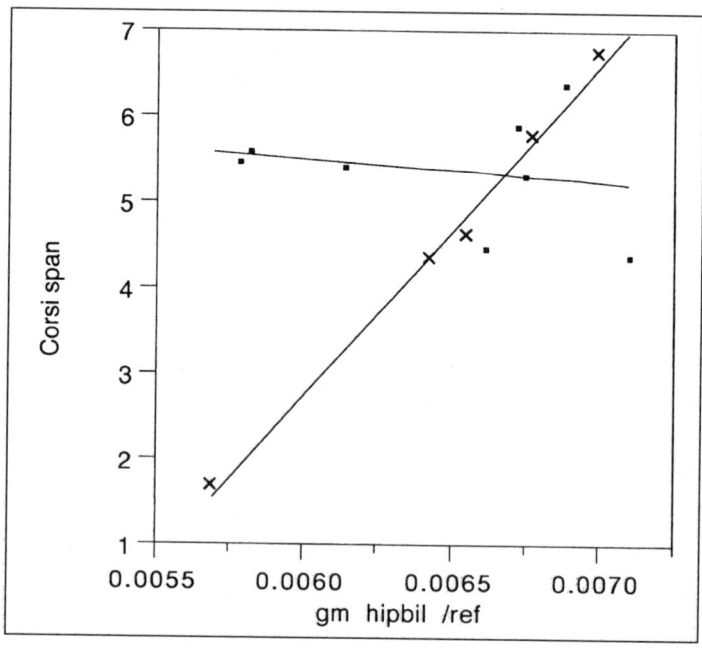

Conclusion

As knowledge about the underlying processes leading to Alzheimer's disease increases, the possibilities to find drugs to halt or slow the disease process in the brains of these patients increases. It is obvious that putative treatments must start early in the disease since the chance to rebuild lost neurons and neuronal connectivity is extremely low. The need for highly sensitive and specific diagnostic methods is of utmost importance since the definitive diagnosis can only be established after the patients death. The evaluation of putative markers as diagnostic tools becomes difficult and time consuming. A number of new diagnostic methods have emerged over recent years most promising of these seem to be the neuroradiological techniques with volumetric measurements of the temporal lobes in combination with physiologic studies of the brain (SPET, PET and EEG). The results of others and our study on familial forms of Alzheimer's disease gives strong support for the fact that structures in the hippocampal formation are early affected in the disease process. Moreover, these structural changes can be detected by using volumetric measurements and they can be used as radiological markers of the disease. However, studies on larger populations including very early cases of Alzheimer's disease are nedeed to support this hypothesis.

References

1. Dahlbeck JW, McCluney KW, Yeakley JW, et al. The interuncal distance: a new MR measurement for the hippocampal atrophy of Alzheimer disease. *AJNR* 1991 ; 12(5) : 931-2.
2. Early B, Escalona PR, Boyoko OB et al. Interunctal distance measurement in healthy volunteers and in patients with Alzheimer disease. *AJNR* 1993 ; 14 : 907-10.
3. de Leon MJ, Colomb J, George AE et al. The Radiologic Prediction of Alzheimer Disease: the Atrophic Hippocampal Formation. *AJNR* 1993 ; 14 : 897-906.
4. Jobst KA, Smith AD, Szatmari M et al. Detection in life of confirmed Alzheimer's disease using a simple measurement of medial temporal lobe atrophy by computed tomography. *Lancet* 1993 ; 340 : 1179-83.
5. Mullan M, Crawford F, Axelman K et al. A pathogenic mutation for probable Alzheimer's disease in the APP gene at the N-terminus of beta-amyloid. *Nat Genet* 1992 ; 5 : 345-7.

59

¹H spectroscopy of the temporal lobes in schizophrenic and bipolar patients

D.A. YURGELUN-TODD, S.A. GRUBER, B.M. COHEN, P.F. RENSHAW

Brain Imaging Center, McLean Hospital, Belmont, MA, USA.
Department of Psychiatry, Harvard Medical School, Boston, MA, USA.

Recent neuroimaging and postmortem studies have reported specific functional and structural changes in a number of cortical regions in patients with schizophrenia. In particular neuropathological studies of schizophrenic brains have demonstrated abnormalities in temporal lobe morphology suggesting localized, non-diffuse changes in this brain area (Bogerts *et al.*, 1985; Falkai *et al.*, 1988). Additional evidence for temporal lobe pathology has come from quantitative measurements of temporal regions using magnetic resonance images (Barta *et al.*, 1990 ; DeLisi *et al.*, 1991 ; Shenton *et al.*, 1992) as well as qualitative ratings of MR images of first-episode schizophrenics (Lieberman *et al.*, 1993).

In vivo magnetic resonance spectroscopy (MRS) permits the direct and non-invasive study of human brain biochemistry. MRS studies have also implicated the temporal lobe in the pathophysiology of schizophrenia. In a study applying phosphorus MRS (PMRS) to the temporal lobes, Calabrese *et al.*, (1992) found asymmetric ratios of PCR/B-ATP in schizophrenics, but not in normal controls. In contrast, O'Callaghan *et al.*, (1991) found no quantitative differences between outpatient schizophrenics and normal control subjects also using ³¹P MRS in the temporal-parietal region, although between-group differences in age and spectral contamination may have obscured the effect of diagnosis. Recent studies applying proton MRS to the temporal regions of schizophrenics and controls also report differences in metabolite concentrations. Nasralah *et al.* (1992) obtained spectra from 12 cm³ voxels localized in the right and left hippocampus. Ratios of N-acetyl aspartate (NAA) to choline plus creatine were found to be 30% lower on the right side for schizophrenics. No significant metabolite changes were reported for the left side. By comparison, proton spectra acquired only in the left temporal and frontal lobes using a localized water suppression technique (Moore *et al.*, 1992) indicated reduced NAA levels, with no decrease in creatine or choline levels in schizophrenic subjects.

The proton spectrum of the human brain has three particularly prominent metabolite peaks; choline, creatine/phosphocreatine, and N-Acetyl aspartate. The relative concentration of these metabolites may reflect changes in disease state due to alterations in cell physiology (Miller, 1991). A decrease in NAA concentration in particular, is associated with reduced neuronal integrity (Behar *et al.*, 1983, Simmons *et al.*, 1991) and has been suggested by some investigators to be associated with decreased neuronal concentration.

Given these findings, we applied single voxel proton MRS to both the right and left temporal lobes of well characterized bipolar patients and clinically stable schizophrenic patients. The study objective was to determine if schizophrenic patients demonstrate lateralized reductions in N-Acetyl-aspartate (NAA), and to assess whether metabolic concentrations differ significantly between schizophrenic and bipolar patients, as well as normal controls.

Methods

Forty-six-subjects, 16 schizophrenic patients, 15 bipolar patients, and 15 normal control subjects were studied at the McLean Hospital Imaging Center. Each subject received a structured clinical interview and diagnosis was made blindly according to DSM-IV criteria. Subjects with a history of organic brain syndrome, head injury, or substance abuse were excluded. All subjects were studied using an integrated MRI/proton MRS protocol performed on a 1.5T Signa whole body imager using a quadrature head coil. Contiguous 6 mm slice thick coronal slices for the entire brain were obtained prior to spectroscopy using an inversion recovery technique (inversion time = 800 ms, echo time (TE) = 20 ms, repetition time (TR) = 2000 ms). These images were used to select a volume of interest (VOI) in each hemisphere.

Proton spectra were obtained from a 3 cm x 2 cm x 2 cm voxel centered in each temporal lobe. A modified STEAM pulse sequence was used for water suppressed, volume localized spectroscopy. (Griffey and Flamig; 1990) MR parameters included TR = 2 sec, TE = 30 ms, 1 024 data points, and 800 Hz spectral width. In a typical experiment, 400 transients were averaged. Data were zero filled to 2 048 points, then an exponential filter resulting in a line broadening of 1 Hz was applied prior to Fourier transformation. A spline function was used to correct for baseline drift caused by incomplete water suppression. The resonances assigned to NAA at 2.0 PPM and to creatine/phosphocreatine (Cr) at 3.0 PPM were fit to a Gaussian lineshape. Quantitative measures were calculated from peak areas.

Results

All metabolite peaks were clearly visible in the study spectra (Figure 1). The metabolite ratios and demographics characteristics of the two study groups are shown in Table I and Figure 2, respectively. The groups were similar in estimated IQ, handedness, and sex. The NAA/Cr ratio did not demonstrate a significant laterality effect in any study group. Schizophrenic patients showed a significant reduction in NAA/Cr in the left temporal lobe when compared with normal controls (.95±.28 vs 1.21±.17, p=.002) or with bipolar patients (.95±.28 vs 1.13 ±.17,p=.019). In the right hemisphere, the only significant group difference between NAA/Cr levels was due to a reduction in metabolites for schizophrenic patients compared with normal controls (.95±.22 vs 1.19 ± .24, p = .002), although a strong trend existed for a reduction in bipolars (.95±.22 vs 1.08±.14, p=.057).

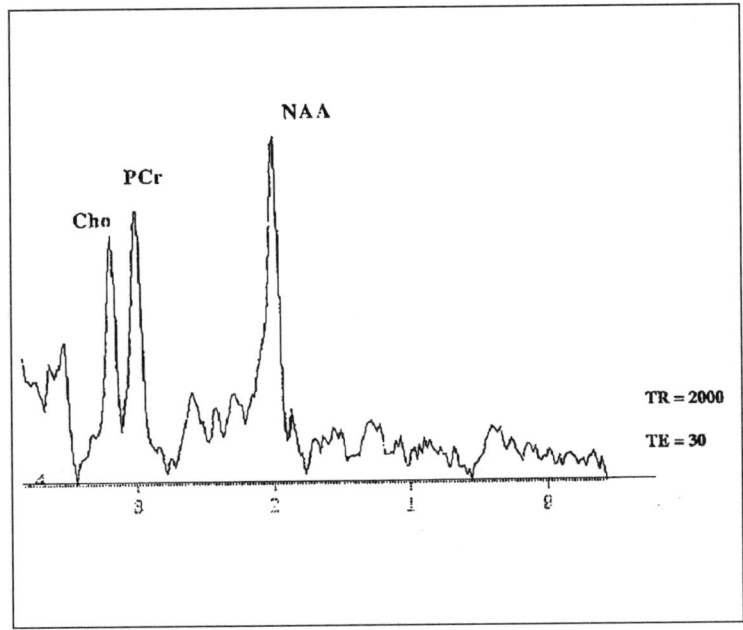

Figure 1. Proton NMR spectrum obtained from the left temporal lobe of a control subject.

Table 1. Demographic information of study subjects.

	EDUCATION (YEARS) COMPLETED	AGE (YEARS)	SEX	HANDEDNESS
NORMAL CONTROLS	17.0+/-2.54 (13-20)	30.9+/-7.06 (20-42)	11M, 4F	13R, 2L
BIPOLAR PATIENTS	14.0+/-2.80 (12-21)	30.1+/-7.30 (19-40)	11M, 4F	13R, 2L
SCHIZOPHRENIC PATIENTS	13.0+/-2.90 (6-18)	31.7+/-5.18 (22-38)	12M, 4F	14R, 2L

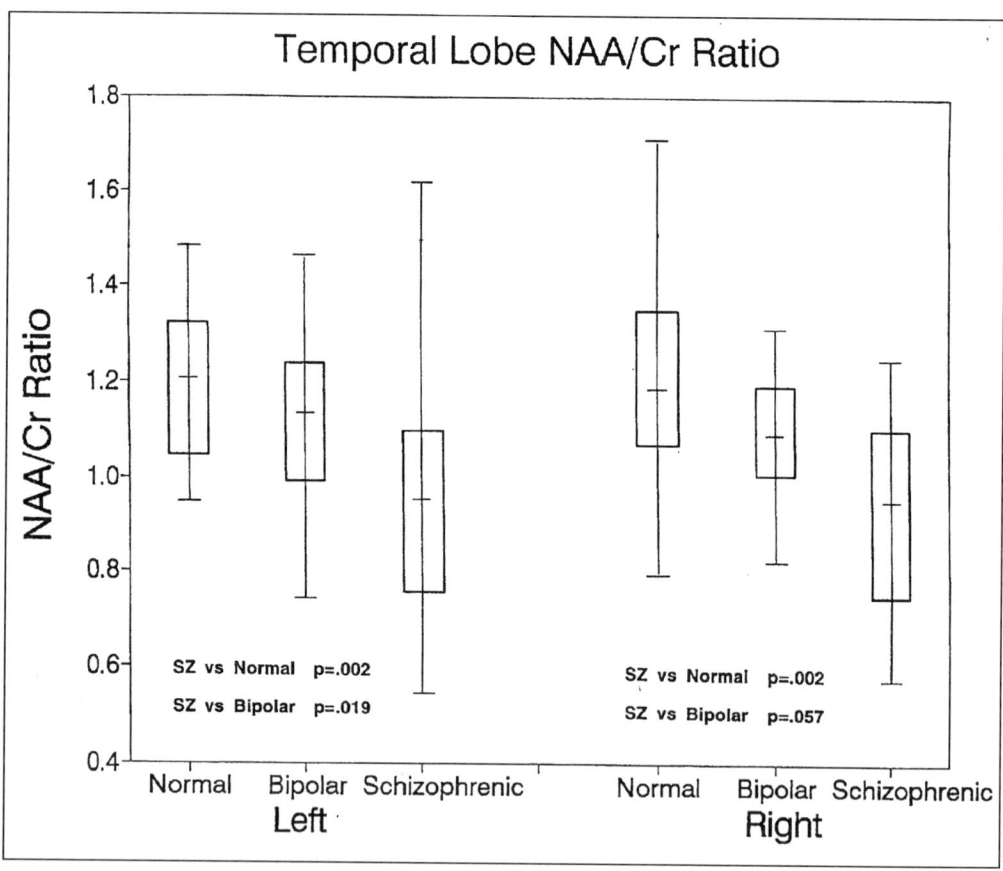

Figure 2

Discussion

These findings demonstrate a bilateral reduction in NAA/Cr in the temporal lobes of chronic schizophrenics, which may reflect a loss of neuronal integrity in this brain region. The meaning of changes in metabolite concentration in these patients is limited by our knowledge of the relation between changes in neurochemistry and in underlying brain morphology. In an attempt to control for heterogeneity of tissue content in the voxel of interest, we have compared ratios of NAA/Cr concentrations for voxels of brain tissue localized in similar temporal lobe regions. The relative amounts of gray matter, white matter, and CSF within the temporal lobes varies for the three diagnostic groups. Clarifying the meaning of these findings will require more extensive investigation of the relation between decreased NAA concentration and variance in brain tissue content for each diagnostic group. Furthermore, additional studies will be required to determine to what extent these results are confounded by patients medications, clinical course, or psychiatric state.

These results strengthen the evidence for biochemical as well as structural abnormalities in the temporal lobes of schizophrenia. The specificity of these metabolite changes for schizophrenia are supported by a unilateral reduction in NAA/Cr in this region compared with bipolar patients. In a study of first episode patients we also found a statistically significant reduction in NAA/Cr in the temporal lobes indicating that differences in metabolite concentrations are present early in the course of psychotic illness. (Renshaw, 1994) Further studies are needed to determine how these metabolite changes relate to function as well as structure.

References

1. Annett M. A classification of hand preference by association analysis. *Br J of Psychol* 1972 ; 61, 303-21.
2. Barta PE, Pearlson GD, Powers RE, Richards SS, Tune E. Auditory hallucinations and smaller superior temporal gyral volume in schizophrenia. *Am J Psychiatry* 1990 ; 147:1457-62.
3. Behar KL, den Hollander JA, Stromski ME *et al*. High-resolution 1H Nuclear magnetic resonance study of cerebral hypoxia in vivo. *Proc Natl Acad Sci USA* 1983 ; 80:4945-8.
4. Bogarts B, Meertz E, Schonfeldt-Bausch R. Basal ganglia and limbic system pathology in schizophrenia: a morphometric study of brain volume and shrinkage. *Arch Gen Psychiatry* 1985 ; 42:784-91.
5. Calabrese G, Deicken RF, Fein G, Merrin EL, Schoefeldt F, Weinger MW. 31Phosphorus magnetic resonance spectroscopy of the temporal lobes in schizophrenia. *Biol Psychiatry* 1992 ; 32:26-32.
6. DeLisi LE, Hoff AL, Schwartz JE, *et al*. Brainmorphology in first episode schizophrenic-like psychotic patients: A quantitative magnetic resonance imaging study. *Biol Psychiatry* 1991 ; 29:159-75.
7. Falkai P, Bogerts B, Rozumek M. Limbic pathology in schizophrenia: The entorhinal region - a morphometric study. *Biol Psychiatry* 1988 ; 24:515-21.
8. Griffey RH, Flamig DP. VAPOR for solvent-suppressed, short echo, volume-localized spectroscopy. *J Magn Reson* 1990 ; 88:161-6.

9. Lieberman J, Bogerts B, Degreef G, Ashtari M, Alvir J. Qualitative assessment of brain morphology in acute and chronic schizophrenia. *Am J Psychiatry* 1993 ; 149:784-94.
10. Miller BL. A review of chemical issues in ^{1}H NMR spectroscopy: N-acetyl-L-aspartate, creatine and choline. *NMR in Biomedicine* 1991 ; 4:47-52.
11. Moore CM, Redmond OM, Buckley P, Larkin C, Stack J, Waddington J, Ennis J. *In vivo* proton NMR spectroscopy (STEAM) in patients with schizophrenia. *Soc Mag Res Med* 1991.
12. Nasrallah HA, Skinner TE, Schmallbrook P, Robitaille PM, ^{1}H Magnetic resonance spectroscopy (MRS) of the hippocampus in schizophrenics and control subjects (Abstract). *Biol Psychiatry* 1992 ; 31:155A.
13. O'Callagahn EM, Redmond O, Ennis R, Stack J, Kinsella A, Ennis JT, Larkin C, Waddington JL. Initial investigation of the left temporoparietal region in schizophrenia by ^{31}P magnetic resonance spectroscopy. *Biol Psychiatry* 1991 ; 29:11-49-1152.
14. Renshaw PF, Yurgelun-Todd DA, Tohen M, Gruber SA, Cohen BM. Temporal Lobe Proton Magnetic Resonance Spectroscopy in Patients with First Episode Psychosis. Submitted for publication 1994.
15. Shenton M, Kikinis R, Jolewsz F, Pollak S, LeMay M, Wible C, Hokama H, Martin J, Metcalf D, Coleman M, McCarly R. Abnormalities of the left temporal lobe and thought disorder in schizophrenia: A qualitative magnetic resonance imaging study. *New Engl J Med* 1992 ; 327:604-612.
16. Silverstein AB. Two and four subtest short forms for the WAIS-R. *J. Consulting and Clinical Psychology* 1982 ; 50:3, 415-8.
17. Simmons ML, Frondoza CG, Coyle JT. Immunocytochemical localization of N-Acetyl-Aspartate with monoclonal antibodies. *Neuroscience* 1991 ; 45:1 : 37-45.
18. Spitzer RL, Williams JBW, Gibbon M. *Structured Clinical Interview for DSM-III-R (SCID)*. New York State Psychiatric Institute, Biometrics Research Department 1989.
19. Wechsler D. Wechsler Adult Intelligence Scale-Revised. New York: Harcourt Brace Jovanovich Inc., 1981 ; 222.

60

Echo planar MRI of schizophrenics and normal controls during word production

D.A. YURGELUN-TODD, P.F. RENSHAW, S.A. GRUBER, B.M. COHEN

Brain Imaging Center at McLean Hospital, Harvard Medical School, Boston, MA, USA.

Abnormal language functions, including difficulties with word association tasks, verbal fluency, and semantic priming have been repeatedly demonstrated in schizophrenic patients. Studies of cerebral activation in normal controls using Positron Emission Tomography suggest that temporal and frontal cortical regions demonstrate the greatest change in metabolism during word production [1, 2]. We have applied echo planar MRI (EPMRI) techniques to study both schizophrenic patients and normal controls using a verbal cognitive challenge paradigm to test the feasibility of using functional MRI to examine language based cognitive functions in psychiatric patients.

Methods

We studied 23 right handed subjects, eleven non-psychiatric controls and twelve DSM-III-R schizophrenic subjects. Activation during word production was examined on a verbal cognitive challenge paradigm which included two tasks: counting and verbal fluency. Scanning was performed on a 1.5 Tesla scanner which had been retrofit with a whole body echo planar coil, using a circular surface coil placed at the left side of the head. A T_1 weighted sagittal image was used to localize a plane parallel to and 7 mm below the AC-PC line. This slice was chosen because it was most comparable to the region activated by PET studies (Figure 1). High resolution images were acquired in the plane of study to allow for anatomic correlation with the functional imaging data.

During each cognitive task condition, a series of 50 sequential images were obtained. Functional images were collected every three seconds using a gradient echo pulse sequence (TE = 40 msec, flip angle = 75 deg.). An image matrix of 64 x 128 was used with a 3 mm x 3 mm in-plane resolution and a 7 mm slice thickness. Each stimulus sequence was divided into five 30 second segments resulting in a total study length of 150 seconds. To visualize signal changes, we used a task-activation paradigm which alternated between resting and stimulated states. The same stimulus was collected twice in each sequence and ten images were obtained consecutively for each of the five segments.

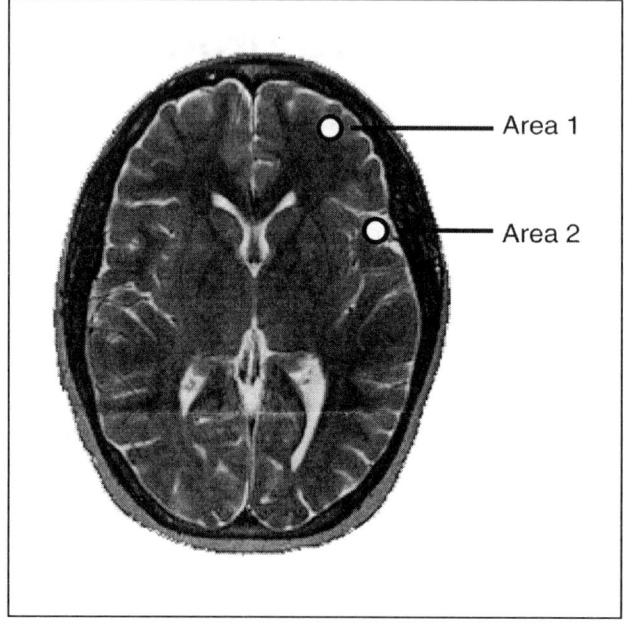

Figure 1. Anatomical image used for fMRI.

Cortical activation was measured using neuroanatomically defined regions of interest based on both conventional MR and EPMR images. We measured activation in the left dorsolateral prefrontal cortex (Brodmann's area 46 and 10), and the superior temporal gyrus (Brodmann's area 22), for the counting and word fluency tasks.

Results

Differences in activation were observed for counting and word fluency tasks relative to the rest condition in each of the subject groups. Figures 2 and 3 illustrate the signal-time plots for the two regions of interest. Subtraction of activation during the counting task from the activation during the fluency task revealed that normal subjects demonstrate a significant increase in activation of the prefrontal cortex while schizophrenic subjects do not. Significance was measured using analysis of variance on the group mean activation data (activation 1, p = .003; activation 2, p=.001). In contrast, schizophrenics were found to display greater activation in the temporal ROI (activation 1, p = .002; activation 2, p =.001). The control group demonstrated increased activation in the frontal region during the recovery periods relative to baseline.

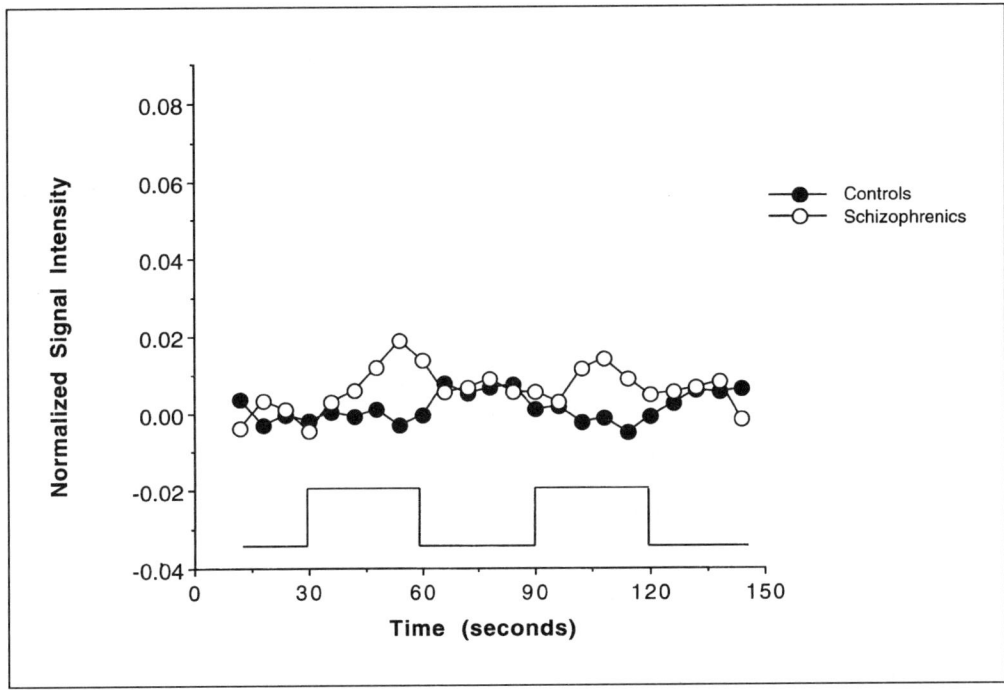

Figure 2. Activation in superior temporal region for controls and schizophrenics (verbal fluency activation - counting activation).

The use of combined fMRI and high resolution MRI permits the examination of regional brain activity in specific neuroanatomical areas with greater temporal and spatial resolution than other functional imaging methods. These preliminary data indicate that fMRI can detect differences in activation between normal controls and schizophrenics during different forms of verbal production. These results are in agreement with PET studies and EPMRI studies of normal subjects which report an increase in left frontal activation during work generation [3,4]. Furthermore, the reduction in frontal activation observed in this study is consistent with PET and SPECT studies which report decreased dorsolateral frontal activation in schizophrenic patients during cognitive challenge paradigms [5].

A second finding in this study is that of increased activation in the temporal region by the schizophrenic patients relative to the non-psychiatric controls during the work production task, results which are similar to the rCBF findings reported by Warkentin [6].

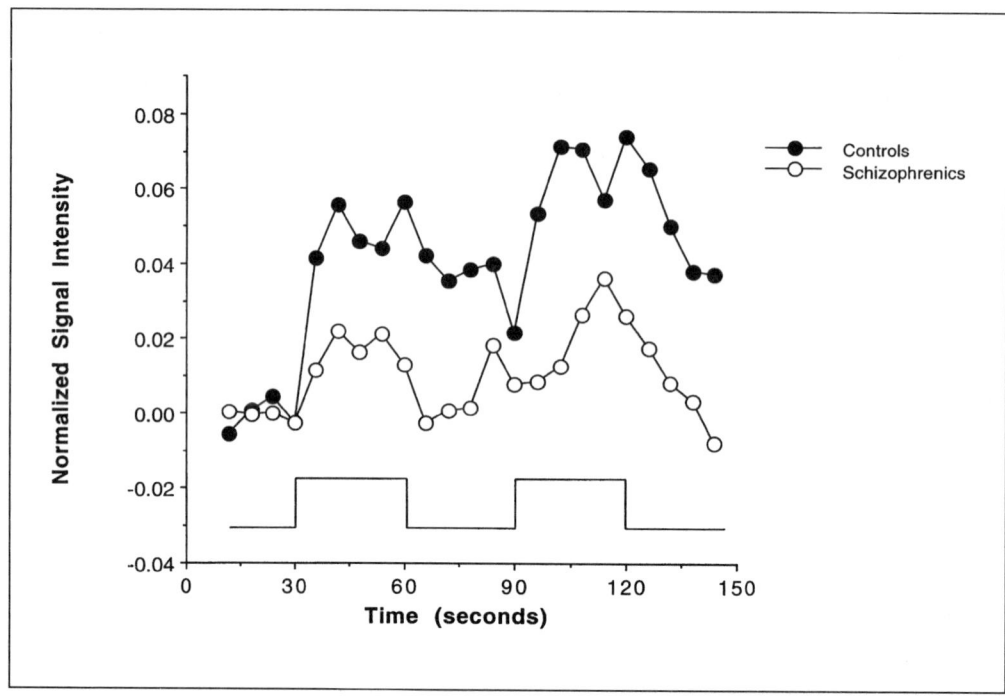

Figure 3. Activation in frontal region for controls and schizophrenics (verbal fluency activation - counting activation).

It has been suggested that both increases and decreases in activation may occur within different brain regions in response to a challenge task due to reciprocal activation networks [2]. This study suggest that functional MR imaging can detect activation during word production and can be applied to studies of higher cortical functioning in psychiatric patients.

References

1. Petersen SE, Fox PT, Posner MI, et al. *Nature* 1988 ; 331 : 585-9.
2. Frith CD, friston KJ, Liddle PF, Frackowiak RS. *Neuropsychologia* 1991 ; 29 : 1137-48.
3. McCarthy G, Blamire AM, Rothman DL, et al. *PNAS*, 1993 ; 90 : 4952-56.
4. Cuenod CA, Bookheimer S, Pannier, et al. *SMRM* 1993 ; 1 : 1414.
5. Weinberger DR, Berman KF, Zec RF. *Arch Gen Psych* 1986 ; 43 : 114.
6. Warkentin S, Nilsson A, Risberg J, Karlson S. *J Cerebral Blood Flow and Metab* 1989 ; 9 :1 : 354.

Achevé d'imprimer par Corlet, Imprimeur, S.A
14110 Condé-sur-Noireau (France)
N° d'Imprimeur : 12756 - Dépôt légal : septembre 1995
Imprimé en C.E.E.